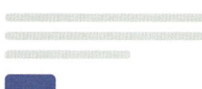

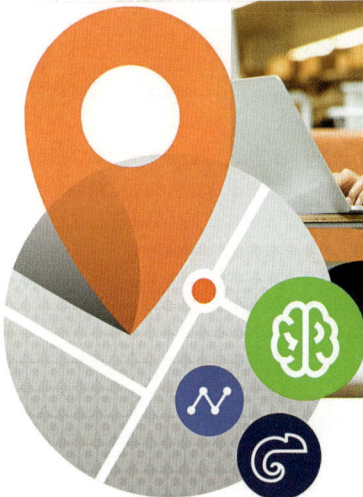

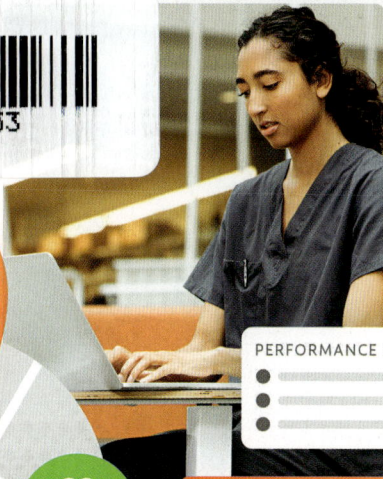

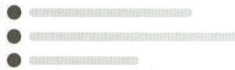

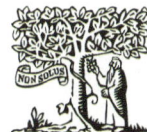

10th EDITION

Radiation Safety AND Radiobiology

IN MEDICAL IMAGING

MARY ALICE STATKIEWICZ SHERER, AS, RT(R), FASRT

PAULA J. VISCONTI, PhD, DABR

E. RUSSELL RITENOUR, PhD, DABR, FAAPM, FACR

KELLI WELCH HAYNES, EdD, RT(R), FASRT

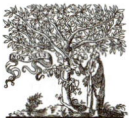

ELSEVIER

Elsevier
3251 Riverport Lane
St. Louis, Missouri 63043

RADIATION SAFETY AND RADIOBIOLOGY IN MEDICAL IMAGING, ISBN: 978-0-443-12353-5
TENTH EDITION

Previous editions copyrighted 2022, 2018, 2014, 2011, 2006, 2002, 1998, 1993, and 1983.

Senior Content Strategist: Luke Held
Senior Content Development Manager: Lisa Newton
Senior Content Development Specialist: Laura Selkirk
Senior Project Manager: Nayagi Anandan
Design Direction: Maggie Reid

Printed in India

Last digit is the print number: 9   8   7   6   5   4   3   2   1

In memory of my parents, Felix J. and Elizabeth M. Krohn,
To my sons, Joseph F. Statkiewicz, Christopher R. Statkiewicz, and Terry R. Sherer, Jr., with love,
And
To all with whom I may share my knowledge.

PREFACE

GOAL OF THE TEXTBOOK AND ACCOMPANYING ANCILLARIES

The title of this edition has been changed to *Radiation Safety and Radiobiology in Medical Imaging*. Its purpose, however, remains unchanged: to offer to new and current radiation science professionals, on multiple educational levels, essential and timely information on the diverse elements of radiation safety while also enlightening and instructing readers about current and new methodologies in both radiographic imaging and radioisotope techniques. The authors feel that meeting these objectives requires extended discussions on radiobiology, cell biology, and relevant radiation physics, all of which are required to educate students and associated professionals in the safe use of X-rays and both common and new radioisotopes for imaging and therapeutic intervention.

CONTENT

This textbook contains extensive introductions to recently developed advanced medical procedures involving the use of ionizing radiation, including an introduction to artificial intelligence (AI), which explains its underlying principles and its current and potential value in radiography. As in the 9th edition, there are 16 chapters, a detailed glossary, and multiple supplementary appendices. The overall format of the book, with the exception of some chapter re-ordering and minor renaming, which is detailed below, has remained the same. In what follows, a brief overview of the contents and purpose of each of the chapters in this textbook will be presented.

Both the 9th and 10th editions reflect a significant update and expansion of imaging technology education and relevant radiation safety aspects. In addition, the therapeutic and diagnostic usage of radioactive isotopes is also treated extensively. The latter subject material has been further extended in the 10th edition.

Several existing chapters have been revised to contain the latest volume of information on both traditional and updated subject matter. New relevant subject matter has been added. As is seen in the table of contents for this edition, the titles of multiple chapters from the 9th edition have been revised to more appropriately delineate their enlarged dedication to specific subject matter. Furthermore, a more suitable chapter reordering has been done.

As with the 9th edition, the individual chapter references are located in one section in the back matter of the book instead of at the end of each chapter. Similar to previous editions, the format of each chapter begins with a list of objectives to be realized by the learner at the conclusion of that chapter. Those objectives are followed by a detailed outline of the chapter that describes the main subject matter included in each section. Subsequently, a catalog of key terms is presented to alert the reader to topics of significant importance.

An introductory paragraph typically begins each chapter to create an immediate awareness of the chapter's content. At the end of the contents of each chapter, there is a comprehensive summary that emphasizes important information to be remembered. Finally, to assess the degree of learning, a set of general discussion questions and multiple-choice review questions is included. A series of appendices that enhance specific topics mentioned throughout the book follows the last chapter. After these appendices, there is a glossary to provide the learner with a quick reference and study guide to important concepts. Lastly, a substantial page index of subject matter topics completes the textbook.

This edition begins with an introduction to radiation protection, followed by reviews of various types and sources of radiation and a beginning presentation of the concepts of radiation dose. Other subject matter includes essential physics concepts relevant to radiation safety, such as X-ray absorption in biologic tissue, X-ray production and energy, and various methods of X-ray interaction with matter. Discussion of traditional and metric radiation quantities and units, the discovery of X-rays, and early radiation-induced injuries are also included. State-of-the-art radiation monitoring for personnel and area monitoring is fully described. A chapter offering an extensive overview of cell biology prepares the reader for the discussions of molecular and cellular radiation biology that follow.

Detailed up-to-date discussions about early tissue reactions and their effects on organ systems, as well as a discourse about stochastic effects and late tissue reactions caused by radiation in organ systems, are presented. Priority is given to the topic of dose limits for exposure to ionizing radiation. Because the designs of diagnostic X-ray and ancillary equipment constantly advance, equipment design for radiation protection is also examined. Major emphasis is placed on management of patient safety during diagnostic X-ray procedures with discussion of effective communication between the radiographer and the patient, use of immobilization, current shielding protocol and revision of patient gonadal shielding policies, technical exposure factors, postprocessing of radiographic images, considerations concerning repeat images, risk of exposure during extended diagnostic imaging procedures, radiation protection for the pregnant or potentially pregnant patient, and various pediatric safety protocols during radiographic imaging. Dual-energy X-ray absorptiometry concepts as applied to bone density examinations are explained as well.

Two chapters are dedicated, respectively, to treating special considerations on radiation safety in computed tomography and radiation safety aspects in X-ray breast imaging. Both traditional mammography and digital breast tomosynthesis (3D mammography) are included in the X-ray imaging of the breast discussion. Because management of imaging personnel radiation dose during diagnostic X-ray procedures is a topic of vital importance, a detailed presentation of relevant subject matter is also included. This features information on annual limits for exposed personnel, the "as low as reasonably achievable (ALARA)" concept, dose reduction methods and techniques, guidance for pregnant personnel, basic principles of radiation protection for personnel exposure reduction, safety during fluoroscopic procedures, protection during mobile X-ray examinations and C-Arm fluoroscopy, caution during high-level control interventional procedures, diagnostic X-ray suite radiation shielding design, and the deployment of radiation caution signs.

To create an opportunity for advancement in other imaging modalities and the special considerations needed in procedures in such disciplines, the last chapter

of the text covers radioisotopes and their associated radiation protection requirements. This chapter includes a section discussing in detail the immune system of the body and a substantial exposition on an important cancer treatment modality called *radioimmunotherapy* (RIT), which, in combination with radioisotope diagnostic techniques, is now known as Theranostics. This final chapter also offers relevant information on radiation emergencies, such as those initiated by the use of radiation as a terrorist weapon, and the appropriate handling and procedures to follow in such situations.

The nine appendices in this textbook provide the reader with a wealth of supplemental material that significantly complements and expands specific information given within various chapters in this textbook. Bullets continue to be used to enhance readability by calling attention to particular information, and key terms, as in previous editions, are identified in bold print. The authors have endeavored to present material in this textbook in a succinct but sensibly complete fashion to meet the initial and, as feasible, ongoing needs of a large number of the various members of the radiation participant health care sector. Historically, with each new edition, the authors have sought to expand the scope of the subject matter covered in the text to provide all readers with a broader base of knowledge. This edition continues this tradition.

New To This Edition

Additional figures, relevant to the new material, are presented throughout the textbook. These and previously existing artworks serve to enhance the visual impact of the text, thereby promoting visual learning and aiding the reader's understanding of various materials throughout the text.

The number of chapters has remained at 16, but three of them have been expanded to accommodate the detailed inclusion of additional relevant material. The arrangement of selective information throughout the text also has been partially altered, as shown in the chapter listing, to improve on the instruction order of all subject matter covered. Similar to its predecessor, this edition contains an expansive glossary of relevant terms associated with radiation protection, radiobiology, and relevant radiation physics. The authors believe that this can serve as a very useful overall quick reference and/ or review tool. All of the new subject matter in both the 9th and now the 10th editions introduces readers to advanced procedures that they may expect to encounter in the modern clinical setting and therefore require an awareness and understanding of the methods of radiation protection needed to ensure safety of patients, themselves, and other personnel while these procedures are being performed.

Chapter Contents

Information covered in **Chapter 1: *Introduction to Radiation Protection*** includes a discussion of the use of ionizing radiation in the healing arts, beginning with the discovery of X-rays in 1895, the fundamental properties of X-rays, the team concept in the medical field, and the control of radiant energy. Goals and concepts of radiation protection are identified, and a simplified introduction to the three main radiation quantities and units of measure (both traditional and metric) is provided to acquaint learners with these concepts earlier in their education. In the sections on the justification and responsibility for imaging procedures, benefit versus risk, diagnostic efficacy, and the ALARA (*as low as reasonably achievable*) principle are explained. The learner is then introduced to the three cardinal rules of radiation protection. A discussion of the responsibility for maintaining ALARA in the medical industry follows.

Other topics covered in this chapter include patient protection and patient education, which bring into consideration the risk of diagnostic imaging procedures versus the potential benefit of such procedures. Ongoing discussion of the use of background equivalent radiation time (BERT) to inform patients of the amount of radiation they will receive during a specific X-ray procedure continues to be an important component of this initial chapter. Discussion on the increased radiation sensitivity of children compared with adults is addressed and is followed by segments on the Image Gently Campaign, and the Monitoring and reporting of radiation dose. The chapter ends with new material that is a detailed introductory discussion on artificial intelligence (AI), what it is, and its increasing assistance in precise radiographic imaging.

Chapter 2: *Radiation: Types, Sources, and Doses* presents generalized information on radiation. Current discussions on the electromagnetic spectrum, ionizing and nonionizing radiation, and particulate radiation are included. An introduction to the concept of radiation dose to create an appreciation of radiation doses that humans can receive and have received is provided. A section covering the topic of biologic damage potential, explaining how this occurs, follows. Updated information on sources of radiation, both natural and human-made, completes this chapter. The second figure in this chapter provides an overview of the Average Annual Effective Radiation Dose Per Person in the United States (mSv) as of 2016. Also, the most recent follow-up data regarding nuclear power plant accidents are covered under the section on human-made (artificial) radiation.

Chapter 3: *X-Ray Interactions with Matter* extensively treats radiation physics relevant to protection and safety to enhance student learning of this subject by providing detailed essential background knowledge of subject matter that intertwines with basic radiation physics concepts. The chapter begins with a discussion on the significance of X-ray absorption in biologic tissue. Subject matter related to X-ray beam production and energy follows. Other topics addressed are radiation attenuation, the probability of interaction of X-rays with matter, and the various types of X-ray interaction, such as coherent scattering, photoelectric absorption, Compton scattering, pair production, and photodisintegration.

Whereas the first and second chapters of the text provided a brief introduction to the topic of radiation quantities and units of measure, **Chapter 4: *Radiation Quantities and Units*** contains a much more detailed discussion of this subject matter. Beginning with the historical evolution of radiation quantities and units of measure, the chapter progresses with the most current information on quantities and units that are the norm today. While some traditional quantities and units are still in use at this time, the main focus on this topic is a much greater emphasis on the standard system, which is employed throughout the world. With the addition and enhancement of information now available in this chapter, the learner will acquire a clearer understanding of the **Système International** (SI) units of measure and terms defining radiation dose.

Chapter 5, in this 10th **edition,** offers a detailed overview of cell biology. Cell chemical composition, cell structure, and cell division are thoroughly treated. Multiple illustrations contribute to enhancing and promoting visual understanding of the material. Selected topics have been updated. Information within this chapter serves as a valuable prerequisite for the subject matter in the following chapter.

Chapter 6 introduces and covers in detail molecular and cellular radiation biology and connected discussions of ionizing radiation. An explanation of radiation energy transfer determinants such as linear energy transfer (LET), relative biologic effectiveness (RBE), and oxygen enhancement ratio (OER) is also given. Molecular effects due to radiation exposure are extensively described. This includes effects of irradiation on somatic and genetic cells, classification of damaging ionizing radiation, direct and indirect action characteristics, the radiolysis of water, specific effects of ionization on DNA and on chromosomes, and target theory. Other significant topics, such as consequences to the entire cell stemming from irradiation, survival curves for mammalian cells, and overall cell radiosensitivity, are also treated. Closely related to all of these are oxygen enhancement effects and the Law of Bergonié and Tribondeau. All topics in this chapter contain the latest information now available.

Chapter 7: *Early Effects of Radiation Exposure* is dedicated to a discussion of the most current information on *early tissue reactions* and their effects on organ systems within a body that was very significantly irradiated. These specific outcomes may occur within minutes, hours, days, or weeks of irradiation. As a result of this, they are termed *early tissue reactions*. A detailed discussion of the acute radiation syndrome (ARS) is presented in this chapter. Examples of human populations affected with ARS are identified and described. Outcomes associated with ARS such as lethality, local tissue damage, detrimental effects on the reproductive and the hematopoietic systems, and cytogenic (cell-producing) effects are examined.

In **Chapter 8:** *Late Effects of Radiation Exposure*, stochastic (random) effects and *late tissue reactions* induced by radiation in organ systems are extensively considered. Effects that occur months or years after exposure to ionizing radiation are the focus of this chapter. These late effects can either be delayed tissue reactions, such as the formation of cataracts, or can be stochastic effects, such as the induction of cancer or genetic alterations. Within this chapter are the most current concepts and terminology that address this subject matter. Other topics of great importance include epidemiology, carcinogenesis, radiation dose-response relationship, and risk models used to predict different types of cancer and various late somatic effects. There is also a substantial discussion of hereditary effects that explains the causes of genetic mutations, both natural and spontaneous. Radiation interactions with DNA macromolecules, mutagens or agents capable of inducing genetic mutations, incapacities of mutant genes, dominant or recessive point mutations, and the doubling dose concept are also treated.

In **Chapter 9:** *Dose Limits for Exposure to Ionizing Radiation*, the basis of the effective dose-limiting system is reviewed, along with the identification and current function of the various radiation protection standards organizations. Existing US regulatory agencies are also identified, and their specific tasks and responsibilities are earmarked. Covered in detail is the necessity for establishing and maintaining a strong radiation safety program, the multiple requirements for such programs, and the identification of qualified persons and/or groups to administer and carry them out. This mandates the formation of a radiation safety committee and the position of qualified radiation safety officer (RSO). Requirements for an RSO are specified.

Also included in this chapter is the Radiation Control for Health and Safety Act of 1968, additional information on the ALARA concept, the position of the US Food and Drug Administration (FDA) as it relates to patient radiation dose, and the value and importance of the Consumer-Patient Radiation Health and Safety Act of 1981. Radiation-induced responses of concern in radiation protection are identified by category, and changes in terminology from the 1970s to the present are addressed. Current radiation protection philosophy, the basics for the effective dose-limiting system, and the latest National Council on Radiation Protection and Measurements (NCRP) recommendations are also described. Action limits for emergency situations involving radiation exposure are identified followed by a discussion on the subject of *radiation hormesis*. At the conclusion of this chapter, occupational and nonoccupational dose limits are considered.

Chapter 10: *Equipment Design for Radiation Protection* includes an extensive treatment of the latest advances in imaging equipment that pertain to radiation safety. Also, other relevant devices and accessories that may be used to provide radiation protection for the patient and the equipment operator are reviewed in detail. Topics presented under the heading of "Radiation Safety Features of Radiographic Equipment, Devices, and Accessories" include discussions of diagnostic-type protective tube housing and functions, the X-ray unit's control panel or console, the radiographic examination table, source-to-image receptor distance indicators, X-ray beam limitation devices for fixed and mobile radiographic equipment, permanent and added filtration, compensating filters, required radiation exposure characteristics, automatic exposure control (AEC), radiographic grids, and mobile or portable radiographic units.

Under the heading of "General Information and Radiation Safety features of Digital Imaging Equipment and Accessories," topics included are digital processed radiographic imaging modes, digital imaging overview, computed radiography (CR), digital radiography (DR), and repeat rates in digital imaging.

The section on "Radiation Safety Features of Fluoroscopic Equipment Devices and Accessories" covers fluoroscopic procedures and patient irradiation rates, non-digital fluoroscopic imaging systems, and mobile fluoroscopic systems. Under the heading of "Radiation Safety Features of Digital Fluoroscopic Equipment," digital fluoroscopy (DF) is treated, followed by an expansive discussion of digital subtraction angiography (DSA) and interventional systems. The chapter concludes with sections on "Radiation Safety for High-Level Control Interventional Procedures," which discusses the rationale for its specialized usage; and on a "Public Health Advisory About the Danger of Overexposure of Patients and Exposure Rate Limits."

Chapter 11: *Management of Patient Radiation Dose* concentrates on attentive control of patient radiation dosage during diagnostic X-ray procedures. Subject matter covered includes the necessity for effective communication between the radiographer and the patient, the need for immobilization of the patient or body part to be imaged, and the types of immobilization available, traditional specific area shielding of the patient, and recently revised protocol of patient gonadal shielding policies by professional and scientific societies. Other areas of radiation safety concern covered in this chapter include discussion of appropriate technical exposure factors and the use of standardized technique charts. Also, the use of high-kVp and low-mAs exposure factors to reduce dose to the patient is explained.

With the widespread adoption of digital imaging and its associated great ease of repetitive imaging, the potential for a large increase in unnecessary repeated digital images to achieve the highest-quality image or to rectify poor technique became a major concern for overexposure of the patient. The consequences of a substantial increase in repeat rates are identified and the benefit of a strong repeat analysis program to remedy this is examined in detail.

The use of the *air gap technique* to reduce scattered radiation and the advantages of high peak kilovoltage radiography for selective procedures are reviewed. Also discussed at length are the avoidance of nonessential radiologic examinations and the ability to accurately specify the amount of radiation received by a patient during a diagnostic imaging procedure.

Reasons why fluoroscopically guided positioning is unacceptable are also treated. Various methods of protecting the pregnant or potentially pregnant patient during radiographic examinations are discussed in detail, and examples of how to calculate an estimate of the approximate equivalent dose to the embryo-fetus are provided. Because children are more vulnerable to radiation exposure, several subtopics are devoted to pediatric protection during radiographic imaging. Although the Image Gently Campaign for reduction of dose in pediatric imaging was described in Chapter 1 of this text it is mentioned again in this chapter to reinforce the importance of lowering radiation doses. The final topic covered in this chapter examines *dual-energy X-ray absorptiometry* (DEXA, or DXA Scan), which is used for patient bone density determinations and monitoring. This is extremely relevant to estimates of potential bone fracture susceptibility in senior citizens.

Chapter 12: *Management of Occupational Radiation Dose* is concerned with methods for limiting imaging personnel radiation exposure during X-ray procedures. This chapter contains the most current radiation safety practices for radiographers. Annual limits for occupationally exposed personnel are identified, and there are included subsections on effective dose limits, annual occupational and nonoccupational dose limits, and a discussion regarding allowance for a larger equivalent dose for radiation workers. The ALARA concept as it pertains to the protection of personnel in the clinical setting, is reviewed. Various methods to achieve lower occupational doses are identified and described, and special attention is given to protection for pregnant personnel. Subtopics in this section include imaging department practices, acknowledgment of counselling and understanding of radiation safety measures, protective maternity apparel, and protocol on work schedule alteration.

Material presented on protection during fluoroscopic procedures includes the following: dose reduction techniques, remote control fluoroscopic systems, protective lead curtains, Bucky slot shielding device, and rotational scheduling of personnel. Radiation safety during mobile X-ray examinations is another topic that is treated. Two subsections are concerned with personnel behaviour guidance, focusing on the use of protective garments and distance as a means of protection. The latter topic explains where a radiographer should stand while performing a mobile radiographic examination.

Protection for the operator during C-Arm fluoroscopy and during high-level control interventional procedures is reviewed in detail. This is followed by a description of diagnostic X-ray suite radiation protection design, which includes information on requirements for radiation-absorbent barriers, reasons for overshielding, and calculation considerations and examples. Lastly, the use of radiation caution signs is discussed.

Chapter 13: *Radiation Monitoring* includes in-depth treatments on state-of-the-art radiation monitoring for personnel and area monitoring. Also presented is detailed information on the various types and methods of usage of current radiation survey instruments.

Chapter 14: *Radiation Safety in Computed Tomography* considers radiation safety in multiple aspects of computed tomography. This extensive and further chapter is not only structured to explain in detail the various aspects, methods, and types of computed tomography, but it is also designed to inform and educate about the numerous methods employed for radiation protection during basic and advanced computed tomography procedures. Specifically included are discussions about the various degrees of CT radiation exposure, concerns related to patient dose that include both skin dose and dose distribution, and the viability of direct patient shielding. Detailed explanations of the methods and characteristics of both axial and spiral or helical computed tomography are presented. Specific methods for the reduction of patient dose in CT are explained in detail. Also included in the chapter are subsections on tube current modulation, iterative reconstruction, optimization of tube voltage, and patient centering. CT dose parameters and effective CT dose are also extensively discussed. Other topics of importance that are comprehensively treated in this edition are multidetector CT (MDCT), CT cardiovascular imaging (CT CVI), and CT CVI radiation dose.

Newly added to this chapter is an introduction to and a detailed treatment of another version of computed tomography initially utilized, for some time, primarily in radiation therapy and dental radiography, but also now employed widely in mobile CT radiography. This technique is known as cone beam computed tomography (CBCT). What it is, its differences with respect to standard CT, its methods of usage, and its importance are explained at length. New illustrations have been added to this chapter to enhance the visual learning of concepts.

Chapter 15: *Radiation Safety in Mammography* begins with a general discussion about mammography and breast compression, followed by a section on patient dose in traditional mammography. Topics extensively discussed in this section include screening mammography, dose reduction, and filtration for mammographic equipment.

A considerable amount of current state-of-the-art material is introduced next in the sections on digital breast tomosynthesis (DBT), also known as 3D mammography. Topics include discussions reviewing tomography in general and digital breast tomography (DBT) in particular. Subtopics under DBT include effects of tomographic angular scan range, lessening of breast compression force, methods of image reconstruction, advantages of DBT, artifacts in DBT, DBT imaging unit characteristics, and DBT procedure steps and details. This section concludes with material on radiation dosage and a digital breast tomography review summary.

Chapter 16: *Radiation Safety in Nuclear Medicine* is the final chapter in the text. This chapter has been further updated and expanded since the previous edition. Consequently, it provides a very strong resource for qualified individuals wanting to advance into other disciplines beyond diagnostic X-ray imaging, such as nuclear medicine or radiation therapy, and related radiation-associated disciplines. Under the main heading of "Medical Usage," the following subtopics are included: radiation therapy, proper handling and disposal of radioactive materials, nuclear medicine, positron emission tomography (PET), radiation protection, and the PET-CT scanner. Besides the extensive treatment of Radioimmunotherapy first covered in the 9th edition, there is now a newly added section on a recent state-of-the-art combined diagnostic and therapeutic cancer treatment-related modality known as Theranostics. Chapter 16 includes multiple illustrations to enhance visual learning in these disciplines. As in the 9th edition, there is a detailed introductory section on the human immune system, its components, and how it functions, and how it can be assisted.

The second half of the chapter discusses radiation emergencies and the use of radiation as a terrorist weapon. Subtopics in this section include radioactive contamination, cleanup of a contaminated urban area, and medical management of persons experiencing radiation bioeffects.

In summary, the tenth edition of this textbook contains a large quantity of vital current and prior radiation safety information, including explanations of multiple additional related topics of importance throughout the book. Also, this edition includes new illustrations and some updated figures and tables. The changes made throughout the textbook, especially the rearrangement of chapters and the revised chapter naming, are intended to make it easier for the learner to gain comprehension of both traditional and newer, more advanced subject matter.

LEARNING ENHANCEMENTS

Each chapter begins with a list of learning objectives to master, followed by a brief chapter outline and a list of key terms that will appear in bold print in each chapter. Following the list of key terms, an introductory paragraph typically provides an overview of the material to be covered. Bullets are used throughout the text to facilitate readability and call attention to specific information.

The chapter content is followed by a bulleted summary that highlights the most important information in the chapter. A list of general discussion questions follows. After that there are multiple-choice review questions that the learners can use to assess their knowledge acquired from completing each chapter. Instructors may use either or both of these categories to stimulate discussion of selected topics of interest.

Bold print has been used to focus attention on the key terms in each chapter. These key terms will also be discussed in the glossary located in the back matter of the textbook. Throughout the text, information boxes are present to direct readers to important information. The back matter of the book also contains a reference section where a listing of references by chapter can be found.

A series of nine well-developed appendices (A through I) provides enhanced supporting material for subject matter contained within various chapters of the text.

Answers to the multiple-choice review questions in this text may be found on the publisher's website, *Evolve*.

Information has been presented in this textbook as clearly and concisely as possible in a style that builds from basic to more complex concepts. Radiographic images, photographs, tables, information boxes, and graphs reinforce and enhance learning and facilitate retention of material. Throughout the textbook useful examples are included after discussion of concepts that may need to be reinforced.

Ancillaries

Workbook. A free-standing workbook to accompany this textbook is also available in printed form. It contains a variety of exercises for each of the 16 chapters in the book. Exercises included in the workbook are matching of terms or phrases with their definitions or other relevant facts, multiple-choice questions, true or false statements, fill-in-the-blank statements, labelling of diagrams or missing information in boxes or charts, short-answer questions, general discussion or opinion questions, and a chapter post-test to assess learning of the subject matter covered in each chapter.

The use of the workbook, in conjunction with the textbook, will provide a challenging but rewarding experience for the learner. It will reinforce comprehension and help students remember important concepts and material covered in each chapter of the textbook. The answers to all of the exercises in the workbook are located separately in the back matter of the workbook. Using both the text and workbook simultaneously will be of significant value in helping radiography students prepare for credentialing examinations such as the American Registry of Radiologic Technologists (ARRT) certification examination for full-scope radiographers. Limited-scope X-ray technologists may also find both the textbook and workbook very helpful in preparing for state licensing examinations.

INSTRUCTOR MATERIALS

Ancillaries for instructors are also available with this tenth edition to assist radiologic technology educators. Ancillaries include a test bank consisting of multiple-choice questions for each chapter, a collection of images from the textbook, and a PowerPoint lecture presentation. These additional materials are available for instructors on the publisher's website, *Evolve*.

The web address is http://evolve.elsevier.com/Sherer/radiationsafety.

USING THE BOOK

The presentation of the tenth edition presumes that the reader has some minor background in elementary physics, human anatomy, and very basic medical and imaging terminology. A knowledge of units of measure [metric and English], atomic structure, the physical concepts of energy, electric charge, the subdivision of matter, electromagnetic radiation, X-ray production (both quality and quantity) and the process of ionization is useful but not mandatory, since these concepts are generously covered in the course of studying the chapter material. The learner will be able to substantially build on any existing knowledge by assimilating information presented in this textbook.

To facilitate a working comprehension of the principles of radiation protection, radiobiology, and physics related to radiation protection, study materials offered in the tenth edition remain sophisticated enough to be true to the subject matter's complexity, yet concise and sufficiently straightforward to permit comprehension by all readers. For student radiographers and radiology residents and other interested new professionals, this text, although quite detailed in every topic considered, is best used in conjunction with formal instruction presented by a qualified instructor.

As mentioned previously, practicing radiographers, new medical physicists, newly appointed radiation safety committee chairs, radiologists, and other physicians interested in the subject matter contained within the textbook may utilize it as a self-learning instrument to reinforce and broaden their knowledge of radiation safety and also acquaint themselves with up-to-date changing imaging and therapeutic concepts and material.

By mastering the material covered in this textbook and its ancillaries, and by applying this knowledge in the performance of radiologic and related procedures in the clinical setting, the reader will help ensure the safety of patients, all diagnostic imaging personnel, and the general public.

Mary Alice Statkiewicz Sherer, AS, RT(R), FASRT

ABOUT THE AUTHORS

Mary Alice Statkiewicz Sherer, AS, RT(R), FASRT, Radiologic Technology Educator/Instructor/Technologist Emeritus, is the primary author of this textbook and the accompanying workbook and ancillary materials. Ms. Sherer continues to be available as a private radiography education, radiation safety, and medical publishing consultant. In the past, she was employed for 6 years as an instructor for the Limited Scope X-Ray Program at High-Tech Institute, Inc. (Anthem College), a career college that was located in Nashville, Tennessee. Before assuming that position in January 2004, Ms. Sherer was employed at Summit Medical Center in Hermitage, Tennessee for 13 years, where she performed diagnostic imaging procedures and served as the department's Compliance/Education Coordinator. Prior to that position, Ms. Sherer was employed at Memorial Hospital of Burlington County (now Virtua Health System Memorial Hospital) in Mount Holly, New Jersey, where she served for over 16 years as radiography program director and then as educational administrative assistant for the Department of Radiology.

After earning an ARRT certification in 1965, Ms. Sherer filled several technical and teaching positions in the New Jersey area and in 1980 graduated with an associate degree in science from the College of Allied Health Professions, Hahnemann Medical College and Hospital of Philadelphia (Hahnemann University). She has been an active and leading member of several professional organizations, having served on committees and task forces of the American Society of Radiologic Technologists, as past president of the 28th Mid-Eastern Conference of Radiologic Technologists, and as president and chairman of the Board of Directors (both district and state levels) of the New Jersey Society of Radiologic Technologists. Services to the ASRT include functioning as chairperson of the *Radiologic Technology* editorial review board for the membership year 1989–1991 and participating as a member of the Committee on Memorial Lectures for the membership years 1989–1991 and 1991–1993.

Other responsibilities fulfilled by Ms. Sherer include: Item Writer for Radiography Certification for the American Registry of Radiologic Technologists (1983), Site Visitor Team Member for the Joint Review Committee on Education on Radiologic Technology (1981–1983), Site Visitor for the State of New Jersey, Bureau of Radiologic Certification for several years, and Critical Textbook Reviewer for unpublished work for WB Saunders Company (1989–1992).

For the services and contributions to the profession of radiologic technology, in June 1990, Ms. Sherer was elevated to the status of Fellow of the American Society of Radiologic Technologists. She continues to hold this professional honor.

Ms. Sherer has also presented lecturers for the New Jersey Society of Radiologic Technologists for a winter seminar in 1978, and an Annual Meeting in 1982. As an author, she has won two first-place awards for technical writing, the 1st place Graduate Essay Award at the 29th Mid-Eastern Conference of Radiologic Technologists in 1976, and the EI DuPont DeNemours Award presented by the Delaware Society of Radiologic Technologists at the 25th Mid-Eastern Conference of Radiologic Technologists in 1974.

In addition to being the primary author of the first edition of *Radiation Protection for Student Radiographers* and the second through ninth editions of *Radiation Protection in Medical Radiography,* as well of this edition, Ms. Sherer is the author of *Q & A: Preparation for Credentialing in Radiography,* published in 1993 by WB Saunders Company. In 1984, she was a coauthor for the textbook, *Radiation Protection for Dental Radiography,* which was published by Multi-Media Publishing, Denver. Articles written by Ms. Sherer have been published in *Radiologic Technology, The Journal of the American Society of Radiologic Technologists,* and *ADVANCE for Imaging and Radiation Therapy Professionals,* a national biweekly newspaper that was published by Merion Publications. She has also previously served as a consultant to ADVANCE.

In 1999, Mosby produced "Radiobiology and Radiation Protection," the fourth program in Mosby's Radiographic Instructional Series, a CD-ROM (and slide series) presentation consisting of eight modules, approximately 1 hour each in duration. A study guide and an instructor's manual accompanied the audiovisual materials. Ms. Sherer served as chief consultant for the development of the program and as a technical reviewer.

More recently, Ms. Sherer served as a member of the advisory board for the second through fifth editions of the textbook, *Radiography Essentials for Limited Practice,* an Elsevier publication.

Paula J. Visconti, PhD, DABR, was the chief of medical physics and radiation safety officer at Virtua Health System Memorial Hospital in Mount Holly, New Jersey, for over 30 years. She had also served for a period as the radiation safety officer for the entire Virtua Health System in southern New Jersey, which comprises four hospitals.

Dr. Visconti received her PhD in experimental atomic physics from the City University of New York in 1971. She served as a full-time instructor in the Physics Department at the City College of New York for several years thereafter. Dr. Visconti began her career in medical physics at Montefiore Hospital and Medical Center in New York City, where she remained for 5 years as an associate physicist. During that time, she lectured extensively in radiologic physics to both therapeutic radiology residents and student radiographers.

Dr. Visconti is a member of the Society of the Sigma Xi, the American Association of Physicists in Medicine, and the American College of Radiology and is certified in therapeutic radiological physics by the American Board of Radiology.

Dr. Visconti has served as an advisor and collaborating author during the development of the second edition of *Radiation Protection in Medical Radiography* published in 1993 and all subsequent editions since that time. She has contributed significantly to the technical content of all these editions and also provided editing support.

E. Russell Ritenour, PhD, DABR, FAAPM, FACR, is currently a Professor in the Department of Radiology and Radiological Science at the Medical University of South Carolina. Dr. Ritenour received his PhD in physics from the University of Virginia in 1980 and completed a postdoctoral fellowship sponsored by the National Institute of Health in medical physics at the University of Colorado Health Sciences Center. He stayed on the faculty at the University of Colorado for 9 years, serving as director of the graduate medical physics training program, until moving to the University of Minnesota in 1989 where he served as Professor and Chief of the physics section in the Department of Radiology, University of Minnesota Medical School, and was Director of Graduate studies in Biophysical Sciences and Medical Physics, University of Minnesota Graduate School, for 25 years.

During his career, Dr. Ritenour has served as radiation safety officer for several hospitals and research facilities. He is a past president of the Rocky Mountain Chapter of the Health Physics Society and a frequent contributor to the national Health Physics Society's website's feature, "Ask the Expert." Dr. Ritenour is a Fellow, past president, and chairperson of the board of the American Association of Physicists in Medicine and a Fellow of the American College of Radiology.

In the area of radiology education and testing, he has authored several other textbooks, audiovisual programs, and educational websites for radiologic technologists, radiology residents, and medical physicists. He has been a consultant to the US Army for resident training programs, and has produced various types of training and testing programs for the American College of Radiology and the American Association of Physicists in Medicine. He has also been involved in volunteer question writing and test production with the American Registry of Radiologic Technologists and the American Board of Radiology since the 1980s.

Dr. Ritenour was a coauthor of the first edition of this text with Mary Alice Statkiewicz Sherer in 1983 and has been a coauthor of all subsequent editions.

Kelli Welch-Haynes, EdD, RT(R), FASRT, FAEIRS is a tenured professor and Program Director for Radiologic Technology Program within the School of Health Sciences at Dallas College in Dallas, Texas. Dr. Welch-Haynes earned her Bachelor of Science degree from Northwestern State University and went on to receive her Master of Science in Radiologic Sciences with a concentration in Administration from Midwestern State University in Wichita Falls, Texas. Dr. Welch-Haynes received her Doctorate of Education in Curriculum and Instruction, specializing in Allied Health Education, from the University of Louisiana at Monroe. Before becoming an educator, Dr. Welch-Haynes served as the Director of Radiology at Promise Hospital in Shreveport, Louisiana, for 5 years, during which she performed diagnostic radiographs examinations and computed tomography.

She has actively participated in several professional organizations, serving on the boards, committees, and task forces of the Association of Educators in Imaging and Radiologic Sciences and the American Society of Radiologic Technologists. Additionally, she was the chapter director for the Louisiana Alpha chapter of Lambda Nu, the national honor society for the radiologic and imaging sciences. Currently, she serves as a Board Member for the Joint Review Committee on Education in Radiologic Technology and is also a member of the Association of College Educators in Radiologic Sciences.

She has created multiple online continuing education modules for the American Society of Radiologic Technologists. Dr. Welch-Haynes serves as a subject matter expert and creates ancillary products for many radiologic sciences textbooks, including *Bushong's Radiologic Science for Technologists: Physics, Biology and Protection, Fauber's Radiographic Imaging and Exposure, Bontrager's*

Radiographic Positioning and Related Anatomy, and Digital Radiography and PACS, She contributes chapters in *Bontrager's Radiographic Positioning and Related Anatomy* and *Radiologic & Imaging Sciences and Patient Care* and *Kinn's The Medical Assistant An Applied Learning Approach.* Dr. Welch-Haynes has conducted over 150 presentations at state, regional, national, and international levels. She has also published articles in *Radiologic Technology, The Journal of the American Society of Radiologic Technologists, Radiologic Science and Education,* and *ADVANCE for Imaging and Radiation Therapy Professionals.*

Currently, Dr. Welch-Haynes serves as a Board Member for the JRCERT. Dr. Welch-Haynes was elevated to Fellow of the ASRT in June of 2021 and Fellow of AEIRS in 2022.

ACKNOWLEDGMENTS

The constant encouragement and support of my family, collaborating authors, professional colleagues, friends, and the competent, supportive staff of Elsevier, Inc., have made the development, updating process, and production of the tenth edition of *Radiation Safety and Radiobiology in Medical Imaging* and all of its ancillaries possible to achieve.

To my family—sons, Joseph, Christopher, and Terry—a very special acknowledgement and sincerest thanks are given. The consistent love, support, and encouragement you provide gives me the strength and determination to accomplish my goals in life. You are my greatest blessing. Also, a special part of my family, are my two, little shih-tzus, Dexter and Roxie, who were always by my side during the writing of this edition, providing companionship, unconditional love and support for me.

The technical integrity of this edition and the amount of new information that has been added to the 10th edition is attributed to the collaborative efforts of two brilliant and exceptional medical physicists, Paula J. Visconti, PhD, DABR, and E. Russell Ritenour, PhD, DABR, FAAPM, FACR, and an extremely competent radiologic technologist educator, Dr. Kelli Welch Haynes, EdD, RT(R), FASRT, whose professional expertise has greatly enhanced this publication.

Each of these individuals has made significant and valuable contributions in terms of technical information, numerous recommendations, reviewing of various subject matter, editing, and development of new materials and illustrations for this new edition, thereby increasing the overall technical accuracy, timeliness, and value of the contents of this textbook. I am sincerely very thankful to Paula, Russ, and Kelli for all their technical contributions and recommendations, and for all the time each has given reviewing, writing, and assisting with editing of material in this and previous editions. Deep appreciation is also given to Dr. Haynes for producing the Test Bank and PowerPoint slide presentation to accompany this textbook. This series is available on the publisher's website, *Evolve*.

Over the years many contributions of information and illustrations have been given by many individuals, companies, and organizations. These materials have helped to enhance the technical value and visual appeal of this and previous editions. We are very grateful for permission to use these materials and acknowledge their use in the book through the process of citation, where applicable.

We acknowledge the continuous use of some photographs and illustrations that were taken for previous editions of the book and continue to be used in this edition. Thanks is given to those persons who participated in earlier photo shoots. The original photos obtained continue to complement various sections of the text and have enhanced the visual appeal of the book.

Sincere gratitude for effective communication, hard work, and ongoing support of our project is given to the highly competent and wonderful staff of Elsevier, Inc. Special acknowledgement and gratitude is given to Senior Content Strategist, Luke Held; Senior Content Development Specialist, Laura Selkirk; and Senior Project Manager, Nayagi Anandan. We applaud your efforts to bring the tenth edition of this textbook, free-standing accompanying workbook, and other ancillaries to publication. We could not have accomplished this enormous task without you! Thank you all.

Those who seek to learn the art and science of medical imaging are the future of the profession. To the radiography students and radiology residents who will use this textbook, it is my hope that the material contained within this edition will greatly contribute to providing you with a foundation in radiation protection/safety and radiation biology and the means to enhance your knowledge in this subject matter. Education is an ongoing process; each person who enters into radiation sciences profession assumes a responsibility to continue learning to enhance their skills and overall knowledge. This growth will enable imaging professionals including American Registered Radiologic Technologists, Radiologists, Medical Physicists, and

Referring Physicians to better serve patients entrusted to their care.

Finally, as I have stated in previous editions of this text, a very special remembrance is given to my parents, the late Felix and Elizabeth (Markovitch) Krohn, for all they did for me. Their many words of wisdom and life-long encouragement remain with me. The education in my chosen profession, they made possible, helped me to gain the knowledge and motivation necessary to prepare these new and previous editions. My personal accomplishments in the field of medical imaging serves as a tribute to them.

Mary Alice (Krohn) Statkiewicz
Sherer, AS, RT(R), FASRT

CONTENTS

Introduction to Radiation Protection

OBJECTIVES

After completing this chapter, the reader will be able to perform the following:

- Define all key terms.
- Identify the consequences of ionization in human cells.
- List the properties or characteristics of x-rays.
- Describe the concept of teamwork in the medical field and state the potential benefit that such an organized collaborative approach can have on radiation safety.
- Give examples of how radiologic technologists and radiologists can exercise control of radiant energy while performing imaging procedures.
- State the goals and discuss the concept of radiation protection.
- List the three types of radiation quantities and identify the unit(s) of measure in which each quantity is specified.
- Explain how the diagnostic efficacy of an imaging procedure can be maximized.

- State the as low as reasonably achievable (ALARA) principle and discuss its significance in diagnostic imaging.
- List the three basic principles of radiation protection.
- List employer requirements for implementing and maintaining an effective radiation safety program in a facility that provides imaging services, and identify the responsibilities that radiation workers must fulfill.
- Describe the importance of patient education as it relates to medical imaging.
- Compare the radiation sensitivity of children with the radiosensitivity of adults.
- Discuss the Image Gently Alliance
- Discuss the reasons for monitoring and reporting radiation dose.
- Understand what artificial intelligence is and how it works, and discuss the reasons for its growing presence and usefulness in radiographic imaging.

CHAPTER OUTLINE

KEY TERMS

absorbed dose
ALARA
alert levels
background equivalent radiation
time
biologic effects
coulomb per kilogram (C/kg)
diagnostic efficacy
effective dose

exposure
gray (Gy)
Image Gently Alliance
ionizing radiation
milligray (mGy)
milliroentgens (mR)
millisievert (mSv)
optimization for radiation
protection (ORP)

radiation
radiation protection
reference values
risk
sievert (Sv)
machine learning (ML)
deep learning (DL)

The phenomenon known as radiation involves the transmission of energy from one point to another and has been present on this planet in its various manifestations since the beginning of time. The use of radiation within the healing arts did not occur until after the discovery of an energetic form of radiation called *x-rays* in 1895. Since the early 1900s, their beneficial and destructive potentials have been known. Ionizing radiation is a type of radiation that has sufficient energy to remove tightly bound electrons from atoms, resulting in the formation of charged particles called *ions*. This high-energy radiation can take various forms, including x-rays, gamma rays, and certain charged particles. Ionizing radiation is capable of penetrating matter and causing changes in the structure of atoms and molecules. Due to its ability to cause biological damage, ionizing radiation is used in cancer treatment and scientific research. Even with this detriment, it is still widely used, but with caution, in medical imaging and in various industrial processes. Thus, it poses potential health risks and requires careful management and control. The consequences of ionization in human cells are listed in Box 1.1.

In the years following their discovery, most of the fundamental properties of x-rays were discovered by experiment. Briefly, they can be described as follows:
- X-rays are invisible.
- X-rays can have varying degrees of penetration in normal tissue, ranging from very superficial (skin

> **BOX 1.1   Consequences of Ionization in Human Cells***
>
> - Creation of unstable atoms
> - Production of free electrons
> - Production of low-energy x-ray photons
> - Creation of highly reactive free molecules (called *free radicals*) capable of producing substances poisonous to the cell
> - Creation of new biologic molecules detrimental to the living cell
> - Injury to the cell that may manifest itself as abnormal function or loss of function

*Each of these consequences is fully discussed in subsequent chapters.

surface) to much deeper (5 cm or greater), depending on their energy.
- X-rays are not deflected from their paths by electric or magnetic fields and are classified as electrically neutral.
- Although visible light may be focused with a lens, x-rays cannot be.
- X-rays travel in straight lines and at the speed of light (300 million meters per second) until they interact with atoms.
- When passing through matter, x-rays can also produce charged particles by interaction with atoms

composing that matter and cause an emission of light known as *fluorescence* in certain crystals.

- X-ray beams generally have a wide range of energies within them; that is, x-ray beams are usually poly-energetic instead of monoenergetic.

TEAM CONCEPT IN THE MEDICAL FIELD

In recent years, there has been an increasing awareness of the value of a "team approach" to patient care. In a team approach, various participants assume responsibility for their areas of expertise, and communication throughout the team is emphasized. The composition of the team will vary with the circumstances of the patient. It will include the physician of record, nursing and other medical assistants, and any specialty care physicians, including radiologists and their support groups. The latter consists of radiologic technologists, radiologic assistants, and medical physicists. The team may further include physical therapists, respiratory therapists, dietary consultants, and language interpreters as well. It is recognized that each team member brings their own unique contributions to a successful medical interaction with the patient and that teamwork reduces the occurrence of medical errors. Such an organized collaborative approach can also benefit from increased radiation safety, both to patients and directly involved members of the imaging team. This model is becoming a standard part of the curriculum at all levels of training for medical schools, residencies, and medical professional training programs.[1-5] Organizations such as The American Registry of Radiologic Technologists (ARRT), The American Society of Radiologic Technologists (ASRT), and The Joint Commission encourage healthcare providers to function as effective team members while establishing a culture of quality and patient safety.

CONTROL OF RADIANT ENERGY

By using the knowledge of radiation-induced hazards gained over many years and employing effective methods to limit or eliminate those hazards, humans can safely control the use of "radiant energy." Radiant energy refers to the energy carried by electromagnetic waves, including visible light, infrared radiation, ultraviolet light, radio waves, microwaves, and x-rays. It is a form of energy that can travel through a vacuum and does not require a medium for transmission. Radiant energy plays a fundamental role in various natural processes, such as the warmth we feel from the sun (which is emitted in the form of sunlight) and the transmission of information through radio waves. In the context of physics, radiant energy is often associated with the energy carried by electromagnetic radiation across the entire electromagnetic spectrum. An example of controllable radiant energy is the radiation produced from an x-ray tube (Fig. 1.1).

Radiologic technologists and radiologists:

- Are educated in the safe operation of x-ray–producing imaging equipment.
- Use protective devices whenever appropriate.
- Follow established procedures.
- Select technical settings that significantly reduce radiation exposure to patients and themselves.

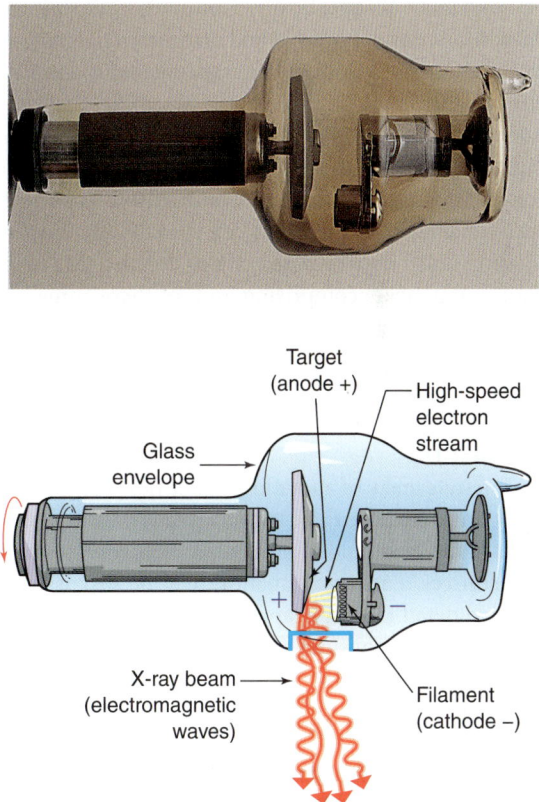

Fig. 1.1 Radiant energy is emitted from the x-ray tube in the form of waves (or particles). This energy made by humans can be controlled by the selection of equipment components and devices made for this purpose and by the selection of appropriate technical settings.

By adhering to these effective practices, technologists and radiologists minimize the possibility of causing damage to healthy biological tissue.

RADIATION PROTECTION

Modern radiation protection programs aim to safeguard individuals from both immediate and long-term radiation effects. Some effects are localized to specific organs or systems, while others, like cancer and genetic changes, can impact the entire body and future generations.

Diagnostic imaging professionals bear the ongoing responsibility of ensuring radiation safety during medical radiation procedures by adhering to established protection programs. **Radiation protection** comprises effective measures implemented by radiation workers to shelter patients, personnel, and the general public from *unnecessary* exposure to ionizing radiation that does not contribute diagnostically. Comprehensive protective actions consider human and environmental factors, technical elements, and procedural considerations. This textbook introduces readers to the scientific principles underlying these measures, emphasizing the common usage of quantities and units, and important concepts such as distance, shielding, and time. Also discussed in much detail are the three existing systems for ionizing radiation units. Appendix A contains detailed lists of the major components comprising each of these three systems and provides the numeric relationships among the corresponding units of each system.

Introduction to Radiation Quantities and Units of Measure

The intricate field of radiation quantities and units is briefly introduced below to help readers understand the varying magnitudes of human exposure to radiation sources. Each such quantity will be discussed in extended detail in later chapters of this textbook. Three key quantities to consider are:

- Exposure
- Absorbed dose
- Effective dose

A brief explanation of these quantities and their commonly specified units follows.

Exposure (coulomb per kilogram [C/kg] or milliroentgen [mR]). In everyday language, *exposure* and *exposed* are commonly used words to describe situations involving human contact with radiation, such as in the statement "The patient was exposed to radiation to obtain a medical image." However, there is also a specific scientific meaning to the term *exposure*. Exposure denotes the production of ions in air resulting from the passage of energetic radiation through the air. When an x-ray tube is activated, some of the air molecules encountered, for example, on the surface of an x-ray room tabletop or within a computed tomography (CT) scanner, can become ionized. Measuring the quantity of this extraneous ionization can be directly accomplished using devices called ionization chambers, which are also used to precisely determine the radiation output of x-ray equipment. Exposure is numerically specified in **coulomb per kilogram (C/kg)** in the metric International System of Units (SI), or historically and still quite commonly, in **milliroentgens (mR)**, a subunit of the nonmetric unit *roentgen*. The milliroentgen is equal to 1/1000th of a roentgen.

Absorbed Dose (milligray [mGy]). The term *dose* is commonly used in everyday language, such as when stating, "Everyone receives a dose of radiation from environmental sources." In the specific technical context, **absorbed dose** refers to the amount of energy due to radiation exposure deposited per unit mass of the material. For living tissue, higher energy radiation deposition generally corresponds to greater disruption of biomolecules, while the reception of lower energy results in less potential damage. Absorbed dose is measured in **milligray (mGy)**, a subunit of the **gray (Gy)** in the SI system of units. One milligray is equal to 1/1000th of a gray.

Effective Dose (ED) (millisievert [mSv]). The term **effective dose** is designed to provide a quantity that seeks to gauge the overall harm caused by radiation exposure in humans, considering factors such as the type of radiation involved, the specific organs irradiated, and the amount of absorbed dose. Effective dose accounts for the differing effects on tissues of ionizing sources such as alpha particles, beta particles, protons, and neutrons at equivalent absorbed dose levels. *Effective dose is thus conceptually the best overall measure of the biological effects of ionizing radiation.* In SI units, ED is typically specified in **millisievert (mSv)**, a subunit of the **sievert (Sv)**. One millisievert is equal to 1/1000th of a sievert.

Ensuring Protection From Harm: Biological Effects of Ionizing Radiation

The imperative to protect against avoidable radiation exposure stems from compelling evidence indicating that ionizing radiation can, and in certain intensities, often does cause nontrivial damage to the living tissue of animals and humans, resulting in potential adverse biological effects. By adhering to radiation safety principles in medical settings, the radiant energy deposited in living tissue during imaging procedures can be restricted, minimizing the risk of adverse biological effects. This textbook concentrates on radiation protection for patients, diagnostic imaging personnel, and the general public.

RATIONALE AND ACCOUNTABILITY IN IMAGING PROCEDURES

Benefit versus Risk

Maintaining minimal radiation exposure is crucial for the general public. However, in instances of illness, injury, or health screening, a patient may willingly assume a relatively small statistical risk to allow physicians to gather vital diagnostic medical information. An illustration of this voluntary acceptance of risk is when women opt for screening mammography to detect early-stage breast cancer. Multiple statistical studies have repeatedly shown that the potential benefits of this exposure to radiant energy significantly outweigh any chance of inducing a radiogenic malignancy or genetic defects.

Diagnostic Efficacy

Diagnostic efficacy is defined as the accuracy of revealing the presence or absence of disease while adhering to radiation safety guidelines, it is maximized by producing essential images with minimal radiation exposure to the patient. This concept is integral to radiation protection in the healing arts, guiding decisions on the justification of imaging procedures (Box 1.2). The referring physician holds the responsibility for determining medical imaging necessity, ordering examinations, and ensuring patient protection from excessive radiation exposure. It is to be strongly emphasized that radiographers and radiologists jointly contribute to maintaining the lowest possible medical radiation exposure by producing

---

BOX 1.2   Achievement of Diagnostic Efficacy

Imaging procedure or practice justified by referring physician	→	Minimal radiation exposure	→	Optimal image(s) produced
		→ Presence or absence of disease revealed	=	Diagnostic efficacy

---

optimal images on the *first* attempt and avoiding repeated examinations due to technical errors or carelessness (Fig. 1.2).

ALARA PRINCIPLE

ALARA, an acronym for "as low as reasonably achievable," is synonymous with the term optimization for radiation protection (ORP). This principle is rooted in evidence compiled by scientists over the past century and remains a cornerstone for radiation protection guidelines.[6] As no *firm* dose limits have been mandated or established for individual imaging procedures, the ALARA philosophy should be a vital component of every healthcare facility's radiation control program (Fig. 1.3). Given the absence of a fixed threshold for radiation-induced cancer, adherence to ALARA principle in selecting exposure factors is crucial for all medical imaging procedures. Regulatory agencies often use the ALARA principle to compare radiation usage among healthcare facilities in particular specific regions.

Cardinal Rules of Radiation Protection

The three cardinal (basic or central) principles of radiation protection are as follows:
- Time
- Distance
- Shielding

These principles are to be applied to both the patient and the radiographer. To reduce the exposure to the patient:
- Reduce the amount of the x-ray "beam-on" time.
- Use as much distance as warranted between the x-ray tube and the patient for the examination.
- Specific area shielding devices may be required under some circumstances.

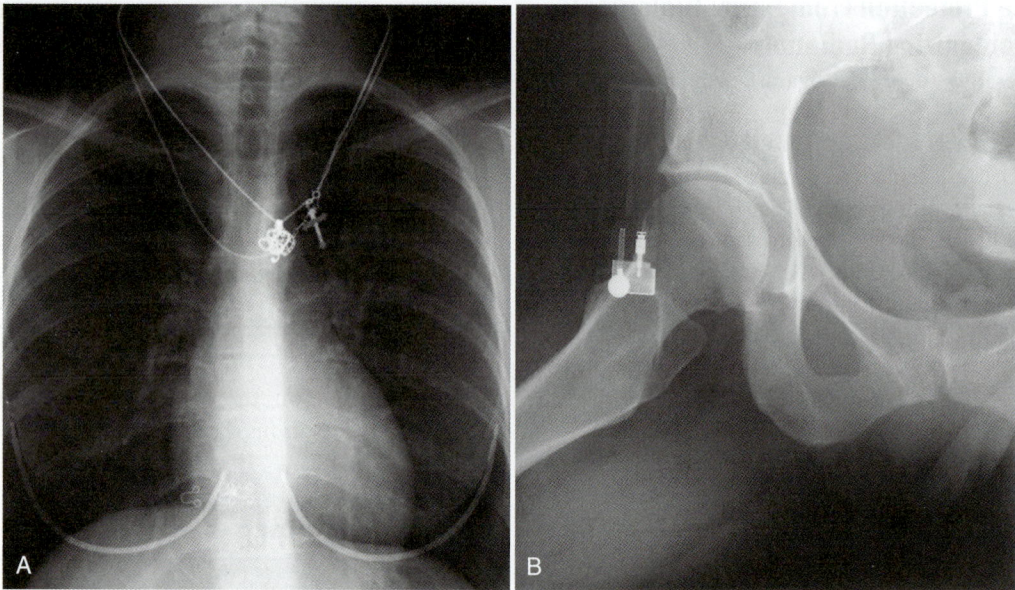

Fig. 1.2 (A) Posteroanterior chest projection requiring repeat examination because of multiple external foreign bodies (several necklaces and an underwire bra) that should have been removed before the x-ray examination. (B) Anteroposterior projection of a right hip requiring a repeat examination because of poor collimation and the presence of an external foreign body (a cigarette lighter) overlying the anatomy of concern. The patient's slacks with the pocket containing the lighter should have been removed before the x-ray examination.

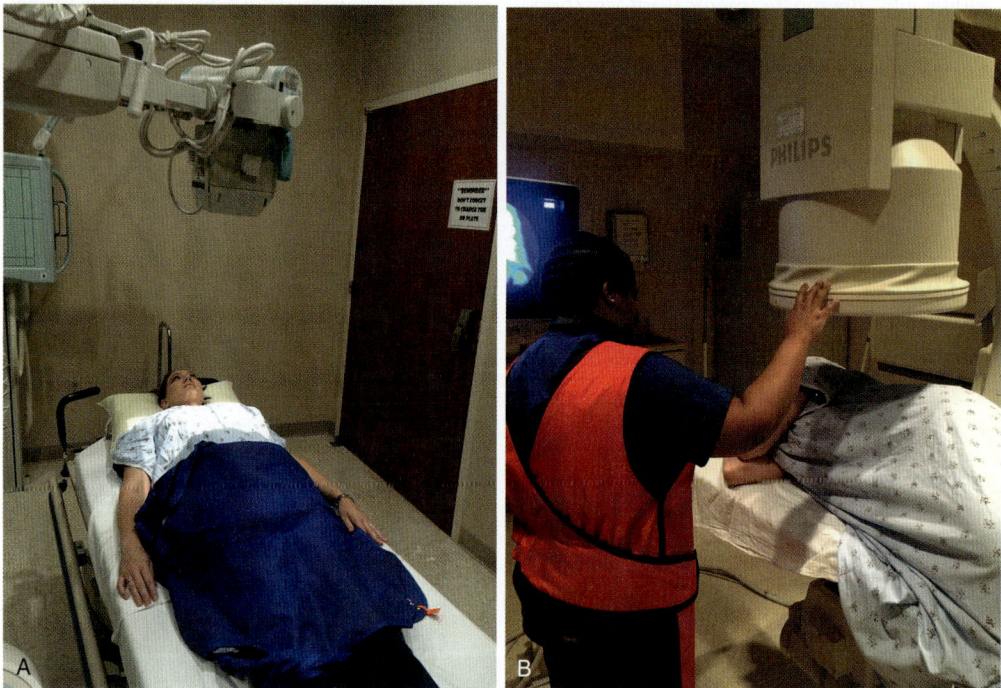

Fig. 1.3 (A) Patient protection. (B) Radiographer protection. Medical radiation exposure should always be kept as low as reasonably achievable (ALARA) for the protection of the patient and for imaging personnel.

Occupational radiation exposures, radiation exposure received by the radiographer while performing their professional responsibilities, can be minimized by the use of these fundamental principles:

- Shorten the time spent in a room where x-radiation is produced.
- Stand at the greatest distance possible from an energized x-ray beam.
- Interpose a radiation-absorbent shielding material between the radiographer and the radiation source.

Maintaining ALARA in the Medical Field: Shared Accountability

Both employers and workers in the medical industry share responsibility for radiation safety. Imaging facilities, prioritizing the welfare of patients and workers, must establish an effective radiation safety program with a firm commitment from all participants. Employers are accountable for providing necessary resources and a conducive environment for implementing an ALARA program, as outlined in a written policy statement available to all employees. In a hospital setting, the *Radiation Safety Officer (RSO)* oversees the execution, enforcement, and maintenance of the ALARA program.

As a significant component of reducing overall radiation exposure in the workplace, management should perform periodic exposure audits to determine whether any large or unusual exposure situations are occurring with any frequency.[7] Radiation workers with proper education and training must consistently adhere to rules, ensuring that their occupational practices align with the ALARA principle (Box 1.3). When utilizing radiation-producing devices in the imaging of patients according to established safeguards, the benefits of exposure can be maximized, minimizing the potential risk of biological damage.

PATIENT PROTECTION AND PATIENT EDUCATION

Educating Patients About Imaging Procedures

Imaging service facilities are tasked not only with ensuring the highest quality of service but also its completeness. A crucial element of the latter involves educating patients about imaging procedures. Patients should be informed not only about the specifics of a particular

---

> **BOX 1.3 Responsibilities for an Effective Radiation Safety Program**
>
> **Employers' Responsibilities**
> - Implement and maintain an effective radiation safety program in which to execute ALARA by providing the following:
>   - Necessary resources
>   - Appropriate environment for the ALARA program
> - Make a written policy statement describing the ALARA program and identifying the commitment of management to keep all radiation exposure ALARA available to all employees in the workplace.
> - Perform periodic exposure audits to determine how to lower radiation exposure in the workplace.
>
> **Radiation Workers' Responsibilities**
> - Be aware of rules governing the workplace.
> - Perform duties consistent with ALARA—as low as reasonably achievable.

---

procedure and their required cooperation but also about any follow-up needed after their examination. Through clear and effective communication, patients can be empowered to actively participate in their own health care (Fig. 1.4).

Risk of Imaging Procedure Versus Potential Benefit

Risk, in general terms, pertains to the likelihood of injury, ailment, or death resulting from an activity. In the medical industry, particularly concerning the use of ionizing radiation, **risk** refers to the possibility of inducing adverse biological effects, such as skin injury, cancer, or genetic defects, after irradiation. People are generally more willing to accept a risk if they perceive that the potential benefit substantially outweighs the risk of injury. Informed patients who understand the medical benefits of imaging procedures are more likely to overcome radiation phobia and accept a small chance of possible biological damage. Knowledge of the biological effects associated with diagnostic radiology has been continually advancing, with the medical imaging industry building on this increased understanding. This information, combined with improved designs of medical imaging equipment and more stringent radiation safety standards, has greatly reduced the risk from imaging procedures for both patients and radiographers.

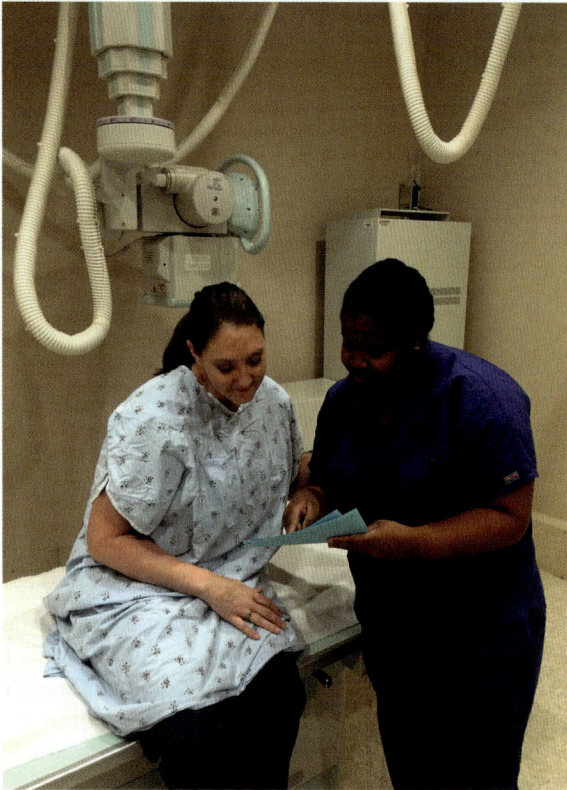

Fig. 1.4 Effective communication is an important part of the patient–radiographer relationship. Patients need to be educated about imaging procedures so that they can understand what the procedure involves and what type of cooperation is required. The radiographer must answer patient questions about the potential risk of radiation exposure honestly. To create understanding and reduce fear and anxiety for the patient, the radiographer can provide an example that compares the amount of radiation received for a specific procedure with natural background radiation received over a given period.

TABLE 1.1   Typical Adult Patient Effective Dose (EfD) and Background Equivalent Radiation Time (BERT) Values

Radiologic Procedure	EfD (mSV)	BERT (Amount of Time to Receive the Same EfD From Nature)
Dental, intraoral	0.06	1 week
Chest radiograph	0.08	10 days
Cervical spine	0.1	2 weeks
Thoracic spine	1.5	6 months
Lumbar spine	3.0	1 year
Upper GI series	4.5	1.5 years
Lower GI series	6.0	2 years
Skull	0.07	11 days
Hip	0.3	7 weeks
Pelvis	0.7	4 months
Abdomen	0.7	4 months
Limbs and joints (except hip)	<0.01	<1.5 days
CT brain	2.0	1 year
CT chest	8.0	3.6 years
CT abdomen/pelvis	10.0	4.5 years

CT, Computed tomography; *GI,* gastrointestinal; *mSv,* millisievert.

Adapted from Wall BF: *Patient dosimetry techniques in diagnostic radiology. New* York, 1988, Institute of Physics and Engineering in Medicine, Vol. 53, p. 117; Cameron JR: Are X-rays safe? *Med Phys World* 15:20, 1999; Stabin MG: *Radiation protection and dosimetry: an introduction to health physics,* New York, 2008, Springer.

Background Equivalent Radiation Time

In addition to providing a standard explanation of a medical imaging procedure, radiographers can further enhance patient understanding and thereby reduce fear and anxiety by employing the **background equivalent radiation time (BERT)** method. Occasionally, radiographers may encounter questions such as "Are x-rays safe?" It is the responsibility of radiologic technologists to offer an honest and understandable response, assuring patients that, for routine diagnostic examinations, there is no documented evidence of unsafe effects from the x-rays used. Addressing queries about the amount of radiation a patient will receive during the procedure can be challenging due to diverse units of measure and the technical nature of radiation dose units. The purpose of this dialogue is not to achieve high scientific accuracy but to relieve radiation-related anxiety by providing an understandable and reasonably correct response.

The BERT method involves comparing the radiation received from a specific x-ray examination to the natural background radiation received over a specified period (Table 1.1). This approach, endorsed by the US National Council on Radiation Protection and Measurements (NCRP), helps radiographers estimate and easily communicate the amount of radiation received during a procedure. For example, the radiographer can respond by estimating the equivalence of the examination to spending approximately 10 days in natural surroundings (see Table 1.1).[8]

The BERT method is based on an annual US population exposure of approximately 3 millisieverts (300 millirems) per year.

Using the BERT method in this context has the following advantages:

- BERT does not imply radiation risk; it is simply a means for comparison.
- BERT emphasizes that radiation is an innate part of the environment.
- BERT provides an answer that is easy for the patient to comprehend.

Patients may mistakenly believe that human-generated radiation is more hazardous than an equal amount of natural radiation. Many patients are unaware that a significant portion of their background radiation originates from natural radioactivity within their own bodies. In summary, alleviating radiation phobia can be achieved by explaining the diagnostic radiation dose to the patients through the BERT method. It is crucial to note that BERT is not a specific radiation quantity but rather a method for public communication, and its name is not ever explicitly mentioned in the explanation.[9]

Increased Radiation Sensitivity of Children

While every patient's received radiation dose is significant, evidence strongly suggests that children exhibit considerably greater radiation sensitivity compared to adults. Exposure to radiation early in life, at the levels found in CT scans or lower, is linked to a measurable increase in cancer incidence as these individuals reach their 50s and 60s. A study done by the Radiation Effects Research Foundation, published in March 2008, followed a specific number "n" of individuals ($n = 2452$ for in-utero exposure and n = 15,288 for childhood exposure) and found a significantly increased risk of fatal cancer in adulthood.[10] This risk persisted even for older children, as seen in a study of patients with scoliosis (mean age at exposure 10.6 years, mean dose received 0.11 Gy, and 4822 persons exposed).[11] The National Academy of Science's latest report on the biological effects of ionizing radiation summarized data indicating that the same radiation exposure in the first year of life poses three to four times the cancer risk for boys compared to exposure between the ages of 20 and 50 years, and six to eight times for girls. Overall, the cancer risk is approximately three times greater in children than in adults.[12]

The Image Gently Alliance

The Image Gently Alliance, a coalition of healthcare organizations, is dedicated to ensuring safe and high-quality pediatric imaging on a global scale. The primary focus of this Alliance is to promote awareness within the imaging community regarding the necessity of adjusting radiation doses when imaging children, with the ultimate aim of bringing about a change in practices.

Originally established as a committee within the Society for Pediatric Radiology in late 2006, the Image Gently Alliance expanded its efforts in 2007 by collaborating with sister societies, including ACR (American College of Radiology), ASRT (American Society of Radiologic Technologists), and AAPM (American Association of Physicists in Medicine), forming what was colloquially known as the "Writers Group." Together, they conceptualized and developed the Alliance's campaign during the summer of 2007. The organization has since launched various campaigns addressing digit'al radiography, fluoroscopy, interventional radiology, nuclear medicine, computed tomography, dentistry, cardiac imaging, and imaging in the context of minor head trauma. As the first in a global network of campaign partners, the Image Gently Alliance has gained recognition at both national and international events.

Monitoring and Reporting Radiation Dose

A significant shift toward more rigorous patient dose reporting in radiologic procedures is currently underway. This trend is particularly pronounced in computed tomography and interventional procedures, where additional measures related to patient dose recording are becoming standard practice. For example, many states now mandate the maintenance of a log for documenting the maximum skin dose for each patient in interventional procedures, while the US Food and Drug Administration (FDA) requires dose measures in CT to be part of each patient's examination record.

The Joint Commission, an independent, not-for-profit organization whose mandate is to accredit healthcare institutions for reimbursement from Medicare and Medicaid, endorses and certifies nearly 21,000 healthcare organizations and programs in the United States, with their guidelines widely accepted by major private healthcare insurance companies. Presently, the Joint Commission requires patient dose monitoring in CT and interventional procedures. However, multiple indications suggest a potential extension of these requirements to all modalities in radiology. The Joint Commission specifies that all ionizing radiation-based imaging equipment undergo detailed annual quality assurance testing by qualified medical physicists and be properly maintained by equipment manufacturers' service personnel. Specifically, for CT scanners, The Joint Commission requires the following.[13]

- Annual staff education in dose-reduction techniques
- Minimum qualifications for medical physicists
- Documentation of CT radiation doses
- Management of CT protocols to minimize radiation dose

The NEXT Program and Reference Values

Various groups have established acceptable **reference values** for patient dose across different procedures, typically derived from extensive surveys of x-ray machines in hospital settings. One notable survey is the Nationwide Evaluation of X-ray Trends (NEXT) project,[14] conducted collaboratively by the FDA and the Conference of Radiation Control Program Directors.[15] State health departments in the United States also provide numerical data based on the latest surveys of existing systems. Dose reference levels (DRLs) are often established as a fraction, such as 75% of the maximum dose values measured. These levels enable individual institutions to assess their degree of adherence to standard practices compared to the majority of institutions.

Given the considerable variation in practice patterns, including the age and health status of the patient population, there are currently no universally dictated values for patient exposures in different examinations and procedures.[16,17] However, this data empowers institutions to evaluate the effectiveness and completeness of their quality assurance programs. Another approach, utilized by the American College of Radiology quality assurance agenda, involves establishing patient dose reference levels through standard required measurements in plastic or tissue-equivalent phantoms as part of the ACR's accreditation programs for acceptable limitations.[18,19]

Protocols for Dose Alerts

Facilities commonly implement **alert levels**. These are protocols to address situations where patient doses are anticipated to or have significantly exceeded normal levels. When this occurs, the staff radiologist is promptly notified, and in certain instances, a medical physicist may be consulted to estimate various patient doses, including effective dose, peak skin dose, or, if applicable, fetal dose.

The radiologic technologist bears the responsibility of ensuring that the radiologist and/or medical physicist receive the necessary information to conduct a dose estimate. This information should include patient size, pregnancy status if relevant, technical factors used for the examination, the anatomical regions imaged, and any available dose measurements recorded through the electronic information system. In cases involving prolonged fluoroscopy, details such as the duration of specific areas of the patient remaining in direct view, as opposed to the fluoroscopic field of view briefly moving through those regions, prove essential in assessing potential substantial radiation dose.

ARTIFICIAL INTELLIGENCE

Artificial Intelligence (AI) is the popular name attached to a rapidly advancing field in computer science that describes the growing ability of computers to realistically simulate human intelligence in performing tasks and/or solving problems. A practical definition of AI is that it represents a computer system that can solve problems without needing detailed, explicit instructions. Many of AI's most dedicated advocates have proposed that the ultimate goal is to create computer models that completely simulate "human intelligence." As intriguing as that may be, the following discussion is not meant to be an artificial intelligence primer. The main intent of this section is to explain what AI is and how AI can be very helpful in providing significant added value to existing imaging modalities in terms of overall medical efficacy. As mentioned at the beginning of this chapter, the team concept of patient care is a well-accepted and significant part of educational curricula across all areas of medical training. There is a growing awareness that in the near future, AI may grow into a role in the medical imaging team that is somewhere beyond a traditional piece of imaging equipment and that will move into a more active advisory role to the human members of the team. There is, of course, significant debate as to how this relationship will evolve, but AI has already established a place in the chain of events leading to diagnosis in areas such as screening exams, where further human oversight will occur prior to any recommendations for treatment.

Specifics of AI

In the sphere of radiographic imaging, AI, simply speaking, is an inclusive shorthand term for *computer-aided diagnostics*. AI has two linked primary subcomponents which are called **machine learning** and **deep learning**. Artificial intelligence is the comprehensive canopy under which both machine learning and deep learning reside. Fig. 1.5 schematically depicts this hierarchy.

Machine Learning

Machine Learning (ML) allows a machine to acquire information and make predictions based on its experience (i.e., its accumulated data in the area of interest). In short, machine learning is a process that allows computers to pursue a task or objective without explicitly being programmed for that task. Thus, ML refers to the enabling of computers to refine their calculation methods *themselves* through experience.

Machine learning begins with previously obtained data which could be numbers, photos, or batches of text. The data are fed into computer memory and subsequently delivered to the CPU (central processing unit) as the raw information which the machine learning model will be *trained on*. The more data that is supplied, the better the ML model's learning efficiency will be. In this situation, the only function of human programmers is to choose a particular machine learning model or algorithm and then sit back and let that computer model train itself via repetitive processes with the supplied data to eventually find patterns or make predictions at an acceptable confidence level. In summary, the function of an ML system can be characterized as:

Descriptive: meaning that the system uses the data to explain what happened, or

Predictive: meaning the system uses the data to predict what will happen, or

Prescriptive: meaning the system will use the data to make suggestions about what action to take.

A descriptive flow chart shown in Fig. 1.6 demonstrates step by step how a machine learning process might take place.

In ML the determinations of *acceptable* and *sufficient* are previously established criteria that help an investigator decide first on what is a decent model from the ML algorithm and second on that model's ability to make predictions or propose actions that are considered to have a desired degree of accuracy. The primary beginning goal is to reduce the difference between model predicted values and the actual values. So, as a starting point, to achieve some rough degree of accuracy, a model is obtained that *reasonably approximates* all of the currently submitted different data points. This is the beginning of the learning process. As more and more data points are collected and associated with more evolutions of the modeling process, significant shrinking of the error or the difference between the actual value and

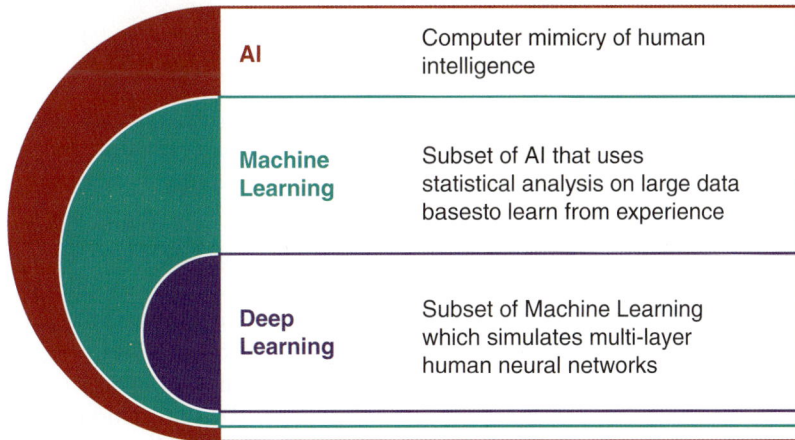

AI	Computer mimicry of human intelligence
Machine Learning	Subset of AI that uses statistical analysis on large data basesto learn from experience
Deep Learning	Subset of Machine Learning which simulates multi-layer human neural networks

Fig 1.5 As noted, deep learning (DL) is taken to be a subset of machine learning (ML), which itself is considered to be a subset of the overall computational technique that is artificial intelligence. So, all three entities: AI, ML, and DL can be thought of as being intrinsically linked. It is helpful to understand how exactly the two sub-components of AI are both different and also related. In what follows, we shall individually consider each in some detail.

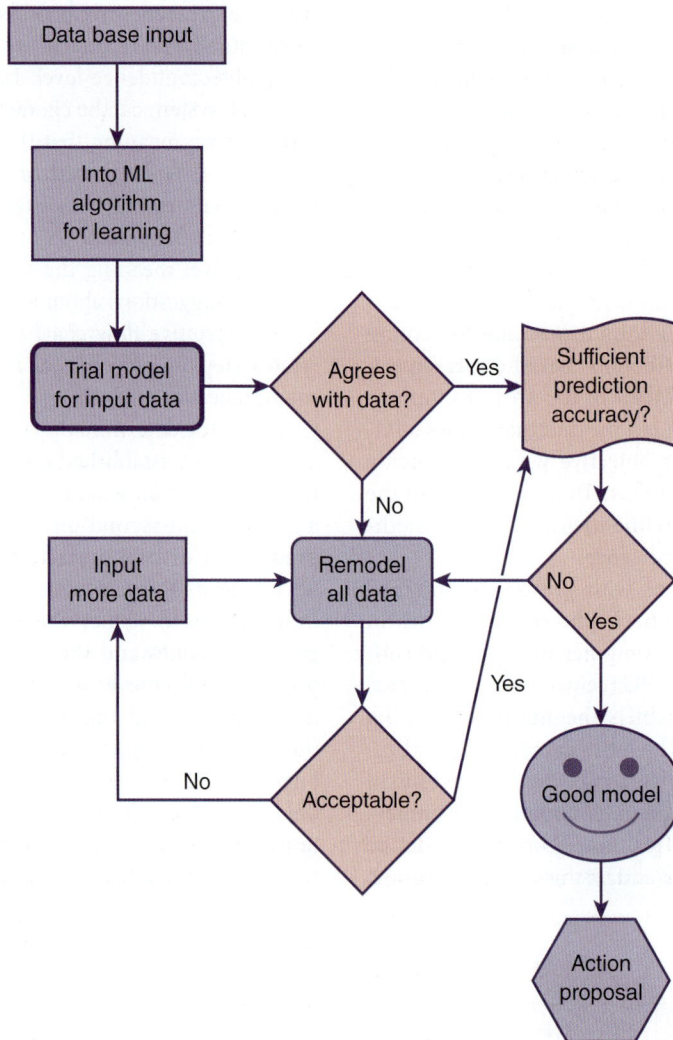

Fig. 1.6 A series of steps or processes depicting how machine learning could be used to evaluate or model a batch of assorted data (e.g., a database) to generate useful predictions, if any exist, from that data.

the model value should occur as a result of the machine learning process *and the better will be the potential predictive ability of our model.* Once a *best-fit model* is judged to be achieved, then, in the future, if a new batch of data is fed into the accepted ML model, it could make new predictions to a satisfactory degree of accuracy.

Deep Learning

Deep learning (DL) is the advance that put artificial intelligence on its rapidly expanding trajectory. Specifically, deep learning is the component of AI that teaches computers to process data in a way that is very

similar to that employed by the human brain. AI systems employing machine learning require very large amounts of data from a specific area to detect potential patterns and correlations linked to a desired outcome. If following a machine learning process, as an example, AI algorithms using deep learning are fed a host of images labeled *cat* and another large quantity of images labeled *not cat*, these DL algorithms will, unlike the ML algorithms, be able to draw on an extensive network of *discovered correlations*, many undetectable by a human being, to determine whether the new image represents a cat or not.

The fundamental structure of a DL machine is a multidimensional grid containing many thousands of, or greater, fundamental processing intersections called *nodes* that are densely interconnected like the neurons in the human brain. In current DL machines, these structures, termed *neural nets*, are usually organized into multiple layers or planes of such nodes (more than 50 in the latest systems), and data moves through them in only one direction. Architecturally, an individual node is connected to several nodes in the layer beneath it or preceding it, from which it receives data, and to several nodes in the layer above it, to which it sends data. As with machine learning algorithms, a deep learning algorithm or machine also requires a *learning process*.

DL Learning Process

Because a DL machine is composed of a large number of networked processing intersections, to successfully employ this complex system to solve problems, a learning procedure must be performed. Prior to starting this, every node of the neural network is structured to have a numerical value or *weight* assigned to each of its incoming connections. When a DL learning process commences, the neural net is activated with each node of the net receiving various numbers or items of data over its connections and subsequently multiplying each connection number by the previously assigned connection weight. The DL algorithm combines all of these weighted values to yield a single number for each node. Only if that number exceeds a predetermined threshold value will data be passed onward from that particular node through all of its outgoing connections to the next layer in the neural net. Data passes through successive layers, as long as predetermined threshold criteria are met, with additional algebraic manipulations being performed and required threshold criteria satisfied until it finally arrives, radically transformed, at the output layer. *Training ceases when the DL machine is judged by a human operator either to have achieved a satisfactory solution to a particular problem or to be ready to tackle some other desired tasks.* Fig. 1.7A and B schematically illustrates a DL process, and the associated captions provide amplified details.

Example

A computer system (machine) is set up to recognize tumors. Imagine that the task of the machine is to diagnose whether a medical image, such as a CT scan of the liver, does or does not contain a tumor. Modern medical images are arrays of picture elements or "pixels." Each pixel value determines the brightness of that part of the image when it is displayed on a monitor. The first step in this AI example is to obtain a set of images with and without tumors. The truth of whether an image contains a tumor would then be established by some independent, well-accepted means, such as pathological testing or review by experienced radiologists. This set of images can be called a "training set." The AI system would be "taught" to find tumors by processing this training set.

Previously, we have explained that in a machine learning (ML) system, a *list of specific image features* in the training set images that contain tumors, such as areas of increased or decreased brightness of an image within a certain size range, are input along with each image as it is processed. In short, some features will have been defined or specified, and then the system will be tasked with identifying which of these features are more important in classifying a particular image.

In a DL system, features which are important for classification of images arise, not from selection by human intervention, but from repeated updates of intermediate states within computer memory called "nodes." These nodes calculate an *activation function* F_x based on inputs, originally from the image and then from each successive node. Each time the system processes the image through all of the levels of nodes an *output function* is calculated. Signal weights among all of the nodes are automatically re-adjusted, and the image data is then processed through all of the nodes to arrive at a different output function. The most successful output function is the one that correlates best with the appearance of tumors in the images!

In ML methods, humans input specific features of the images that are suspected to correlate with the presence of tumors, whereas in DL, the computer selects patterns of node input weights that most closely correlate with the presence of tumors. *This is the essence of the difference between DL and ML.* Both types of AI require the input of a training set. In ML, human operators must decide on some schemes to clearly differentiate two types of images (such as tumor vs. nontumor) within the training set. In DL, an initial set of intermediate node weights and filter functions is selected by technicians that, after

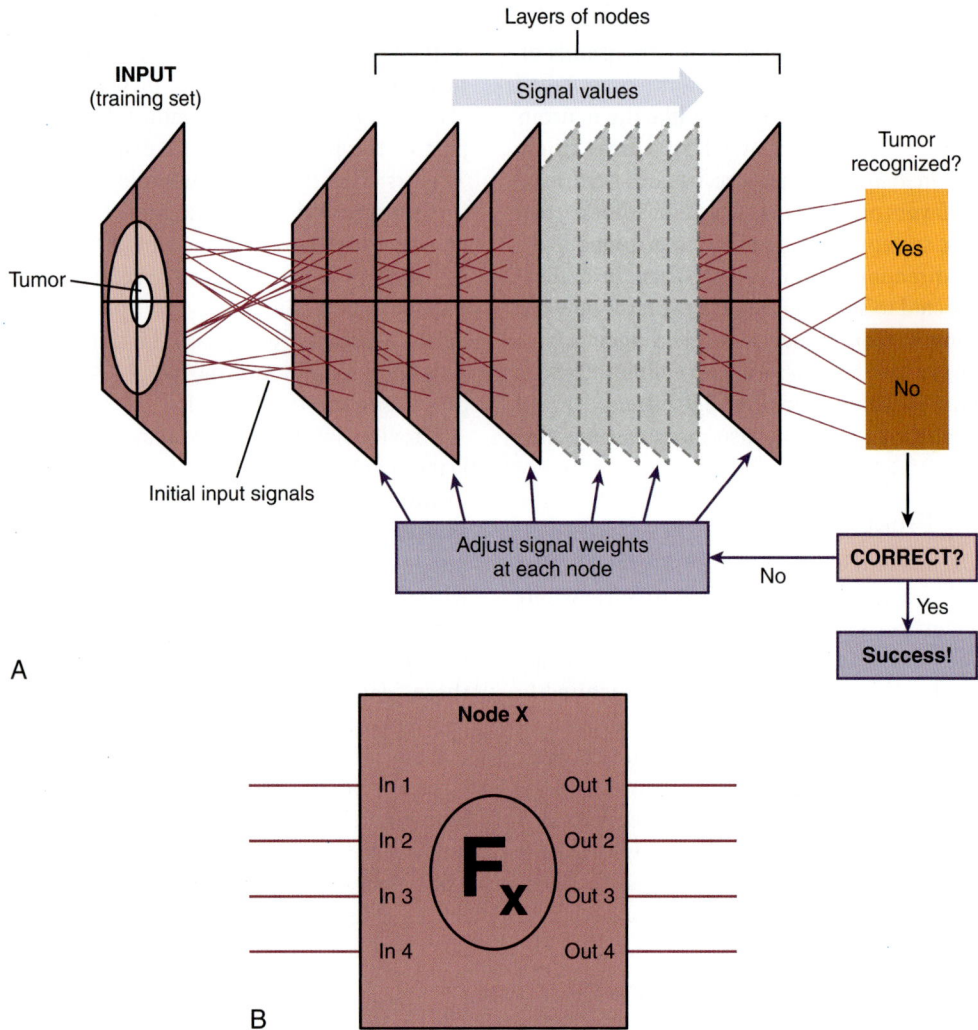

Fig. 1.7 (A) A medical imaging Deep Learning AI system is trained using a set of medical images for which the correct diagnosis (e.g., the presence or absence of a tumor) is known. Each image in a training set serves as *input*. Pixel values from an image are employed as initial input signals, which are subsequently passed on to *arrays or layers of nodes*. From then onwards, each node receives signals from all elements of the preceding layer. (B) Signals are processed at each node according to an *activation function* F_x. This function is a mathematical operation that takes input signal values from a previous layer of nodes (e.g., immediately prior to the Node X group) and provides corresponding outputs to the next nodal layer. F_x's actions may be as simple as plain addition or can involve more complex transformations that depend on the Input's location or depth within the node group. Initially, in the DL process, the signals are all equally weighted, but, and this is the crucial training part, according to the final output, the weights of each signal can be changed until the correct answer *tumor or no tumor,* is achieved. The ultimate objective is to obtain a system that, if presented with an unknown image, uses the signal weights and activation functions to predict a correct result.

repeated exposure to training sets, are adjusted until the system can be used to best differentiate the training set. Once "trained," the system is then used to predict the presence or absence of tumors in new, unknown images.

Utility of AI in Medical Imaging

Throughout the expanse of medical imaging, AI has repeatedly shown excellent accuracy, sensitivity, and specificity for the detection of small radiographic abnormalities. Outcome assessment in AI imaging studies is currently commonly defined just by lesion or abnormality detection while saying little, however, about the type and biological aggressiveness of that discerned irregularity. Moreover, the additional detectability offered by AI techniques could detrimentally lead to an increase in *overdiagnoses* because of detecting and then highlighting minor changes in either size or architecture that may reflect just subclinical or indolent disease. Even with these caveats, deep learning networks have shown a higher sensitivity for pathological findings, particularly for subtle lesions.

In review, where do these conflicting statements leave us in judging the efficacy of AI in medical imaging? Below are listed the multiple significant current contributions of AI systems to successful diagnostic medical imaging.

- *Image Analysis and Interpretation*: Analysis of brain CT and MRI studies using machine learning has exhibited the potential to identify tissue changes suggestive of early ischemic stroke (i.e., interruption of blood supply to the brain) in a timeline from symptom onset that is briefer than that of a human reader. Dedicated studies, however, are still needed to determine whether such AI-detected cerebral changes accurately correlate with clinically proven neurological disability.
- *Efficiency*: AI has proven very useful in selecting among various protocols for the most efficient methods to radiographically scan patients and to conduct subsequent image processing after scans are acquired.
- *Second Reads*: A major additional diagnostic benefit in imaging from the use of artificial intelligence methods is successful *second reads* of screening mammograms. This latter aid suggests that the most immediate role for AI here is in *partnership with human radiologists*, providing quality and safety checks while prompting review and final judgment by the radiologist.[20]

- *Image Reconstruction*: AI algorithms contribute to advanced image reconstruction techniques, improving the quality of images and considerably reducing artifacts. This is especially beneficial in low-dose imaging and in faster image acquisition.
- *Quantitative Analysis*: AI facilitates quantitative analysis of medical images, allowing for precise measurements of size, volume, and other parameters. This is significant in monitoring disease progression and treatment effectiveness.
- *Training and Education*: AI is employed in medical imaging education by providing simulations, tutorials, and interactive learning experiences for healthcare professionals to enhance their diagnostic skills.

Synopsis

AI enables a machine (computer) to make independent decisions when faced with new data. AI systems are trained by exposure to sets of data for which the outcome is known. After this preparation, the AI system can receive new data sets and make decisions about the new data on the basis of its experience with the training data. In ML systems, specific identifiable features of data that are expected to correlate well with correct decisions are input along with the teaching set. In DL systems, more abstract and global schemes are used for processing data into nodes and adjusting weights of intermediate inputs to achieve the best correlation with the training set's known results.

It is expected that DL systems will discover analysis pathways that are not as easily specified by simple rules but are more analogous to the mental processes of trained and experienced observers. Even with all of the cited actual and potential benefits, it is essential to reiterate that "at present, the most successful applications in medical imaging involve using the AI system as a "second read" that alerts the radiologist to a need for further human review of the image."[20]

SUMMARY

- Radiation is the transfer of energy from one location to another.
- X-rays have several unique properties.
- X-rays are a form of ionizing radiation.
- Ionizing radiation has both a beneficial and a destructive potential.

- A team approach to patient care is an organized, collaborative approach that can produce increased radiation safety for patients and directly involved members of the imaging team.
- Radiant energy can be controlled by using the knowledge of radiation-induced hazards gained over many

years and by employing effective methods to limit or eliminate those hazards.

- Radiologic technologists and radiologists should adhere to good safety practices that minimize the possibility of causing damage to healthy biological tissue.
- The goal of modern radiation protection programs is to protect persons from both short-term and long-term effects of radiation.
- To safeguard patients, personnel, and the general public from *unnecessary* exposure to ionizing radiation, effective radiation protection measures should always be employed when diagnostic imaging procedures are performed.
- Living tissue of animals and humans can be damaged by exposure to ionizing radiation; therefore, it is necessary to safeguard against unnecessary exposure.
- Radiation protection may be defined simply as effective measures by radiation workers to safeguard patients, personnel, and the general public from *unnecessary* exposure to ionizing radiation.
- The main descriptors of radiation quantities are exposure, absorbed dose, and effective dose.
- The realized benefits of exposing patients to ionizing radiation should far outweigh any slight chance of inducing radiogenic cancer or any genetic defects.
- Referring physicians should justify the need for every radiation procedure and accept basic responsibility for protecting patients from unnecessary radiation exposure.
- Radiographers should select the smallest radiation exposure settings that produce the most useful radiographic results and avoid errors resulting from *repeated* x-ray exposures.
- The three basic principles of radiation protection are time, distance, and shielding.
- Imaging facilities must have in place an effective radiation safety program that provides patient protection and education.
- A significant understanding of the biologic effects of ionizing radiation, ever-improving designs of medical x-ray equipment, and more stringent radiation safety standards have greatly reduced the risk from imaging procedures for patients and radiographers.
- BERT is a method used to compare the amount of radiation a patient receives from a radiologic procedure with natural background radiation received over a specific period.
- Children are significantly more radiation sensitive than adults, and exposure to radiation early in life, at levels found in CT and even lower, leads to a measurable increase in cancer incidence as these individuals age into their 50s and 60s.
- The Image Gently Alliance advocates lowering patient dose by "child sizing" the kV and mA settings, by scanning only the indicated area, and by removing multiphase scans from pediatric protocols.
- In CT- and x-ray guided interventional procedures, various measures related to patient dose recording are becoming the norm. The US FDA mandates that measures of dose in computed tomography be available as part of the record of each examination. At present, The Joint Commission only requires monitoring of patient dose in CT and in interventional procedures; however, there are indications that it is also moving toward requirements for all modalities in radiology.
- Reference values for patient dose are usually based on large-scale surveys of actual measurements of x-ray machines in hospitals.
- Alert levels are sometimes used when a patient's dose is predicted to or has substantially exceeded normal dose levels.
- Artificial intelligence systems are being developed to find features within medical images that are difficult to describe with specific instructions. By repeated exposure to "training sets" an AI system can refine its ability to find potentially medically significant features without specific instructions.
- AI systems have demonstrated some valuable utility as secondary readers that may indicate a need for further human analysis of images.

GENERAL DISCUSSION QUESTIONS

1. What are the consequences of ionization in the human cell?
2. When is medical radiation exposure considered unnecessary?
3. How can the BERT method be used to eliminate a patient's fears about medical radiation exposure?
4. Describe how radiographers can use the ALARA concept in the performance of their daily responsibilities.

5. Why is a team approach of significant value in patient care?
6. How will a patient benefit from monitoring and reporting of radiation dose?
7. Why should the ALARA philosophy be maintained as a main part of every healthcare facility's radiation safety program?
8. When are patients more likely to suppress any radiation phobia and be willing to assume a small chance of possible biologic damage?
9. On what premise is BERT based?
10. In the medical industry, with reference to the radiation sciences, how is risk defined?
11. What is the first goal of the Alliance for Radiation Safety in Pediatric Imaging?
12. Describe the Image Wisely Campaign, Pause and Pulse: Image Gently in Fluoroscopy Campaign, and the Image Gently Campaign.
13. Describe how machines (computers) can process images to find objects such as tumors without specific descriptions of the objects.

REVIEW QUESTIONS

1. A patient may choose to assume a relatively small statistical risk of exposure to ionizing radiation for a physician to obtain essential diagnostic medical information when:
   1. Illness occurs
   2. Injury occurs
   3. A specific imaging procedure for health screening purposes is called for
   A. 1 and 2 only
   B. 1 and 3 only
   C. 2 and 3 only
   D. 1, 2, and 3
2. Effective measures employed by radiation workers to safeguard patients, personnel, and the general public from *unnecessary* exposure to ionizing radiation defines:
   A. Diagnostic efficacy
   B. Optimization
   C. Radiation protection
   D. Reference values
3. Which of the following is a method that can be used to answer patients' questions about the amount of radiation received from a radiographic procedure?
   A. ALARA concept
   B. BERT
   C. PULSE
   D. EPA
4. The term *optimization for radiation protection* (ORP) is synonymous with which of the following?
   A. As low as reasonably achievable (ALARA)
   B. Background equivalent radiation time (BERT)
   C. Effective dose (EfD)
   D. Diagnostic efficacy (DE)

5. Monitoring and reporting of patient dose for CT and interventional procedures can lead to:
   A. An invasion of patient privacy
   B. An increase in patient radiation dose
   C. A reduction in patient radiation dose
   D. Elimination of the need for imaging equipment radiation safety features
6. The amount of ionization produced in the air when ionizing radiation is present is known as:
   A. Absorbed dose
   B. Effective dose
   C. Efficacy
   D. Exposure
7. The degree to which the diagnostic study accurately reveals the presence or absence of disease in the patient while adhering to radiation safety guidelines defines which of the following terms?
   A. Radiation protection
   B. Radiographic pathology
   C. Effective diagnosis
   D. Diagnostic efficacy
8. The millisievert (mSv) is equal to:
   A. $\frac{1}{10}$ of a sievert
   B. $\frac{1}{100}$ of a sievert
   C. $\frac{1}{1000}$ of a sievert
   D. $\frac{1}{10,000}$ of a sievert
9. An effective radiation safety program requires a firm commitment to radiation safety by:
   1. Facilities providing imaging services
   2. Radiation workers
   3. Patients

A. 1 and 2 only
B. 1 and 3 only
C. 2 and 3 only
D. 1, 2, and 3

10. If a child receives a dose of radiation in a CT scan where adult protocols are used, the child, because of being smaller in size, will receive a:

A. Lethal dose of radiation
B. Higher effective dose than would an adult, but the image produced will appear to be of acceptable quality
C. Lower effective dose than would an adult, and the image produced will be of acceptable quality
D. Severe radiation burns

Radiation: Types, Sources, and Doses

OBJECTIVES

After completing this chapter, the reader will be able to perform the following:

- Define all key terms.
- Provide examples of different types of radiation.
- Draw a diagram to illustrate the electromagnetic spectrum, and explain how the spectrum can be divided for the purpose of studying radiation protection.
- List the different forms of electromagnetic and particulate radiations, and identify those forms that are classified as ionizing radiation.
- Identify the unit of measure in which radiation absorbed dose is most commonly specified.
- Explain the concepts of equivalent dose and effective dose, and identify the unit of measure in which each of these radiation quantities is most often specified.
- Explain how ionizing radiation can cause biologic damage in body tissue.
- List and describe three sources of natural background ionizing radiation and six sources of human-made, or artificial, ionizing radiation.
- Discuss the local and global consequences of radiation exposure resulting from accidents in nuclear power plants.
- Discuss the general responsibility for radiation safety and the need for radiation protection in medical imaging.
- Discuss the modalities used in medical imaging that have caused an increase in radiation dose for patients from 1980 until the present time.

CHAPTER OUTLINE

Radiation
  Types of Radiation
  The Electromagnetic Spectrum
  Ionizing and Nonionizing Radiation
  Particulate Radiation

An Introduction to the Concept of Radiation Dose
Biologic Damage Potential
Sources of Radiation
Summary

KEY TERMS

absorbed dose
biologic damage
cellular damage
effective dose (EfD)
electromagnetic radiation
electromagnetic spectrum
electromagnetic wave
equivalent dose (EqD)

human-made, or artificial, radiation
ionization
isotopes
milligray (mGy)
millisievert (mSv)
natural background radiation
organic damage

particulate radiation
radiation
radiation dose
radioactive decay
radioisotope
radionuclides
radon

Radiation is the emission of energy in the form of electromagnetic waves or as moving subatomic particles (protons, neutrons, beta particles, etc.) passing through space from one location to another. Some types of radiation produce damage to biological tissue, whereas others do not. Some sources of radiation are considered **natural** because they are always present in the environment. However, other sources are created by humans for specific purposes and therefore are classified as **human-made** (historically called "man-made" radiation), or **artificial**, **radiation**. This chapter presents an overview of the various types and sources of radiation, as well as the doses that are typically received from both categories.

RADIATION

Types of Radiation

Some examples of different types of radiation are presented in Box 2.1. When radiation is in the form of subatomic particles that have mass, such as neutrons, protons, or electrons, then its energy is given by the mass and velocity of the particles through the equation for kinetic energy, $KE = \frac{1}{2} mv^2$. When radiation is in the form of subatomic particles that have no mass and always travel at the speed of light, then its energy E is given by the *frequency* of the photon "v" multiplied by a fundamental constant of nature, called Planck's constant "h," with: $E = hv$. Some examples of different types of radiation are presented in Box 2.1.

The Electromagnetic Spectrum

The full range of frequencies* and wavelengths* of **electromagnetic waves** is known as the **electromagnetic spectrum**. Each grouping on this scale represents a type or category of radiation generated by varying electric and magnetic fields. Table 2.1

---

*To understand the concepts of wavelength and frequency, consider ocean waves. The distance between successive highpoints or crests of the water waves is called the wavelength of the water waves and the rate (e.g., number per second) at which successive crests flow past a specific location is called the frequency of the water waves. This description directly carries over to the waves associated with **electromagnetic radiation**, namely λ (wavelength) = c (speed of light) / v (frequency) or more commonly written as: c = λv.

BOX 2.1   Examples of Different Types of Radiation

Example 1. Mechanical Vibrations of Materials
Such mechanical vibrations can travel through the air or other materials to interact with structures in the human ear and produce the sensation known as *sound*. *Ultrasound* is the mechanical vibration of a material in which the rate of vibration does not stimulate the human ear sensors and therefore is beyond the range of human hearing.

Example 2. The Electromagnetic Wave
Radio waves, microwaves, visible light, and *x-rays* are all representatives of the **electromagnetic wave**. In these waves, electric and magnetic fields fluctuate rapidly as they travel through space. A limited range of frequencies of this fluctuation is interpreted by its interaction with the human system as visible light. Within this range, small variations in frequency—the number of cycles or wavelengths of a simple harmonic motion per unit of time—are interpreted as different colors. However, frequencies both above and below the visible range exist and have many uses. Electromagnetic waves are also characterized by their wavelength, which is simply the physical distance between successive maximum values of oscillating wavelike electric and magnetic fields.

At the beginning of the 20th century, leading scientists first realized that electromagnetic radiation appears to have a dual nature, referred to as *wave–particle duality*. This means that this form of radiation travels or propagates through space in the form of a wave but can interact with matter as a particle of energy called a *photon*. For this reason, x-rays may be described as both waves and particles.

---

demonstrates the electromagnetic spectrum in terms of *frequency* (given in units of hertz [Hz], i.e., cycles per second), *wavelength* (in meters), and *energy* (specified in electron volts [eV], a unit of energy equal to the quantity of kinetic energy an electron acquires as it moves through a potential difference of 1 volt). Each frequency within the spectrum has a characteristic wavelength and energy. Some of the practical uses of these different frequency ranges are listed. Note that higher frequencies are associated with shorter wavelengths and higher energies; therefore as the wavelength ranges from largest to smallest, frequencies and energy cover the corresponding smallest to largest ranges.

TABLE 2.1	The Electromagnetic Spectrum*		
Use	**Frequency**	**Wavelength**	**Energy**
AM radio	0.54–1.6 MHz	0.6–0.2 km	2–7 neV
FM radio	88–108 MHz	3.4–3 m	370–440 neV
Television	54 MHz–0.8 GHz	5.6–0.4 m	220 neV–3.3 µeV
Microwaves	0.1–100 GHz	3 m–3 mm	0.4 eV–0.4 meV
Infrared	100 GHz–400 THz	3 mm–0.7 m	0.4 meV–1.6 eV
Visible	400–700 THz	0.7–0.4 m	1.6–2.8 eV
Ultraviolet	1–100 PHz	300–3 nm	4–400 eV
X-rays	100 PHz–100 EHz	3 nm–3 am	0.4–400 keV
Gamma rays	100 EHz–infinity	3–0 am	400 keV–infinity

*Frequency (in units of hertz [Hz] or cycles per second), wavelength (in meters), and energy (in electron volts [eV]). Each member of the spectrum has a characteristic wavelength and frequency. Some of the uses of different frequency ranges are listed. Note that higher frequencies are associated with shorter wavelengths and higher energies. The values shown here are typical representations. See Appendix C for an explanation of the abbreviations (M, G, T, P, µ, etc.).

Precise frequency intervals attributed to different parts of the electromagnetic spectrum may vary in different references, and there is a substantial overlap of ranges (note that FM radio falls completely within the television range). Box 2.2 demonstrates the calculation of the wavelength and energy of electromagnetic radiation. All forms of electromagnetic radiation have one common characteristic: their velocity. It is equal to the speed of light. The speed of light (or any type of electromagnetic radiation) is 3×10^8 meters per second in space (a vacuum) and is slightly less in transparent materials such as glass or plastic.[1]

Ionizing and Nonionizing Radiation

To study radiation protection, the electromagnetic spectrum (Fig. 2.1) can be divided into two categories:
1. Ionizing radiation
2. Nonionizing radiation

Of the entire span of types of radiation included in the electromagnetic spectrum, only the following radiations are classified as ionizing radiations[1]:
- X-rays
- Gamma rays
- Ultraviolet radiation with an energy greater than 10 eV

Because they do not have sufficient kinetic energy to eject electrons from the atom, the following radiations are considered nonionizing:
- Ultraviolet radiation with energy less than 10 eV
- Visible light
- Infrared rays
- Microwaves
- Radio waves

BOX 2.2   Calculation of the Wavelength and Energy of Electromagnetic Radiation

The speed of light (c), wavelength (λ), and frequency (v) are related by the following equation:

$$c = \lambda v$$

where c = 3×10^8 m/sec.

Therefore, if the frequency of an electromagnetic wave is known, the wavelength may be calculated as follows:

$$\lambda = \frac{c}{v}$$

Example: Find the wavelength of a 0.5-MHz radio wave.

$$\lambda = \frac{3 \times 10^8 \, m/sec}{0.5 \times 10^6 \, sec^{-1}} = 6.0 \times 10^2 m = 0.6 \times 10^3 m = 0.6 \, km$$

The energy (in electron volts, eV) of an electromagnetic wave may be calculated using the frequency (n) and Planck's constant (h) as follows:

$$E = hv$$

where h = 4.14×10^{-15} eV-sec.

Example: Find the energy of an x-ray having a wavelength of 1 picometer (1 pm = 10^{-12} m).

Solution: The energy is given by the following relation:

$$E = hv = hc/wavelength$$
$$= (4.14 \times 10^{-15} eV - sec)(3 \times 10^8 m/sec)/(1 \times 10^{-12} m)$$
$$= 12.42 \times 10^5 eV$$
$$= 1.242 \times 10^6 eV$$
$$= 1.24 \, MeV$$

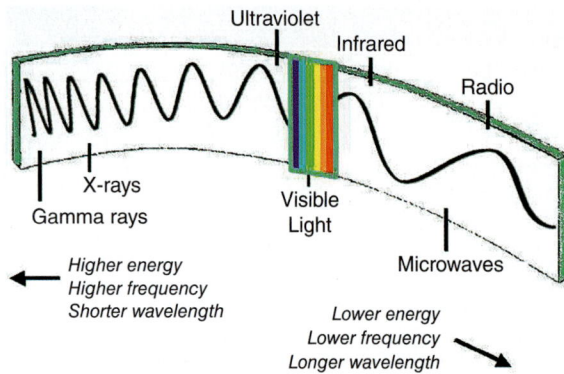

Fig. 2.1 The electromagnetic spectrum.

If **electromagnetic radiation** is of a high enough frequency, it can transfer sufficient energy to some orbital electrons to remove them from the atoms to which they were attached. As mentioned in Chapter 1, this process, called **ionization**, is the foundation of the interactions of x-rays with human tissue. It makes them valuable for creating images but has the undesirable result of potentially producing some damage to the biological material.

Particulate Radiation

In addition to electromagnetic radiation, there is another category of ionizing radiation, called **particulate radiation**. This form of radiation includes the following:
- Alpha particles
- Beta particles
- Neutrons
- Protons

All of these are subatomic particles that are ejected from the nucleus of atoms at high speeds. They possess sufficient kinetic energy to be capable of causing ionization by direct atomic collision. However, no ionization occurs when the subatomic particles are at rest relative to a potential target atom.

Alpha particles, also known as *alpha rays,* are emitted from nuclei of very heavy elements, such as uranium and plutonium, during their radioactive decay. **Radioactive decay** is a naturally occurring process in which unstable nuclei relieve that instability by various types of spontaneous nuclear emissions, one of which is the emission of charged particles. Alpha particles contain two protons and two neutrons. They are simply helium nuclei or helium atoms minus their electrons. Alpha particles have a mass that is

approximately four times the mass of a hydrogen atom and a positive charge twice that of an electron, which permits them to have the potential to transfer very substantial amounts of kinetic energy to orbital electrons of other atoms.[2]

Particulate radiations vary in their ability to penetrate matter. Compared with beta particles, which are just fast electrons, alpha particles are much less penetrating (i.e., they have a large interaction cross-section or scattering probability). Because they lose energy quickly as they travel a short distance—for example, into the superficial layers of the skin—they are considered virtually harmless as an external source of radiation. Several pieces of ordinary paper can significantly attenuate them and therefore serve as a shield. However, as an internal source of radiation, the reverse is true. If emitted from a **radioisotope** that was deposited in the body—for example, in the lungs—alpha particles will be absorbed in the relatively radiosensitive epithelial tissue and be extremely damaging to that tissue. The process is in a way analogous to what a bowling ball does to a set of pins.

Beta particles, also known as *beta rays,* are identical to high-speed electrons except for their origin. Electrons originate in atomic shells (Appendix F) outside of the nucleus, whereas beta particles, like alpha particles, are emitted from within the nuclei of radioactive atoms. This process, called *beta decay,* occurs when a nucleus relieves instability by a neutron transforming itself into a combination of a proton and an energetic electron (called a *beta particle*). There is also the emission of another particle called a *neutrino,* which has negligible mass and no electric charge but carries away any excess energy. Beta particles are 8000 times lighter than alpha particles and have only one unit of electrical charge (−1) as compared with the alpha's two units of electrical charge (+2). These attributes mean that beta particles will not interact as strongly with their surroundings as do alpha particles. Therefore, they are capable of penetrating biologic matter to a much greater depth than alpha particles, with far less ionization along their paths. Not all high-speed electrons, however, are beta radiation. Alternative sources of high-speed (high energy) electrons are commonly produced in a radiation oncology treatment machine called a *linear accelerator.* These nonnuclear electrons are most often used to treat superficial skin lesions in small areas or to deliver radiation boost treatments to breast tumors at tissue depths typically not exceeding 7 to 8 cm. As previously stated, alpha rays can be absorbed by a few pieces of ordinary paper because they interact so readily with matter and consequently lose their kinetic energy quite rapidly. Beta rays or accelerator produced electrons, however, with a noticeably lesser probability of interaction with atoms of matter, will penetrate more deeply and therefore cannot be stopped by ordinary pieces of paper. Very high-energy electrons require either millimeters of lead or multi centimeter-thick slabs of wood to absorb them. For energies of less than 2 million electron volts (MeV), either a 1-cm-thick piece of wood or a 1-mm-thick lead shield would be sufficient for absorption.

Protons are positively charged components of an atom. An isolated proton, which is simply identical to an ionized hydrogen atom, has a mass that exceeds the mass of an electron by a factor of 1800. Therefore protons are generally also significantly less penetrating than high energy electrons. The number of protons in the nucleus of an atom constitutes its atomic number, or "Z" number. The atomic number identifies an element and determines its placement in the periodic table of elements (see Appendix D).

Neutrons are the electrically neutral components of an atom and have approximately the same mass as a proton. If two atoms have the same number of protons but a different number of neutrons in their nuclei, they are referred to as isotopes. If one of these combinations of Z protons and some number of neutrons leads to an unstable nucleus, then that combination is called a **radioisotope**.

An Introduction to the Concept of Radiation Dose

In the remainder of this chapter, radiation doses that humans can receive and have received are described. To appreciate the relative magnitude of these exposures, it is necessary to become familiar with the quantities and units that are used to specify radiation dose. Therefore, at this time, this section provides a brief discussion of important radiation units. They will be discussed in much greater detail in succeeding chapters.

The radiation quantity, absorbed dose (often just called "dose"), is defined to be the amount of energy per unit mass that has been absorbed in a material due to its interaction with ionizing radiation. It is usually measured in units called **gray (Gy)** or fractions of a gray called centigray (cGy). 1 cGy = .01 Gy.

The amount of energy absorbed by human tissue is an important determinant of the extent of biologic harm that may occur. However, other factors must be considered when attempting to predict how much actual biologic harm might be caused by a dose of radiation. The equivalent dose (EqD) takes into account the *type of ionizing radiation* that was absorbed. In diagnostic radiology, this absorption is caused by x-rays. Exposure to radioisotopes in the environment or to radioactive materials released from nuclear reactors or radioisotopes used in radiotherapy treatments (Brachytherapy) involves other types of ionizing radiation, such as neutrons, protons, electrons, etc. The EqD provides an overall dose value that includes the different degrees of tissue interaction that could be caused by the different types of ionizing radiation. The most common unit of measure of EqD is the millisievert (mSv). 1 mSv = 1/1000th of a Sievert.

Another factor that plays a role in determining the degree of biologic damage that may be caused by ionizing radiation is the organ or organ systems irradiated. For example, irradiation of internal organs has very different, and generally much more severe, consequences than irradiation of extremities. Therefore, the contribution of radiation absorbed dose that affects different organs and organ systems, as well as the type of ionizing radiation that caused the dose, is considered in deriving the dosimetric quantity called the effective dose (EfD). The effective dose is intended to be the best estimate of overall harm that might be produced by a given absorbed dose of radiation in human tissue. It takes into account both the type of radiation and the part of the body irradiated. The standard unit of effective dose is the same as that of the equivalent dose, the mSv. *This signifies that when a dose value is given in mSv, the unit should be defined as either Effective or Equivalent and, if Equivalent, the type of radiation quantity that is being expressed needs to be identified.*

Biologic Damage Potential

While penetrating body tissue, ionizing radiation primarily causes biologic damage by ejecting electrons from the atoms, composing the tissue. Destructive radiation interaction at the atomic level results in molecular

TABLE 2.2   Radiation Equivalent Dose and Subsequent Biologic Effects Resulting From Acute Whole-Body Exposures*

RADIATION EqD	
Sv	**Subsequent Biologic Effects**
0.25	Blood changes (e.g., measurable hematologic depression, substantial decreases within a few days in the number of lymphocytes or white blood cells that are the body's primary defense against disease)
1.5	Nausea, diarrhea
2.0	Erythema (diffuse redness over an area of skin after irradiation)
2.5	If a dose is to gonads, temporary sterility
3.0	50% chance of death; lethal dose for 50% of the population over 30 days (LD 50/30)
6.0	Death

*Radiation exposures are delivered to the entire body over a time period of less than a few hours.
Adapted from *Radiologic health*, unit 4, slide 17, Denver, Multi-Media Publishing (slide program).

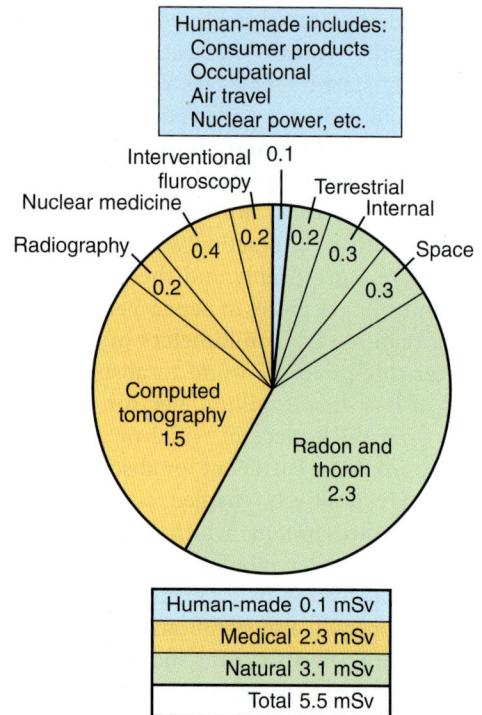

Fig. 2.2 Contribution of various sources to the average annual effective dose per person in the United States. (Data from National Council on Radiation Protection and Measurements [NCRP]: *Medical radiation exposure of patients in the United States*. Report No. 184, Bethesda, 2019; National Council on Radiation Protection and Measurements [NCRP]: *Ionizing radiation exposure of the population of the United States*. Report No. 160, Bethesda, 2009, NCRP).

change, and this, in turn, can cause **cellular damage**, leading to abnormal cell function or even complete loss of cell function. If excessive multicellular damage occurs, the living organism will have a significant possibility in various locations of exhibiting genetic or somatic changes such as the following:

- Mutations
- Cataracts
- Leukemia

Changes in blood count are classic examples of **organic damage** that results from nonnegligible exposure to ionizing radiation. An EqD of 250 mSv delivered to the *whole body* may cause a substantial decrease within a few days in the number of lymphocytes or white blood cells that are the body's primary defense against disease. Table 2.2 provides some basic information on the known biologic effects that result when radiation exposures of various EqDs are delivered to the whole body over a time period of less than a few hours (acute exposures). This emphasizes that the use of ionizing radiation should be limited whenever possible.

Sources of Radiation

Human beings are continuously exposed to sources of ionizing radiation. Sources of ionizing radiation may be one of the following:

- Natural
- Human-made (artificial)

For simplification purposes Fig. 2.2 shows a pie chart that provides an overview of the contribution of various sources to the average annual effective dose per person in the United States in 2016. All EfD values on the pie chart are given in mSv. The dose from **natural background radiation** is approximately 3.1 mSv, medical radiation exposure is approximately 2.3 mSv, and human-made radiation contributes approximately 0.1 mSv. Collectively, from all-natural, medical, and human-made sources, the total dose per year is approximately 5.5 mSv. Table 2.3 presents the

TABLE 2.3   Average Annual Radiation Equivalent Dose (EqD) per Person in the United States in 2016

Category	Type of Radiation	DOSE (mSv)
Natural[1]	Radon and Thoron (inhaled)	2.28
	Cosmic	0.33
	Terrestrial (environmental radionuclides)	0.21
	Internal (from ingested sources)	0.29
	Subtotal	3.11
Medical imaging[2]	Computed Tomography	1.45
	Radiography	0.22
	Nuclear medicine	0.41
	Interventional* procedures	0.25
	Subtotal	2.33
Human-made[2]	Consumer Products, Occupational, Air Travel, Nuclear Power, etc.	
	Subtotal	0.11
	Total annual EqD from all sources	5.55

*Interventional includes cardiac procedures.
[1]Data from National Council on Radiation Protection and Measurements (NCRP): Ionizing *radiation exposure of the population of the United States. Report No. 160,* Bethesda, 2009, NCRP.
[2]Data from National Council on Radiation Protection and Measurements (NCRP): *Medical radiation exposure of Patients in the United States. Report No. 184,* Bethesda, 2019, NCRP.

information on the Average Annual Radiation EqD Per Person in the United States in 2016 in a more detailed manner.

Natural Radiation. Natural sources of ionizing radiation have always been a part of the human environment. They are a consequence of this planet's geology and its location relative to the sun and the solar system's position in the galaxy. Ionizing radiation from planetary and extra-planetary sources is called natural background radiation and has the following three components:

- Terrestrial radiation from radioactive materials in the crust of the Earth
- Cosmic radiation from the sun (solar) and beyond the solar system (galactic)

- Internal radiation from radioactive atoms, also known as radionuclides, which make up a small percentage of the body's tissue

If radiation from any of these natural sources grows more substantial because of accidental or deliberate human actions such as mining radioactive elements, the causes are termed *enhanced natural sources.*

Terrestrial radiation. Long-lived radioactive elements such as uranium-238, radium-226, and thorium-232 (all emitters of densely ionizing radiation) are present in variable quantities in the crust of the Earth. These sources of ionizing radiation are classified as *terrestrial radiation.* The amount of terrestrial radiation present in any area depends on the composition of the soil or rocks in that geographic region. The most recent data show that 2.3 mSv of natural background radiation exposure comes primarily from the gaseous radionuclide, radon (^{222}Rn), and to a much lesser degree from the radionuclide *thoron** (see Fig. 2.2). Both these gases emit alpha particle radiation. Radon initially does not join or interact with the atoms of other particles. Because of this property, it is sometimes colloquially referred to as a *noble gas.* It behaves as a free agent that floats around in the soil. As a consequence, the natural flow of air can draw radon gas into the lower levels of homes through cracks or holes in the foundation, and then the gas may permeate upward as it decays and becomes solid particles.[3,4,2]

Geologic formations or soils containing granite, shale, phosphate, and pitchblende produce higher concentrations of radon than other commonly encountered materials. Radon is by far the most significant contributor to background radiation. The average US resident receives approximately 2.0 mSv per year from indoor and outdoor levels of radon. Radon is the first decay product of radium (^{226}Ra), a metallic chemical element, and is produced as radium decays in soil. It is a colorless, odorless, invisible, dense radioactive gas that, along with its decay products, polonium-218 (^{218}Po) and polonium-214 (^{214}Po, solid form), is always present to some

---

*Thoron is the name given to a radioactive isotope of radon, namely radon-220, which has a half-life of 54.5 seconds as compared with the much longer 3.8-day half-life of radon. It is given the name thoron because radon-220 was itself derived from the radioactive decay of thorium-232, a naturally occurring material.

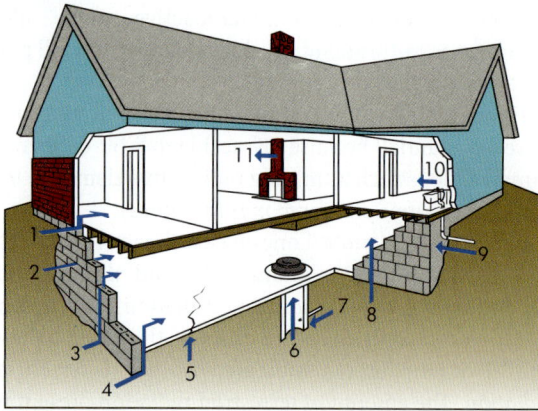

Fig. 2.3 Radon gas can percolate up through the soil and enter a home through holes or cracks in its framework, crawl spaces under the living areas, floor drains, sump pumps, and porous cement block foundations. *1,* Spaces behind brick veneer on top of block foundation; *2,* pores and cracks in concrete block foundation; *3,* open top of block foundation walls; *4,* floor to wall joints; *5,* cracks in concrete floor; *6,* exposed soil as in basement sump; *7,* weeping drain tile draining into open sump; *8,* mortar joints; *9,* loose-fitting pipe wall penetration; *10,* well water from some wells; *11,* building materials such as stone. (From US Environmental Protection Agency, Washington, DC.)

degree in the air. Radon has a half-life of 3.825 days.[4] To summarize, in homes radon may gain access through the following areas (Fig. 2.3):

- Crawl spaces under the living areas
- Floor drains
- Sump pumps
- Porous cement block foundations

Typically, a pressure gradient exists between a house and the soil on which it rests so that the house draws on the ground like a vacuum cleaner. Commonly used building materials such as bricks, concrete, and gypsum wallboard naturally contain some radon. These construction materials are classified as Earth-based materials.[2]

Radon concentrations in a particular structure vary across days and seasons. In the colder months, when homes and buildings are tightly closed, radon levels are usually higher, so this is the best time to perform tests for radon.*

High indoor concentrations of radon and radon decay products, which are solid particles that have attached

themselves to dust, have the potential to cause serious health hazards for humans.[3] After being inhaled, these airborne radioactive gases and decay products produce daughter radioactive isotopes that remain for lengthy periods in the epithelial tissue of the lungs. As these secondary isotopes decay, they give off alpha radiation that will injure lung tissues, thereby increasing the risk for lung cancer. The severity of risk depends on the concentration of radon and the length of time to which the person is exposed to the gas and solid particles.[5] Smokers exposed to high radon levels face a higher risk of lung cancer than do nonsmokers. One reason for this may be that smokers have already been exposed to higher concentrations of radioactivity from the lead-210 (^{210}Pb) and polonium-210 (^{210}Po) isotopes contained in tobacco and tobacco smoke. *The Environmental Protection Agency (EPA) considers radon to be the second leading cause of lung cancer in the United States.* It is estimated that radon is responsible for approximately 20,000 cancer deaths per year. The EPA recommends that action be taken to reduce elevated levels of radon to a concentration *less than* 4 picocuries* per liter (pCi/L) of air (the number of radioactive emissions per second that occur on average in 1 liter of air). A radon air activity density of 4 pCi/L results in a yearly EqD to the lung of approximately 0.05 mSv.[6] A presence of radon below this level is considered statistically safe by the EPA. The EPA estimates that 1 in every 15 homes in the United States exceeds the recommended action limit of 4 pCi/L.[7] Hence, accurate radon testing and appropriate structural repair, if required, are essential to reducing the risk of lung cancer from radon. In actuality, radiation exposure to radon cannot be entirely eliminated, but with suitable structural correction, it can be significantly reduced.[4]

Cosmic radiation. Cosmic rays are of extraterrestrial origin and result from nuclear interactions that have taken place in the sun and other stars. The number of cosmic rays varies with altitude relative to the Earth's surface. The greatest intensity occurs at high altitudes where there is less attenuation due to the low atmospheric density, whereas the most moderate-intensity occurs at sea level. The considerable reduction at sea level happens because the cosmic rays that are not deflected by the Earth's magnetic field must traverse the entire

---

*Detection kits are relatively easy to use and may be purchased at retail stores or obtained at minimal cost from the National Safety Council in Washington, DC, by calling 1-800-SOS-RADON.

---

*1 picocurie = 10^{-12} curie. 1 Ci = 3.7 $(10)^{10}$ nuclear disintegrations per second. So, 1 pCi = .04 dps.

thickness and steadily increasing density of the Earth's atmosphere before reaching the surface. The average US inhabitant received an EqD of approximately 0.3 mSv per year from extraterrestrial radiation (see Fig. 2.2). Cosmic radiations consist predominantly (about 90%[†]) of high-energy protons that have estimated mean energy of 300 MeV. As a result of interactions with molecules in the Earth's atmosphere, these protons may be accompanied by alpha particles, atomic nuclei, mesons[*], gamma rays, and high-energy electrons as they approach the Earth's surface. These other forms of radiation are collectively referred to as *secondary cosmic radiation*. The gamma rays among them can be energetic enough to penetrate several meters of lead.[5,6]

Terrestrial and internal radiation. The tissues of the human body contain many naturally existing radionuclides that have been ingested in minute quantities from various foods or inhaled as particles in the air. The types of ionizing radiation released by these radionuclides may include the following:
- Alpha particles (helium nuclei)
- Beta particles (electrons)
- Gamma rays (similar to x-rays, but usually of higher energy, in the range of a MeV)
- Emission of x-rays due to some types of radioactive decay affecting the distribution of electrons around atoms

Examples of radioactive nuclides that exist in small quantities in the human body are as follows:
- Potassium-40 (^{40}K)
- Carbon-14 (^{14}C)
- Hydrogen-3 (^{3}H; tritium)
- Strontium-90 (^{90}Sr)

Radionuclides in the soil and air also add to the human radiation dose burden. The average member of the general population received approximately 0.5 mSv per year from combined exposure to radiations from the Earth's surface (terrestrial) and radiation within the human body (see Fig. 2.2).

Radon and Thoron (2.3 mSv), cosmic ray radiations (0.3 mSv), terrestrial, and internally deposited radionuclides (0.5 mSv) comprise the natural background radiation in the United States and result in an estimated average annual individual EqD of approximately 3.1 mSv (see Fig. 2.2).

Human-made (Artificial) Radiation. Ionizing radiation created by humans for various uses is classified as **human-made, or artificial, radiation**. Sources of artificial ionizing radiation include the following:
- Consumer products containing radioactive material
- Nuclear fuel for the generation of power
- Atmospheric fallout from nuclear weapons testing
- Nuclear power plant accidents
- Nuclear power plant accidents as a consequence of natural disasters
- Medical radiation

Human-made radiation contributes about 0.1 mSv to the average annual radiation exposure of the US population. Medical radiography provides 0.2 mSv, nuclear medicine procedures contribute 0.4 mSv, 1.5 mSv is due to computed tomography (CT), and 0.2 mSv comes from interventional fluoroscopy (see Fig. 2.2). Thus, human-made and medical radiation procedures contribute a total of 2.4 mSv to the average annual individual background radiation in the United States as of 2016. These figures represent an "average share" of dose to members of the population that would be so if the total human-made and medical radiation dose were pooled equally among all individuals in the population. A qualified medical physicist can calculate an individual's actual medical radiation exposure and consequent equivalent dose from x-ray examinations if provided with the essential technical details (e.g., X-ray tube voltage used, exposure time, tube current [mA], patient dimensions, number of x-ray projections, etc.) pertaining to the studies.

Consumer products and devices containing radioactive material or producing radiation exposure. These include the following:
- Airport surveillance scanning systems
- Electron microscopes
- Ionization-type smoke detector alarms
- Industrial static eliminators

[†]The remaining 10% are composed mostly of alpha particles and heavier nuclei.
[*]Mesons are short-lived (only a few hundredths of a microsecond) subatomic particles smaller in size than a proton but much more massive than an electron and are generated as by-products from very high-energy collisions between protons and protons or between protons and neutrons. They can carry an electric charge of the same value as that of an electron or be neutral.

These items contribute a tiny fraction of the total average EqD to each member of the general population. As a result of technological advances since the 1970s and strict regulations imposed within the United States by the Food and Drug Administration regarding such devices, the radiation exposure of the general public from consumer products and devices as a whole may now be considered negligible.

Air travel. Commercial airline flights bring many humans to higher elevations and therefore in closer contact with high-energy extraterrestrial radiation (e.g., cosmic radiation) and consequently increases their exposure. A flight on a typical commercial airliner result in an EqD rate of 0.005 to 0.01 mSv/hour.

Sunspots sometimes play a role in increased radiation exposure during air travel. Sunspots are dark spots that every so often appear on the surface of the sun. They indicate regions of increased electromagnetic field activity and are occasionally responsible for ejecting particulate radiation into space. This radiation typically constitutes a small fraction of the dose from cosmic radiation here on Earth. However, the solar contribution to the cosmic ray background increases substantially during periods of high sunspot activity. It will then potentially contribute a nonnegligible added radiation dose to airplane passengers and crew. If a person spends 10 hours flying aboard a commercial aircraft during a period of regular sunspot activity, that individual will receive a radiation EqD that is about equal to the dose received from one chest x-ray. During irradiation from a *solar flare,* "a tremendous explosion on the surface of the sun,"[8] however, this dose can be 10 to as much as 100 times higher. Awareness of these potentially significant increases in radiation exposure at high altitudes is essential information for pilots and airline crews and the general public. An increase in radiation exposure, typically, carries an immeasurably small health risk for those individuals who travel by air infrequently. However, for pilots, flight attendants, and the general public who are "very frequent flyers," the possibility exists that they "may unknowingly be exposed to excessively large doses of radiation."[9] With adequate knowledge, a person choosing air travel during periods of high sunspot activity and solar flares can make an intelligent decision about whether the potential benefit of air travel outweighs any increased health risk.

A commercial flight crew's (pilot, flight attendants, etc.) actual radiation exposure sometimes exceeds that of workers at nuclear power plants. The Federal Aviation Administration (FAA) and other organizations maintain ongoing programs of monitoring and evaluation of radiation risks to maintain the safety of occupational exposed airline workers.[9]

Nuclear fuel for the generation of power. Nuclear power plants that produce nuclear fuel for the generation of power do not contribute significantly to the annual EqD of the US population during their regular operating cycles. The nuclear fuel cycle provides only a small portion of 0.1 mSv to the total average annual EqD for persons living in the United States.

Atmospheric fallout from nuclear weapons testing. An accurate estimate of the total annual EqD from fallout cannot be made because actual radiation measurements do not exist. The *dose commitment,* a dose that may ultimately be delivered from a given intake of radionuclides,[10] may be estimated by using a series of approximations and simplistic models that are subject to considerable speculation. The actual radiation dose to the global population from atmospheric fallout from nuclear weapons testing is not received all at once. Instead, it is delivered over a period of years at changing dose rates. The changes in the dose rates depend on factors such as characteristics of the fallout field and the elapsed time since the test occurred. No atmospheric nuclear testing has happened since 1980.

When spread over the inhabitants of the United States, the fallout from nuclear weapons tests (Fig. 2.4) and other environmental sources, along with other human-made radiation, contributes only a small portion of 0.1 mSv to the EqD of each person.

Nuclear power plant accidents. Although nuclear power benefits humans by creating a needed supply of electricity, unfortunate accidents involving nuclear reactors can occur. Such events may lead to substantial incidental radiation exposures for humans and the environment. Examples of two nuclear power plant accidents are addressed in the discussions that follow.

Three Mile Island Unit 2. It has been over 40 years since the Three Mile Island Unit 2 (TMI-2) pressurized water reactor, situated on an island in the Susquehanna River near Harrisburg, Pennsylvania, underwent an accidental loss of coolant, leading to severe overheating of the highly radioactive reactor core that resulted in a partial meltdown and significant radiation leak. This mishap on March 27, 1979 created considerable concern and stress among people living in nearby areas surrounding the plant. The most significant unease resulting from this

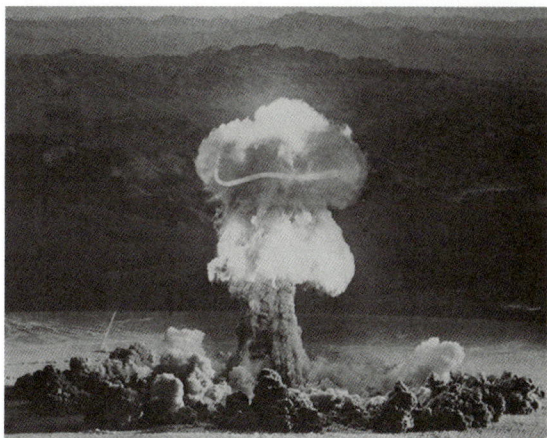

Fig. 2.4 The United States performed aboveground nuclear weapons tests before 1963. During the Priscilla Test, this atomic cloud resulted when a 37-kiloton testing device exploded from a balloon at the Nevada test site on June 24, 1957. The atomic cloud top, which contained human-made ionizing radiation, ascended approximately 43,000 feet. (From US Department of Energy, Nevada Operations Office, Las Vegas, Nevada.)

commercial accident was the possibility of developing adverse biologic effects. The welfare of animals, and the environment was also of great concern.

The cause of the accident at TMI-2 was a combination of human error, design deficiencies, and equipment failure.[11] Steam generators that received water operated by a pump were used to remove heat from the nuclear reactor's radioactive core. Unfortunately, when the pump malfunctioned, heat ceased to be carried away, resulting in severe overheating of the core, ultimately leading to the destruction of the reactor.[11]

Several highly regarded organizations have, over many years following the accident, conducted extensive studies and evaluations of immediate area populations but have not yet found conclusive proof of adverse health effects resulting from the nuclear accident at TMI-2.[12]

The World Nuclear Association has stated that "the average radiation dose to people living within 10 miles of the plant was 0.08 mSv, with no more than 1 mSv to any single individual. A radiation dose of 0.08 mSv is comparable to that of a chest x-ray for an adult and 1 mSv is about a third of the average background level of radiation received by US residents in a year."

TMI-2 "has been dormant since the accident in 1979 and it is estimated to close in 2036."[13] TMI-1 "was shutdown at noon on September 20, 2019."[14]

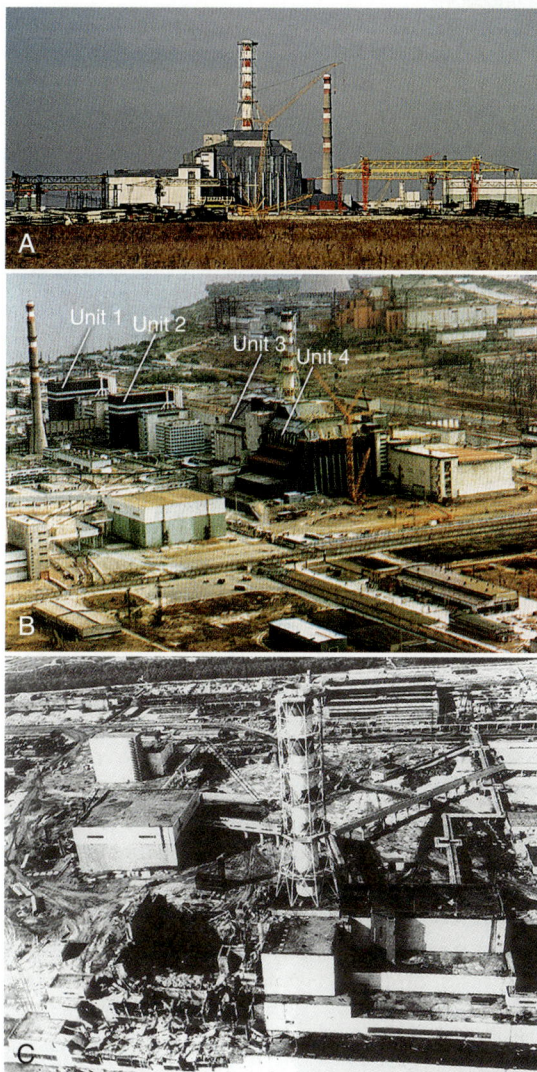

Fig. 2.5 (A) Nuclear power plant in Chernobyl, former Soviet Union, site of the 1986 radiation accident. (B) Aerial view of the four identical units of the Chernobyl nuclear power plant before the accident. Graphics point out each of the reactors. (C) Chernobyl nuclear power plant after the explosion of unit 4 on April 26, 1986. (A, Ken Graham Photography. B and C, US Department of Energy, Nevada Operations Office, Las Vegas, Nevada.)

Chernobyl. Over 30 years have passed since a steam explosion at the nuclear power plant in Chernobyl occurred in 1986 (Fig. 2.5). At the time of the accident, dynamically and for an extended period, radionuclides plumed upward from the reactor into the atmosphere and subsequently contaminated extensive areas surrounding the plant. The government was compelled to fully evacuate all people living in communities within a 30-km radius of the plant. In the days that followed the explosion, winds carried the released radioactive smoke and dust from the crippled reactor throughout Europe, exposing many additional areas to fallout.

The quantity of radioactive material that was released from the ruptured reactor was more than 1 million times the amount of radioactive material released at TMI or "30 to 40 times as much radioactivity as Hiroshima and Nagasaki atomic bombs in 1945."[15] It was later determined that in excess of 200 plant workers received a whole-body EqD exceeding 1 Sv. More than two dozen workers died as a result of explosion-related injuries and the destructive effects of receiving whole-body doses greater than 4 Sv. The average EqD to the approximately quarter of a million individuals living within 200 miles of the reactor was eventually calculated to be as high as 0.2 Sv. In some individuals, thyroid doses resulting from drinking milk contaminated with radioactive iodine exceeded several Sv. Adverse health effects from radiation exposure continue to be expected for many years as a consequence of the total collective EqD received by the affected population.

Thyroid cancer, leukemia, and breast cancer as a result of the chernobyl disaster. Thyroid cancer continues to be the most harmful health effect of the Chernobyl nuclear power plant accident. Children and adolescents living in the Ukraine, where the radiation dose was heaviest, continue to be the focus of the disease. After 30 years have gone by, "it is now conclusive that around 5000 cases of thyroid cancer—most of which were treated and cured—was caused by the contamination."[16]

Since the 1986 Chernobyl accident, there has also been an increase in the incidence of breast cancer directly attributed to the generated radiation exposure.[17,18] The World Health Organization (WHO)* Expert Group revealed that "reports indicated a small increase in the incidence of premenopausal breast cancer in the most contaminated areas, which appeared to be related to radiation dose.[20] However, follow-up epidemiologic studies are still needed to confirm these findings. Other types of cancer may also have occurred or could arise in the affected population, but this has not as yet been proven. "Determining an accurate number of excess cancer deaths caused by the radiation fallout from Chernobyl,"[21] has been extremely difficult because of many variables.[7]

Some early research indicated no other increases in the effects that are generally associated with radiation exposure (leukemia, congenital abnormalities, or adverse pregnancy outcomes[22]). For example, the WHO found no increase in leukemia incidence by 1993 in the population hit hardest by fallout from Chernobyl.[23] Later studies began to show some of the expected effects. For example, it was reported that there had been a 50% increase in leukemia cases in children and adults in the Gomel region (located within Belarus) since the Chernobyl disaster.[24,25] Also reported in June 2001 at the Third International Conference on Health Effects of the Chernobyl accident held in Kiev, Ukraine, the Russian personnel who worked to clean up radioactive contamination during 1986 and 1987 at the plant had a statistically significant rise in the number of leukemia cases.[26,27] At that time the WHO had reported that their "investigations suggested a doubling of the incidence of leukemia* among the most highly exposed Chernobyl liquidators.[20] However, this organization also revealed that "no such increase had been clearly demonstrated among children or adults in any contaminated areas."[23,8]

Interestingly, "some research from Ukraine has documented a staggering increase in cases of diabetes and other noncancer endocrine disorders."[28] "Scientists from Ukraine reported in 2017 that levels of diabetes in radiation-exposed survivors (including site clean-up workers) remain noticeably higher than in the rest of the population."[28] It is conceivable that radiation exposure may have a more significant effect on the endocrine system, particularly the pancreas, than previously believed.[28]

Although there has been considerable concern about the possibility of genetic effects from radioactive fallout,

---

*The World Health Organization is the authority that directs and coordinates International Health within the United Nations health system. One of their most significant concerns is global public health security. In situations such as a nuclear power plant accident, the mandate of the WHO is to determine and respond to public health risks. This organization also "conducts a program on radiation and health that aims to promote safe and appropriate use of radiation to protect patients, workers and the general public in planned, existing and emergency exposure situations."[19]

---

*"Leukaemia" is a variation of the spelling of "leukemia" that is used in some countries and by the WHO. This European spelling can differ from the US spelling, as in, for example, "aluminum" (US spelling) and "aluminium" (British spelling).

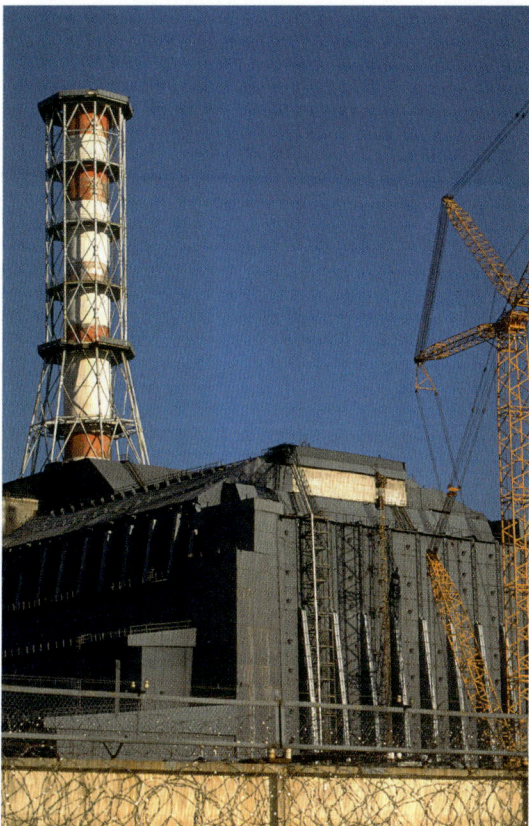

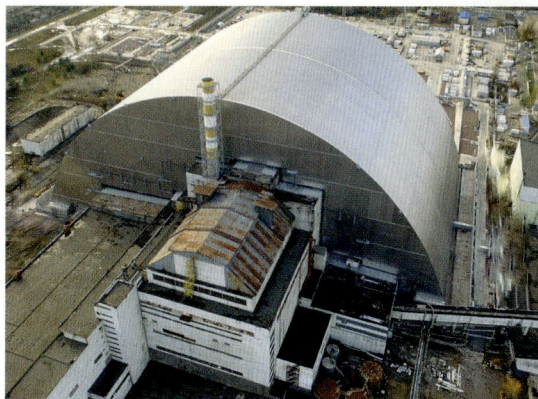

Fig. 2.7 Photograph of the New Safe Confinement structure that now covers Chernobyl reactor unit 4 and the concrete sarcophagus that entombs it. (From Sergey Koshelev.)

Fig. 2.6 The large concrete "sarcophagus," encasing the remains of Chernobyl reactor unit 4. Within 10 years after the shelter's construction the walls weakened, leaving the sarcophagus in danger of collapsing. (© Clive Shirley/Signum/Greenpeace.)

research studies have not provided conclusive evidence that the fallout from the destroyed reactor caused congenital defects.[18,21] Research on potential hereditary effects is expected to continue.

Confinement of radioactive material from the destroyed nuclear reactor. During the 6 months after the Chernobyl nuclear power plant disaster, a large concrete shelter known as the "sarcophagus" (Fig. 2.6) was constructed by the Soviets atop the remains of the reactor 4 building so that the other reactors could continue operating to provide nuclear power.

Because of severe deficiencies subsequently occurring with the sarcophagus, plans were made to cover the remains of the Chernobyl reactor unit 4 and the concrete sarcophagus that entombs it, with a weatherproof, massive steel vault. Construction of this new structure

began in April 2012 and it was slid in place in November 2016. The shelter is an arch-type steel-shaped enclosure with a 100-year designed lifetime, referred to as the *New Confinement Shelter* (Fig. 2.7) and is now fully operational. The new structure provides a much more substantial protection for both the environment and the population.

Nuclear power plant accidents as a consequence of natural disasters. Accidents can also occur in nuclear power plants as a consequence of severe damage from natural disasters. This devastation can generate widespread environmental and health effects on the affected population of the surrounding area. Discussed below is such a catastrophic event.

Fukushima Daiichi Nuclear Plant Disaster. Over 9 years ago a 9.0-magnitude earthquake off the northeast coast of Japan triggered a tsunami that slammed into the island's coast, causing 914-cm (30 foot) high waves that traveled 9.66 kilometers (6 miles) inland, wrecking everything in their path within minutes,[29] including the Fukushima Daiichi Nuclear Plant located in the town of Naraha 93 miles southwest of the epicenter. The 2011 earthquake also caused the *entire Japanese coastline to drop as much as 90 centimeters (3 feet)*, making it easier for the tsunami to cause severe destruction at the nuclear plant. Even though the plant survived the earthquake, its 5.5-meter (18 foot) protection walls were not high enough to stop 9-meter waves from flooding the diesel generators powering the pumps enabling the cooling of the nuclear reactor cores. Eventually the backup batteries to the diesel generators also failed, leaving nothing to generate power to operate the cooling pumps. Their absence allowed uncontrolled rising temperatures in the reactors. The fuel rods subsequently overheated, resulting in the production of hydrogen gas, which eventually exploded. Three reactors were destroyed and others were severely damaged, leading to the release of a considerable amount of radiation into the atmosphere and surrounding areas.[29]

Because it is challenging to measure the amounts of radiation people received, long-term effects such as an increased incidence of cancer in the exposed population cannot be precisely determined. In 2018 it was reported by Time.com that the Japanese government recognized that a male Fukushima power plant worker in his 50s died of lung cancer attributed to radiation exposure. However, it is not known exactly when his death occurred.[30] Previously the WHO estimated that the lifetime risk for development of some cancers may be somewhat higher "above baseline rates in certain age and sex groups that were in areas with the highest estimated doses."[31] Increased health risks were not expected to be observed beyond the borders of Japan.[31] Areas of Fukushima Prefecture that were less affected by radiation exposure from the accident were also not expected to demonstrate an increase in cancer risk as a consequence of the combined accident.[31]

As in recent studies of radiation-exposed Chernobyl survivors, survivors of the Fukushima nuclear power plant disaster, and people living in surrounding areas closest to the plant, have demonstrated an increase in the number of cases of type 2 diabetes.[28] Additional research is needed to understand these findings.

Clean up of the disaster zone around the plant continues to be a demanding task, even though the immediate danger has been eliminated. Robotic units have been used to pick up small pieces of radioactive debris lying on the bottom of reactor Unit 2 that melted down following the earthquake and tsunami.[32] Fuel rods in reactors 1, 2, and 3 need to be carefully removed over the course of time. In addition, removal and storage of contaminated water continues to be a major concern because the amount of contaminated water can still increase. It should also be noted that soon after the accident, substantial volumes of contaminated water containing radioactive debris were dumped into the Pacific Ocean. Trace amounts of radioactive tritium and cesium linked to Fukushima reactors have since been detected in the Bering Sea and in the waters off of the California coast. However, any radiation doses resulting from exposure to the levels detected are far below natural background dose levels.

Medical radiation. The National Council on Radiation Protection (NCRP) Report No. 160 was released on March 3, 2009 and has been, since its publication, an important and much referred to compendium of medical usage data extending up to 2006. However, the patterns of medical usage of radiation have changed significantly in recent times due to manifest advances in technology and a much heavier reliance on and use of CT scans. NCRP Report No. 184 is now the latest publication to present medical usage data. It was published on November 15, 2019 and reflects usage data up to 2016. Data from this newer report are presented in Table 2.4.

Medical radiation accounts for approximately 2.3 mSv of the average annual individual EfD of ionizing radiation received (see Fig. 2.2). The total average annual EfD from human-made and natural radiation, including radon, is not associated with any measurable level of harm.[33]

Although the average amount of natural background radiation remains fairly constant from year to year at 3.1 mSv, the frequency of exposure to human-made radiation in medical applications *continues to increase rapidly* among all age groups in the United States for several reasons. Among the main instigators of this are medicolegal considerations. Physicians, to protect

TABLE 2.4 **Medical Radiation Exposure: 2016**					
Modalities	**Number of Procedures**	**Percentage (%)**	**Collective Dose (Person-Sv)**	**Percentage (%)**	**Per Capita (mSv)**
Computed tomography	74 million	20	444,000	63	1.50
Nuclear medicine	14 million	4	106,000	15	0.4
Radiography and fluoroscopy	275 million	74	71,000	10	0.2
Interventional	8.1 million	2	82,000	12	0.2
Total	**371 million**	100%	**703,000**	100%	**2.3**

TABLE 2.5 Representative Entrance Skin Exposures, Bone Marrow Dose, and Gonadal Dose From Various Diagnostic X-Ray Procedures

Examination	Exposure Factors (kVp/mAs)	Entrance Skin Dose (mGy,)*	Bone Marrow Dose (mGy,)	Gonad Dose (mGy,)
Skull	76/50	2.0	0.10	<1
Chest	110/3	0.1	0.02	<1
Cervical spine	70/40	1.5	0.10	<1
Lumbar spine	72/60	3.0	0.60	2.25
Abdomen	74/60	4.0	0.30	1.25
Pelvis	70/50	1.5	0.20	1.50
Extremity	60/5	0.5	0.02	<1
CT (head)	125/300	40.0	0.20	0.50
CT (pelvis)	125/400	20.0	0.50	20.0

*Milligray in tissue.
CT, Computed tomography.
Adapted from Bushong SC: *Radiologic science for technologists: physics, biology, and protection,* 12 ed, St. Louis, 2021, Elsevier.

themselves from malpractice lawsuits, rely more on unneeded, expensive, sophisticated technology to assist them in making diagnoses for patient care rather than prescribing much less expensive and much lower radiation dose procedures, such as basic x-ray projections that may well be just as informative. To reduce the possibility of genetic damage in future generations, this increase in the frequency of radiation exposure in medicine must be counterbalanced by controlling the amount of patient exposure in specific imaging procedures. For example, this can best be accomplished by limiting the widespread substitution of unnecessary CT scans or repetitive CT scans by many emergency departments for convenience, in place of using alternative, less costly diagnostic procedures. In areas such as interventional procedures, radiation doses to the public can be kept in check through efficient application of radiation lessening measures (e.g., use of pulsed not continuous operation, lower mA settings, use of the last image hold feature, and other less radiation beam-on time methods) on the part of the radiographer, radiologist, and physicians using fluoroscopy. Because of the large variety of radiologic equipment and differences in imaging procedures and in individual radiologist and radiographer technical skills, the patient dose for each examination varies according to the facility and the staff providing imaging services. The amount of radiation received by a patient from a diagnostic x-ray procedure may be indicated in terms such as the following:
1. Entrance skin exposure (ESE), which includes skin and glandular dose

TABLE 2.6 Representative Fetal Doses for Radiographic Examinations

Examination	Fetal Dose (mGy)
Skull (lateral)	0
Cervical spine (AP)	0
Shoulder	0
Chest (PA)	0
Thoracic spine (AP)	0.10
Lumbosacral spine (AP)	0.80
Abdomen (AP)	0.770
Intravenous urogram (IVP)	0.60
Hip*	0.50
Extremity	0

*Gonadal shields should be used if appropriate.
AP, Anteroposterior projection; *IVP,* intravenous urogram; *PA,* posteroanterior projection.
Adapted from Bushong SC: *Radiologic science for technologists: physics, biology, and protection,* 11 ed, St. Louis, 2021, Elsevier.

2. Bone marrow dose
3. Gonadal dose

Table 2.5 provides some examples of patient ESEs (skin and glandular), bone marrow, and gonadal doses. For pregnant women undergoing radiological imaging procedures, the fetal dose also may need to be estimated. Table 2.6 provides some representative fetal doses for several different radiologic examinations.

Because humans are unable to control natural background radiation, exposure from artificial sources that can be controlled must be limited to protect the general population from further biologic damage.

SUMMARY

- Radiation is the emission of energy in the form of electromagnetic waves or as moving subatomic particles (protons, neutrons, beta particles, etc.), passing through space from one location to another.
- Natural radiation is always present in the environment.
- Human-made, or artificial, radiation is created by humans for specific goals.
- To study radiation protection, the electromagnetic spectrum can be divided into two categories: ionizing radiation and nonionizing radiation.
- X-rays, gamma rays, and ultraviolet radiation with an energy greater than 10 eV are classified as ionizing radiations.
- Low-energy ultraviolet radiation with energy less than 10 eV, visible light, infrared rays, microwaves, and radio waves are classified as nonionizing radiations.
- Energy transfer through the process of ionization is used to create medical images. However, it is also the mechanism of potential biological harm for the patient.
- Alpha particles, beta particles, neutrons, and protons are particulate radiations. They vary in their ability to penetrate matter.
- Radiation absorbed dose is usually measured in units of Gray (Gy) and commonly specified in fractions of a Gray, namely centigray (1 cGy = .01 Gy) or **milligray** (1 mGy = .001 Gy).
- Equivalent dose (EqD) takes into account the type of radiation that was absorbed. It provides an overall dose value that includes the different degrees of tissue interaction that could be caused by the different types of radiation. The millisievert (1 mSv = .001 Sv) is the most commonly used measure of equivalent dose.
- An equivalent dose enables the calculation of the effective dose.
- The effective dose (EfD) is intended to be the best estimate of overall harm that might be produced by a given dose of radiation in human tissue. It takes into account both the type of radiation and the part of the body irradiated. The millisievert (mSv) is also the unit of measure for the effective dose.
- Ionizing radiation produces electrically charged particles that can cause biologic damage on molecular, cellular, and organic levels in humans.
- Sources of ionizing radiation may be natural or human-made.
- Natural sources include radioactive materials in the crust of the Earth, cosmic rays from the sun and beyond the solar system, internal radiation from radionuclides deposited in humans through natural processes, and terrestrial radiation in the environment.
- Human-made sources include consumer products containing radioactive material, nuclear fuel, atmospheric fallout from nuclear weapons testing, nuclear power plant accidents whatever their origin, and medical radiation from diagnostic x-ray machines and radiopharmaceuticals in nuclear medicine procedures.
- Although there has not been much change in the amount of natural background radiation to the US population since 1987, there have been significant increases in the amount of radiation exposure resulting from increased usage of medical imaging procedures, such as CT scanning, cardiac nuclear medicine examinations, and interventional fluoroscopic procedures.
- The most recently available data show that 2.3 mSv of natural background radiation exposure comes primarily from the gaseous radionuclide, radon, and to a much lesser degree from the radionuclide thoron.
- The Environmental Protection Agency (EPA) considers radon to be the second leading cause of lung cancer in the United States.
- The recommended action limit for radon in homes is 4 pCi/L of air.
- As of 2016 natural background radiation in the United States results in an estimated average annual individual EqD of 3.1 mSv.
- Human-made radiation exposure contributes about 0.1 mSv to the average annual radiation exposure per person in the United States as of 2016.
- The total average annual EqD from the natural background, medical, and human-made radiations combined as of 2016 is about 5.5 mSv.
- Thyroid cancer continues to be the main adverse health effect of the 1986 Chernobyl nuclear power plant accident.
- The amount of ionizing radiation actually received by a patient from a diagnostic x-ray procedure may be indicated in terms such as entrance skin exposure (ESE) which includes skin and glandular exposure, bone marrow dose, and gonadal dose. In pregnant women, fetal dose also may be estimated.

GENERAL DISCUSSION QUESTIONS

1. How do different types of radiation, both natural and human-made, interact with biological tissues, and what are the potential consequences of such interactions?

2. Explain the concept of ionizing and nonionizing radiation. What are the key differences between them, and how does ionization form the basis of x-ray interactions with human tissue?

3. Discuss the characteristics of particulate radiations, such as alpha particles, beta particles, neutrons, and protons. How do these particles differ in terms of penetration capabilities and potential harm to biological tissues?

4. Explore the significance of absorbed dose, equivalent dose, and effective dose in measuring and understanding radiation exposure. How do these quantities contribute to assessing potential biologic damage?

5. What are the natural sources of ionizing radiation, and how do they contribute to the overall background radiation exposure for individuals? Explain the components of natural background radiation, including terrestrial, cosmic, and internal radiation.

6. Describe the potential health hazards associated with radon exposure, particularly in indoor environments. How can individuals reduce the risk of radon-related health issues?

7. Compare the radiation exposure from commercial airline flights to other sources of radiation. How do sunspots and solar flares contribute to variations in radiation exposure during air travel?

8. Discuss the role of nuclear power plants in generating power and the potential health implications of accidents, using examples such as Three Mile Island, Chernobyl, and Fukushima. How are these incidents managed to protect the environment and population?

9. Explore the balance between the benefits and risks of medical radiation procedures. What measures can be taken to minimize unnecessary exposure during diagnostic imaging, especially with the increasing frequency of medical applications?

10. Considering the ongoing advancements in technology, how has the understanding and management of radiation exposure evolved over time? What future developments or challenges might impact radiation protection practices in various fields?

REVIEW QUESTIONS

1. What is the primary factor that determines the energy of subatomic particles with mass, such as neutrons, protons, or electrons?
   A. Frequency of the particle
   B. Wavelength of the particle
   C. Mass and velocity of the particle
   D. Planck's constant

2. Which of the following radiations is considered ionizing?
   A. Microwaves
   B. Ultraviolet radiation with energy less than 10 eV
   C. X-rays
   D. Visible light

3. What is the primary mechanism through which ionization occurs in x-ray interactions with human tissue?
   A. Detachment of electrons from atoms
   B. Scattering of photons
   C. Changes in atomic structure
   D. Molecular changes in DNA

4. Among alpha particles, beta particles, neutrons, and protons, which particle is derived from the decay of heavy elements and resembles helium nuclei?
   A. Alpha particles
   B. Beta particles
   C. Neutrons
   D. Protons

5. What unit is commonly used to measure absorbed dose?
   A. Hertz (Hz)
   B. Joule (J)
   C. Gray (Gy)
   D. Electron volt (eV)

6. What is the standard unit for measuring effective dose in radiobiology?
   A. Centigray (cGy)
   B. Sievert (Sv)
   C. Millisievert (mSv)
   D. Electron volt (eV)

7. What contributes the most to natural background radiation exposure in the average US resident?
   A. Cosmic radiation
   B. Terrestrial radiation
   C. Internal radiation
   D. Radon exposure

8. Which nuclear power plant accident involved a partial meltdown and radiation leak but did not definitively prove adverse health effects?
   A. Chernobyl
   B. Fukushima
   C. Three Mile Island
   D. None of the above

9. What is the primary reason for fluctuations in cosmic radiation intensity at high altitudes?
   A. Earth's magnetic field
   B. Solar activity
   C. Atmospheric density
   D. Presence of lead shielding

10. How can individuals reduce the risk of radon-related health issues in indoor environments?
   A. Increasing ventilation
   B. Using lead shielding
   C. Avoiding sunlight exposure
   D. Regularly performing chest x-rays

3

X-ray Interactions With Matter

OBJECTIVES

After completing this chapter, the reader will be able to perform the following:

- Define all key terms.
- Explain the meaning and significance of peak kilovoltage (kVp) and milliampere-seconds (mAs) as technical exposure factors.
- Describe the process of absorption and explain why absorbed dose in atoms of biologic matter should be kept as small as possible.
- Differentiate among the following: primary radiation; exit, or image-formation, radiation; and scattered radiation.
- List two types of x-ray photon transmission and explain the difference between them.
- Discuss the way x-rays are produced and detail the range of energies present in the x-ray beam.
- Catalog the events that occur when x-radiation passes through matter.
- Explain what determines the probability of photon interaction with matter.
- Describe and illustrate by diagram the x-ray photon interactions with matter that are important in diagnostic radiology.
- List the x-ray photon interactions with matter that occur above the energy range used in diagnostic radiology.
- Explain how the introduction of positive contrast media affects the appearance and the absorbed dose of body structures that contain it.
- Describe the effect of kVp on radiographic image quality and patient absorbed dose.

CHAPTER OUTLINE

KEY TERMS

absorbed dose (D)
absorption
attenuation
Auger effect
characteristic photon
characteristic x-ray
coherent scattering

Compton scattered electron, or secondary, or recoil, electron
Compton scattering
contrast media
effective atomic number (Z_{eff})
exit, or image formation, photons
fluorescent radiation

fluorescent yield
image receptor (IR)
mass density
milliampere-seconds (mAs)
pair production
peak kilovoltage (kVp)
photodisintegration

Fundamental physics concepts that relate to radiation absorption and scatter are reviewed in this chapter. The processes of interaction between radiation and matter are emphasized because a basic understanding of the subject is necessary for radiographers to optimally select the following technical exposure factors:

- **peak kilovoltage (kVp)**, the highest energy level of photons in the x-ray beam, equal to the highest voltage established across the x-ray tube
- **milliampere-seconds (mAs)**, the product of electron tube current and the amount of time in seconds that the x-ray tube is activated

Peak kilovoltage controls the quality, or penetrating power, of the photons in the x-ray beam and to some degree also affects the quantity, or number of photons, in the beam. The product of milliamperes (mA), which is the x-ray tube current, and time (seconds [s] during which the x-ray tube is activated) is the main determinant of how much radiation is directed toward a patient during a selected x-ray exposure. Because the level of energy (beam quality) and the number of x-ray photons are controlled by technique factors selected by the radiographer, the radiographer is responsible for the radiation dose the patient receives during an imaging procedure. With a suitable understanding of these factors, radiographers will be able to select appropriate techniques that can minimize that dose to the patient while producing optimal-quality images.

SIGNIFICANCE OF X-RAY ABSORPTION IN BIOLOGIC TISSUE

X-rays are carriers of human-made electromagnetic energy. If x-rays enter a material such as biologic tissue, they may:

1. Interact with the atoms of the biologic material in the patient and be absorbed
2. Interact with the atoms in the biologic material and be scattered, causing some indirect transmission
3. Pass through without interaction

   If an interaction occurs, electromagnetic energy is transferred from the x-rays to the atoms of the patient's biologic tissue. This process is called **absorption** (Fig. 3.1), and the amount of energy absorbed per unit mass is referred to as the **absorbed dose (D)**. The more electromagnetic energy that is received by the atoms of the patient's body, the greater is the possibility of biologic damage in the patient. Therefore the amount of electromagnetic energy transferred should be kept as small as possible. However, without absorption and the differences in the absorption properties of various body structures, it would not be possible to produce diagnostically useful images,

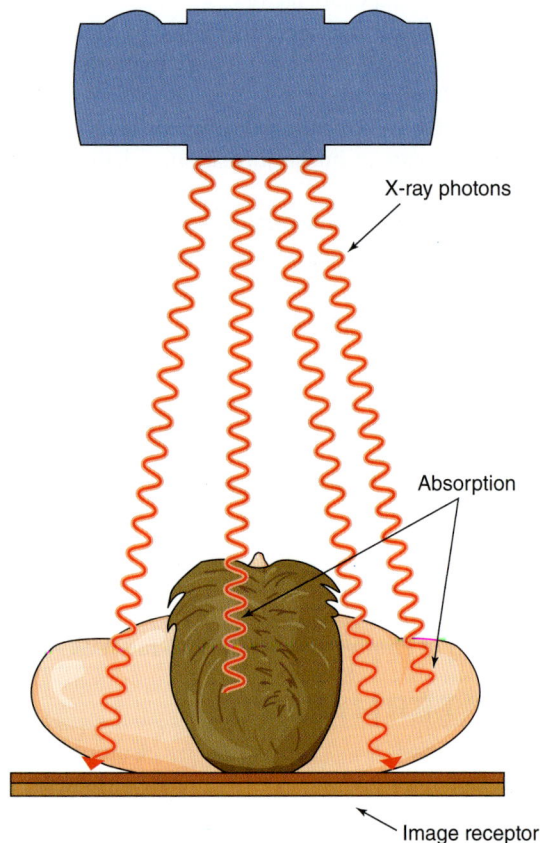

Fig. 3.1 X-ray photons can interact with atoms of the patient's body and transfer energy to the tissue. This transference of electromagnetic energy to the atoms of the material is called *absorption*.

that is, images in which different anatomic structures could be perceived and distinguished. Thus, some small amount of radiation dose is necessary. The radiographer also benefits when the patient's dose is minimal because less radiation is scattered from the patient.

X-RAY BEAM PRODUCTION AND ENERGY

Production of Primary Radiation

A diagnostic x-ray beam is produced when a stream of very energetic electrons bombards a positively charged target in a highly evacuated glass tube. In general radiography, this target, also known as the *anode*, is usually made of tungsten or an alloy of tungsten and rhenium. These materials have:

- High melting points
- High atomic numbers (tungsten [74] and rhenium [75])

As the electrons interact with the atoms of the tube target, x-ray photons are produced. Photons are particles associated with electromagnetic radiation that have neither mass nor electric charge and travel at the speed of light. X-ray photons exit from the tube target with a broad range, or spectrum, of energies and leave the x-ray tube through a glass window. The glass window permits passage of all but the lowest-energy components of the x-ray spectrum. It therefore acts as a filter by removing diagnostically useless, very-low-energy x-rays. In addition to this, a certain thickness of added aluminum is placed within the collimator assembly to intercept the emerging x-rays before they reach the patient. This aluminum "hardens" the x-ray beam (i.e., raises its effective energy) by removing low-energy components that would serve only to increase patient dose. The combination of the x-ray tube glass wall and the added aluminum placed within the collimator is called the *permanent inherent filtration* of the x-ray unit. This filtered x-ray photon beam is collectively referred to as **primary radiation** (Fig. 3.2).

Energy of Photons in a Diagnostic X-ray Beam

Although all photons in a diagnostic x-ray beam do not have the same energy, the most energetic photons in the beam can have no more energy than the electrons that bombard the target. The energy of the electrons inside the x-ray tube is generally specified in

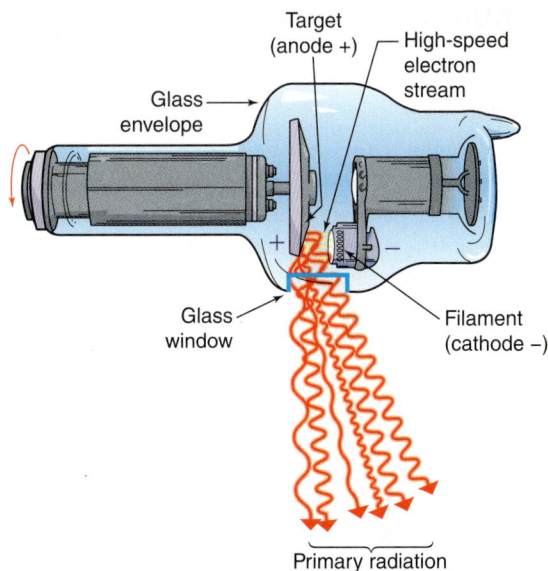

Fig. 3.2 Primary radiation emerges from the x-ray tube target and consists of x-ray photons of various energies. It is produced when the positively charged target is bombarded with a stream of high-speed electrons and these electrons interact with the atoms of the target.

terms of the electrical voltage applied across the tube. In diagnostic radiology, this voltage is expressed in thousands of volts, or kilovolts (kV). Because the voltage across the tube is not fully constant but fluctuates a bit, it is usually characterized by the kilovolt peak value (kVp).

If an electron is drawn across an electrical potential difference of 1 volt, it has acquired an energy of 1 electron volt (eV). Therefore a technique factor setting of 100 kVp (i.e., establishing a peak potential difference of 100,000 volts between cathode and anode of the x-ray tube) means that the electrons bombarding the tube target have acquired a maximum energy of 100,000 eV, or 100 keV. X-rays of various energies, comprising a spectrum, are produced, but the most energetic x-ray photon can have no more energy than 100 keV. For a typical diagnostic x-ray unit, the mean photon energy in the x-ray beam is about one-third the energy of the most energetic photon. Therefore a 100-kVp beam contains photons having energies of 100 keV or less, with an average or effective energy of approximately 33 keV. In summary, the units kVp or kV refer to the voltage on the x-ray tube, and keV refers to the energy of specific x-rays.

ATTENUATION

Direct and Indirect Transmission of X-ray Photons

In radiography, x-rays travel from an x-ray tube to an **image receptor**, a type of digital device that can convert the spatial pattern of the photons that emerge from the patient (the patient's x-ray "shadow") into electrical signal values that can be stored in a computer and displayed as an image. A number of terms are used to refer to the behavior of x-ray photons as they interact or else simply pass through the patient. The atomic processes that produce the behaviors of the x-ray photons will be discussed later in this chapter.

Absorption vs. Scatter. X-rays sometimes interact with atoms of a patient such that they give up all of their energy and cease to exist. These photons are said to be *absorbed*. Other photons interact with atoms of the patient, but only surrender part of their energy. They will continue to exist but will emerge from the interaction at a different angle (somewhat like a billiard ball colliding with another billiard ball). These photons are said to be *scattered*.

Attenuation vs. Transmission. Photons that strike the image receptor are called *transmitted photons*. These are photons that either did not interact with the atoms of the patient or else interacted through scatter but still struck the receptor, although at a different spot than they would have struck the image receptor if they had not interacted. *Attenuated photons* are the photons that have undergone either absorption or scatter and do not strike the image receptor. This terminology can be connected to absorption and scatter as follows: If a person were counting photons that were emitted from the x-ray tube, the total number of photons attenuated would equal the total number of photons absorbed plus the total number that scattered away from the image receptor.

Direct Transmission vs. Indirect Transmission. If photons pass through the patient without interacting with the atoms of the patient, they are referred to as *direct transmission photons*. If they interacted but still happened to strike the image receptor, they are termed *indirect transmission photons*. To connect to the previous terminology, indirect transmission is always the result of scatter. However, all scatter does not result in indirect transmission. The goal of radiographic imaging is to use the directly transmitted photons to construct the final image and to eliminate as much indirect transmission as possible. The latter detracts from the sharpness or quality of the image. Unfortunately, indirect transmission is always present. A number of techniques, however, have been devised to substantially reduce the influence of indirect transmission or scattered photons upon the final image.

Primary, Exit, and Attenuated Photons

Fig. 3.3 illustrates the passage of four x-ray photons through a patient. Before the four photons produced by the x-ray source enter human tissue, they are referred to as *primary photons*. Only two photons emerge from the tissue and strike the x-ray detector below it. They are referred to as **exit, or image-formation, photons**. The two that miss the detector are classified as attenuated. The term *attenuation* is rather broad. With respect to x-rays, attenuation may be used to refer to any process decreasing the intensity of the primary photon beam (i.e., the number of photons crossing unit area per second) directed toward a particular destination. In Fig. 3.3 that end point is the image receptor. Therefore photon 3, which has deviated from its path (i.e., it has been "scattered") to the extent that it will not strike the detector is said to have been attenuated. Photon 4 seems to disappear. It has transferred all its energy to the atoms of the patient and has therefore been eliminated. This occurs because a photon has no mass, only energy, which implies that it ceases to exist when it gives up its energy. *Attenuation*, then, refers to both absorption and scatter processes that prevent photons from reaching a predefined location. Fig. 3.3 shows that the path of photon 2 was bent, but not so much that the photon missed its target. Since photon 2 reaches the **image receptor (IR)**, it is part of the exit, or image-formation, radiation, but the bending of its path represents what is called **small-angle scatter**. Scattered photons in this category have essentially the same energy as the incoming, or "incident," photons. As mentioned previously, small-angle scatter degrades the appearance of a completed radiographic image by blurring the sharp outlines of dense structures. Because many billions of such scatter events happen, a greater

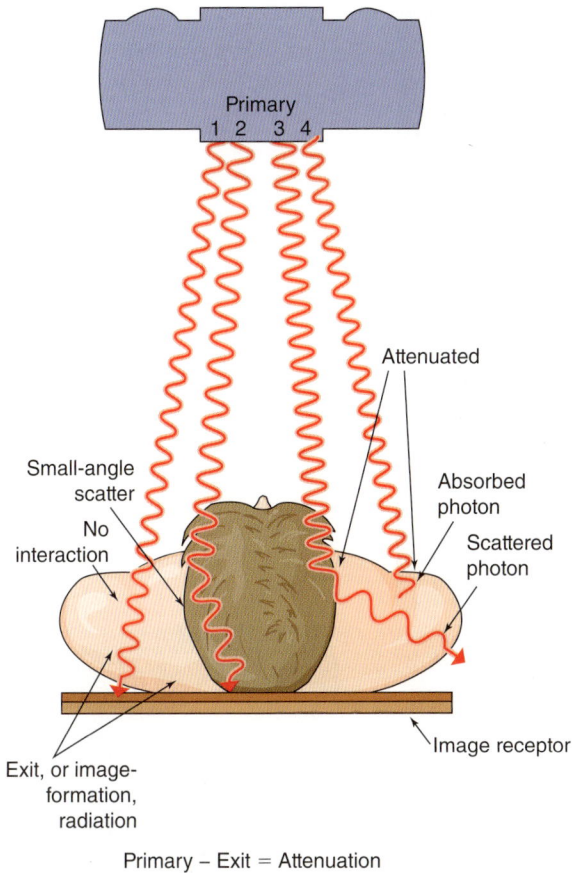

Fig. 3.3 Primary, exit, and attenuated photons. Primary photons (photons 1, 2, 3, and 4) are photons that emerge from the x-ray source. Exit, or image-formation, photons (photons 1 and 2) are photons that pass through the patient being radiographed and reach the radiographic image receptor. Attenuated photons (photons 3 and 4) are photons that have interacted with atoms of the patient's biologic tissue and been scattered or absorbed such that they do not reach the radiographic image receptor.

overall exposure of the IR occurs than is needed. This additional, undesirable exposure is commonly called **radiographic fog**. It interferes with the radiologist's ability to distinguish different structures in the image. Reducing the amount of tissue irradiated decreases the amount of fog produced and is therefore another method of limiting the number of indirectly transmitted photons. The radiographer can achieve this by confining, or collimating, the x-ray beam as much as possible to include only the region of interest (Fig. 3.4).

PROBABILITY OF PHOTON INTERACTION WITH MATTER

Because the interaction of photons with biologic matter is random, it is impossible to predict with certainty what will happen to any single photon when it enters human tissue. When dealing with a very large number of photons, however, it is possible to predict what will happen on the average, and this is more than adequate to determine the characteristics of the image that results from these numerous interactions. Table 3.1 provides a short description of the characteristics of each of the various types of radiation interactions with tissue.

Table 3.2 shows the factors that influence the probability of interactions in matter. In the remainder of this chapter, the different interactions of photons with individual atoms and the effect of a particular type of interaction on the radiographic image are examined.

PROCESSES OF INTERACTION

Five types of interactions between x-radiation and matter are possible:
1. Coherent scattering
2. Photoelectric absorption
3. Compton scattering
4. Pair production
5. Photodisintegration
   Of these, only two are important in diagnostic radiology:
1. Compton scattering
2. Photoelectric absorption
   Box 3.1 presents an overview of the various interactions between x-radiation with matter and where they are important.

Coherent Scattering

Coherent scattering is sometimes also called by the following names:
- Classical scattering
- Elastic scattering
- Unmodified scattering
  It is a simple process that results in no loss of energy as x-rays scatter.

Process of Coherent Scattering. When a low-energy (typically less than 10 keV) photon interacts with an atom, it may transfer its energy by causing some or all of the electrons of the atom to momentarily vibrate. This

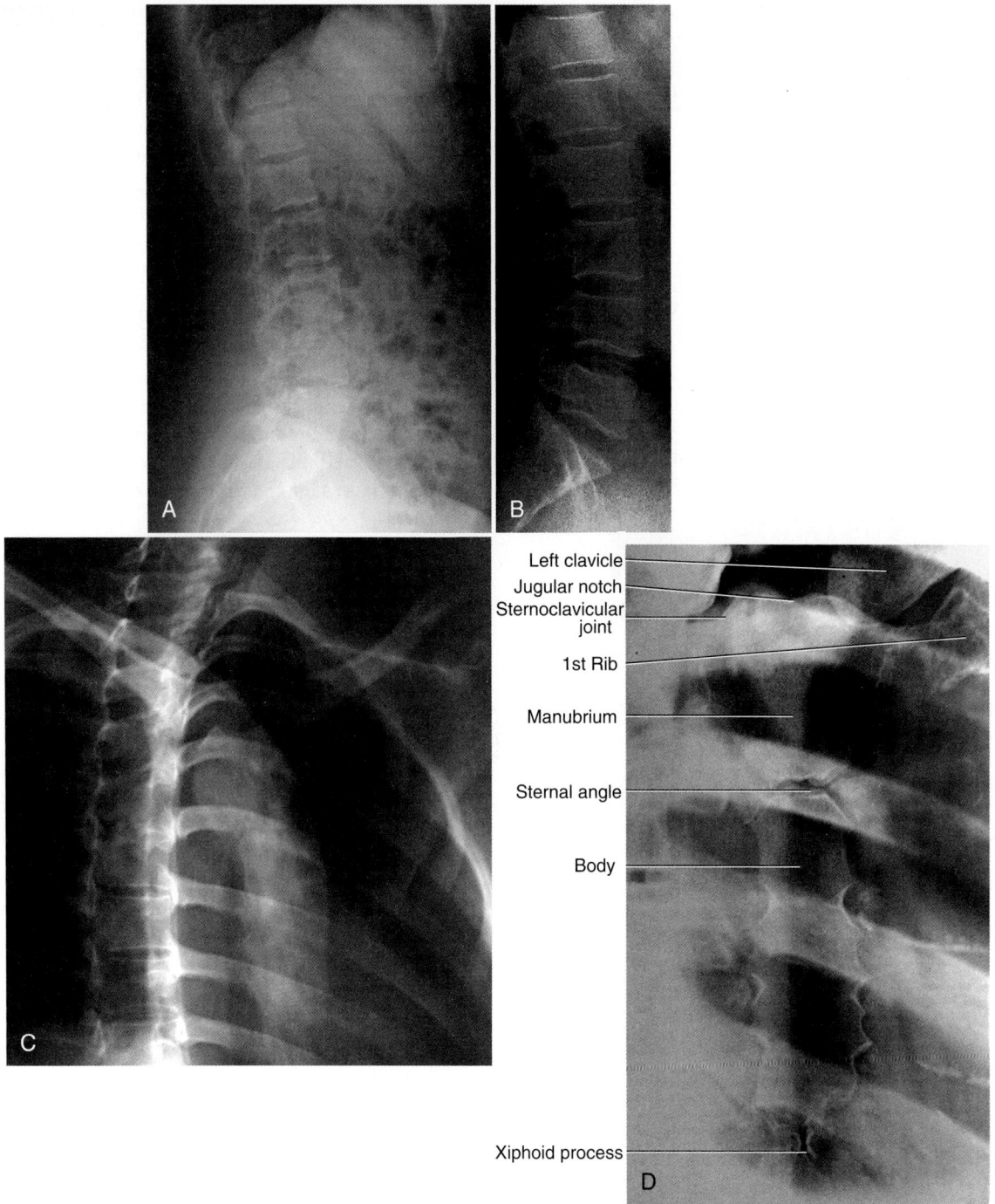

Fig. 3.4 (A) Lateral image of the lumbar vertebrae showing improper collimation, which results in the production of radiographic fog and a consequent lack of radiographic clarity. (B) Lateral image of the lumbar vertebrae showing adequate collimation, which eliminates radiographic fog and consequently increases radiographic clarity. (C) PA oblique projection (right anterior oblique [RAO] position) of the sternum, demonstrating poor collimation. (D) PA oblique projection (RAO position) of the sternum, demonstrating good collimation. (D, From Rollins JH, Long BW, Curtis T: *Merrill's Atlas of radiographic positioning and procedures,* ed 15, St. Louis, 2023, Elsevier.)

TABLE 3.1	Interaction of X-Radiation With Soft Tissue: Overview			
X-ray Photon Energy Range	**Site of Interaction**	**X-ray Photon**	**Typical Interaction**	**By-Products of Interaction**
1–50 kVp	An atom	Energy: unchanged; direction after interaction: slight change (<20 degrees)	Coherent scattering*	None
1–50 kVp	Inner-shell electron (usually K or L shell)	Energy: absorbed; direction after interaction: not applicable	Photoelectric absorption[†]	Photoelectron (characteristic photon)
60–90 kVp	Outer-shell electron	Energy: reduced; direction after interaction: changed (x-ray photon energy partially absorbed)	Compton scattering[‡] — Photoelectric absorption[†]	Compton scattered electron — Compton scattered photon
90–120 kVp	Outer-shell electron	Energy: reduced after interaction: changed (x-ray photon energy partially absorbed)	Compton[‡] scattering — Photoelectric absorption[†]	Compton scattered electron — Compton scattered photon
200 kVp–2 MeV	Outer-shell electron	Energy: reduced; direction after interaction: changed	Compton scattering[§,‖]	Compton scattered electron — Compton scattered photon
Begins at about 1.022 MeV; becomes important at 10 MeV; becomes predominant at 50 MeV and greater	Nucleus of atom	Energy: disappears after interaction with nucleus; transformed into two new particles that annihilate each other; at photon energy 1.022 MeV, after interaction: energy reappears in the form of two 0.511-MeV photons moving in opposite directions	Pair production	Positive electron (positron); ordinary electron (negatron); two 0.511-MeV photons a 1.022 MeV initial energy
Greater than 10 MeV	Nucleus of atom	Energy: absorbed by nucleus after collision with high-energy photon; excess energy in nucleus creates instability that is usually alleviated by emission of a neutron; other emissions possible	Photodisintegration	Neutron; other types of emissions possible if sufficient energy is absorbed by the nucleus: proton or proton–neutron combination (deuteron) or even an alpha particle

*This scattering occurs mostly in this energy range, but it is still much less probable than photoelectric absorption.
[†]The interaction most responsible for radiation dose in this energy range.
[‡]Both Compton and photoelectric interactions occur in this energy range.
[§]Compton interaction is predominantly responsible for radiation dose in this energy range.
[‖]In this energy range, the scattered particles go on to produce many more Compton and photoelectric interactions on their own.

TABLE 3.2   Factors That Influence the Probability of Interaction of Photons With Energy E in Materials With Density ρ

Interaction	Photon Energy Dependence	Atomic Number Dependence	Electron Density ρe (e/g)	Physical Density ρ (g/cm³)
Photoelectric	$1/E^3$	Z^3	Independent	ρ
Compton	$1/E$	Independent	ρ_e	ρ
Pair production	E	Z	Independent	ρ

BOX 3.1   Importance of Various Interactions of X-Radiation With Matter

Interaction	Where Important
Coherent scattering	Not significant in any energy range
Photoelectric absorption	Diagnostic radiology
Compton scattering	Diagnostic radiology and therapeutic radiology
Pair production	Therapeutic radiology
Photodisintegration	Therapeutic radiology

is analogous to the behavior of electrons in the antenna of a receiver intercepting a radio signal. Because they are charged particles, each of the atom's now *vibrating* electrons radiates energy in the form of electromagnetic waves. These waves combine with one another, as multiple water waves would similarly merge, to form a resultant scattered wave, or photon. Because the wavelengths of both incident and scattered waves are the same, no net energy has been absorbed by the atom (see Appendix E). However, a small change in direction for the emitted photon is very likely. In general, this change in direction is less than 20 degrees with respect to the initial direction of the original photon. This is the net effect of coherent, or unmodified, scattering. Although coherent scattering is most likely to occur at less than 10 keV (energies that will be eliminated by the inherent filtration), some of this unmodified scattering occurs throughout the diagnostic energy range and can result in small amounts of radiographic fog (Fig. 3.5). This source of fog, however, is not significant in general diagnostic imaging. In breast imaging or mammography, which of necessity involves many low-energy photons and therefore utilizes much less inherent filtration, coherent scattering also does not contribute noticeably to radiographic fog because during this imaging procedure, breast tissue is gently but firmly compressed. As a result of this compression, the breast

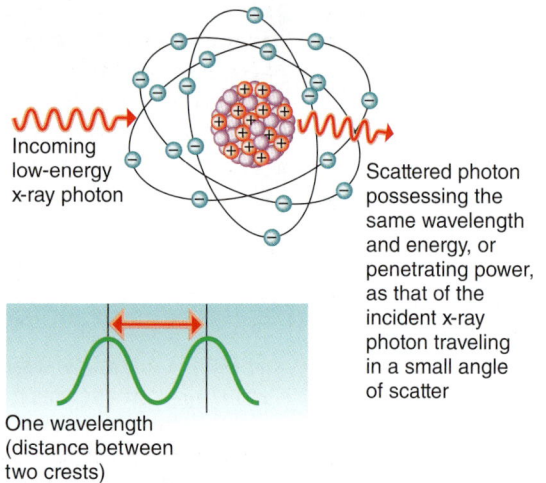

Incoming low-energy x-ray photon

Scattered photon possessing the same wavelength and energy, or penetrating power, as that of the incident x-ray photon traveling in a small angle of scatter

One wavelength (distance between two crests)

Fig. 3.5 Coherent scattering. The incoming low-energy x-ray photon interacts with an atom and transfers its energy by causing some or all of the electrons of the atom to momentarily vibrate. The electrons then radiate energy in the form of electromagnetic waves. These waves nondestructively combine with one another to form a scattered wave, which represents the scattered photon. Its wavelength and energy, or penetrating power, are the same as those of the incident photon. Generally, the emitted photon may change in direction less than 20 degrees with respect to the direction of the original photon. (Wavelength is the distance from one crest to the next.)

becomes relatively much thinner. This eliminates the production of a large amount of scatter radiation.

Small angle coherent scattering does not have much of an effect on radiographic imaging, but it does have a noticeable effect on visible light. This is why the sky is blue and sunsets are red.[1] Photons of much longer wavelengths than those of x-rays, especially "visible" wavelengths such as those belonging to blue light, are far more likely to be scattered and to scatter over a greater angle. Therefore when people look up in the sky in any direction, they tend to see the blue light scattered toward them. At sunset and at sunrise, as a person looks toward the sun, the blue light is mainly scattered away from them, so the sun appears to consist of mostly longer wavelength visible light, that is, mostly red.

A summary of facts about the process of coherent scattering is presented in Box 3.2 for quick reference.

Photoelectric Absorption

Within the energy range of diagnostic radiology (23 to 150 kVp), which also includes mammography, photoelectric absorption is the most important mode of interaction between x-ray photons and the atoms of the patient's body for producing useful images.

Process of Photoelectric Absorption. Photoelectric absorption is an interaction between an x-ray photon and an inner-shell electron (usually in the K or L shells [Fig. 3.6, Table 3.3; and for a detailed explanation see Appendix F]). To dislodge an inner-shell electron from its atomic orbit, the incoming x-ray photon must be able to transfer a quantity of energy as large as or larger than the amount of energy that holds the electron in its orbit. On interacting with an inner-shell electron, the x-ray photon surrenders all its energy to the orbital electron and ceases to exist. The electron escapes from its inner shell, thus creating a vacancy. The now unbound orbital electron, called a **photoelectron**, possesses energy equal to the energy of the incident photon minus the binding energy of its electron shell. This photoelectron may interact with other atoms in the vicinity, thereby causing excitation (promotion of electrons from lower energy shells to higher energy shells) or ionization (complete ejection of the electron from an atom), until all of its energy has been spent. The photoelectron is usually absorbed within a few micrometers of the medium through which it travels. In the human body, this energy transfer results in increased patient absorbed dose and does not contribute to the radiographic image.

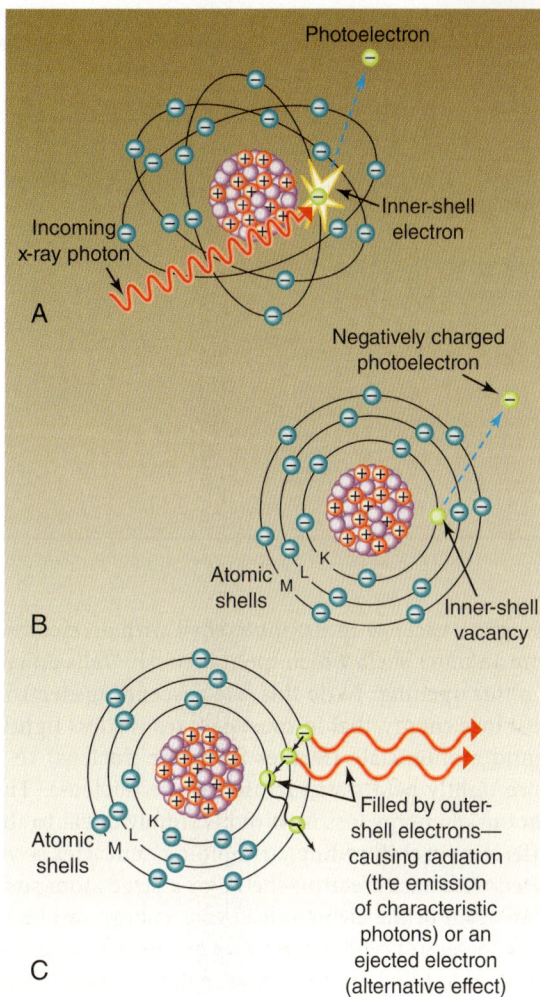

Fig. 3.6 Photoelectric absorption. (A) On encountering an inner-shell electron, usually in the K or L shell, the incoming x-ray photon surrenders all its energy to the electron, and the photon ceases to exist. (B) The atom responds by ejecting the electron, called a *photoelectron*, from its inner shell, thus creating a vacancy in that shell. (C) To fill the opening, an electron from an outer shell drops down to the vacated inner shell by releasing energy in the form of a characteristic photon. Then, to fill the new vacancy in the outer shell, another electron from the shell next farthest out drops down and another characteristic photon is emitted and so on until the atom regains electrical equilibrium. There is also some probability that instead of a characteristic photon, an Auger electron will be ejected.

As a result of the photoelectric interaction, a vacancy is created in an inner shell of the target atom. For the ionized atom, this represents an unstable energy situation. The instability is alleviated by

TABLE 3.3   Electron Shell Occupancies for Some Common Atoms*

Atom	Symbol	Atomic Number	K	L	M	N	O	P
Hydrogen	H	1	1					
Helium	He	2	2					
Lithium	Li	3	2	1				
Carbon	C	6	2	4				
Oxygen	O	8	2	6				
Sodium	Na	11	2	8	1			
Aluminum	Al	13	2	8	3			
Calcium	Ca	20	2	8	8	2		
Copper	Cu	29	2	8	18	1		
Molybdenum	Mo	42	2	8	18	13	1	
Tungsten	W	74	2	8	18	32	12	2
Lead	Pb	82	2	8	18	32	18	4
Radon	Rn	86	2	8	18	32	18	8

*For a detailed discussion of electron shell structure, please see Appendix F.

filling the vacancy in the inner shell with an electron from an outer shell, which spontaneously "falls down" into this opening. To do this, the descending electron must lose energy, that is, must pass from a less tightly bound atomic state (farther from the nucleus) to a more tightly held status (closer to the nucleus). The amount of energy loss involved is simply equal to the difference in the binding, or "holding," energies associated with each electron shell. For a large atom such as an atom of the element lead, this energy can be in the kiloelectron volt range, whereas for the small or low atomic number atoms that make up most of the human body, the energy is on the order of 10 eV. The "released" energy is carried off in the form of a photon that is called a **characteristic photon**, or **characteristic x-ray**, because its energy is directly related to the shell structure of the atom from which it was emitted. Those photons generated from photoelectric interactions within human tissue are low enough in energy that they are predominantly absorbed within the body. In general, ensuing vacancies in other electron shells are successively filled, and associated characteristic photons are emitted until the atom achieves an electronic equilibrium.

One additional process can occur as a result of photoelectric interactions. It is called the **Auger effect** (pronounced "awzhay"), named after the French scientist, Pierre Victor Auger, who discovered it in 1925. When an inner electron is removed from an atom in a photoelectric interaction, thus causing an inner-shell vacancy, the energy liberated when this vacancy is filled can be transferred to another electron of the atom, thereby ejecting that electron, instead of emerging from the atom as characteristic radiation. Such an emitted electron is called an *Auger electron*. Its energy is equal to the difference between that released by an outer electron in filling the initial created vacancy and the binding energy of the emitted or Auger electron. Because this process does not include any x-ray emission, it is called a *radiationless effect*. It reduces the total amount of characteristic radiation produced by photoelectric interactions. The term **fluorescent yield** refers to the number of x-rays emitted per inner-shell vacancy. Because the Auger effect is more prevalent in materials with higher atomic number atoms, the fluorescent yield per photoelectron is generally lower in such materials than for substances with low atomic numbers (see Fig. 3.6C).

In summary, the by-products of photoelectric absorption include the following:

1. Photoelectrons (those induced by interaction with external radiation and the internally generated Auger electrons)
2. Characteristic x-ray photons (**fluorescent radiation**)

When the energy of these by-products is locally absorbed in human tissue, both the dose to the patient and the potential for biologic damage increase.

A summary of facts about the process of photoelectric absorption is presented in Box 3.3 for quick reference.

BOX 3.3   Summary of the Process of Photoelectric Absorption

Photoelectric absorption is the most important mode of interaction between x-radiation and the atoms of the patient's body in the energy range used in diagnostic radiology because this interaction is responsible for both the patient's dose and contrast in the image. During the process of photoelectric absorption, the total energy of the incident photon is completely absorbed as it interacts with and ejects an inner-shell electron of an atom within human tissue or bone from its orbit. The newly ejected *photoelectron* has appreciable energy and thus can subsequently ionize other atoms it encounters until its energy is sufficiently depleted. After losing an electron, the original ionized atom is unstable and attempts to re-stabilize. This occurs as an electron from a higher shell drops down and fills the vacancy in the inner shell by releasing energy as a characteristic photon. This cascading effect of electrons dropping down to fill existing shell vacancies continues until the original atom regains its stability.

Probability of Occurrence of Photoelectric Absorption. The probability of occurrence of photoelectric absorption per atom within a particular material depends on the energy (E) of the incident x-ray photons and the atomic number (Z) of the atoms comprising the irradiated object; it increases markedly as the energy of the incident photon decreases and the atomic number of the irradiated atoms increases. Experimentally, the probability is observed to vary approximately as Z^3/E^3. Thus, in the radiographic kilovoltage range, compact bone with an effective atomic number* of 13.8 undergoes much more photoelectric absorption than an equal mass of soft tissue (Z_{eff} approximately = 7.4) and air (Z_{eff} = 7.6). Consequently, because of the greater "x-ray shadow" that it casts, bone can be exceptionally well delineated from soft tissue and air in diagnostic imaging.

Since air has only a slightly higher effective atomic number than soft tissue, the *photoelectric interaction occurrence probability* for either substance is virtually identical. Thus, this interaction alone, for equal amounts or volume densities of each substance, will not yield an imaging difference between the two media.

*Effective atomic number [Z_{eff}] is a composite Z value by weight for a material that is composed of multiple chemical elements.

Mass Density and Effective Atomic Number of Different Body Structures. Since the density of air is approximately 1000 times smaller than that of soft tissue, a given volume of air will interact with far fewer x-ray photons than adjacent regions of soft tissue, thereby permitting more radiation to reach the image receptor. This results in a greater exposure to the phosphor plate or the digital radiography receptor than from the denser expanses of tissue. The outcome is more adequate image contrast. As discussed with "air," dissimilar densities (**mass density** measured in grams per cubic centimeter) of different body structures influence attenuation. A density increase leads to a corresponding increase in the number of atoms in a given volume with which x-ray photons can interact and therefore to an increased probability of photon absorption. Therefore in any given sample of biologic material, both density and atomic number are important in determining attenuation and ultimately imaging contrast. As an example, if radiography is performed on an equal thickness of bone and soft tissue, the bone, which is approximately twice as dense as soft tissue, would absorb twice as much radiation due to the density difference alone. Furthermore, bone would absorb 6.5 times as much radiation because of the difference in effective atomic numbers since $(13.8)^3 / (7.4)^3 = 6.5$. So, for equal thicknesses of bone and soft tissue, bone will absorb 13 times as many x-ray photons as soft tissue in the diagnostic energy range (Fig. 3.7A).

Body Part Thickness and Density Differences. Thickness of body parts also plays a role in absorption. The thickness factor is approximately linear. If two structures have the same density and atomic number but one is twice as thick as the other, the thicker structure will absorb twice as many photons. Consider now the situation when there are different thickness and density values for adjacent structures: if a 2-cm-thick bone sample is radiographed next to a 4-cm-thick tissue sample, because the bone is half as thick in this example but is approximately twice as dense, the density and thickness factors will cancel each other out (Fig. 3.7B). The effective atomic number difference remains, however, so that there will be 6.5 times as many x-ray photons absorbed in the bone, and it will still cast a noticeable "shadow" or produce directly a darker gray effect on a digital detector image.

Effects of Attenuation on Radiographic Images. The less a given structure attenuates radiation, the brighter its appearance will be on a raw digital detector image, and

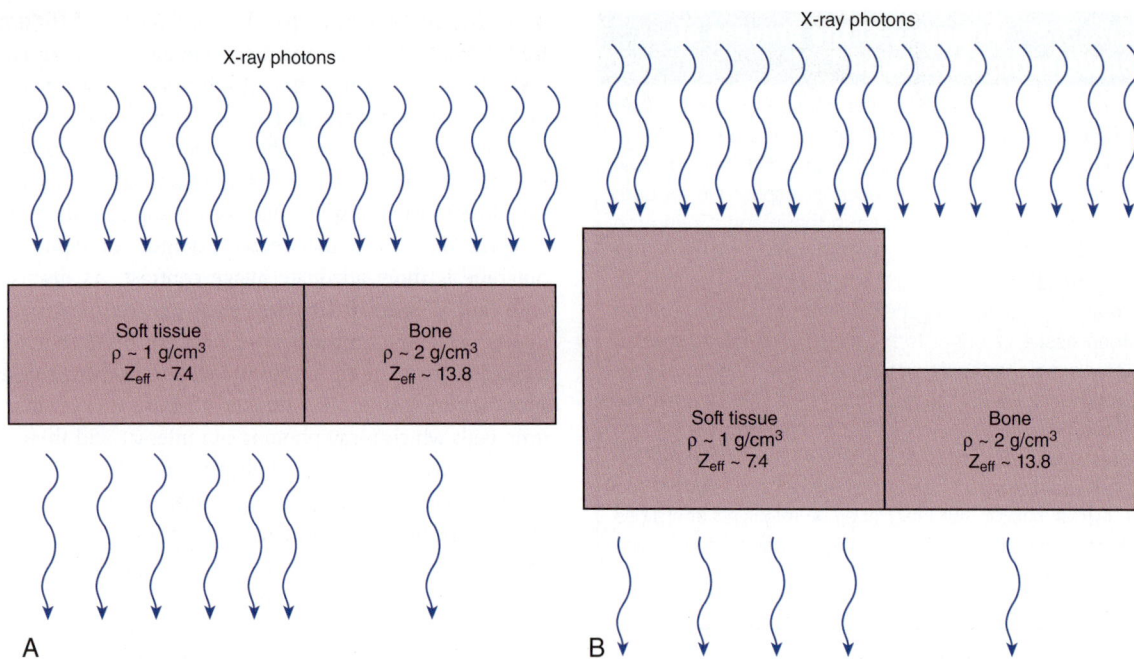

Fig. 3.7 (A) Equal thickness of bone and soft tissue are shown here. The bone absorbs 13 times as many photons as the soft tissue. A factor of 2 is the result of bone's being approximately twice as dense as soft tissue. A factor of 6.5 is the result of the higher atomic number of bone compared with that of soft tissue. Both factors together result in 2 × 6.5 = 13 times more absorption in this sample of bone. (B) In the example shown here, the soft tissue is twice as thick as the bone. This thickness difference approximately cancels out the density difference between the bone and soft tissue. However, because the difference in atomic number still exists, in this example the bone would absorb 6.5 times as many photons as the soft tissue. NOTE: The curved arrows shown in this figure are only for general illustrative purposes and are not calculational.

the more it absorbs radiation, the less radiation will be received by the detector and consequently the darker a shade of gray it will display as a raw image. A generated radiographic image, overall, must have a sufficient amount of variation in shades of gray for an observer to clearly visualize anatomic structures of interest. These principles are illustrated in Fig. 3.8.

In Fig. 3.9, two finalized posteroanterior (PA) hand projections illustrate age-related changes in bone density resulting from changes in calcium content.

1. Image A exhibits substantial quantities of calcium in the bones of a young person.
2. Image B exhibits the demineralized bones of an elderly person. The lesser amount of x-ray absorption results from the decrease in bone calcium. Hence the elderly person's bones are almost nonattenuating in radiographic appearance. Pathologic conditions such as degenerative arthritis also contribute to differences in absorption. Technical radiographic

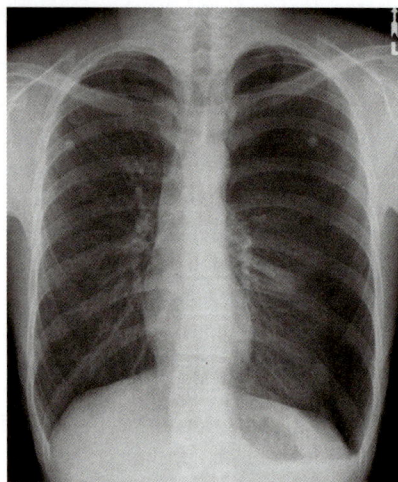

Fig. 3.8 Structures within the patient that are more attenuating (because of their physical density, thickness, and atomic number) will be displayed as brighter on the *finalized* image. (From Lampignano J, Kendrick LE: *Bontrager's textbook of radiographic positioning and related anatomy*, ed 11, St. Louis, 2025, Elsevier.)

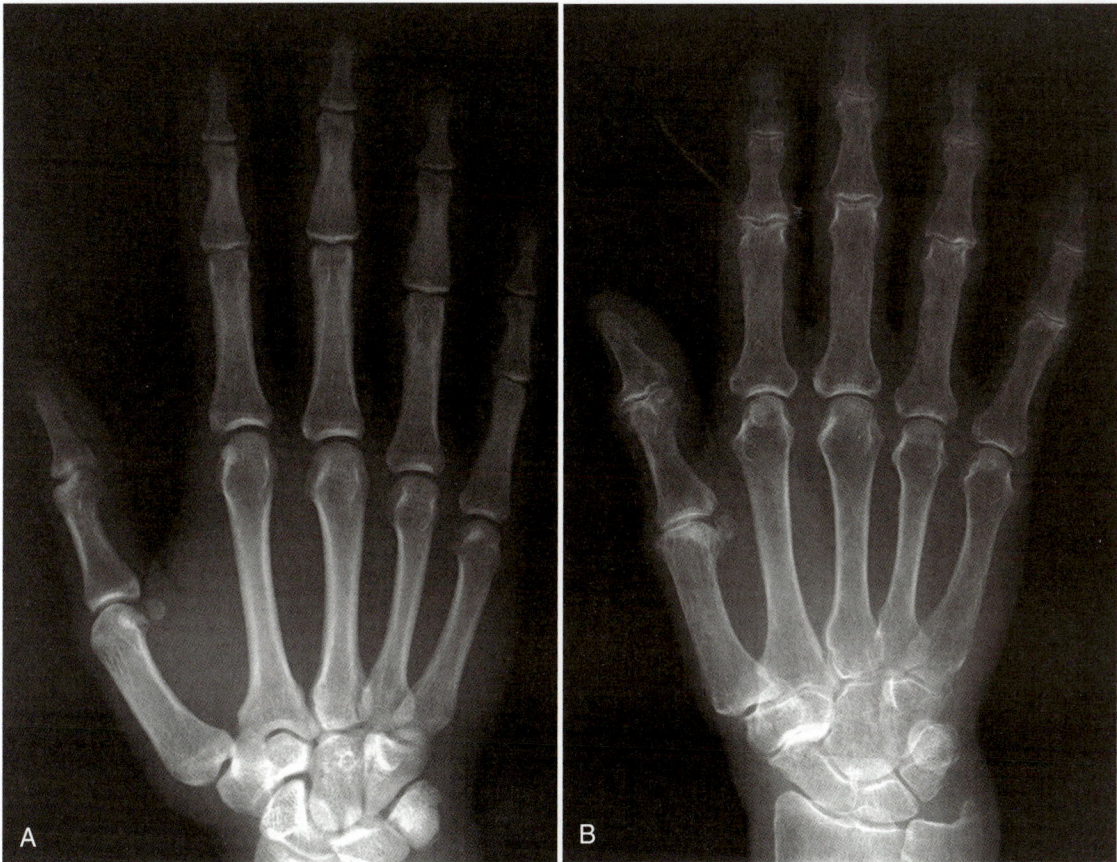

Fig. 3.9 (A) Posteroanterior (PA) image of a young person's hand exhibiting substantial quantities of calcium in the bones. (B) PA image of an elderly person's hand exhibiting demineralized bone as a consequence of a decrease in bone calcium. This and other degenerative changes account for the almost transparent appearance of the bones.

exposure factors must be adjusted to compensate for such changes.

Impact of Photoelectric Absorption on Radiographic Contrast. Within the energy range of diagnostic radiology, the greater the difference there is in the amount of photoelectric absorption, the greater the contrast in the radiographic image will be between adjacent structures of differing atomic numbers. However, as absorption by structures increases, so does the potential for biologic damage. To ensure both radiographic image quality and patient safety, the radiographer should choose the technical factors that permit adequate **radiographic contrast** while delivering the smallest dose to the patient. Usually, the selection of technique factors is predetermined by the equipment manufacturer. However, the manufacturer's technical factors are only a guide for the radiographer. Ultimately, the radiographer must make the decision as to what technical factors to use for a particular patient based on patient conditions such as existing disease processes. Often, with the aid of an experienced radiographer and a medical physicist, the manufacturer's protocols can be modified at the time of commissioning of a new x-ray unit. Even with this, there will be some occasions when the radiographer may be called upon to manually adjust techniques. One of the simplest and best ways of reducing patient dose through technique adjustment is to raise the kVp (never the opposite, which would substantially increase patient dose). The higher energy x-ray beam will be more penetrating, thereby permitting a lower mAs setting. This higher energy will, however, lead to a slight but still acceptable lessening of image contrast because of a decrease in the amount of photoelectric interactions at the higher beam energy.

Use of Contrast Media to Ensure Visualization of Anatomic Structures. If tissues or structures that are similar in atomic number and mass density must be distinguished, the photoelectric interaction by itself will not be sufficient to produce the imaging differences needed in those tissues or structures to visually differentiate them in the radiographic image. To resolve the problem, the use of contrast media has been adopted. Very simply, positive contrast media consist of solutions (e.g., barium or iodine based) containing elements having a higher atomic number than surrounding soft tissue. These solutions are either swallowed to enhance the GI tract or directly injected into the other tissues or structures to be visually enhanced. The high atomic number of the contrast media (barium, Z = 56; iodine, Z = 53) significantly increases the occurrence of photoelectric interaction relative to adjacent similar structures that do not have the contrast media. In addition, the inner-shell electrons of iodine and barium have a binding energy that is in the energy range of the x-ray photons that are most commonly used in general-purpose radiography (30 to 40 keV). This means that photoelectric absorption of the photons in the x-ray beam is further increased. In the radiographic image, positive contrast–enhanced structures therefore appear lighter than adjacent structures that did not receive the contrast. Fig. 3.10A presents an anteroposterior (AP) projection of the abdomen without the aid of a positive contrast medium to visualize the urinary system, whereas Fig. 3.10B presents an AP projection of the abdomen with a positive contrast medium that shows each contrast-filled structure in the urinary system to be distinguished.

Caution must be exercised in the use of contrast media because some patients may have adverse reactions to its presence. The use of a positive contrast medium also leads to an increase in absorbed dose in the body structures that contain it. A negative contrast medium such as air or gas can be used for some

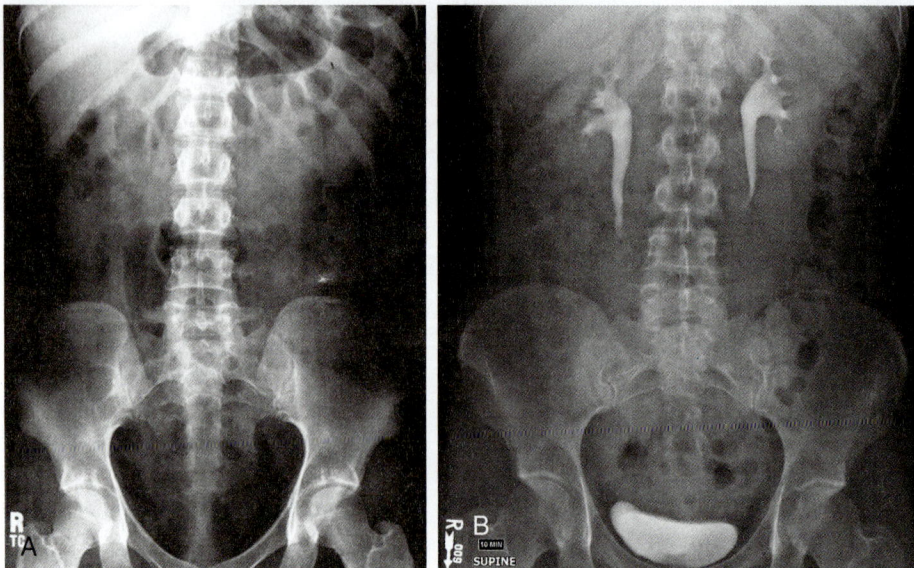

Fig. 3.10 (A) Anteroposterior (AP) projection of an abdomen without the aid of a positive contrast medium. Parts of the urinary system other than the kidneys, which have their own unique density, are not radiographically demonstrated. (B) AP projection of an abdomen, following intravenous injection of an appropriate positive contrast medium that permits visualization of the entire urinary system, thereby allowing each contrast-filled structure to be distinguished. (From Lampignano J, Kendrick LE: *Bontrager's textbook of radiographic positioning and related anatomy*, ed 11, St. Louis, 2025, Elsevier.)

radiologic examinations. These negative agents which are far easier to penetrate result in areas of decreased brightness on the radiographic image.

Compton Scattering

Compton scattering is also known by the following terms:

- Incoherent scattering
- Inelastic scattering
- Modified scattering

It is responsible for most of the scattered radiation produced during radiologic procedures. This scatter may be directed forward as small-angle scatter, to the rear as backscatter, and laterally as side scatter. The intensity of radiation scatter in various directions is a major factor in planning protection for medical imaging personnel during a radiologic examination.

Process of Compton Scattering in a Patient. In a typical Compton interaction event within a patient, an incoming x-ray photon interacts with a loosely bound outer electron of an atom (Fig. 3.11). On encountering the electron, the incoming x-ray photon surrenders a portion of its energy in dislodging the electron from its outer-shell orbit, thereby ionizing the biologic atom (see Appendix G for an extended discussion of this type of interaction). The freed electron, called a **Compton scattered electron, or secondary, or recoil, electron**, possesses excess energy and thus is potentially capable

of ionizing other biologic atoms. In general, it loses its energy by a series of collisions with nearby atoms and finally recombines with an atom that needs another electron. This usually occurs within a few micrometers (10^{-6} meters) of the site of the original Compton interaction.

The incident x-ray photon that surrendered some of its energy (see Appendix G) to free the loosely bound outer-shell electron from its orbit continues on its way, but in a new direction, and is now called a *Compton scattered photon*. It has the potential to interact with other atoms, either by the process of photoelectric absorption or by subsequent Compton scattering. The photons can also emerge from the patient, possibly contributing to degradation of the radiographic image by adding to it an additional multidirectional off-focus exposure (radiographic fog). In fluoroscopy, these deflected exit photons may also expose personnel who are present in the room to scattered radiation. This scattering therefore mandates that such personnel wear protective lead shielding. If the presence of personnel is not immediately required in the x-ray room, they should stand behind a protective barrier (Figs. 3.12 and 3.13).

The Compton interaction's probability of occurrence has no explicit dependence on atomic number. Instead, it shows something of an energy and density dependence. Density dependence just means that the more atoms or targets per unit volume, the greater the likelihood of an interaction occurring in that volume. With increasing x-ray photon energy however, the chance for a billiard ball–like interaction between the photon and an outer atomic electron decreases. What must be strongly emphasized is that the Compton interaction's

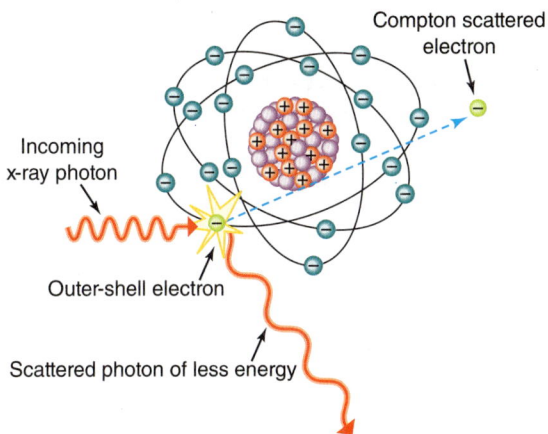

Fig. 3.11 Compton scattering. On encountering a loosely bound outer-shell electron, the incoming x-ray photon surrenders a portion of its energy to dislodge the electron from its orbit. The energy-degraded x-ray photon then continues on its way, but in a new direction. The high-speed electron ejected from its orbit is called a *Compton scattered electron, or secondary, or "recoil" electron.*

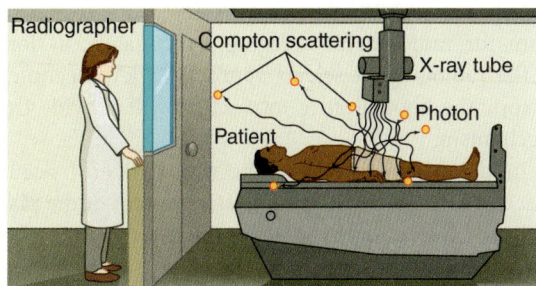

Fig. 3.12 Compton interactions are responsible for most of the scattered radiation produced during a radiologic procedure. (From *Radiobiology and radiation protection: Mosby's radiographic instructional series*, St. Louis, 1999, Mosby.)

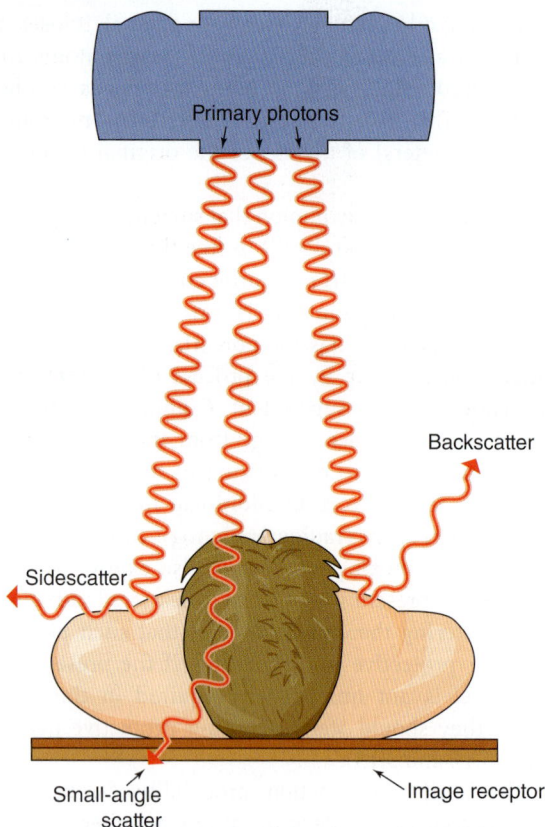

Fig. 3.13 Compton scattering results in all-directional scatter. This scatter may be directed forward as small-angle scatter, to the rear as backscatter, and laterally as side scatter. The intensity of radiation scatter in various directions is a major factor in planning the protection for medical imaging personnel during a radiologic examination.

BOX 3.4 **Summary of the Process of Compton Scattering**

Compton scattering is also important in the energy range used in diagnostic radiology. Because the scattered x-ray photon produced from the interaction of the incoming photon with an outer-shell electron of an atom of human tissue results only in a partial transfer of energy to that biologic atom, the scattered photon now traveling in a different direction can exit the patient and become a potential health hazard for imaging personnel by increasing their occupational radiation exposure. In the event that Compton scattered photons reach the image receptor, they can decrease contrast of the image by adding an undesirable additional off focus exposure called *radiographic fog*. Because its energy dependence decreases much more slowly with increasing energy than does the photoelectric interaction, Compton scattering is very important even at therapeutic energies.

lack of Z dependence implies that it does not differentiate between *equal amounts* of bone and soft tissue and thus does not serve as a useful contrast mechanism for radiographic imaging. Fortunately, as long as the radiographer selects appropriate kVp technical factors, the photoelectric interaction will provide that mechanism.

In diagnostic radiology, the probability of occurrence of Compton scattering relative to that of the photoelectric interaction escalates as the energy of the x-ray photon increases because of the $1/E^3$ energy dependence of the photoelectric interaction as contrasted to the approximate $1/E$ dependence for Compton scattering. It is found that Compton scattering and photoelectric absorption in tissue are equally probable at

approximately 35 keV x-ray photon energy. Therefore in a 100-kVp x-ray beam, where the photons will normally have an average energy in the range of 30 to 40 keV, significant numbers of Compton events occur.

A summary of facts about the process of Compton scattering is presented in Box 3.4 for quick reference.

Pair Production

Pair production is a process that does not occur unless the energy of the incident x-ray photon is at least 1.022 million electron volts (MeV). Although this energy range is far higher than that used in diagnostic radiology, a brief and very elementary description of the pair production interaction is included in this chapter to provide the reader with a broadscale understanding of the possible interactions of x-radiation with matter.

Process of Pair Production. In pair production, the incoming x-ray photon strongly interacts with the electric field surrounding the nucleus of an atom of the irradiated biologic tissue and subsequently disappears (Fig. 3.14). In the process, the energy of the photon is absorbed and transformed into matter composed of two particles: a negatron (an ordinary electron) and a positron (a positively charged electron). The negatron and the positron have the same mass and magnitude of charge; the only difference is in the "sign" of their electrical charges. The incoming photon

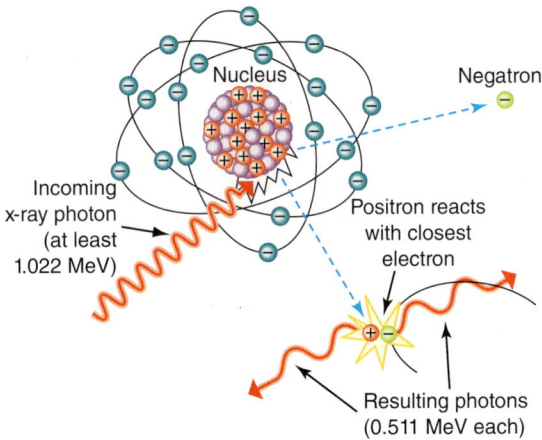

Fig. 3.14 Pair production. Pair production occurs when incoming x-ray photons with energy of at least 1.022 MeV interact with the nucleus of an atom. For a 1.022-MeV event, the end result of this interaction is the annihilation of a positron and an electron with their rest masses converted into energy, which appears in the form of two 0.511-MeV photons moving in the opposite direction.

BOX 3.5 Mass–Energy Equivalent

[Mass (electron or positron) = 9.1 × 10⁻³¹ kg, c = 3 × 10⁸ m/s, 1 MeV = 1.602 × 10⁻¹³ j]

E(total) = E(electron) + E(positron) = sum of rest mass energy of each particle

= 2 × m_0c^2

= 2 × (9.1 × 10⁻³¹) × (9 × 10¹⁶)

= 16.38 × 10⁻¹⁴ joules

= 1.022 MeV

---

must have enough energy to supply the combined rest mass* of these two particles; otherwise, the process does not happen. The minimum energy required to produce an electron–positron pair is 1.022 MeV (Box 3.5). For this reason, pair production does not influence ordinary diagnostic x-ray imaging. The electron of the pair loses energy by exciting and ionizing atoms in its path. It eventually loses enough energy that it may be captured by an atom in need of another electron. Regarding the

*Rest mass is a term associated with the mass a particle possesses or would be measured to have when it is at rest relative to the frame of measurement. According to the theory of special relativity, the mass of an object is in general not a fixed value but rather is dependent on the magnitude of its velocity "v" according to the relation:

$$m = m0 / (1 - v^2/c^2)$$

where m0 is the rest mass value of the particle and c is the speed of light in a vacuum. As can be seen from this expression, if the speed of the object is zero, then its mass is equal to m0, but if the speed is not zero, then the mass of the particle will be substantially increasing as its speed approaches a significant fraction of the speed of light. The expression also shows that a particle with a nonzero rest mass can never be brought to the speed of light, for then its mass m would become infinite, and the amount of energy required to achieve this would also be infinite.

generated positron, as far as is known, no large quantities of positrons freely exist in the universe. A positron is classified as a form of *antimatter* because it is seen to interact destructively with any nearby ordinary matter that it may be attracted to, such as an atomic electron. During such an interaction, the positron and the electron will annihilate each other, in the process converting matter into energy. This energy is called annihilation energy. This is the reverse of a pair production event in which energy (that of a photon) is converted to matter. Both types of processes happen in accordance with Albert Einstein's famous concept of mass–energy equivalence, mathematically expressed as $E = mc^2$ (c is the speed of light in a vacuum). The energy that appears from the annihilation of the electron and positron does not disappear but rather, in accordance with the conservation laws of energy and momentum, is carried off by two 0.511-MeV photons moving in opposite directions when a pair production event occurs at 1.022 MeV. Although pair production does not occur unless the energy of the incoming photon is at least 1.022 MeV, its probability of occurrence starts to become significant (i.e., noticeably greater than zero) at 10-MeV x-ray energies and higher.

Use of Annihilation Radiation in Positron Emission Tomography. Annihilation radiation is used in an imaging modality employed in Nuclear Medicine called *positron emission tomography (PET)*. Briefly, in the PET scanning of patients, the source of the positrons are injected radionuclides, whose atomic nuclei are unstable because they contain too many protons relative to their number of neutrons. To relieve this instability, a surplus proton is converted in the nucleus into a neutron, and a positron and another particle called a *neutrino* are ejected from the nucleus. Within a very short distance (several micrometers or less), the emitted positron interacts with a local electron, and the two mutually annihilate, yielding a pair of photons emerging in opposite directions from the electron–positron interaction site. These *annihilation photons* are intercepted by a ring of detectors surrounding the patient. The positional information from these detectors is then used to build a cross-sectional image of the radioactivity distribution within the patient. Some examples of radionuclides used in PET scanning are:

- Fluorine-18 (^{18}F)
- Carbon-11 (^{11}C)
- Nitrogen-13 (^{13}N)

Photodisintegration

Photodisintegration is another interaction that becomes important at x-ray energies exceeding 10 MeV during the operation of high-energy radiation therapy treatment machines. Because this energy range is also far higher than useful diagnostic energies, only a brief account of this interaction process of radiation with matter is included. With this discussion and those directly preceding it, the reader will have been introduced to all of the important types of radiation and matter encounters.

Process of Photodisintegration. In photodisintegration, a high-energy photon collides with the nucleus of an atom, which directly absorbs all the photon's energy. This energy excess in the nucleus creates an instability that in most cases is alleviated by the emission of a neutron by the

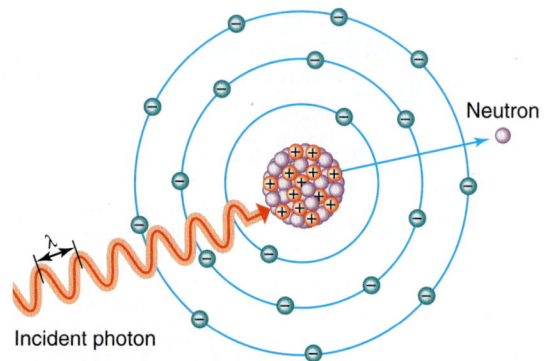

Fig. 3.15 Photodisintegration. An incoming high-energy photon collides with the nucleus of an atom and absorbs all the photon's energy. This energy excess in the nucleus creates an instability that is usually alleviated by the emission of a neutron. In addition, if sufficient energy is absorbed by the nucleus, other types of emissions will be possible, such as a proton or proton–neutron combination (deuteron), or even an alpha particle.

nucleus. Other types of emissions—a proton or proton–neutron combination (deuteron) or even an alpha particle (two protons and two neutrons bound together)—are possible if sufficient energy is absorbed by the nucleus. Because emission of charged and/or uncharged particles has occurred from a previously inactive nucleus, it can be said that the photodisintegration interaction has made a nucleus partially break apart. Fig. 3.15 demonstrates one type of photodisintegration event.

SUMMARY

- Peak kilovoltage (kVp) controls the quality, or penetrating power, of the photons in the x-ray beam and to some degree also affects the quantity, or number of photons, in the beam.
- Because radiographers select the technical exposure factors, they are responsible for the radiation dose the patient receives during an imaging procedure.
- The amount of energy absorbed by the patient per unit mass is called the *absorbed dose*.
- Biologic damage in the patient may result from the absorption of x-ray energy. However, some small amount of radiation dose is necessary to produce a diagnostic image.
- Variations in x-ray absorption properties of various body structures make radiographic imaging of human anatomy possible.

- Radiographers receive less radiation exposure when the patient's dose is minimal because less radiation is scattered from the patient during an imaging procedure.
- The anode of an x-ray tube is usually made of tungsten or an alloy of tungsten and rhenium.
- The units kVp and kV refer to the voltage on the x-ray tube, and keV refers to the energy of specific x-rays.
- Attenuation results when, through the processes of absorption and scatter, the intensity of the primary photons in an x-ray beam decreases as it passes through matter.
- Scattered radiation can result in diminished contrast of the image by adding additional undesirable exposure to the image receptor (radiographic fog). In fluoroscopy, Compton scattered photons may expose personnel who are present in the room to scattered radiation.

- Two interactions of x-radiation are central in diagnostic radiology: photoelectric absorption and Compton scattering. The photoelectric absorption is the basis of useful radiographic imaging, whereas Compton scattering is its bane.
- For each radiographic procedure, an optimal peak kilovoltage (kVp) and milliampere-seconds (mAs) combination exists that minimizes the dose to the patient and produces an acceptable image.
- Within the energy range of diagnostic radiology (23 to 150 kVp), which also includes mammography, when kVp is decreased, the number of photoelectric interactions increases and the number of Compton interactions decreases; however, the patient absorbs more energy, and therefore the dose to the patient increases.
- When kVp is increased, the patient receives a lower dose, but image quality may be compromised.
- kVp selection is usually based on type of procedure and body part imaged.
- Radiographers must balance other variables, such as the type of image receptor used, patient thickness, and degree of muscle tissue, to arrive at technical exposure factors that will provide an acceptable image yet stay within the standards of radiation protection.
- Coherent scattering is most likely to occur at less than 10 keV; pair production and photodisintegration occur far above the range of diagnostic radiology.

GENERAL DISCUSSION QUESTIONS

1. How does peak kilovoltage (kVp) influence both the quality (penetrating power) and quantity (number of photons) of the x-ray beam, and why is it crucial for radiographers to understand this relationship?

2. Explain the role of milliampere-seconds (mAs) in determining the radiation directed toward a patient during an x-ray exposure. How can radiographers use mAs to optimize both image quality and patient dose?

3. Discuss the significance of x-ray absorption in biological tissue. How does absorption contribute to the absorbed dose (D), and why is minimizing the transferred energy important for patient safety?

4. Describe the process of x-ray beam production, including the generation of primary radiation. Why is it essential to filter out low-energy x-rays, and how does added aluminum contribute to "hardening" the x-ray beam?

5. What is the relationship between the electrical voltage applied across the x-ray tube (kVp) and the energy of the most energetic x-ray photon in a diagnostic x-ray unit? Why is the effective energy of the x-ray beam important for imaging?

6. Explain the concepts of attenuation, direct transmission, and indirect transmission of x-ray photons in radiography. How do these processes influence the quality of radiographic images?

7. Discuss the five possible interactions between x-radiation and matter, focusing on the importance of Compton scattering and photoelectric absorption in diagnostic radiology.

8. How does the probability of photon interaction with matter vary, and why is it essential for predicting the average outcome when dealing with a large number of photons?

9. Explore the impact of photoelectric absorption on radiographic contrast. How does the mass density and effective atomic number of different body structures affect the interaction of x-ray photons?

10. In what scenarios would radiographers manually adjust technique factors, and why is it crucial to balance patient dose and image quality? How does raising the kilovoltage peak (kVp) influence patient dose and image contrast?

REVIEW QUESTIONS

1. How does peak kilovoltage (kVp) influence the x-ray beam?
   A. It controls exposure time.
   B. It affects image sharpness.
   C. It influences both the quality (penetrating power) and quantity (number of photons).
   D. It determines the tube current.

2. What is the role of milliampere-seconds (mAs) in x-ray exposures?
   A. Controls beam energy.
   B. Regulates tube voltage.
   C. Determines radiation direction.
   D. Governs the amount of radiation produced.

3. Why is minimizing transferred energy important in x-ray absorption in biological tissue?
   A. To increase patient comfort.
   B. To improve image resolution.
   C. To reduce the risk of biologic damage.
   D. To speed up the imaging process.

4. What is the purpose of filtering out low-energy x-rays in x-ray beam production?
   A. To reduce exposure time.
   B. To decrease image contrast.
   C. To enhance image quality.
   D. To increase patient dose.

5. How does the electrical voltage applied across the x-ray tube (kVp) relate to the most energetic x-ray photon?
   A. Higher kVp results in lower photon energy.
   B. Lower kVp results in higher photon energy.
   C. kVp and photon energy are unrelated.
   D. kVp affects only the quantity of photons.

6. Which interaction is crucial for diagnostic radiology, causing small-angle scatter and potentially degrading image quality?
   A. Pair production.
   B. Compton scattering.
   C. Coherent scattering.
   D. Photodisintegration.

7. Why is predicting the average outcome important in dealing with a large number of photons interacting with matter?
   A. To minimize patient dose.
   B. To enhance image contrast.
   C. Due to the random nature of photon interactions.
   D. To increase exposure time.

8. How does photoelectric absorption impact radiographic contrast?
   A. It reduces image sharpness.
   B. It increases image brightness.
   C. It decreases image contrast.
   D. It enhances image contrast.

9. What influences the probability of photoelectric absorption in specific materials?
   A. Thickness of the material.
   B. Atomic number (Z) and incident photon energy (E).
   C. Mass density.
   D. Density and effective atomic number.

10. When might radiographers manually adjust technique factors, and how does raising kilovoltage peak (kVp) affect patient dose and image contrast?
    A. To increase patient dose, decrease image contrast.
    B. To decrease patient dose, increase image contrast.
    C. To increase patient dose, increase image contrast.
    D. To decrease patient dose, decrease image contrast.

4

Radiation Quantities and Units

OBJECTIVES

After completing this chapter, the reader will be able to perform the following:

- Define all key terms.
- Explain how x-rays were discovered.
- Describe some of the early acute biologic damage to humans that resulted from exposure to x-rays.
- Explain the concepts of skin erythema dose, tolerance dose, and threshold dose.
- Differentiate between somatic and genetic (hereditary) effects.
- List five examples of radiation responses recognized in modern times as early tissue reactions, three examples of late tissue reactions, and two examples of stochastic effects.
- Differentiate among the following radiation quantities: exposure, air kerma, absorbed dose, equivalent dose, and effective dose, and identify the appropriate symbol for each quantity.
- List and explain the International System (SI) units for radiation exposure, air kerma, absorbed dose, equivalent dose, and effective dose.
- Define the term *dose area product (DAP)*.
- State the formula for determining the equivalent dose.
- Determine the equivalent dose in terms of SI units when given the radiation weighting factor and the absorbed dose for different ionizing radiations.
- Describe the function of a tissue weighting factor.
- State the formula for determining the effective dose.
- Given the absorbed dose of radiation to an organ, the radiation weighting factor for the energy and type of radiation in question, and the tissue weighting factor, determine the effective dose to that organ.
- Explain the concept of effective dose when used for radiation protection purposes.
- State the purpose of the radiation quantity, collective effective dose, and list its SI unit.
- Explain the importance of linear energy transfer as it applies to biologic damage resulting from irradiation of human tissue.
- State the whole-body total effective dose equivalent (TEDE) for occupationally exposed personnel and for the general public.

CHAPTER OUTLINE

KEY TERMS

absorbed dose (D)
air kerma
collective effective dose (ColEfD)
committed effective dose
   equivalent (CEDE)
coulomb (C)
coulomb per kilogram (C/kg)
dose area product (DAP)
early tissue reactions

effective dose (EfD)
equivalent dose (EqD)
exposure (X)
genetic, or hereditary, effects
gray (Gy)
International System of Units (SI)
late tissue reactions
linear energy transfer (LET)
occupational exposure

radiation weighting factor (W_R)
Sievert (Sv)
somatic damage
stochastic effects
tissue weighting factor (W_T)
total effective dose equivalent
   (TEDE)

As the potentially harmful effects of ionizing radiation became known, the medical community sought to reduce these effects throughout the world by developing standards for measuring and limiting radiation exposure. To control patient and personnel exposure in a consistent and uniform manner, diagnostic imaging personnel must become familiar with the radiation quantities and units discussed in this chapter.

HISTORICAL EVOLUTION OF RADIATION QUANTITIES AND UNITS

Discovery of X-rays

On November 8, 1895, while working in a modest laboratory at the University of Wurzburg in Bavaria, German physics professor Wilhelm Conrad Roentgen (Fig. 4.1) discovered a mysterious ray. During an experiment investigating the nature of cathode rays and fluorescent materials, Roentgen passed electricity through a partially evacuated pear-shaped glass tube known as a *Crookes tube* (Fig. 4.2) that he had covered with black cardboard. As he passed a charge through this tube, the Professor observed light emanating (a fluorescence effect) from a piece of paper coated with a material compound of barium, platinum, and cyanide that was lying on a bench several feet away. Roentgen hypothesized that some type of radiant energy, or "rays," had been emitted from the Crookes tube that caused the barium platinocyanide to glow. To determine whether any object had the ability to obstruct the mysterious rays, Roentgen held various items between the Crookes tube and the fluorescent-coated paper and found that most materials would allow some degree of transmission. Roentgen called his

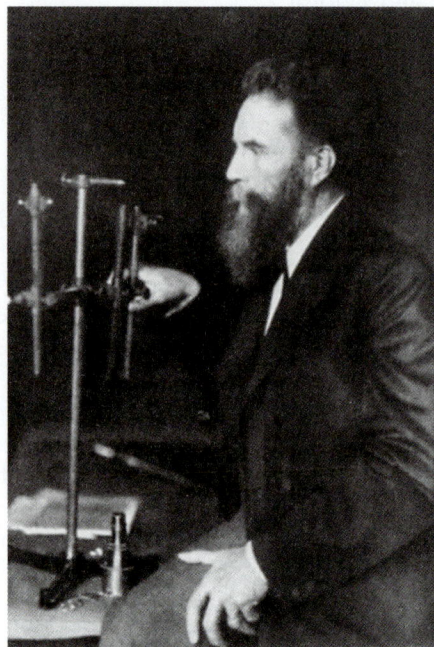

Fig. 4.1 Wilhelm Conrad Roentgen, the discoverer of x-rays. (US National Library of Medicine.)

momentous discovery *x-rays*. Very soon thereafter he produced an x-ray image on a glass plate "coated with a light-sensitive emulsion of silver salts. The emulsion consisted of silver halide crystals dispersed in gelatin."* Glass plates used to produce x-ray images only had emulsion on one side to avoid blurring of the image. The

---

*Personal communication, Dr. Uwe Busch, Director, Deutsches Roentgen Museum, Schwelmer Str. 41, Remscheid D - 42897, Germany, 03/16/2017 and 03/17/2017.

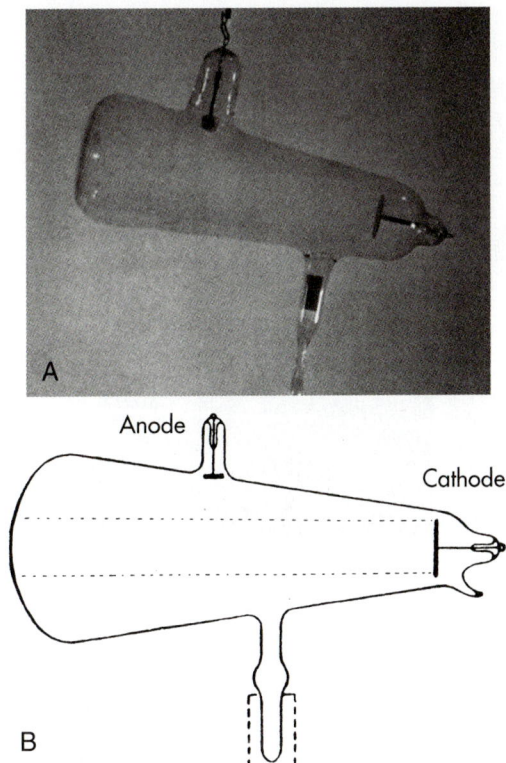

Fig. 4.2 Photograph (A) and diagram (B) of the original type of x-ray tube. The cathode stream produced x-rays by impinging on the large area of the glass wall of the tube. (Courtesy Carestream Health, Inc.)

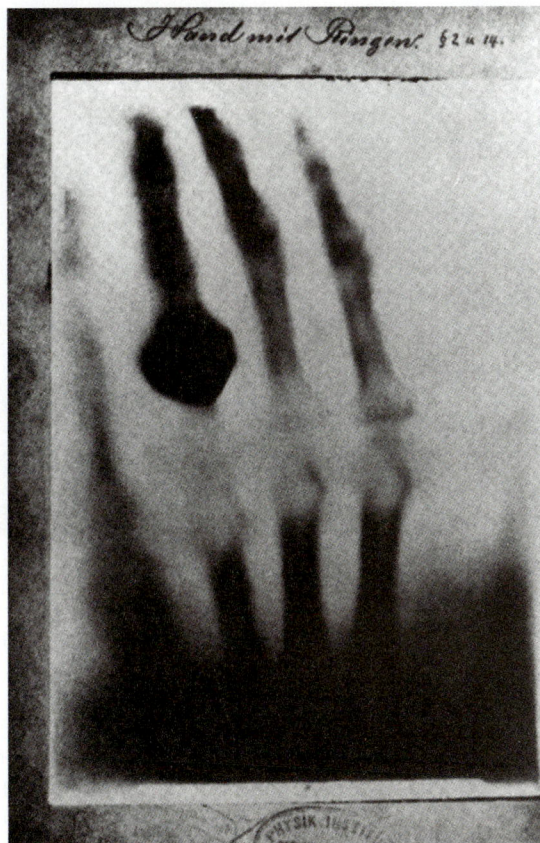

Fig. 4.3 Photograph of the first x-ray picture on a glass plate: Mrs. Roentgen's hand. (From Glasser O: *William Conrad Roentgen and the early history of the Roentgen rays,* London, 1933, John Bale, Sons and Danielsson, Ltd.)

first x-ray image the Professor produced was an image of his wife's hand that clearly showed her bones (Fig. 4.3). In December 1895 Roentgen announced his scientific findings in an abbreviated manuscript titled "On a New Kind of Ray, a Preliminary Communication," which was presented to the Physical Medical Society of Würzburg.

First Reports of Injury

In the months that followed the announcement of Roentgen's findings, unguarded experimentation with the new "wonder rays" unfortunately resulted in acute biologic damage to some investigators and their human subjects. Cases of **somatic damage** (from the Greek term *soma*, meaning "of the body") were reported in Europe as early as 1896. In the United States, Clarence Madison Dally (Fig. 4.4A), glass blower, tube maker, assistant, and long-time friend of fluoroscope inventor, Thomas A. Edison (Fig. 4.4B), became the first American radiation fatality.

Dally died of radiation-induced cancer in October 1904 at the age of 39 years. Because of Clarence Dally's severe injuries and death, Thomas Edison discontinued his x-ray research.

Among physicians, cancer deaths attributed to x-ray exposure were reported as early as 1910. As a result of **occupational exposure**, radiation exposure received in the course of exercising professional responsibilities, many radiologists and dentists using the new penetrating rays developed a reddening of the skin called *radiodermatitis*. A substantial number of these skin lesions on the hands and fingers of these radiation workers eventually became cancerous as a consequence of continued exposure to what was soon found to be ionizing radiation (Fig. 4.5). Blood disorders such as aplastic anemia, which results from bone marrow failure, and

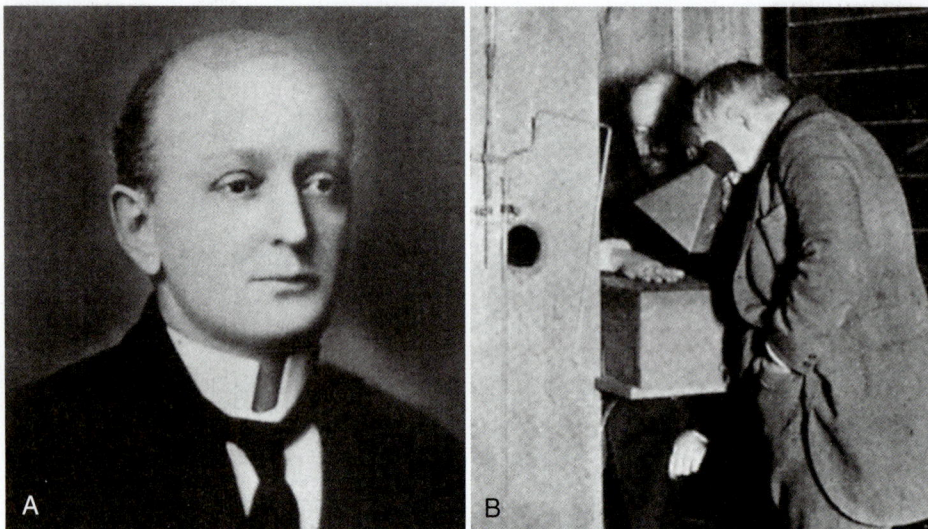

Fig. 4.4 (A) Clarence Madison Dally (1865–1904), the first American radiation fatality. (B) Dally, assistant to Thomas A. Edison, is seen holding his hand over a box containing an x-ray tube while Edison examines the hand through a fluoroscope that he invented. (A, From Brown P: *American martyrs to science through the Roentgen rays,* Springfield, IL, 1936, Charles C Thomas. B, From Eisenberg RL: *Radiology: an illustrated history,* St. Louis, 1995, Mosby.)

leukemia, an abnormal overproduction of white blood cells, were also more common among early radiologists than among nonradiologists.

Investigation of Methods for Reducing Radiation Exposure

Alarmed by the increasing number of radiation injuries reported, the medical community decided to investigate methods for reducing radiation exposure from all sources of radiation. In 1921 the British X-Ray and Radium Protection Committee was created to perform this task. The committee planned to formulate guidelines for the manufacture and use of radium and x-ray equipment and devices to reduce the chance of occupational injury. Even though the committee members recognized the danger of excessive radiation exposure, they were handicapped because they did not have accurate measurement techniques or adequate background knowledge of radiobiology. Ultimately, because they could not agree on a workable unit of radiation exposure, the members of the committee were unable to fulfill their responsibility.

Skin Erythema Dose

From 1900 to 1930, the unit in use for measuring radiation exposure was called the *skin erythema dose,* defined as the received quantity of radiation that causes diffuse redness over an area of skin after irradiation. This amount of absorbed radiation corresponds roughly to a skin dose that would be specified as several gray today. The radiation unit, **gray (Gy)**, is discussed later in this chapter. Because the amount of radiation required to produce an erythema reaction varied from one person to another, the skin erythema dose was often a crude and inaccurate way to quantify radiation exposure. Scientists felt compelled to continue searching for a more reliable unit. The new unit selected was to be based on some exactly assessable effect produced by radiation, such as ionization of atoms or energy absorbed in the irradiated object.

Early Definition of Quantities and Units

The First International Congress of Radiology was held in London, England, in 1925. This meeting allowed radiologists from all over the world to collaborate. Unfortunately, no definite decisions for quantifying the effects of ionizing radiation were made based on the recommendations presented. The International Commission on Radiation Units and Measurements (ICRU) was also formed in 1925. In 1928 a Second International Congress of Radiology was held in Stockholm, Sweden.

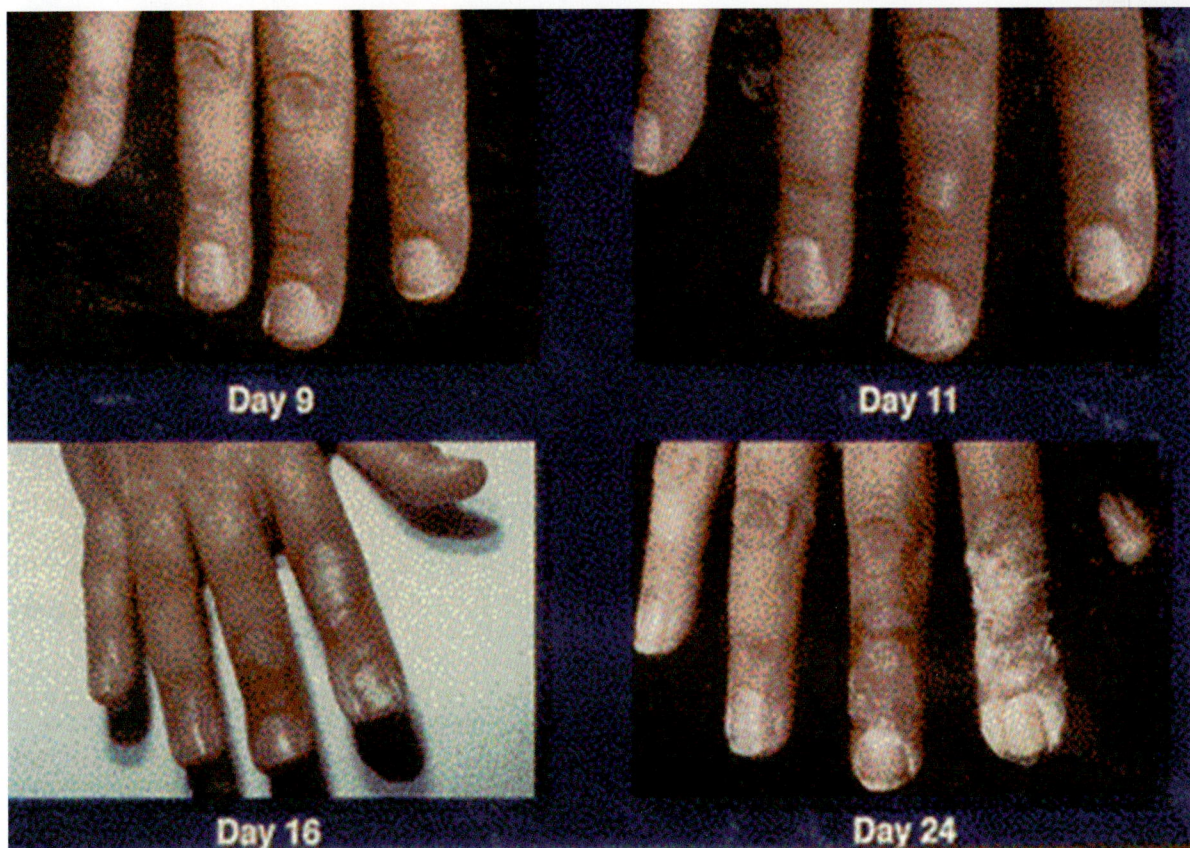

Fig. 4.5 Lesions of the fingers induced by ionizing radiation. (From Gusev IA, Guskova AK, Mettler FA, Jr., editors. *Medical management of radiation accidents*, ed 2, New York, 2001, CRC Press, Inc.)

Although at this time a unit of measure, the "roentgen," was in place as a unit associated with a certain degree of exposure, it was not as yet by any means scientifically well defined. The 1928 congress charged the ICRU with precisely defining this unit of exposure. The congress also established the International X-Ray and Radium Protection Commission, predecessor of the International Commission on Radiological Protection (ICRP).

Since the early days of radiology, biologic effects in humans caused by exposure to ionizing radiation were only too apparent. These **early tissue reactions** (Box 4.1), which appeared within minutes, hours, days, or weeks of the time of radiation exposure, were believed to be preventable if doses to radiation workers were limited.

A *tolerance dose* is a radiation dose to which occupationally exposed persons could be subjected without any apparent harmful acute effects, such as erythema of the skin. The general belief was that no adverse effects from radiation exposure would be demonstrated at doses lower than this level. Alternatively, this tolerance exposure level could be regarded as a *threshold dose*, that is, a dose of radiation lower than which an individual has a negligible chance of sustaining specific biologic damage. At the time of the 1928 International Congress, the tolerance dose was specified in *roentgen* units, which were then an imprecise measure of the quantity called *exposure*. Even with this uncertainty, the roentgen remained the principal guideline for occupational radiation exposure tolerance levels during the 1930s. Neither tolerance dose nor threshold dose is presently used for the purposes of radiation safety.

In 1934 the International X-Ray and Radium Protection Commission recommended a tolerance dose daily limit of 0.2 roentgen. In the United States, the Advisory Committee on X-Ray and Radium Protection, which was formed in 1931 to formulate recommendations for

BOX 4.1   Effects of Ionizing Radiation

Early Tissue Reactions
- Nausea
- Fatigue
- Diffuse redness of the skin
- Loss of hair
- Intestinal disorders
- Fever
- Blood disorders
- Shedding of the outer layer of skin

Late Tissue Reactions
- Cataract formation
- Fibrosis
- Organ atrophy
- Loss of parenchymal cells
- Reduced fertility
- Sterility

Stochastic Effects
- Cancer
- Genetic (hereditary) effects

radiation control, also recommended a tolerance dose equal to 0.2 roentgen per day.

In 1936 the committee reduced this dose to 0.1 roentgen per day. As scientists began to recognize the late tissue reactions and stochastic effects of ionizing radiation that appeared months or years after exposure and the possibility of genetic, or hereditary, effects, they began to focus on finding ways to minimize the risk of sustaining such damage (see Box 4.1). The search was on for a more reliable unit to replace the tolerance dose.

In 1937 the ICRU finished its assignment from the Second International Congress of Radiology, and, although still not accurately defined but now much better quantified, the roentgen became internationally adopted as the unit of measurement for exposure to x-radiation and gamma radiation (short-wavelength, higher-energy electromagnetic waves emitted by the nuclei of radioactive substances). In 1962 the roentgen was conceptually revisited and more rigorously defined in scientific terms.

In 1946 the US Advisory Committee on X-Ray and Radium Protection became known as the National Committee on Radiation Protection. The name of this radiation standards organization underwent another change in 1956 and again in 1964, when it became the National Council on Radiation Protection and Measurements (NCRP).

The General Conference of Weights and Measures, which was responsible for the development and international unification of the metric system, assigned its International Committee for Weights and Measures the responsibility of developing guidelines for the units of measurement in 1948. To fulfill this responsibility, the committee developed the International System of Units (SI), from the French "Système International d'Unités." This system makes possible the interchange of units among all branches of science throughout the world.

The Modern Era of Radiation Protection

By the early 1950s, maximum permissible dose (MPD) replaced the tolerance dose for radiation protection purposes. MPD essentially indicated the largest dose of ionizing radiation that an occupationally exposed person was allowed within a certain period that was not anticipated to result in major adverse biologic effects according to the best available data. However, the concept of an MPD did not mean that some small risk of damage would not exist with radiation doses at the MPD level. MPD was initially expressed in a unit called *rem** (an acronym for *radiation equivalent man,* also historically known as *Roentgen equivalent man*), the traditional British unit used for radiation protection purposes at that time. The rem has since been replaced by the SI unit, **sievert**. Please refer to Appendix A for all relationships between original, or traditional, units and the current standard SI units.

Removing the notion of "tolerance dose" and adopting the statistical MPD concept in its place ultimately meant that *no amount* of radiation was considered *completely* safe. The probability of long-term harm, such as the development of cancer, was expected to decrease as the dose decreased, but *it was not expected to become zero at any dose level!* This raised a dilemma: If no amount of radiation exposure was safe, and if it was impossible to design a work environment where the dose was zero, and still be able to perform procedures that unavoidably included some degree of exposure, then *what would determine the maximum allowed occupational exposure?*

---

*One rem is defined as the dose that is equivalent to any type of ionizing radiation that produces the same biologic effect as 1 rad (radiation absorbed dose) of x-radiation. One rad corresponds to an energy transfer of 100 ergs per gram to an irradiated object. The rad is identical to the subunit centigray or cGY.

The solution was to compare rates of death and accident among various occupations. Insurance companies had been using this actuarial method of comparison for many years to determine insurance rates. Some occupations are very hazardous. Examples of such occupations are:

- Deep sea diving
- Professional mountaineering
  Some nonhazardous occupations are:
- Trade
- Government desk work

However, even in nonhazardous occupations, there is still a small risk of fatality or serious injury, approximately one chance in 10,000 each year.[1] With this in mind, the decision was made to base recommendations for dose limits on the concept that the probability of harm associated with typical dosimeter readings should be no more than the amount of harm in industries that are generally considered reasonably safe.

By the 1970s dosimetry and risk analysis had become quite sophisticated. Radiation units were developed that contained factors that accounted for the varied bioeffects of different types of radiation, namely:

- Alpha
- Beta
- Gamma
- X-radiation
- Neutrons

There was also growing recognition that the consequences from radiation exposure to the health of a human as a whole depended on which organs and organ systems had been irradiated. For example, irradiation of the bone marrow was found to be much more significant to the whole-body health of an individual than irradiation of the skin. Equal doses of radiation to bone marrow and to skin had very different penalties! In the late 1970s, using these concepts of different organ radiosensitivity expressed numerically in terms of tissue-specific weighting factors, dose limits were calculated and established to ensure that the overall risk from radiation exposure acquired on the job did not exceed risks encountered in "safe" occupations, such as clerical work, in which the risk is approximately 10^{-4} (one chance in 10,000) per year.[1]

In 1991 the ICRP revised the values of the tissue radiosensitivity weighting factors. The revision was based on data from more recent epidemiologic studies of the atomic bomb survivors. The ICRP also adopted the term **effective dose (EfD)**. Based on the energy

deposited in biologic tissue by ionizing radiation, it takes into account both of the following:

1. The type of radiation (e.g., x-radiation, gamma, neutron)
2. The variable sensitivity of the tissues exposed to the radiation

This quantity, EfD, is therefore the best measure of the overall risk arising from the simultaneous irradiation of various biologic tissues and organs within an individual. EfD is expressed in the SI unit, **sievert (Sv)**, or in subunits of the sievert. The Sv is discussed further in the next section.

Quantities and Units in Use Today

In 1980 the ICRU adopted SI units, a unified system of metric units, for use with ionizing radiation and urged full implementation of the units as soon as possible. Many developed countries, particularly in Europe, have already made a complete transition to SI units. In the United States, SI units, such as the Gy and the centigray (cGy), are now used routinely in therapeutic radiology to specify absorbed dose. Even though the NCRP adopted the internationally accepted SI units for use in 1985, traditional units, older units associated with radiation protection and dosimetry, such as the roentgen (R)* and its subunit the milliroentgen (mR), are being utilized. In addition, the rem, the traditional unit for the radiation quantity **equivalent dose (EqD)** currently remains a used quantity. This is especially so in radiation dosimetry reports for occupationally exposed personnel. In the SI system of units, the Sv has replaced the rem for radiation protection purposes. Like the *rem*, it provides a common scale whereby varying degrees of biologic damage caused by equal absorbed doses of different types of ionizing radiation can be compared with the degree of biologic damage caused by the same amount of x-radiation or gamma radiation. One Sv is the same as 100 rem.

Fluoroscopic patient entrance radiation levels are now specified in milligray per minute (mGy-/min), but in many facilities they are still measured as exposure rates in roentgens per minute (R/min), and essentially all radiation survey instruments, even the newer SI-oriented devices, continue to also provide readings

---

*One roentgen is the photon exposure that under standard conditions of pressure and temperature produces a total positive or negative ion charge of 2.58×10^{-4} coulombs per kilogram of dry air.

BOX 4.2   Historical Evolution of Radiation Quantities and Units

Year	Event
1895	X-rays are discovered, and the discovery is announced.
1896	Initial cases of somatic damage caused by exposure to ionizing radiation are reported in Europe.
1900	Skin erythema dose becomes the unit for measuring radiation exposure.
1904	Clarence Madison Dally becomes the first American radiation fatality.
1910	First cancer deaths among physicians that are attributed to x-ray exposure are reported.
1921	The British X-Ray and Radium Protection Committee is formed to investigate methods for reducing radiation exposure.
1925	The First International Congress of Radiology is held in London, England; radiologists from all over the world collaborate, but no definite system for measuring ionizing radiation exposure is identified. The International Commission on Radiation Units and Measurements (ICRU) is formed.
1928	The ICRU is charged by the Second International Congress of Radiology (Stockholm, Sweden) with defining a unit of exposure. The International X-Ray and Radium Protection Commission (predecessor of the ICRP) is established by the Second International Congress of Radiology.
1930	Tolerance dose is used for radiation protection purposes.
1931	The US Advisory Committee on X-Ray and Radium Protection is formed to formulate recommendations for radiation control.
1934	A tolerance dose of 0.2 R per day is recommended.
1936	The tolerance dose is reduced to 0.1 R per day.
	The Bragg–Gray theory is introduced.
1937	The roentgen (R) becomes internationally accepted as the unit of measurement for exposure to x-radiation and gamma radiation.
1946	The US Advisory Committee on X-Ray and Radium Protection becomes known as the National Committee on Radiation Protection and Measurements (NCRP).
1948	The International System of Units (SI) is developed.
Early 1950s	Maximum permissible dose (MPD) replaces the tolerance dose for radiation protection purposes.
1962	The roentgen (R) is redefined to increase accuracy and acceptability.
1963	The National Committee on Radiation Protection and Measurements becomes the National Council on Radiation Protection (NCRP).
1977	The International Commission on Radiological Protection (ICRP) recommends that the dose equivalent limit or effective dose equivalent replace the MPD.
1980	The ICRU adopts SI units for use with ionizing radiation.
1985	The National Council on Radiation Protection (NCRP) adopts SI units for use.
1991	The ICRP replaces effective equivalent dose with the term *effective dose (EfD)*.

History of Terminology Used to Determine Radiation Dose Limitation

1900–1930	Skin erythema dose (SED)
1930–1950	Tolerance dose (TD)
1950–1977	Maximum permissible dose (MPD)
1977–1991	Effective dose equivalent
1991–present	Effective dose (EfD)

in traditional units. Furthermore, many regulatory criteria are given in terms of traditional units. In this text, in an effort to advance the full conversion to SI units, all dosimetry information will be presented as much as possible in terms of SI units. Appendix A contains a complete discussion of both SI and traditional units and the relationship between them. Examples of conversion between various units are also included.

Box 4.2 presents an overview of the important dates in the historical evolution of radiation quantities and units and an overview of terminology used in a given time period to describe radiation dose limitation.

The SI unit of absorbed dose, the **gray (Gy)**, was named after the English radiobiologist, Louis Harold Gray (1901–1965), who was instrumental in developing what is arguably the most important theory in all of radiation dosimetry. The Bragg–Gray theory (1936) *relates the ionization produced in a small cavity within an irradiated medium or object to the energy absorbed in that medium as a result of its radiation exposure.* With the use of appropriate correction factors, the theory essentially links the determination of the absorbed radiation dose in a medium to a relatively simple measurement of ionization charge.

RADIATION QUANTITIES AND THEIR SI UNITS OF MEASURE

Diagnostic imaging professionals must have a clear understanding of the following basic radiation quantities:

- Exposure (X)
- Air kerma
- Absorbed dose (D)
- Equivalent dose (EqD)
- Effective dose (EfD)

In everyday usage, it is commonly said that an "exposure" has occurred when ionizing radiation strikes an object such as a human body. However, the quantity, "exposure," has a rigorous scientific meaning related to ionization produced in air. Absorbed dose is the deposition of energy per unit mass in any material from exposure to ionizing radiation. EqD is a quantity that builds upon D but then takes into account the type of radiation striking an object. Different types of radiation affect molecules and cells of the body in different ways. EfD builds upon EqD by adding an attempt to take into account the different harmful degrees of radiation effects on the parts of the body that are being irradiated to arrive at an index of overall harm to a human (Box 4.3). Each radiation quantity has its own special unit of measure. These quantities and units are discussed in detail in the following sections.

Exposure

When a volume of air is irradiated with x-rays or with gamma rays, the interaction that occurs between the

> **BOX 4.3   Difference Between Equivalent Dose and Effective Dose**
>
> The quantity *equivalent dose* uses radiation weighting factors (W_R) to adjust the value of the *absorbed dose* to reflect the different capacity for producing biologic harm by various types and energies of ionizing radiation.
>
> The quantity *effective dose* uses tissue weighting factors (W_T) to adjust the quantity *equivalent dose* to reflect the difference in harm to the person as a whole depending on the tissues and organs that have been irradiated. Therefore effective dose takes into account both the type of radiation and the part of the body irradiated.

radiation and neutral atoms in the air causes some electrons to be liberated from those air atoms as they are ionized. Consequently, the ionized air can function as a conductor and carry electricity because of the negatively charged free electrons and positively charged ions that have been created. As the intensity of x-ray exposure of the air volume increases, the number of electron–ion pairs produced also increases. Thus, the amount of radiation responsible for the ionization of a well-defined volume of air may be determined by measuring the number of electron–ion pairs, or charged particles of either sign, in that volume of air. This radiation ionization in air is termed *exposure*.

Exposure (X) is defined as the total electrical charge of one sign, either all plus or all minus, per unit mass that x-ray and gamma ray photons with energies up to 3 million electron volts (MeV) generate in dry (i.e., nonhumid) air at standard temperature and pressure (760 mm Hg or 1 atmosphere at sea level and 22°C). It is a radiation quantity "that expresses the *intensity of radiation* delivered to a specific area, such as the surface of the human body."[2]

As it is defined, the exposure quantity, X, is based on a response produced when radiation interacts with air. For a precise measurement of X, the total amount of ionization (charge) an x-ray beam produces in a known mass of air must be obtained. This type of *direct* measurement is normally accomplished in an accredited dosimetry calibration laboratory (ADCL) by using a standard, or free-air, ionization chamber (Fig. 4.6). The chamber contains a known quantity of

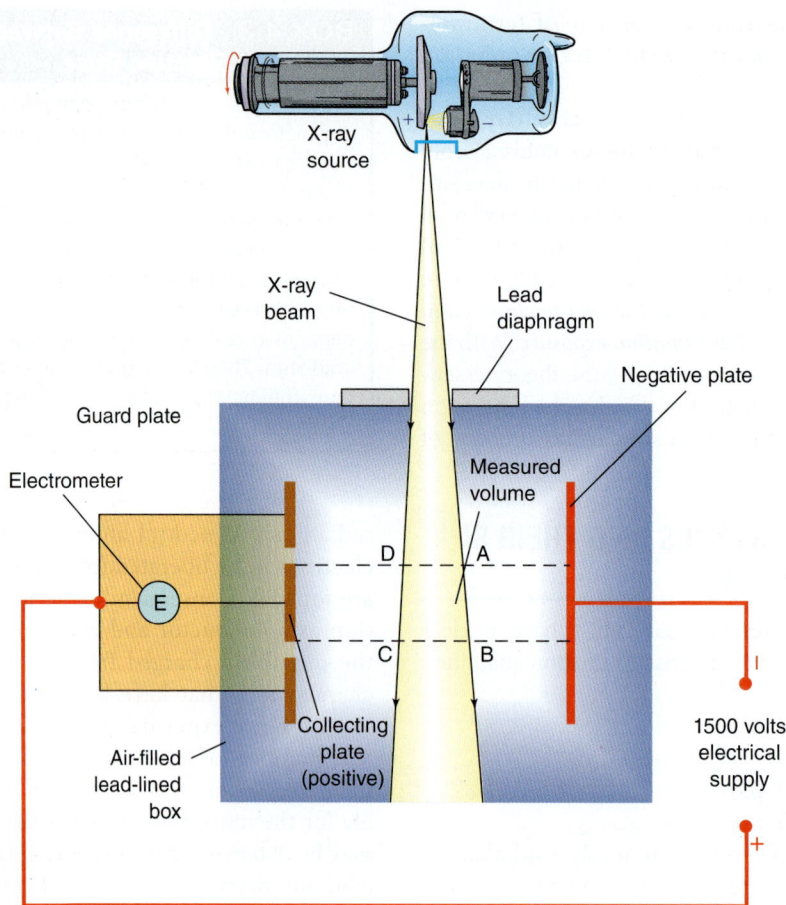

Fig. 4.6 This device determines radiation exposure by measuring the amount of ionization (charge) an x-ray beam produces within its air collection volume. The instrument consists of a box containing a known quantity of air, two oppositely charged metal plates, and an electrometer, an instrument that measures the total amount of charge collected on the positively charged metal plate. The chamber measures the total amount of electrical charge of all the electrons produced during the ionization of a specific volume of air at standard atmospheric pressure and temperature. The electrical charge is measured in units called *coulombs (C)* (charge of an electron = 1.6×10^{-19} C). A collected electrical charge of 2.58×10^{-4} C/kg of irradiated air constitutes an exposure of 1 roentgen (R).

air with precisely measured temperature, pressure, and low humidity. If in that specified volume of dry air the total charge of all the ions of one sign (either all plus or all minus) produced is collected and measured, the total amount of radiation exposure may be accurately determined. Lastly, the free-air chamber response is modified to correspond to standard temperature and pressure of dry air in accordance with the definition of exposure.

Such an instrument, however, is not a practical device at locations other than a standardization laboratory. As a result, much smaller and less complicated instruments have been developed for use away from the laboratory. Although very convenient, these instruments must be periodically recalibrated in an ADCL against a free-air chamber.

The **coulomb (C)** is the basic unit of electrical charge. It is equal to the "amount" of electrical charge

"Q" moving past a point in a conductor in 1 second when an electrical current "I" amounting to 1 ampere is used. The *ampere** is the SI unit of electrical current. Current consists of moving electrical charges, the most common of which is the electron (the charge carried by an electron is equal to: -1.6×10^{-19} C). Essentially, the ampere quantifies the flow rate of electric charge and mathematically is simply given by: $I = Q/t$ where Q is the total net electrical charge in coulombs moving past a location in a conductor in a time t (given in seconds).

In the International System, the exposure unit is **coulombs per kilogram (C/kg)**. No special name for this SI quantity has been assigned. This exposure unit is simply equal to an electrical charge of 1 C produced in a kilogram of dry air by ionizing radiation. Appendix A provides examples of numeric conversions between C per kilogram and the roentgen traditional unit. Both of these remain very useful for x-ray equipment calibration because x-ray output intensity is measured directly with an ionization chamber.

Air Kerma

Air kerma is another SI quantity that is used to express how energy is transferred from a beam of radiation to air. It is mostly replacing the traditional quantity, *exposure*. Because of this, "x-ray tube output and inputs to image receptors are now often given in air kerma."[3] A standard, or free-air, ionization chamber is the instrument that can be calibrated to read air kerma.[2] "A conversion factor can also be used to change between air kerma and exposure values."[2]

"Kinetic energy released in air," "kinetic energy released in material," and "kinetic energy released per unit mass" all use the word *kerma* as an acronym. In simple terms, *air kerma* is the total kinetic energy released in a unit mass (kilogram) of air and is expressed in metric units of joules per kilogram (J/kg).[2] In a similar way *tissue kerma* can be

defined as the total kinetic energy released in a unit mass of tissue. Tissue kerma is also given in units of joules per kilogram. This unit for kerma is in fact the same radiation unit, the Gy, which was previously defined as the SI unit for the radiation quantity, absorbed dose. With respect to radiographic and fluoroscopic units, however, "air" kerma, not "tissue" kerma, is the primary concept because in these situations the main concern is with exposure and the patient's resulting entrance dose.

Modern radiographic and fluoroscopic units have incorporated an ability to determine the entire amount of energy delivered to the patient by the x-ray beam. This quantity is often referred to as the **dose area product (DAP)**. It is the sum total of air kerma over the exposed area of the patient's surface or, in other words, a measure of the amount of radiant energy that has been thrust into a portion of the patient's body surface. DAP is usually specified in units of mGy-cm^2. As an illustration of this concept, consider a patient whose irradiated surface receives an air kerma dose of 20 mGy. If the area of the irradiated surface is 100 cm^2, then the DAP will be 20 mGy $\times$ 100 cm^2 = 2000 mGy-cm^2.

Absorbed Dose

As ionizing radiation passes through an object such as a human body, some of the energy of that radiation is absorbed by the body and stays within it. The quantity **absorbed dose (D)** is defined as the amount of energy per unit mass absorbed by an irradiated object. Therefore D indicates the energy that the patient actually receives from an exposure to ionizing radiation. This absorbed energy is what causes damage in biologic tissues of the patient.

Because many x-ray examinations require relatively small radiation doses, smaller units, which are only a fraction of a specific unit, may frequently be used to indicate D values. Examples of some of these subunits are provided in Box 4.4. Box 4.5 demonstrates

BOX 4.4   Subunits of the Gray

Smaller fractions of measured quantities such as the gray (Gy) will have a prefix. Examples follow.

Prefix	Subunit	Symbol	Fraction	Factor
centi-	centigray (cGy)	c	1/100	10^{-2}
milli-	milligray (mGy)	m	1/1000	10^{-3}
micro-	microgray (µGy)	µ	1/1,000,000	10^{-6}

TABLE 4.1   Quality Factors for Different Types of Ionizing Radiation

Type of Ionizing Radiation	Quality Factor
X-ray photons	1
Beta particles	1
Gamma photons	1
Thermal neutrons	5
Fast neutrons	20
High-energy external protons	1
Low-energy internal protons*	20
Alpha particles	20
Multiple charged particles of unknown energy	20

*Protons produced as a result of neutrons interacting with the nuclei of tissue molecules.
Data from National Council on Radiation Protection and Measurements (NCRP): *Limitation of exposure to ionizing radiation, Report No. 116,* Bethesda, MD, 1993, NCRP.

conversion between decimal values of gray and the numerically smaller units: centigray (cGy) and milligray (mGy). It is also easy to convert milligray or centigray to gray. This is done just by dividing the number of milligray by 1000 or the number of centigray by 100. SI subunits can also facilitate conversion from traditional units of D to SI units of absorbed dose, especially in therapeutic radiology (see Appendix A for an example).

Equivalence of Radiation-Produced Damage From Different Sources of Ionizing Radiation

Equal absorbed doses of different types of radiation produce different amounts of biologic damage in body tissue. For example, in laboratory experiments it has been shown that a 1-Gy D of fast neutrons causes much more biologic damage than a 1-Gy D of x-rays. A 1-Gy dose of neutrons would kill a laboratory rat, but a 1-Gy dose of x-rays would not. The concept of dose equivalence takes this varied biologic impact into consideration by using a specific modifying factor termed a *quality factor.* The quality factor (Q) is an adjustment multiplier that is employed in the calculation of dose equivalence to detail the specific ability of a dose of any kind of ionizing radiation to cause biologic damage.

X-rays, beta particles (high-speed electrons), and gamma rays produce virtually the same biologic effect in body tissue for equal absorbed doses. In terms of quality factor, these radiations have been given a numeric adjustment value of 1 (i.e., Q = 1) and are the basis, or standard, against which to compare the effectiveness of other types of ionizing radiation in producing biologic damage. The quality factors of different kinds of ionizing radiations are listed in Table 4.1. The concept of **linear energy transfer (LET)** helps explain the need for a quality, or modifying, factor. LET is the amount of energy transferred on average by incident radiation to an object per unit length of track, or passage, through the object and is expressed in units of kiloelectron volts per micrometer (keV/μm)

(see Appendix C). Radiation with a high LET transfers a large amount of energy into a small area and can therefore potentially do much more biologic damage than radiation with a low LET. As a result, a high-LET radiation has a quality factor that is noticeably greater than the quality factor for a low-LET radiation.

Equivalent Dose

EqD is the product of the average D in a tissue or organ in the human body and its associated **radiation weighting factor (W_R)** chosen for the type and energy of the radiation in question. X-radiation and gamma radiation have a W_R of 1, whereby 1 Gy equals 1 Sv. Other types of radiation have different radiation weighting factors.

The W_R takes into consideration the fact that some types of radiation are more efficient at causing biologic damage than other types of radiation for a given dose. Values for the radiation weighting factors are selected by national and international scientific advisory bodies (NCRP, ICRP) and are based on quality factors and LET. The NCRP, in Report No. 116, described the W_R as "a dimensionless factor" (a multiplier) that was chosen for radiation protection purposes to account for differences in biologic impact among various types of ionizing radiations.[1] This factor places risks associated with biologic effects on a common scale. Each type and energy of radiation has a specific radiation weighting factor, the numeric value of which may be found in Table 4.2. The

TABLE 4.2 Radiation Weighting Factors for Different Types and Energies of Ionizing Radiation

Radiation Type and Energy Range	Radiation Weighting Factor (W_R)
X-ray and gamma ray photons and electrons (every energy)	1
Neutrons, energy <10 keV	5
10 keV–100 keV	10
>100 keV–2 MeV	20
>2 MeV–20 MeV	10
>20 MeV	5
Protons	2
Alpha particles	20

Data adapted from International Commission on Radiological Protection (ICRP): *Recommendations,* ICRP Publication No. 60, New York, 1991, Pergamon Press.

BOX 4.7 Determining and Expressing Equivalent Dose Using Gray and Sievert

Example: An individual received the following absorbed doses: 0.1 Gyt of x-radiation, 0.05 Gyt of fast neutrons, and 0.2 Gyt of alpha particles. What is the total equivalent dose (EqD)?

$$EqD = (D \times W_R)_1 + (D \times W_R)_2 + (D \times W_R)_3$$

(The radiation weighting factor for each radiation in question may be obtained from 4.2.)
Answer:

Radiation Type	D	×	W_R	=	EqD
X-radiation	0.1 Gyt	×	1	=	0.1 Sv
Fast neutrons	0.05 Gyt	×	20	=	1.0 Sv
Alpha particles	0.2 Gyt	×	20	=	4.0 Sv
	Total EqD			=	5.1 Sv

BOX 4.6 Subunits of the Sievert

Smaller fractions of measured quantities such as the sievert (Sv) will have a prefix. Examples follow.

Prefix	Subunit	Symbol	Fraction	Factor
centi-	centisievert (cSv)	c	$1/100$	10^{-2}
milli-	millisievert (mSv)	m	$1/1000$	10^{-3}
micro-	microsievert (µSv)	µ	$1/1,000,000$	10^{-6}

W_R actually has the *same numeric value as the quality factor* that was previously used for determining dose equivalence.

EqD is used for radiation protection purposes when a person receives exposure from various types of ionizing radiation. EqD is expressed in sieverts or in a subunit of the Sv (Box 4.6). EqD is obtained by multiplying the D by the W_R as follows:

$$EqD = D \times W_R$$

which in terms of units corresponds to:

$$Sv = Gy \times W_R$$

An example of determining and expressing EqD using gray and Sv is provided in Box 4.7. Because radiation doses for radiation workers employed in diagnostic radiology are normally relatively small, they may be specified in terms of millisievert. To change Sv to millisievert, multiply the number of Sv by 1000, whereas millisievert can be converted to Sv by dividing the number of millisievert by 1000.

Effective Dose

EfD is the best measure of the overall risk of exposure to humans from ionizing radiation. The NCRP, in Report No. 116, defines it as "the sum of the weighted equivalent doses for all irradiated tissues or organs."[1] EfD incorporates both the effect of the type of radiation used (e.g., x-radiation, gamma, neutron, alpha) and the variability in radiosensitivity of the specific organ or body part irradiated through the use of appropriate weighting factors. These factors quantify the overall potential harm to those biologic components and the risk of developing a radiation-induced cancer or, for the reproductive organs, the risk of genetic damage. The term that specifically takes into account the relative detriment to each specific particular organ and tissue is called the **tissue weighting factor (W_T)**. More precisely, each W_T value (Table 4.3) denotes the percentage ratio of the summed stochastic (cancer plus genetic) risk stemming from irradiation of a specific tissue or organ to the all-inclusive risk when the entire body is irradiated in a uniform fashion. As a result, EfD accounts for the risk to the entire organism brought on by all types of irradiation of individual tissues and organs. The ICRP originally introduced the

TABLE 4.3 Organ or Tissue Weighting Factors

Organ or Tissue	Weighting Factor (W_T)
Gonads	0.08
Active marrow	0.12
Colon	0.12
Lungs	0.12
Stomach	0.12
Bladder	0.05
Breast	0.05
Liver	0.04
Esophageal wall	0.04
Thyroid	0.04
Skin	0.01
Bone surface	0.01
Urinary bladder wall	0.04
Brain	0.01
Remainder*†	0.12

*The remainder takes into account the following additional tissues and organs: adrenals, brain, small intestine, large intestine, kidney, muscle, pancreas, spleen, thymus, and uterus.
†In extraordinary circumstances in which one of the remainder tissues or organs receives an equivalent dose in excess of the highest dose in any of the 12 organs for which a weighting factor (W_T) is specified, a W_T of 0.025 should be applied to that tissue or organ and a W_T of 0.025 to the average dose in the other remainder tissues or organs.
Data from National Council on Radiation Protection and Measurements (NCRP): *Medical radiation exposure of patients in the United States, Report No. 184*, Bethesda, Md, 2019, NCRP. Reprinted with permission of the National Council on Radiation Protection and Measurements, http://NCRPonline.org.

BOX 4.8 Determining and Expressing Effective Dose in Sievert

Example: The W_R for alpha particles is 20 (see Table 4.2), and the W_T for the lung is 0.12 (see Table 4.3). If the lungs receive an absorbed dose (D) of 0.5 Gyt from exposure to alpha radiation, what is the effective dose (EfD) in Sv?
Answer:

$$EfD = D \times W_R \times W_T$$
$$= 0.5 \times 20 \times 0.12$$
$$= 1.2\,Sv$$

TABLE 4.4 Typical Values for Radiation Doses Associated With an Anteroposterior Lumbar Spine Examination

Absorbed dose to skin at entrance surface	6.4 mGy
Absorbed dose to bone marrow	0.6 mGy
Absorbed dose to a fetus	3.5 mGy
Equivalent dose to a fetus	3.5 mSv
Effective dose to a fetus	3.3 mSv

W_T concept because uniform, whole-body irradiation seldom occurs, causing different organs and body tissues to vary considerably in the amount of D received and, consequently, the intensity of their response.

To determine EfD, an D is multiplied by a W_R to obtain EqD and that product is multiplied by a tissue weighting factor (W_T) to give:

$$EfD = D \times W_R \times W_T$$

EfD is expressed in sieverts or millisieverts. An example of determining and expressing EfD in Sv is provided in Box 4.8.

EfD can be used to compare the average detrimental amount of radiation received by the entire body from a specific radiologic examination with that from natural background radiation (see Table 1.1). By using the background equivalent radiation time (BERT) method as discussed in Chapter 1, it is possible to describe the examination's *significant* radiation dose in terms of the length of time it would take to acquire a comparable amount from environmental sources.

Table 4.4 gives some typical values for radiation doses that are associated with a radiographic examination of the lumbar spine, and it illustrates some of the principles of the different ways to specify radiation dose. The dose to the patient is highest at the "entrance skin surface," the surface of the patient that is toward the x-ray tube. This surface will be exposed to the unattenuated primary beam of x-rays. Absorbed doses to various organs may be calculated from standard tables. Two organ absorbed doses are given in Table 4.4, namely, bone marrow and fetus. The EqD to the fetus is also given and is the same as the D to the fetus because the W_R is 1. Finally, the EfD to the fetus is given. It was calculated from the various tissue weighting factors and organ absorbed doses for fetal organs in the field of view of this examination.

BOX 4.9 Determining Collective Effective Dose Using the Radiation Unit Person-Sievert

Example: If 200 people receive an average effective dose of 0.25 Sv, the collective effective dose (ColEfD) is 200 × 0.25 = 50 person-sieverts.

Collective Effective Dose

In addition to EqD and EfD, another dosimetric quantity has been derived and implemented for use in radiation protection. It takes into account both internal and external dose measurements. Collective Effective Dose (ColEfD) represents an attempt to describe the radiation exposure of a population or group from low doses of different sources of ionizing radiation. It is determined as the product of the average EfD for an individual belonging to the exposed population or group and the number of persons exposed. The radiation unit for this quantity is *person-sievert*. An example using this unit is provided in Box 4.9. With respect to the validity of this concept, the ICRP states: "Collective effective dose is an instrument for optimization, for comparing radiological technologies and protection procedures. ColEfD is not intended as a tool for epidemiological studies, and it is inappropriate to use it in risk projections. This is because the assumptions implicit in the calculation of ColEfD (e.g., when applying the LNT* model) conceal large biological and statistical uncertainties. Specifically, the computation of cancer deaths based on collective effective doses involving trivial exposures to large populations is not reasonable and should be avoided."[4]

Total Effective Dose Equivalent

Total Effective Dose Equivalent (TEDE) is a radiation dosimetry quantity that was defined by the Nuclear Regulatory Commission (NRC) to monitor and control human exposure to ionizing radiation. Essentially, as described by NRC regulations, it is the sum of EfD equivalent from external radiation exposures and a

*LNT, which stands for linear nonthreshold, is a dose model that implies there is no dose value below which there is no risk of biologic damage and that the degree of risk is directly proportional to the dose at any level.

TABLE 4.5 SI Unit Equivalents

1 SI exposure unit equals	$\dfrac{1}{(2.58\times10^{-4})}$R
1 coulomb equals	1 ampere-second
1 coulomb per kilogram of air equals	1 SI unit of exposure
	$C/kg = \dfrac{1}{(2.58\times10^{-4})}F$
1 gray equals	1 J/kg
	100 cGy
	1000 mGy
	1 J/kg (for x-radiation, Q = 1)
1 sievert equals	100 centisievert (cSv)
	1000 mSv
	1 J/kg
	107 erg/kg = 104 erg/gm
1 joule equals	1 newton-meter
1 joule equals	6.24 × 1018 eV

quantity called Committed Effective Dose Equivalent (CEDE)* from internal radiation exposures. Thus TEDE is designed to take into account all possible sources of radiation exposure. It is a particularly useful dose monitor for occupationally exposed personnel such as nuclear medicine technologists and interventional radiologists, who are likely to receive possibly significant radiation exposure during the course of a year. Traditionally, the whole-body TEDE regulatory limit is 0.05 Sv for occupationally exposed personnel and 0.001 Sv for the general public. Radiation monitoring services can provide annual TEDE values for individuals.

Table 4.5 and Table 4.6 summarize radiation quantities, units, and equivalents. An additional table emphasizing relationship between traditional units and SI units is also found in Appendix A.

*The "committed dose" in radiation protection is a measure of the probabilistic health effect on an individual as a result of an intake of radioactive material into the body. A "committed dose" from an internal source takes into account the total amount of radiation dose delivered by radioactive material in the body until it is eliminated (exhaled, excreted, physically decays away). This is the origin of the name "committed effective dose equivalent." For nuclear medicine technologists who, through certain procedures (e.g., thyroid ablations, using iodine-131), have a possibility of radioisotope absorption and consequent internal exposure, committed dose is certainly an appropriate measure.

TABLE 4.6 Summary of Radiation Quantities and Units

Type of Radiation	Quantity	SI Unit	Measuring Medium	Radiation Effect Measured
X-radiation or gamma radiation	Exposure (X)	Coulombs per kilogram (C/kg)	Air	Ionization of air
	Air kerma	Gray (Gy-a)	Air	Kinetic energy deposited in air
All ionizing radiations	Absorbed dose (D)	Gray (Gyt)	Any object	Amount of energy per unit mass absorbed by object
	Air kerma	Gray (Gyt)		
All ionizing radiations	Equivalent dose (EqD)	Sievert (Sv)	Body tissue	Biologic effects
All ionizing radiations	Effective dose (EfD)	Sievert (Sv)	Body tissue	Biologic effects

SUMMARY

- German physics professor Wilhelm Conrad Roentgen discovered "x-rays" on November 8, 1895, during an experiment investigating the nature of cathode rays and fluorescent materials.
- Many individuals who were exposed to substantial doses of x-rays in the early years after their discovery developed somatic damage from the exposure.
- Skin erythema dose was used from 1900 to 1930 as the unit for measuring radiation exposure. Eventually a tolerance dose was established for occupationally exposed individuals that could be regarded as a threshold dose. MPD replaced the tolerance dose in the early 1950s. In 1977 dose equivalent or effective dose equivalent replaced the MPD. In 1991 the ICRP replaced effective dose equivalent with the term *effective dose,* which is still in use today.
- Effective dose is based on the energy deposited in biologic tissue by ionizing radiation. It takes into account both the type of radiation and the variable sensitivity of the tissues exposed to the radiation. EfD is expressed in the SI unit sievert (Sv) or in subunits of the sievert.
- In 1980 the ICRU adopted SI units for use with ionizing radiation. Many developed countries, particularly in Europe, have already made a complete transition to SI units. In the United States, this transition is not as yet fully complete, and some conventional units are still broadly in use.
- SI radiation units are preferred for specifying radiation quantities because the traditional system of units does not fit into the metric system that provides "one unified system of units for all physical quantities."[2]

- Coulomb per kilogram (C/kg) is used for specifying x-ray or gamma ray exposure in air only. This exposure unit is equal to an electrical charge of 1 coulomb produced in a kilogram of dry air by ionizing radiation.
- Air kerma is an SI quantity that is used to express how energy is transferred from a beam of radiation to air.
- DAP is the sum total of air kerma multiplied by the exposed area of the patient's surface.
- Absorbed dose (D) is the amount of energy per unit mass absorbed by an irradiated object.
- The gray (Gy) is used for measuring absorbed dose in air (Gya) or for measuring absorbed dose in tissue (Gyt).
- The number of gray times 1000 equals the number of milligray. The number of gray times 100 equals the number of centigray.
- LET is the amount of energy transferred on average by incident radiation to an object per unit length of track, or passage, through the object and is expressed in units of kiloelectron volts per micrometer (keV/μm).
- Equivalent dose (EqD) and effective dose (EfD) are the quantities of choice for measuring biologic effects when all types of radiation must be considered.
- EqD specifies how the potential for biologic damage from different types and doses of radiation will be equivalent if correct weighting factors are included. To calculate equivalent dose: $EqD = D \times W_R$.

- EfD describes the total biologic damage to a human that is caused by equivalent doses received by specific organs. To calculate effective dose: $EfD = D \times W_R \times W_T$.
- In the SI system, sievert (Sv) or the subunits millisievert and microsievert are used to specify EqD and EfD. These units are used for occupational radiation exposure.
- ColEfD represents an attempt to describe the radiation exposure of a population or group from low doses of different sources of ionizing radiation. Person-sievert is the radiation unit used to calculate this quantity. According to the ICRP it is not a valid method for computing the potential number of deaths from cancer.

- The radiation dosimetry quantity, TEDE, is designed to take into account all possible sources of radiation exposure and is used for dose monitoring for occupationally exposed personnel who are likely to receive possibly significant radiation exposure during the course of a year. The whole-body TEDE regulatory limit for exposed personnel is 0.05 sievert and 0.001 sievert for the general public.
- The CEDE in radiation protection is the total effective dose to an individual resulting from an intake of radioactive material into the body. Such material may remain in the body for some time, resulting in a dose that accumulates over time.

GENERAL DISCUSSION QUESTIONS

1. How did early discoveries in radiobiology and radiation impact the development of safety guidelines and standards for radiation exposure in the medical field?
2. In the early 20th century, how did the unfortunate incidents involving individuals like Clarence Madison Dally shape the approach towards occupational radiation exposure, leading to the discontinuation of Thomas Edison's x-ray research?
3. What challenges did the British X-Ray and Radium Protection Committee face in formulating guidelines for radium and x-ray equipment, and how did the lack of accurate measurement techniques hinder their efforts?
4. How did the concept of tolerance dose evolve over time, and why was it eventually replaced by the maximum permissible dose (MPD) in radiation protection?
5. What factors contributed to the adoption of SI units in radiation measurement, and how did this transition impact the field of radiology, particularly in the United States?
6. In the mid-20th century, how did the recognition of late tissue reactions and stochastic effects influence the establishment of dose limits for radiation workers, and what role did the International X-Ray and Radium Protection Commission play in this process?
7. What were the key reasons behind revisiting and redefining the roentgen in 1962, and how did this contribute to the evolution of radiation measurement standards?
8. How did the development of the International System of Units (SI) in 1948 contribute to the international unification of metric units in radiation dosimetry and measurement?
9. Explore the rationale behind replacing the tolerance dose with the concept of the maximum permissible dose (MPD) in the 1950s, and how did this shift impact the understanding of radiation safety?
10. In the 1980s, what challenges and benefits were associated with the adoption of SI units in radiation protection, and how did this impact the coexistence of traditional units in dosimetry reports and regulatory criteria?

REVIEW QUESTIONS

1. What was the primary reason for the creation of the British X-Ray and Radium Protection Committee in 1921?
   A. To develop new X-ray technologies
   B. To investigate methods for reducing radiation exposure
   C. To promote the use of radium in medical treatments
   D. To establish guidelines for manufacturing X-ray equipment
2. What unit of measurement was in place for quantifying radiation exposure during 1900–1930?
   A. Gray (Gy)
   B. Skin erythema dose
   C. Roentgen
   D. Sievert (Sv)

3. In the 1930s, what was the principal guideline for occupational radiation exposure tolerance levels?
   A. Sievert (Sv)
   B. Gray (Gy)
   C. Roentgen (R)
   D. Rem

4. What concept replaced the tolerance dose in the early 1950s for radiation protection purposes?
   A. Gray (Gy)
   B. Roentgen (R)
   C. Tolerance Equivalent Dose (TED)
   D. Maximum Permissible Dose (MPD)

5. When did the International Commission on Radiation Units and Measurements (ICRU) adopt SI units for ionizing radiation?
   A. 1925
   B. 1948
   C. 1962
   D. 1980

6. What was introduced as the unit to express radiation exposure in the SI system?
   A. Coulomb per kilogram (C/kg)
   B. Roentgen (R)
   C. Gray (Gy)
   D. Rem

7. Which term represents the product of the average absorbed dose and the radiation weighting factor?
   A. Equivalent dose (EqD)
   B. Effective dose (EfD)
   C. Air kerma
   D. Exposure (X)

8. What is the primary purpose of the tissue weighting factor (W_T) in radiation protection?
   A. To measure exposure in air
   B. To calculate effective dose (EfD)
   C. To convert traditional units to SI units
   D. To determine air kerma values

9. Which dosimetric quantity attempts to describe the radiation exposure of a population from various sources?
   A. Equivalent dose (EqD)
   B. Total Effective Dose Equivalent (TEDE)
   C. Collective Effective Dose (ColEfD)
   D. Air kerma

10. What is the purpose of the Total Effective Dose Equivalent (TEDE)?
    A. To monitor external radiation exposure only
    B. To measure absorbed dose in tissues
    C. To account for all possible sources of radiation exposure
    D. To calculate radiation weighting factors

Overview of Cell Biology

OBJECTIVES

After completing this chapter, the reader will be able to perform the following:

- Define all key terms.
- State the purpose for acquiring a basic knowledge of cell structure, composition, and cell function as a foundation for understanding the effects of radiation in biology.
- Identify and describe some important roles of the major classes of organic and inorganic compounds that exist in the cell.
- List the essential tasks of water in the human body.
- Name and describe a landmark event pertaining to the human genome that occurred in 2001, and explain the progress that has been made since then as a result of this project.
- Describe the molecular structure of deoxyribonucleic acid, and explain the way it operates in the cell.
- Describe the structural differences between DNA and RNA.
- List the various cellular components, and identify their physical characteristics and functions.
- Distinguish between the two types of cell divisions, mitosis and meiosis, and describe each process.

CHAPTER OUTLINE

KEY TERMS

amino acids
anaphase
carbohydrates
cell division
cell membrane
centrosome
chromosomes
cytoplasm
cytoplasmic organelles
deoxyribonucleic acid (DNA)

endoplasmic reticulum (ER)
genes
human genome
inorganic compounds
interphase
lipids
meiosis
messenger RNA (mRNA)
metaphase
mitochondria

mitosis (M)
nucleic acids
nucleus
organic compounds
osmosis
oxidation
prophase
proteins
protein synthesis
protoplasm

Biology is a science that explores living things and life processes. Cells are the basic units of all living matter. The cell is the fundamental element of structure, development, growth, and life processes in the human body. Before imaging professionals can comprehend the effects of ionizing radiation on the human body, they must acquire a basic knowledge of how cells are assembled, what they are made of, and how they operate. This chapter is designed to provide an understanding of cellular biology, which ultimately will help the learner appreciate the effects of radiation in the body.

THE CELL

The human body is composed of trillions of cells. These cells exist in a multitude of different forms and perform many diverse functions for the body, such as the following:

- Conduction of nerve impulses
- Contraction of muscles
- Support of various organs
- Transportation of body fluids, such as blood

Some cells are freely moving, independent units (e.g., leukocytes), whereas others remain in one position as part of the tissues of larger organisms throughout their lifetimes (e.g., bone marrow cells). Every mature human cell is highly specialized and has predetermined tasks to perform in support of the body.

Cells:

- Move
- Grow
- React
- Protect themselves
- Repair damage
- Regulate life processes
- Reproduce

To ensure efficient cell operation, the body must have food as a source of raw material for the release of energy, be supplied with oxygen to help break down the food, and have enough water to transport inorganic substances such as calcium and sodium into and out of the cell. In turn, proper cell function enables the body as a whole to maintain homeostasis or equilibrium, which is the ability to operate in a normal manner despite any changes the body may undergo due to outside influences, such as stress, exercise, injury, or disease.

In summary, cells are engaged in an ongoing process of obtaining energy and converting it to support their vital functions. Cells absorb molecular nutrients through the cell membrane and use these nutrients to produce energy and synthesize molecules. If exposure to outside influences, such as ionizing radiation, damages the components involved in molecular synthesis beyond repair, then cells either behave abnormally or die.

CELL CHEMICAL COMPOSITION

Protoplasm

Cells are made of **protoplasm**, the living contents of a cell surrounded by a plasma membrane. The *protoplasm is the chemical building material for all living things*. This substance carries on the:

- Complex process of metabolism
- Reception and processing of food and oxygen
- Elimination of waste products

Metabolism enables the cell to synthesize proteins and produce energy. Protoplasm, which includes both small and very large molecules, called macromolecules, consists of:

- Organic compounds (those compounds that contain carbon, hydrogen, and oxygen)
- Inorganic materials (compounds that do not contain carbon)

These are either dissolved or suspended in water.

The biomolecules that constitute protoplasm are formed from many elements, among which there are four primary components:

- Carbon
- Hydrogen
- Oxygen
- Nitrogen

When combined with phosphorus and sulfur, they comprise the essential major *organic* compounds:

- Proteins
- Carbohydrates

- Lipids
- Nucleic acids
  These compounds are discussed later in this chapter. The most important *inorganic* substances are:
- Water
- Mineral salts (electrolytes)

Water plays a fundamental role in sustaining life and is the most abundant inorganic compound in the body. The essential functions of water are listed in Box 5.1 and are also discussed later in this chapter. Depending on cell type, water normally accounts for 80% to 85% of protoplasm (Fig. 5.1). Mineral salts exist in smaller quantities but are of vital importance in sustaining cell life because they help produce energy and aid in the conduction of nerve impulses.

BOX 5.1   Life-Sustaining Role of Water in the Human Body

- Acts as the medium in which acids, bases, and salts are dissolved
- Functions as a solvent by dissolving chemical substances in the cell
- Functions as a transport vehicle for material the cell uses or eliminates
- Maintains a constant body core temperature of 98.6°F (37°C)
- Provides a cushion for vital organs, such as the brain and lungs
- Regulates concentration of dissolved substances
- Lubricates the digestive system
- Lubricates skeletal articulations (joints)

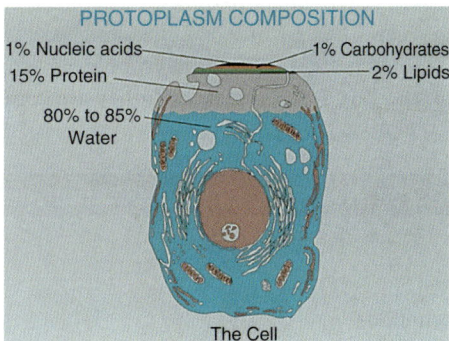

PROTOPLASM COMPOSITION

1% Nucleic acids
15% Protein
1% Carbohydrates
2% Lipids
80% to 85% Water

The Cell

Fig. 5.1 Depending on cell type, water normally accounts for 80% to 85% of protoplasm. (From *Radiobiology and radiation protection: Mosby's radiographic instructional series*, St. Louis, 1999, Elsevier.)

Mineral salts are also instrumental in the prevention of muscle cramping.

Organic Compounds

The four major classes of **organic compounds** (proteins, carbohydrates, lipids [fats], and nucleic acids) all contain carbon as a fundamental constituent (Box 5.2). By combining with:

- Hydrogen
- Nitrogen
- Oxygen

carbon makes life possible. Of the four classes of organic compounds, proteins contain the most carbon.

Proteins. **Proteins** are the most elementary building blocks of cells, and they make up approximately 15% of cell content (see Fig. 5.1). Proteins are essential for growth, the construction of new body tissue (including acellular tissue such as hair and nails), and the repair of injured or debilitated tissue. Proteins are formed when organic compounds called **amino acids** combine into long, chainlike molecular complexes. Amino acids are essentially composed of combinations of NH_2 (called *amine*) and COOH (carboxyl group) molecules. Thus nitrogen, hydrogen, carbon, and oxygen are the key constituents of amino acids, of which approximately 500 different types are currently known, although humans require only 22 specific amino acids. To summarize, proteins are macromolecules made up of strings of amino acids. When proteins are produced within a cell, a process known as **protein synthesis**, the order of arrangement of amino acids, determines the precise function of each protein molecule, and the types of proteins that any given cell contains determine the characteristics, or genetics, of that cell. Key components of genetic material, called *chromosomes* and *genes*, which organize the amino acids into different orderings to make different types of proteins, are discussed later in this chapter (Fig. 5.2).

Structural and enzymatic proteins. Structural proteins, such as those found in muscle, provide the body with its shape and form and are a source of heat and

BOX 5.2   Major Classes of Organic Compounds That Compose the Cell

Proteins	Lipids (fats)
Carbohydrates	Nucleic acid

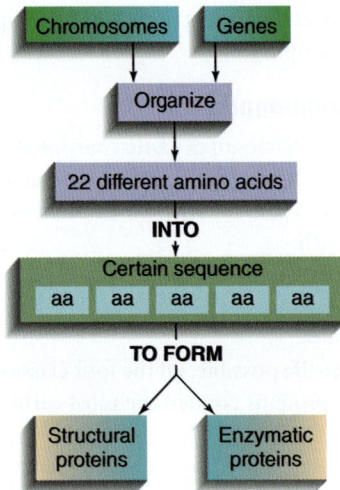

Fig. 5.2 Chromosomes and genes organize the 22 different amino acids into certain sequences to form the different structural and enzymatic proteins.

energy. Enzymatic proteins function as organic catalysts, that is, agents that affect the rate or speed of chemical reactions without being altered themselves. As a result of this, enzymatic proteins (commonly called *enzymes*) moderate or control the cell's various physiologic activities. Among other tasks, enzymes can cause an increase in cellular activity that in turn causes biochemical reactions to occur more rapidly to meet the needs of the cell in stressful situations. In general, proper cell functioning depends heavily on enzymes.

Repair enzymes. Many of the proteins produced in the cell, by necessity, are enzymes, initiating vital chemical reactions within the cell at the appropriate time. Some of the enzymes produced, called *repair enzymes,* can also mend damaged molecules and are therefore capable of helping the cell recover from a small amount of radiation-induced damage. Both the catalytic (i.e., reaction facilitator) and repair capabilities of enzymes are of vital importance to the survival of the cell.

Repair enzymes work effectively in radiation induced cell injury associated with both diagnostic and therapeutic radiation energy ranges. However, if the radiation damage is excessive because of a large delivered equivalent dose, the cellular harm will be too severe for repair enzymes to have enough positive effect. Thus, when ionizing radiation is used for therapeutic purposes to destroy malignant cells, a very significant effort using the latest advances in imaging and treatment planning

algorithms is always made to minimize the absorbed dose to healthy surrounding tissue. In radiation therapy, this concept is referred to as a *therapeutic ratio,* wherein the intent is to deliver enough radiation to kill cancerous cells in a tumor (i.e., damage them sufficiently so that they are irreparable) while delivering a much less-than-cell-killing equivalent dose to any surrounding noncancerous tissue structure. This concept is the foundation on which successful radiation therapy rests.

Hormones and antibodies. In addition to providing structure and support for the body, proteins may function as hormones and antibodies. Hormones are chemical secretions manufactured by various endocrine glands (i.e., organs that secrete substances into the blood stream) and carried by the bloodstream to influence the activities of other parts of the body. For example, hormones produced by the thyroid gland located in the neck control metabolism throughout the body. Hormones also regulate body functions, such as growth and development.

Antibodies are protein molecules created by specialized cells in the bone marrow called *B lymphocytes.* Lymphocytes are white blood cells involved in the body's immune reactions. Antibodies are produced when other lymphocytes in the body, known as *T lymphocytes,* detect the presence of molecules that do not belong to the body. These foreign objects (e.g., bacteria, flu viruses) are called *antigens.* Although the skin of the body is the initial barrier to any outside invasion by pathogens or the like, once it has been penetrated, the body's primary defense mechanism against infection and disease are the antibodies that chemically attack any foreign invaders.

Carbohydrates. Carbohydrates, also referred to as saccharides, make up approximately 1% of cell content (see Fig. 5.1). They include starches and various sugars. Carbohydrates range from simple to complex compounds (Box 5.3), even though they are composed

---

BOX 5.3   Simple to Complex Carbohydrates

Monosaccharides
$C_6H_{12}O_6$

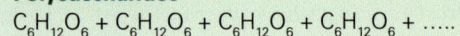

Disaccharides
$C_6H_{12}O_6 + C_6H_{12}O_6$

Polysaccharides
$C_6H_{12}O_6 + C_6H_{12}O_6 + C_6H_{12}O_6 + C_6H_{12}O_6 + \ldots$

of only carbon, hydrogen, and oxygen. Simple sugars such as glucose, fructose, and galactose, have six carbon atoms and six molecules of water (e.g., glucose has the chemical formula $C_6H_{12}O_6$). Glucose is the primary energy source for the cell. Because it is a simple sugar, it is called a *monosaccharide*. Other sugars that have two units of a simple sugar linked together are called *disaccharides*. Sucrose (cane sugar) and lactose are examples of disaccharides. Both monosaccharides and disaccharides are relatively small molecules. *Polysaccharides* contain several or many molecules of simple sugar. Plant starches and animal glycogen* are the two most important polysaccharides. Through the process of metabolism, the body breaks these down into simpler sugars for energy.

Carbohydrates, simply described as chains of sugar molecules, function as short-term energy warehouses for the body. Their primary purpose is to provide fuel for cell metabolism. Although carbohydrates are found throughout the human body, they are most abundant in the liver and in muscle tissue. They also are important structural parts of intercellular materials.

Lipids. Lipids can simply be defined as substances such as fats and fatty acids, oil, or wax that dissolve in alcohol but not in water. Lipids are organic macromolecules, in general containing carbon, hydrogen, and oxygen. In their simplest form, they are made up of a molecule of glycerin† and three molecules of fatty acid** (Box 5.4). Lipids are *the structural parts of cell membranes*, constituting approximately 2% of cell content (see Fig. 5.1). Therefore, lipids are present in all body tissue. The functions they perform for the body are listed in Box 5.5.

> ### BOX 5.4   Lipid Formation
>
> Fats or lipids
> ↑
> 1 molecule of glycerin + 3 molecules of fatty acid
> ↑
> Carbon, oxygen, hydrogen

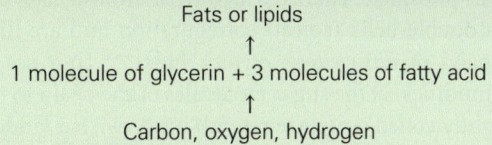

> ### BOX 5.5   Functions That Lipids Perform for the Body
>
> 1. Act as reservoirs for the long-term storage of energy
> 2. Insulate and guard the body against the environment
> 3. Support and protect organs such as the eyes and kidneys
> 4. Provide essential substances necessary for growth and development
> 5. Lubricate the joints
> 6. Assist in the digestive process

Nucleic Acids. Nucleic acids are complex macromolecules comprising approximately 1% of the cell (see Fig. 5.1). The much smaller structures that are the building blocks of nucleic acids are called *nucleotides*. Each nucleotide is a unit formed from a nitrogen-containing *organic base*,* a five-carbon sugar molecule (deoxyribose), and a *phosphate molecule*.**

Deoxyribonucleic and ribonucleic acids. Cells contain two types of nucleic acids that *are of primary importance* to all life:

- Deoxyribonucleic acid (DNA)
- Ribonucleic acid (RNA)

---

*Glycogen, also known as animal glycogen, is a polysaccharide that is the main storage form for glucose in both animals and humans. In humans, it is mainly concentrated in the liver, comprising about 10% of the liver mass.
†Glycerin is a clear, odorless, syrupy liquid that is a simple sugar and alcohol compound. It has the chemical formula C3H8O3.
**When glucose is broken down in the body during respiration, fats are among the generated intermediate products. When a fat combines with an acidic group of atoms (e.g., the carboxyl group, COOH), a fatty acid is formed. An example of a fatty acid is CH_3COOH, which is commonly known as *acetic acid*. Fatty acids are constituents of amino acids from which proteins are built.

*In general, a base is a substance that, among other characteristics, is slippery to the touch in aqueous solutions, tends to accept protons (i.e., ionized hydrogen atoms) from any proton donor, and reacts with acids to neutralize them, forming salts in the process. If the base contains one or more carbon and hydrogen bonded components, it may be classified as an organic base.
**A phosphate molecule has the chemical description *PO4* and therefore consists of one phosphorus atom bonded to four oxygen atoms. It is a negative ion carrying a charge of −3 produced by the dissolution of phosphoric acid H3PO4. Excluding the phosphate molecule, Fig. 5.3 displays the molecular structure of the sugars and the organic bases. The latter are divided into two categories called *purines* and *pyrimidines*.

The DNA macromolecule is composed of two long sugar–phosphate chains, which twist around each other in a double-helix (spiral) configuration and are linked by pairs of *nitrogenous organic bases**** (purines and pyrimidines) at the sugar molecules of the chain to form a tightly coiled structure resembling a twisted ladder or spiral staircase. The sugar–phosphate compounds are the rails, and the pairs of nitrogenous bases, which consist of complementary chemicals, are the steps, or rungs, of the DNA ladder-like structure (Fig. 5.3). Hydrogen bonds attach the bases to each other and join the two side rails of the DNA ladder.

Nitrogenous organic bases in DNA. The four nitrogenous organic bases (Fig. 5.4) in DNA macromolecules are as follows:

- Adenine (A)
- Cytosine (C)
- Guanine (G)
- Thymine (T)

Adenine and guanine are *purines,* and the compounds cytosine and thymine are classified as *pyrimidines.* As can be seen in the figure, a primary difference between the two classes of compounds is the number of carbon–nitrogen rings, with purines always having two rings and pyrimidines only one. A unique characteristic of these organic bases in DNA is that purines link with pyrimidines only in *certain specific combinations*; more precisely, adenine always bonds only with thymine, and cytosine bonds only with guanine. This property is the reason the two strands of DNA are described as complementary.

DNA: The master chemical substance. DNA, which is a very large conglomeration of complex molecules, is regarded as the master chemical substance because it contains all of the information a cell needs to function. DNA carries the genetic information necessary for cell replication and regulates all cellular activity needed to direct protein synthesis. DNA establishes an individual's personal characteristics by *regulating the ordering of amino acids* in the person's constituent proteins

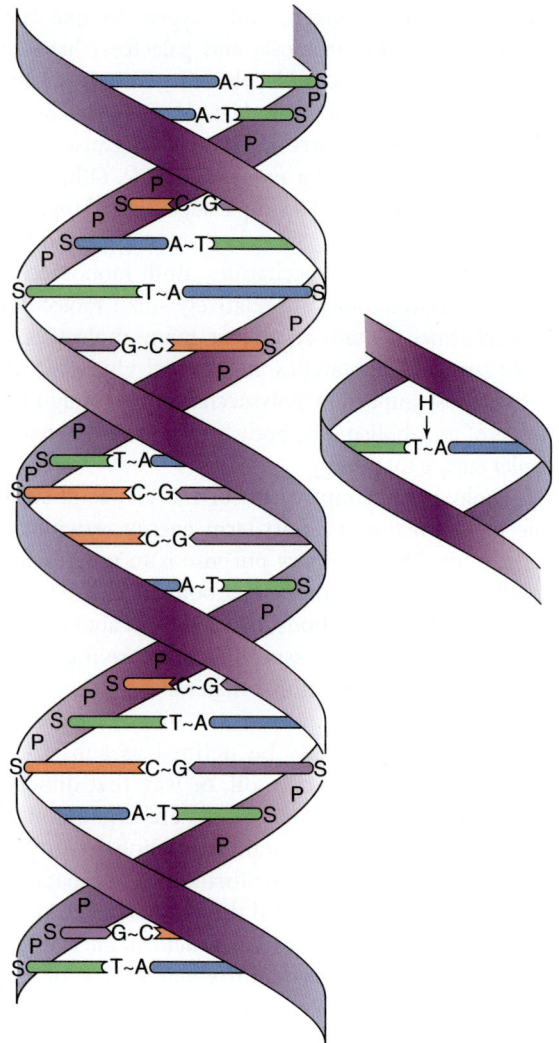

Fig. 5.3 Diagram of a DNA macromolecule that illustrates its twisted ladder-like or spiral staircase–like configuration. Alternating sugar and phosphate molecules form the side rails of the ladder, and the nitrogenous organic bases, which consist of the complementary chemicals adenine (A), thymine (T), guanine (G), and cytosine (C), form the rungs, or steps. A hydrogen bond joins the bases together.

***If an organic base is covalently bonded (i.e., a chemical union formed when electrons are shared between two atoms wherein each atom typically contributes one electron to form a pair of electrons that are shared by both atoms) to one or more nitrogen atoms, this chemical combination is called a *nitrogenous base.* A nitrogenous base may also contain oxygen atoms that form bonds with carbon.

during the synthesis of these proteins. These arrangements of amino acids are determined by the succession of adenine–thymine and cytosine–guanine base pairs in the DNA macromolecules. Therefore the sequence of nitrogenous base pairs in the DNA molecule constitutes a genetic code. Different sequences of amino acids produce proteins with different functions. Protein characteristics determine cell characteristics, and cell

SUGARS

D-ribose   D-2-deoxyribose

PURINES

Adenine (A)   Guanine (G)

PYRIMIDINES

Cytosine (C)   Thymine (T)

Uracil (U)

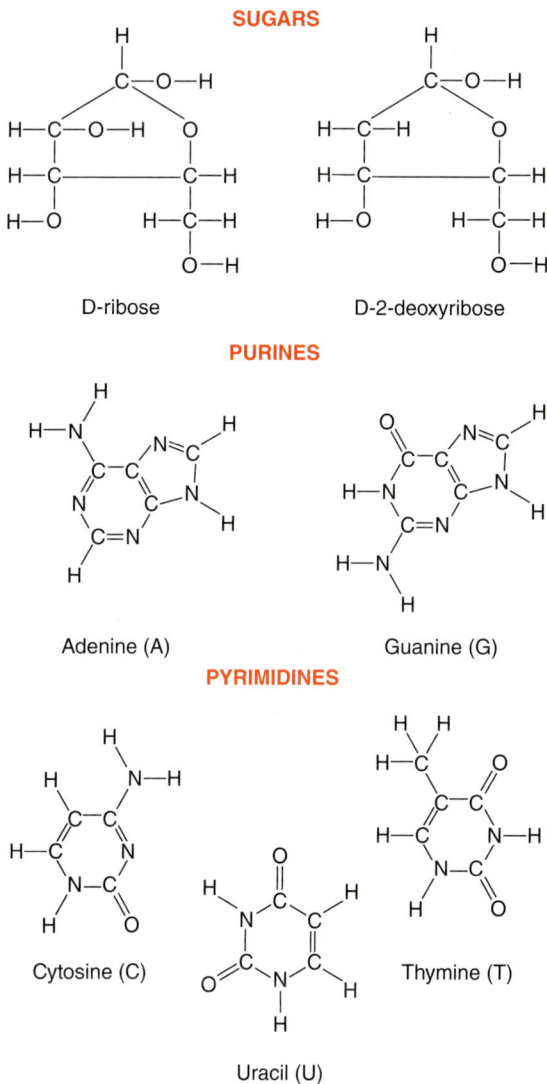

Fig. 5.4 The components of nucleic acid (H, hydrogen; C, carbon; N, nitrogen; O, oxygen). Sugars are strung together with phosphate groups, and a base is attached to each sugar. DNA uses d-2-deoxyribose sugar, and RNA uses d-ribose. Both nucleic acids use the same two purines, but thymine (T) in DNA is replaced by uracil (U) in RNA.

characteristics ultimately determine the characteristics of the entire individual. All of the information necessary to construct and maintain a living organism is written in the "genetic code book" of DNA—*the letters, words, and sentences are the arrangements and groupings of the nitrogenous organic bases.* Why is one person's DNA different from another's? Small differences in base pair

layouts are responsible for variations in human beings because such slightly altered base pair configurations lead to changes in the proteins produced, how much are produced, and when they are produced.

Structural differences between DNA and RNA. RNA is a long, single-stranded chain of cells that processes protein. The nucleic acid polymer (a macromolecule containing many repeated subunits) RNA plays an essential part in the translation of genetic information from DNA into protein products. To do this, RNA functions as a messenger between DNA and the ribosomes, or "protein factories," where synthesis occurs. RNA differs structurally from DNA in several ways, some of which are as follows:

- RNA is a single-strand macromolecular structure, whereas DNA is a double-strand macromolecular structure. Both have spiral ladder-like arrangements of their bases.
- RNA contains ribose,* whereas DNA contains deoxyribose.*
- RNA has the nitrogenous base uracil (see Fig. 5.4) as a component of its ladder steps, whereas DNA has thymine instead in its ladder steps. Both also contain the bases adenine, guanine, and cytosine as elements of their spiral structure. Unlike with DNA, where thymine forms a bond with adenine, for RNA, uracil links with an adenine base.
- RNA performs many different biologic functions (e.g., acts as an enzyme), but DNA carries the genetic information.
- RNA has a much shorter chain of nucleotides than DNA.

Messenger RNA. Because DNA is found mostly in the cell nucleus, it cannot directly influence cellular activity such as growth and differentiation, which occur in the cytoplasm (the part of the cell that lies outside the nucleus). Instead, DNA regulates cellular activity indirectly, transmitting its genetic information outside the cell nucleus by reproducing itself in the form of messenger RNA (mRNA), which is able to leave the cell nucleus. Once in the cytoplasm, mRNA directs the process of making proteins from amino acids.

*Ribose is an organic compound classified as a simple sugar. Chemically, ribose is made up of a bonded pentagon-shaped arrangement of 5 carbon atoms, 10 hydrogen atoms, and 5 oxygen atoms. If a ribose molecule should lose one of its oxygen atoms, it is called *deoxyribose*.

DNA serves as a prototype for mRNA, but mRNA differs from DNA in two important ways:

1. mRNA contains in its backbone the sugar molecule, ribose, which differs only in the presence of an extra O–H bond from the sugar molecule, deoxyribose, found in the backbone or side rails of DNA (see Fig. 5.3).
2. In mRNA, the pyrimidine base *uracil* (U) replaces the thymine that is found in DNA (Fig. 5.5).

An mRNA macromolecule, as does any type of RNA, resembles one half of a DNA macromolecule. RNA therefore appears as a single strand of the DNA ladder-like configuration, with the ladder being severed in half lengthwise (see Fig. 5.5).

Transfer RNA. Macromolecules of mRNA carry their genetic codes in their sequences of nitrogenous organic bases (e.g., U, U, C, C, A, U, G, etc.) from the cell nucleus to the *ribosomes.** Proteins are manufactured in the ribosomes. Within the ribosome, both mRNA and **transfer RNA (tRNA)** macromolecules are present. The mRNA delivers its genetic code to tRNA. This encoded tRNA combines with individual amino acids from different areas of the cell and attaches them to the ribosomes, where the amino acids are subsequently arranged in specific orders to form chainlike protein molecules. Each tRNA molecule is specifically coded for a particular amino acid. Because each of the 22 different amino acids has an associated tRNA, at least 22 different types of tRNAs exist. The ribosomes travel along the mRNA and link tRNA and its corresponding amino acids in the correct order so that the proteins necessary to provide for the needs of the cell are produced (Fig. 5.6).

Ribosomal RNA. **Ribosomal RNA (rRNA)** is yet another type of RNA. Ribosomal RNA's function is to assist in the linking of mRNA to the ribosome to facilitate protein synthesis.

Chromosomes and genes. **Chromosomes** are tiny, rod-shaped bodies that under a microscope appear to be long, threadlike structures that become visible only in dividing cells (Fig. 5.7). Chromosomes are composed of:

- Protein
- The genetic material DNA

---

*Ribosomes: small, spherical organelles (subunits of a cell that perform a specific function) that are the assembly sites (similar to an auto assembly line) where mRNA and tRNA combine amino acids into proteins. A further discussion of ribosomes is provided later in this chapter.

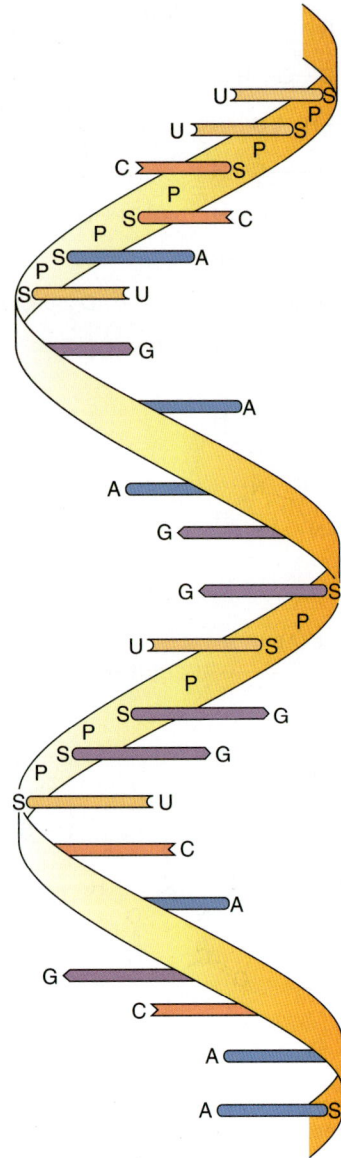

Fig. 5.5 Messenger RNA (mRNA) resembles one half of a DNA macromolecule. It appears as a single strand (one side rail) of the DNA ladder-like configuration, with the ladder being severed in half lengthwise. Uracil (U) replaces thymine (T) as one of the nitrogenous organic bases in the mRNA molecule.

A normal human being has 46 different chromosomes composed of *23 pairs* in each somatic (nonreproductive) cell. Individual male and female reproductive cells, also known as *germ cells,* do not have this pairing. Instead, each of these germ cells has only 23 chromosomes, which pair up to form a full set of 46 chromosomes

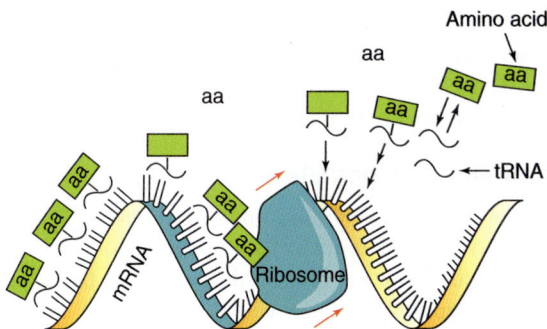

Fig. 5.6 Ribosomes, the cell's protein factories, travel along the messenger RNA (mRNA) rails, linking transfer RNA (tRNA) and its corresponding amino acids in the proper sequences to produce the proteins appropriate for the needs of the cell.

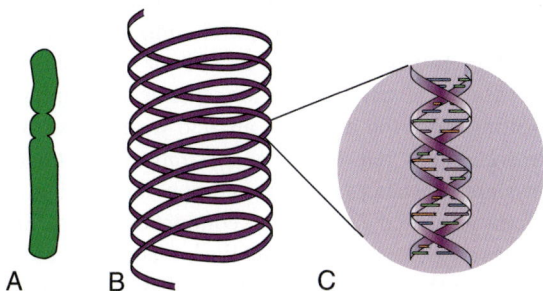

Fig. 5.7 (A) A chromosome viewed under a microscope appears rod shaped; (B) when further magnified, a chromosome appears as a tightly wound spiral structure composed of hundreds of genes—(C) a segment of the DNA macromolecule.

when a sperm cell fertilizes an egg cell. The DNA that makes up every chromosome is divided into many hundreds of segments or subunits called **genes**. Each gene, because of the ordering of its nitrogenous base pairs, contains information responsible for or related to one or more of the following:

- Directing cytoplasmic activities
- Controlling growth and development of the cell
- Transmitting various aspects of hereditary information (e.g., hair color, blood type, general body characteristics, etc.)

Thus, genes are the *basic units of heredity*. Taken as a whole, they control the formation of proteins in every cell through the intricate process of parentally shared genetic coding.

The human genome. The total amount of genetic material (DNA) contained within the chromosomes of a human being is called the **human genome**. The human

genome is the blueprint for each person's body. The process of locating and identifying the genes in the genome is called *mapping*. A landmark event occurred in 2001, when after years of intense effort two rival groups succeeded in deciphering the human genome.[1] Essentially, they uncovered the entire sequence of DNA base pairs (i.e., all of the "rungs" of the DNA ladder structure) on all 46 chromosomes. This major milestone in biology and medicine was accomplished by Celera Genomics, a private company in Rockville, Maryland, and the International Human Genome Sequencing Consortium, a group of academic centers funded mostly by the National Institutes of Health and the Wellcome Trust of London.[2]

The groups found that there are 2.9 billion base pairs in the human genome and that these base pairs are arranged into approximately 30,000 genes. It is estimated that these genes are capable of producing at least 90,000 different proteins.

According to the National Institutes of Health (2010), the Human Genome Project has already led to the discovery of more than 1800 disease genes. In addition, with the knowledge gained from the project, today's researchers can find a gene suspected of causing an inherited disease in a matter of days, rather than the years it took before the genome sequence was discovered. There are now more than 2000 genetic tests for human conditions. These tests enable patients to learn their genetic risks for disease and help health care professionals diagnose disease. As of 2013 at least 350 biotechnology-based products resulting from the Human Genome Project have been placed in clinical trials. Possessing the complete sequence of the human genome is similar to owning all the pages of a manual needed to create the human body. The challenge now is to determine how to read the contents of these pages and understand how all of these many complex parts function together in human health and disease.[3] The potential gain from this effort is to be able to eventually both predict a person's risk of disease and provide that person with specific drugs for targeting and stopping the disease.

Interpreting the map of the human genome is similar to that of a building contractor discovering a list of all the items that are needed to build a house but not a blueprint that demonstrates how often or in what order the steps should be performed. Presymptomatic testing, carrier screening, workplace genetic screening, and testing by insurance companies pose significant ethical issues. Second, the burgeoning ability to manipulate human genes raises a number of important ethical questions. Ethical, legal and social issues raised by genomic research include: possible discrimination by employers or health insurers, the need for ethical standards for work with human research subjects or tissues, and consideration of social, cultural and religious perspectives on genetics and health. Over the next few decades, the great tasks will be to answer questions such as the following:

1. What determines when genes will produce proteins and when genes will not?
2. In what order are various proteins produced during development and throughout life?
3. What genes cause some individuals to be susceptible to a certain disease?
4. Is it possible to learn how to deactivate those genes and turn on other genes that provide resistance?
5. Are there genes that make some people more or less sensitive to the effects of ionizing radiation?
6. Can the newly acquired insight into the human genome be used to both detect and properly correct the defective genes that are the root of genetically transmitted disease?

Gene therapy raises another group of challenging ethical issues. Gene therapy is an experimental technique that uses genes to treat or prevent disease. Bioethicists and researchers generally believe that human genome editing for *reproductive purposes* should not be attempted at this time, but that studies which would make gene therapy safe and effective should continue. Once the consent, safety, and scientific issues are resolved, there is probably nothing ethically unique about conducting somatic cell gene therapy or fetal gene therapy to correct genetic diseases. In the future, this technique may allow doctors to treat a disorder by inserting a gene into a patient's cells instead of using drugs or surgery. Researchers are at this time testing several approaches to gene therapy, including:

- Replacing a mutated gene that causes disease with a healthy copy of the gene.
- Inactivating, or "knocking out," a mutated gene that is functioning improperly.
- Introducing a new gene into the body to help fight a disease.

Although gene therapy is a promising treatment option for a number of diseases (including inherited disorders, some types of cancers, and certain viral infections), the technique remains risky and is still under study to make sure that it will be safe and effective. Gene therapy is currently being investigated only for diseases that have no other cures.[4]

Inorganic Compounds

Inorganic compounds are compounds that do not contain carbon. The inorganic compounds found in the body occur in nature independent of living things and are made up of three categories:

- Inorganic acids
- Inorganic bases
- Salts (electrolytes)

Inorganic acids are hydrogen-containing compounds such as HNO_3 (nitric acid) that can attack and dissolve metal. *Inorganic bases* are alkali or alkaline-earth (see Appendix D, first 2 columns) OH compounds such as $Mg(OH)_2$ (otherwise known as *milk of magnesia*) that can neutralize acids. *Salts* are chemical compounds resulting from the action of an acid with a base. Salts are sometimes referred to as *electrolytes*. Chemically, they "are substances that become ions in solution and thereby acquire the capacity to conduct electricity. Electrolytes are present throughout the human body, and the balance of the electrolytes in our bodies is essential for normal function of our cells and our organs."[5] A list of some of the important electrolytes in the body may be found in Box 5.6.

Water is the primary inorganic substance contained in the human body; it comprises approximately 80% to 85% of the body's weight (Fig. 5.8). If water content within a cell is too low, the cell will collapse, resulting in a lack of ability to continue normal biologic function. Conversely, if water content is excessive, the cell most likely will rupture. Therefore it is imperative that the correct amount of water in a cell be maintained.[6]

Function of Water Within and Outside of the Cell. Within the cell, water is indispensable for metabolic activities since it is the medium in which the chemical reactions

---

BOX 5.6   Some of the Important Electrolytes in the Body

Sodium (Na^+)	Chloride (Cl^-)
Potassium (K^+)	Bicarbonate (HCO_3^-)
Calcium (Ca^{++})	Phosphate (HPO_4^-)
Magnesium (Mg^{++})	Sulfate (SO_4^{-2})

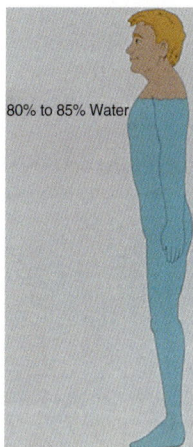

Fig. 5.8 Water constitutes approximately 80% to 85% of the body's weight. (From *Radiobiology and radiation protection: Mosby's radiographic instructional series,* St. Louis, 1999, Elsevier.)

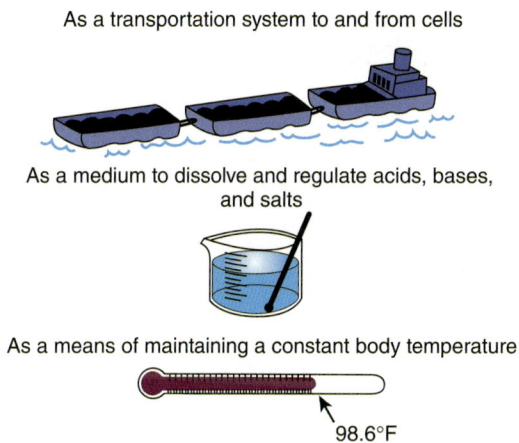

As a transportation system to and from cells

As a medium to dissolve and regulate acids, bases, and salts

As a means of maintaining a constant body temperature

98.6°F

Fig. 5.9 Water's role outside the cell. (From *Radiobiology and radiation protection: Mosby's radiographic instructional series,* St. Louis, 1999, Elsevier.)

that are the basis of these activities occur. Cellular water also acts as a solvent, keeping compounds dissolved so they can more easily interact and their concentration be regulated. Outside the cell, water functions as a transport vehicle for materials the cell uses or eliminates. In addition, water is responsible for maintaining a constant body core temperature of 98.6°F (37°C) (Fig. 5.9) while at the same time serving to lubricate both the digestive system and skeletal articulations (joints). Organs such as the brain and lungs are also protected by a cushion of compounds composed primarily of water.

Function of Mineral Salts Within the Cell. Salts resulting from acid/base reactions, predominantly involving sodium (Na) and/or potassium (K) (e.g., potassium chloride, sodium iodide, potassium nitrate, and the like) preserve the correct proportion of water in the cell. Because salts are inorganic (i.e., no carbon is present) and have a crystalline atomic structure, they are classified as *mineral salts*. Their presence is vital for:

- Proper cell performance
- Creation of energy
- Conduction of impulses along nerves

Within an aqueous solution, these salts can be broken down, with their constituents existing as ions (particles carrying either a positive or negative electric charge) in the cell. The resulting medium is called a *solute*. The ions within the solute, via chemical reactions, cause materials to be altered, fragmented, and recombined to form new substances. Potassium (K) contributes most of the positive ions (K^+ also known as *cations*) present in cells, whereas phosphorus (P^-) contributes the majority of negative ions (*anions*). Potassium is of primary importance in maintaining adequate amounts of intracellular fluid. This is because water, a solvent, will preferentially move across cell surfaces or membranes into areas with a high concentration of ions, also known as *high solute regions*. This motion is referred to as **osmosis**. Thus, by controlling its concentration of potassium ions (as well as the ever-present sodium [Na] and chloride [Cl] ions resulting from the intake of table salt), the cell regulates the amount of water passing through its membrane and consequently the amount of fluid it contains. Osmotic pressure is the external pressure required to be applied so that there is no net movement of solvent, typically water, across the cell membrane. Retaining the correct proportion of water in the cell causes osmotic pressure to be maintained. Potassium also aids in maintaining acid–base balance, a state of equilibrium, or stability, between acids and bases.

CELL STRUCTURE

The normal cell has the following components (Fig. 5.10):
1. Cell membrane
2. Cytoplasm
3. Cytoplasmic organelles (organelles are subcellular structures)
   a. Endoplasmic reticulum
   b. Golgi apparatus or complex

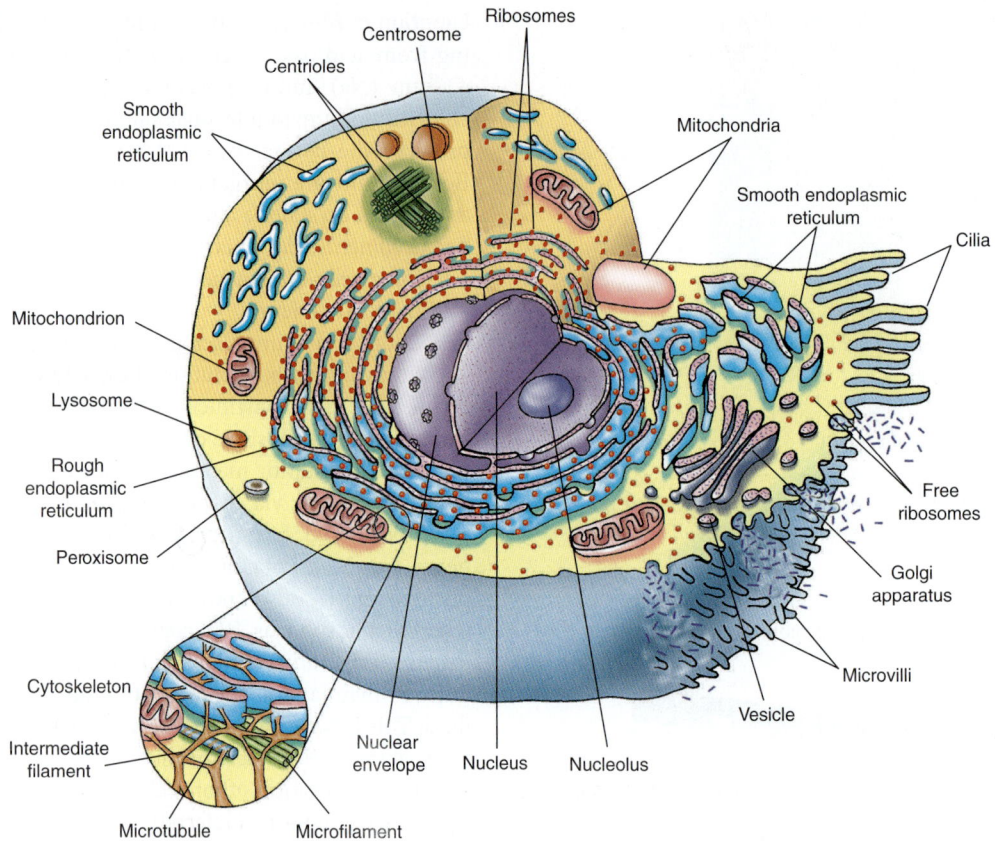

Fig. 5.10 Diagram of a typical cell, demonstrating its basic components. (From Thibodeau A: *Anatomy and physiology*, ed 9, St. Louis, 2016, Elsevier.)

c. Mitochondria
d. Lysosomes
e. Ribosomes
f. Centrosomes
4. Nucleus

Cell Membrane—a "Plastic Storage Bag" to Contain the Cell

The **cell membrane** is a frail, semipermeable, flexible structure encasing and surrounding the human cell. The cell membrane, shown in blue in Fig. 5.10:

- Is made of lipids and proteins.
- Functions as a barricade to protect cellular contents from the outside environment.
- Controls the passage of water and other materials into and out of the cell.

Because the cell membrane allows penetration only by certain types of substances and regulates the speed at which these substances travel within the cell, it plays a primary role in the cell's transport system. When a substance moves through the cell membrane by osmosis, the transport system is classified as passive because the cell uses no energy to maintain the concentration. When the movement of a substance across a cell membrane is controlled more by the properties and powers of the cell membrane than it is by the relative concentrations of particles in fluid, the transport system is classified as active. In *active transport*, the cell must expend energy to pump substances into and out of it.

Cytoplasm

Cytoplasm is the protoplasm that exists outside the cell's nucleus and is primarily composed of water, but also contains:

- Proteins
- Carbohydrates

- Lipids
- Salts
- Minerals

Cytoplasm comprises the majority of the cell and contains large amounts of the cell's molecular components, with the exception of DNA. All cellular metabolic functions occur in the cytoplasm. The major functions of the cytoplasm are listed in Box 5.7.

Cytoplasmic Organelles

The cytoplasm contains all the miniature cellular components that enable the cell to function in a highly organized manner. These small organs of the cell are collectively referred to as **cytoplasmic organelles**, which consist of the following:

- Tubules (small tubes)
- Vesicles (small cavities or sacs containing liquid)
- Granules (small insoluble, nonmembranous particles found in cytoplasm)
- Fibrils (minute fibers or strands that are frequently part of a compound fiber)

Together these structures perform the major functions of the cell in a systematized manner. DNA, which is located in the cell nucleus, separated from the cytoplasm, determines the function of each cytoplasmic organelle; mRNA carries the DNA code from the nucleus into the cytoplasm.

Endoplasmic Reticulum—the "Highway" of the Cell.

The **endoplasmic reticulum (ER)** is a vast, irregular network of tubules and vesicles spreading and interconnecting in all directions throughout the cytoplasm. The ER enables the cell to communicate with the extracellular environment and transfer food and molecules from one part of the cell to another. Thus, it functions as the highway system of the cell. For example, mRNA travels from the nucleus to different locations in the cytoplasm through the ER, and lipids and proteins are also routed into and out of the nucleus through the ER tubular network.

Cells have two types of endoplasmic reticulum:

- Rough surfaced (granular)
- Smooth (agranular)

When numerous ribosomes (the sites where mRNA and tRNA assemble amino acids into proteins) are present on the surface of the ER, the surface is rough or granular. If they are not present, the surface is smooth or agranular. The "smooth" or "rough" distinction refers to the endoplasmic reticulum's appearance when viewed with an electron microscope. The cell type determines the type of ER. For example, cells that actively manufacture proteins for export, such as the pancreatic cells, which produce insulin, need more ribosomes and therefore have an extensive rough or granular endoplasmic reticulum. A lesser amount of rough or granular ER is found in cells that synthesize proteins mainly for their own use.

Golgi Apparatus or Complex—Hauls "Freight" Within and Out of the Cell.

The Golgi apparatus contains minute vesicles that extend from the nucleus to the cell membrane. The vesicles consist of tubes and a tiny sac located near the nucleus. This structure unites large carbohydrate molecules (i.e., various types of sugars) and then combines them with proteins, which are typically found floating in or around the membrane of cells, to form *glycoproteins*. Glycoproteins are involved in nearly every process in cells. Glycoproteins have diverse functions throughout the body within the immune system, in communication between cells, and in the reproductive systems. In addition, when the cell manufactures glycoproteins that function as enzymes and hormones, the Golgi apparatus concentrates, packages, and transports them through the cell membrane so they can exit the cell, enter the bloodstream, and be carried to the areas of the body where they are required.

Mitochondria—the "Power-Generating Station" of the Cell.

The large, double-membranous, oval or bean-shaped structures called **mitochondria** function as the "powerhouses" of the cell because they supply the energy for all cellular function. They contain highly organized enzymes in their inner membranes that produce this energy for cellular activity by breaking down nutrients such as:

- Carbohydrates
- Fats
- Proteins

This breakdown of nutrients occurs through the process of oxidative metabolism. **Oxidation** is any chemical reaction in which atoms lose electrons. The substance that loses electrons is said to have been oxidized, and chemical energy is released in the process. The oxidation of iron, for example, which occurs in a moist environment in the presence of oxygen, produces iron oxide (Fe_2O_3) commonly known as *rust*. In the case of rust, the iron atoms give up electrons to oxygen atoms, creating a bond between iron and oxygen.

Destructive metabolism (also known as *catabolism*) is the breaking down of large molecules (e.g., polysaccharides, lipids, proteins) into smaller molecules. Oxidative metabolism is the oxidation of these smaller molecules to release energy. Some of this energy is lost as heat, and the remainder is primarily used with the assistance of the enzymes contained within the mitochondria to produce the compound *adenosine triphosphate (ATP)*.* ATP is the prime energy-containing molecule in the cell. ATP is essential for sustaining life and performs a significant role in active transport within the cell. As mentioned previously, in active transport molecules are moved or pumped through cell membranes. This happens regardless of the relative concentrations of particles on either side of the membrane. This process will therefore often require energy. The needed energy is supplied by ATP. ATP functions by losing its endmost phosphate group (Fig. 5.11) when instructed to do so by enzymes. This reaction releases a large amount of energy, which the organism can then also use to build proteins, contract muscles, etc. When the organism is resting and energy is not immediately needed, the reverse reaction takes place

***

*The ATP molecule is composed of three molecular subgroups. At the center is a sugar molecule, ribose (the same sugar that forms the basis of RNA). Attached to one side of this is a base (a group consisting of linked rings of carbon and nitrogen atoms); in this case the base is adenine. The other side of the sugar is attached to a string or chain of phosphate groups. These phosphates are the key to the energy activity of ATP (see Fig. 5.11).

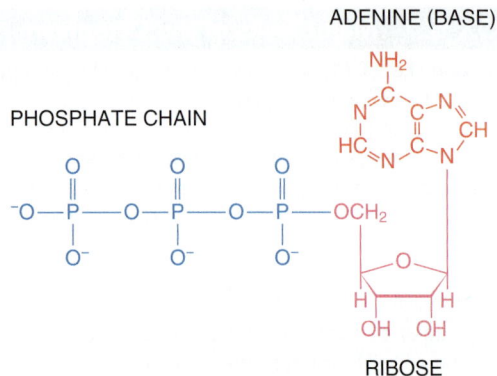

Fig. 5.11 Molecular structure of adenosine triphosphate (ATP).

and the phosphate group is reattached to the molecule, using energy obtained from food or sunlight. Thus, the ATP molecule acts as a chemical "battery," storing energy when it is not needed, but is able to release it instantly when the organism requires it. The number of mitochondria in cells varies from a few hundred to several thousand. The greatest number of mitochondria is found in cells exhibiting the greatest activity.

Lysosomes—"Garbage Bags" With "Poison Pills." Lysosomes are small, pea-like sacs or single-membrane spherical bodies that are of great importance for digestion within the cytoplasm. Lysosomes contain a group of different *digestive enzymes* that target proteins, and their primary function appears to be the breaking down of unwanted large molecules that either penetrate into the cell through microscopic channels or are drawn in by the cell membrane itself. If lysosomes fail in their cellular "garbage disposal" tasks, the resulting accumulation of large molecules can ultimately obstruct normal functions in organs. Lysosomes are sometimes referred to as *suicide bags*, because their enzymes break down and digest not only proteins and certain carbohydrates, but also will do the same to the cell itself should the lysosome's surrounding membrane rupture. Exposure to radiation may induce such a rupture. When this occurs, the cell is likely to die.

Ribosomes—"Manufacturing Facilities" of the Cell. **Ribosomes** are very small, spherical organelles that attach to the endoplasmic reticulum. They consist of:

- Two-thirds RNA
- One-third protein

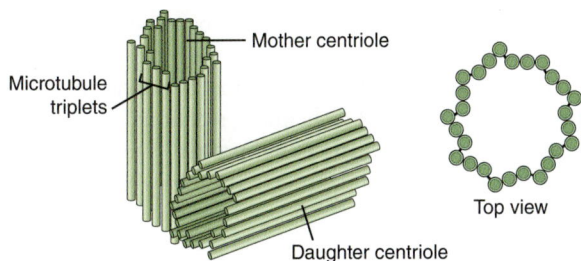

Fig. 5.12 Centriole configuration. The centrioles are cylindrical-shaped cellular organelles that occur in pairs. Each centriole is made up of groups of microtubules that are arranged in a pattern, forming a ring of nine trio microtubules known as *triplets*. As shown, the centrioles are arranged at right angles to one another. In human cells, the centrioles facilitate the organizing and assembly of microtubules during the process of cell division.

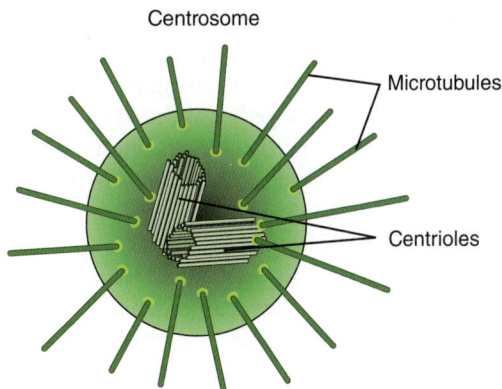

Fig. 5.13 Centrosome structure.

Ribosomes are commonly referred to as the cell's *protein factories* because their role is to manufacture (synthesize) the various proteins that cells require by using the blueprints provided by mRNA. Ribosomes' role in the assembly of amino acids into proteins was detailed earlier in this chapter.

Centrosomes—"Weavers of the Spindle." Centrosomes are located in the center of the cell near the nucleus. Centrosomes contain *centrioles*, which are a pair of small, hollow, cylindrical structures within each centrosome (Fig. 5.12) oriented at right angles to each other and embedded in a material mass of more than 100 proteins.

When a cell divides and produces two new identical cells, first, the cell must create two copies of its DNA. Each copy of DNA will subsequently travel to a new cell so that the new cells have the identical DNA as the original cell.

The centrosome and centrioles have crucial roles in this process: during cell division, two centrioles combine together with some other special proteins and form the **centrosome**. Fig. 5.13 is an image of a centrosome, comprised of two centrioles and microtubules. The centrosome serves as the main microtubule-organizing center of the cell, as well as a regulator of cell-cycle progression.

The centrioles' pair duplicates within a cell, and the resultant two pairs migrate to the opposite ends of the cell to form and organize the mitotic spindle.* The stages of cell division are discussed in detail later in this chapter.

---

*The mitotic spindle is essentially a protein machine that segregates chromosomes into two daughter cells during the cell division process.

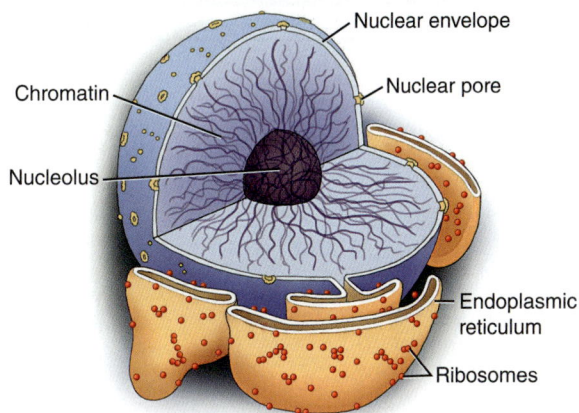

Fig. 5.14 Anatomy of the cell nucleus.

Nucleus—information-processing and administrative center

Separated from the other parts of the cell by a double-walled membrane with pores, called the *nuclear envelope,* the **nucleus** is a highly specialized cellular component that is the information-processing and administrative center of the living cell (Fig. 5.14). The nucleus consists of a spherical mass of semifluid protoplasm, known as *nucleoplasm*, which contains the genetic or hereditary material, DNA (the blueprints, or instructions, for building proteins in the cell), and proteins. The pores in the nuclear envelope allow molecules of specific types and sizes to pass back and forth between the nucleus and the cytoplasm.

Proteins and DNA within the nucleoplasm are arranged in long threads called *chromatin*. Chromatin is essentially a less condensed or less tightly packed form of the cell's DNA that, together with various proteins, during the division of a cell contracts into the tiny rod-shaped bodies that are called *chromosomes*. The genetic history of the cell is contained within the chromosomes in the *segments of DNA called genes.*

The cell nucleus also contains at least one very small, rounded body called the *nucleolus*. The nucleolus is the RNA copy center. This nuclear organelle manufactures and contains a large amount of RNA and protein. The nucleolus synthesizes ribosomes, which are protein-producing machines.

In summary, the nucleus controls cell division, multiplication, and the biochemical reactions that occur within the cell. By directing protein synthesis, the nucleus plays an essential role in the following:

- Active transport
- Metabolism
- Growth
- Heredity

A summary of cell components is presented in Table 5.1.

TABLE 5.1   Summary of Cell Components

Component	Site	Activity
Cell membrane	Cytoplasm	*Plastic storage bag*—Functions as a barricade to protect cellular contents from their environment and controls the passage of water and other materials into and out of the cell; performs many additional functions, such as elimination of wastes and refining of material for energy through breakdown of the materials.
Endoplasmic reticulum	Cytoplasm	*The highway*—Enables the cell to communicate with the extracellular environment and transfers food from one part of the cell to another.
Golgi apparatus	Cytoplasm	*Freight hauling*—Unites large carbohydrate molecules and combines them with proteins to form glycoproteins; transports enzymes and hormones through the cell membrane so that they can exit the cell, enter the bloodstream, and be carried to areas of the body in which they are required.
Mitochondria	Cytoplasm	*Power-generating stations*—Produce energy for cellular activity by breaking down nutrients through a process of oxidation.
Lysosomes	Cytoplasm	*Garbage bags with poison pills*—Dispose of large particles such as bacteria and food, as well as smaller particles; also contain hydrolytic enzymes that can break down and digest proteins, certain carbohydrates, and the cell itself if the lysosome's surrounding membrane breaks.
Ribosomes	Cytoplasm	*Manufacturing facilities*—Manufacture the various proteins that cells require.
Centrosomes	Cytoplasm	*Spindle weaver*—Plays an important role in organizing the formation of the mitotic spindle during cell division.
Nucleus	Nucleus	*Information-processing and administrative center of the cell*—Contains the genetic, or hereditary, material, DNA, and proteins. Also contains the nucleolus. The nucleus controls cell division and multiplication and the biochemical reactions that occur within the cell. Also directs protein synthesis.
DNA	Nucleus	*The blueprints*—Contains the genetic material; controls cell division and multiplication and biochemical reactions that occur within the living cell.
Nucleolus	Nucleus	*RNA copy center*—Holds a large amount of RNA and synthesizes ribosomes.

CELL DIVISION

Cell division is the multiplication process whereby one cell divides to form two or more cells (Fig. 5.15). The two types of cell divisions that occur in the body are:

- Mitosis
- Meiosis

When somatic cells (all cells in the human body other than the germ cells) divide, they undergo mitosis, a process in which the nucleus first divides, followed by the division of the cytoplasm. Genetic cells (the oogonium, or female germ cell, and the spermatogonium, or male germ cell), however, undergo meiosis, a process of reduction division.

Mitosis

When **mitosis (M)** (Fig. 5.16) occurs, a parent cell divides to form two daughter cells identical to the parent cell. Mitosis results in an approximately equal distribution of all cellular material between the two daughter cells. The entire cellular life cycle may be depicted as shown in Fig. 5.17. Differing degrees of cell growth, maturation, and division occur in each phase. Four distinct phases of the cellular life cycle are identifiable:

- G_1 (pre-DNA synthesis)
- S (synthesis)
- G_2 (post-DNA synthesis)
- M (mitosis)

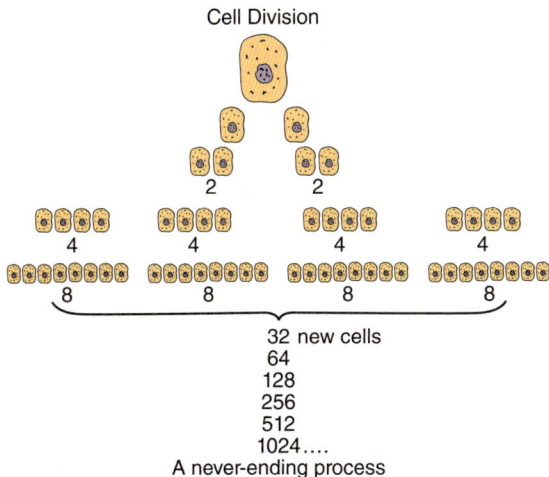

Fig. 5.15 Cell division is the multiplication process whereby one cell divides to form two or more cells. (From *Radiobiology and radiation protection: Mosby's radiographic instructional series,* St. Louis, 1999, Elsevier.)

In addition, the M phase, itself, can be divided into four subphases:

- Prophase
- Metaphase
- Anaphase
- Telophase

Mitosis should be thought of as the division phase of the cellular life cycle and therefore is actually the last phase of the cycle. After mitosis has commenced, it takes about 1 hour to complete division in all cells. Just prior to mitosis, however, there is a relatively brief time of cell growth. This interval is called *Interphase* and is itself composed of three phases:

1. G_1
2. S
3. G_2

G1 is the earliest period among reproductive events. *G1* is the gap in the growth of the cell that occurs between mitosis and DNA synthesis. Depending on the types of cells involved, this phase may take a few minutes, or it may take several hours. *G1* is designated as the pre-DNA synthesis period. During G_1, a form of RNA is manufactured in the cells that are to reproduce. This RNA is needed before actual DNA creation can efficiently begin. *S* is the actual DNA synthesis period. While in S phase, each DNA molecule contained within the chromosome (Fig. 5.18) is first copied (replicated) and then is divided into two individual sister components called *chromatids,** each containing DNA molecules. By the end of the S phase these chromatids will join together to form a new chromosome that has an X-shaped structure (see Fig. 5.18). Thus, each of the identical genetic pieces has now become one half of a new chromosome. The region of this chromosome where the two chromatids join together is the *centromere* (see Fig. 5.18). Note, that during the anaphase portion of Mitosis (described later), the paired sister chromatids separate from one another to form individual daughter chromosomes.

When compared with G_1 and G_2, the S portion of Interphase is relatively long, lasting up to 15 hours. *G2* is the post-DNA manufacturing interval in the cellular life cycle. G_2 is of comparatively short duration, lasting

---

*A chromatid is a highly coiled strand; one of the two duplicated portions of DNA in a replicated chromosome that appear during cell division.

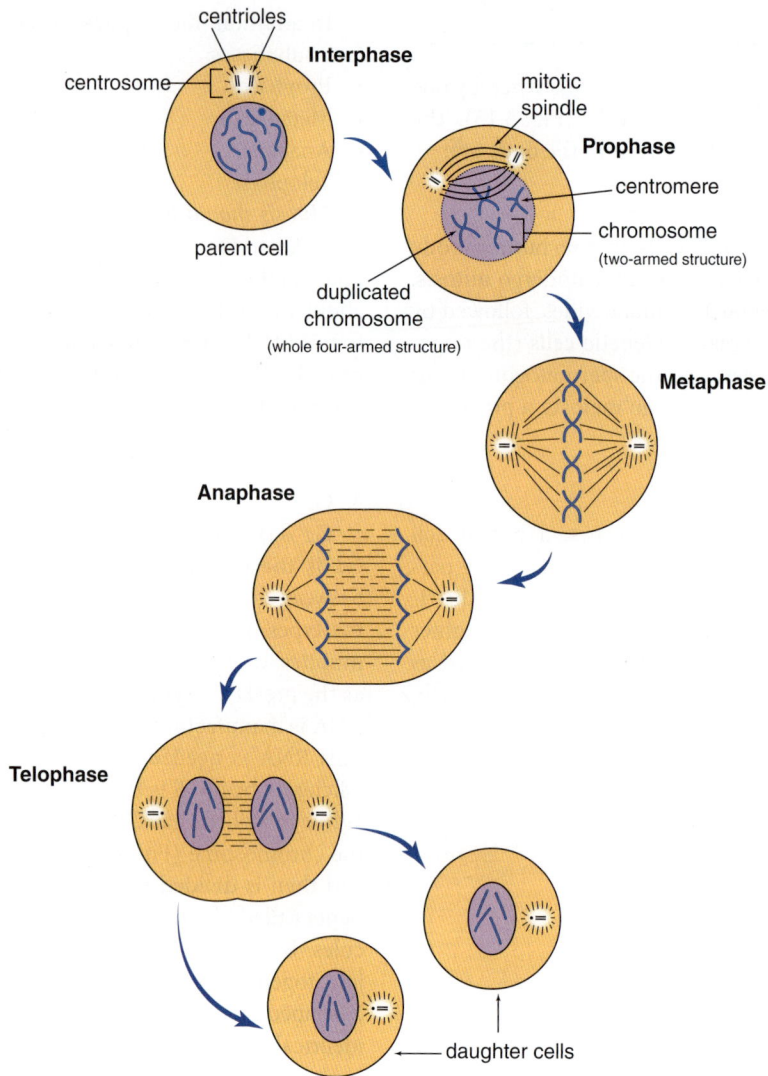

Fig. 5.16 Diagram of mitosis. An animal cell with four chromosomes first multiplies (duplicates its DNA) and then divides, forming two new daughter cells, each of which contains exactly the same genetic material as the parent cell.

approximately 1 to 5 hours. During G_2, cells manufacture certain proteins and RNA molecules, which are needed for initiating and completing the subsequent Mitosis process. Directly after G_2, cells enter the first phase of Mitosis, and the process of division commences.

The Four Phases of Mitosis. In the discussion which follows, it will be helpful to the reader to refer to Fig. 5.16.

Prophase. During prophase, the first phase of cell division, the nucleus enlarges, the DNA complex (the chromatid network of threads) coils up tightly, and the chromatids become visible on stained microscopic slides. Chromosomes enlarge, and the DNA begins to assume structural form. Next, the nuclear membrane disappears, and the centrioles (small hollow, cylindrical structures) migrate to opposite sides of the cell and begin to regulate the formation of the *mitotic spindle,* the delicate fibers that are attached to the centrioles and extend from one side of the cell to the other across the equator of the cell.

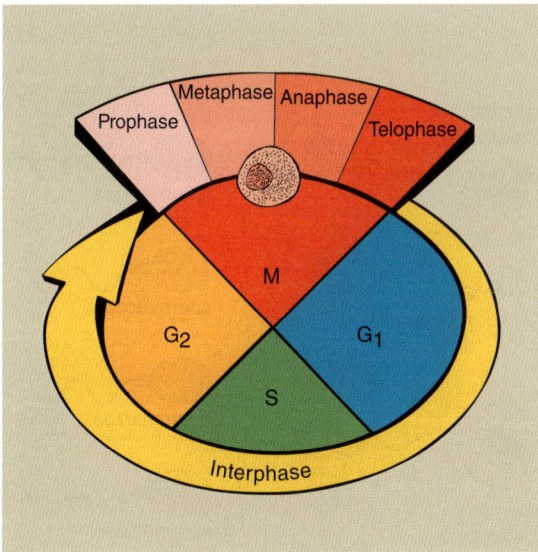

Fig. 5.17 The entire cellular life cycle may be depicted as four distinct, identifiable phases: G$_1$, S, G$_2$, and M. M may be divided into four subphases: prophase, metaphase, anaphase, and telophase. (From Bushong SC: *Radiologic science for technologists: physics, biology and protection*, ed 12, St. Louis, 2021, Elsevier.)

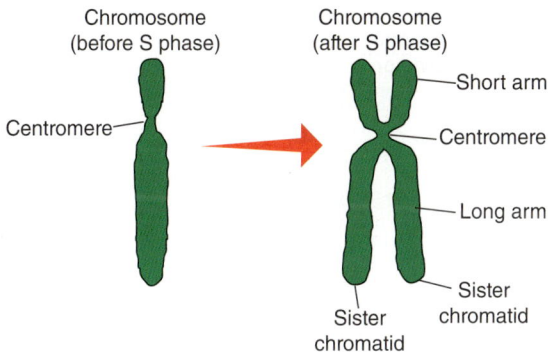

Fig. 5.18 A single-strand chromosome gets duplicated during S phase, and the duplicates are joined together in an X-shape configuration to form a new chromosome. Each crossed arm of this new chromosome is called a *sister chromatid*.

Metaphase. As **metaphase** begins, the *mitotic spindle* forms between the centrioles. Each chromosome which now consists of two chromatids, lines up in the center, or equator, of the cell attached by its centromere to the mitotic spindle. This configuration establishes the equatorial plate (see Fig. 5.16). During metaphase, cell division can be stopped, and visible chromosomes can be examined under a microscope. Chromosome damage caused by radiation can then be evaluated.

Anaphase. **Anaphase** begins with the breakdown of a protein called *securing,* which maintains chromosome stability by inhibiting the action of a protein called *separase,* whose primary function is to break down the protein complex *cohesin.* Cohesin proteins hold sister chromatids together after DNA replication by maintaining the integrity of the centromeres attached to the microtubules forming the mitotic spindle. In anaphase, dissolution of cohesin by active separase proteins leads to the separation of sister chromatids. With the removal of active cohesion, the centromeres are severed and the sister chromatids move apart and are subsequently pulled toward opposite poles of the spindle. During this progression, the chromatids acquire a shape that is similar to a V placed on its side (see Fig. 5.16). This process causes the cell to stretch or elongate into an oval shape. The cell is now ready to begin the last phase of its division process.

Telophase. During **telophase**, the chromatids undergo changes in appearance by uncoiling and becoming long, loosely spiraled threads. Simultaneously, the nuclear membrane forms anew, and two nuclei (one for each new daughter cell) appear. The cytoplasm of the parent cell then divides into two daughter cells (cytokinesis) near its equator to separately surround each new nucleus. After this cell division is complete, each daughter cell has a whole cell membrane and contains exactly the same amount of genetic material (46 chromosomes) as the parent cell.

Meiosis

Meiosis is a special type of cell division that reduces the number of chromosomes in each daughter cell to half the number of chromosomes in the parent cell (Fig. 5.19). Box 5.8 provides terms associated with the female reproductive cell. Male and female germ cells, or sperm and ova, of sexually mature individuals each begin meiosis with 46 chromosomes. However, before the male and female germ cells unite to produce a new organism, the number of chromosomes in each must be reduced by one half to ensure that the daughter cells (called *zygotes*) formed when they unite will contain only the standard number of 46 chromosomes. Hence meiosis is actually a process of reduction division (Fig. 5.20).

Meiosis begins with a doubling of the amount of genetic material. This doubling of DNA is called

MEIOSIS

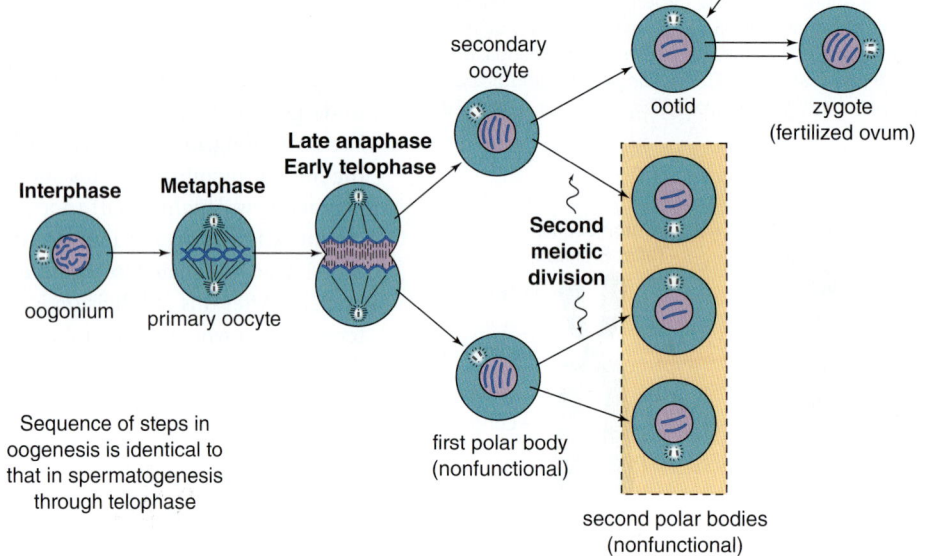

Fig. 5.19 Diagram of meiosis. Four cells result from one germ cell. In spermatogenesis, four spermatids become mature spermatozoa. In oogenesis, one ootid may be fertilized, and three second polar bodies remain nonfunctional.

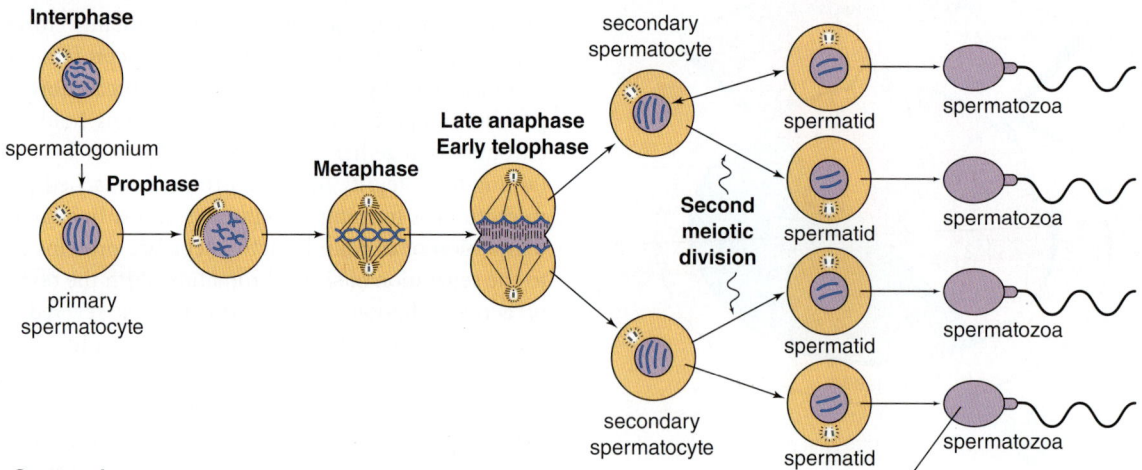

replication and occurs during interphase. As a result of DNA replication, each one-chromatid chromosome duplicates, thus forming a two-chromatid chromosome. This indicates that sperm and egg cells begin meiosis with twice the amount of genetic material as the original parent cell. Thus, at the beginning of meiosis, the number of chromosomes increases from $2n$ to $4n$ ($n = 23$).

The various phases of meiosis are similar to those of mitosis. The main difference between the two types of cell division begins at the end of telophase. In meiosis, after the parent germ cell has formed two daughter cells, each of which (in human beings) contains 46 chromosomes, the daughter cells divide without DNA replication. Chromosome duplication does not occur at this phase of division. These two successive divisions result in the formation of four granddaughter cells, each of which contains 23 chromosomes. This ensures that the proper number of 46 chromosomes will be produced when a female ovum containing 23 chromosomes is fertilized by a male sperm containing 23 chromosomes.

During meiosis, the sister chromatids exchange certain chromosomal material (genes). This process, called *crossover,* results in changes in genetic composition and traits that can be passed on to future generations.

Multiple Births. Multiple births can occur during a pregnancy in one of two instances. The first method is if an ovum, or egg cell, splits after fertilization and two separate offspring develop. The two offspring would be referred to as *monozygotic* (coming from one zygote) *twins.* Monozygotic twins are also known as *identical twins* because they contain exact replicas of genetic material. Another method to achieve a multiple birth is if more than one ootid (see Box 5.8) is available for fertilization and the separate ootids are fertilized by separate spermatozoa. In this case the children have no more resemblance to each other than other children born at different times from the same parents. Such dizygotic twins are also known as *fraternal twins.* More than two such twins would be known as *polyzygotic siblings.* Fraternal twins or multiple siblings, as with siblings born in different pregnancies, sometimes bear a striking resemblance

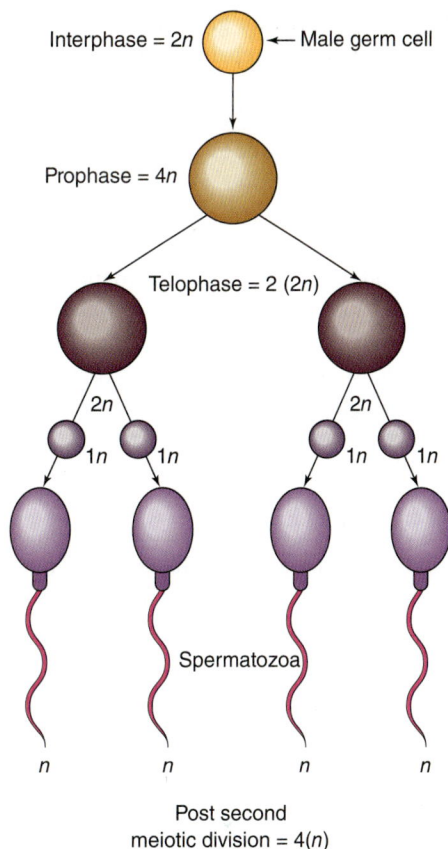

Fig. 5.20 This figure indicates the total amount of genetic material at different stages of meiosis of a male germ cell. Twenty-three chromosomes, half the amount needed to produce a new human organism, are needed in the spermatozoa. If 23 chromosomes are referred to as an amount of genetic material n, then before meiosis (during interphase) the germ cell has $2n$. During prophase, this number doubles to $4n$. There then follows two reduction divisions to form the final $1n$ (23 chromosomes) in the spermatozoa. An egg cell, or ovum, undergoes a similar process, but only one of the four resulting germ cells at the end of the process is functional.

to one another. However, unless they were monozygotic, they are not identical twins and do not have exact copies of all their chromosomes.

SUMMARY

- The cell is the fundamental component of structure, development, growth, and life processes in the human body.

- Cells are made of protoplasm, which consists of proteins, carbohydrates, lipids, nucleic acids, water, and mineral salts (electrolytes).

- Proteins are essential for growth, the construction of new body tissue, and repair of injured or debilitated tissue; they may function as hormones and antibodies.
- The primary purpose of carbohydrates is to provide fuel for cell metabolism.
- Lipids act as a reservoir for long-term storage of energy, insulate and guard the body against the environment, and protect organs.
- Nucleic acids (DNA, RNA) carry genetic information necessary for cell replication.
- RNA has the nitrogenous base uracil as a component of its ladder steps, whereas DNA has thymine instead in its ladder steps.
- Genes are segments of DNA that are the basic units of heredity.
- The Human Genome Project has mapped the entire sequence of DNA base pairs on all 46 chromosomes. This project has led to the discovery of more than 1800 disease genes.
- There are 2.9 billion base pairs arranged into approximately 30,000 genes.
- Water, the primary inorganic substance contained in the human body, comprises approximately 80% to 85% of the body's weight, is essential to sustaining life, and serves as the transport vehicle for materials the cell uses or eliminates.
- Mineral salts keep the correct proportion of water in the cell, support proper cell function, assist in the creation of energy, aid in the conduction of impulses along nerves, and prevent muscle cramping.
- Cells have multiple components or subunits called *organelles*.

- The cell membrane surrounds the human cell, functions as a barricade, and controls passage of water and other materials into and out of the cell.
- Cytoplasm is the portion of a cell outside the nucleus in which all metabolic activity occurs.
- The Endoplasmic Reticulum transports food and molecules from one part of the cell to another. It functions as the highway system of the cell.
- The Golgi apparatus unites large carbohydrate molecules with proteins to form glycoproteins.
- Mitochondria, the powerhouses of the cell, contain enzymes that produce energy for cellular activity.
- Lysosomes break down unwanted large molecules; they may rupture when they are exposed to radiation, with resulting cell death.
- Ribosomes synthesize the various proteins that cells require.
- Centrosomes contain the centrioles.
- The nucleus controls cell division, multiplication, and biochemical reactions.
- Somatic cells divide through the process of mitosis.
- The cellular life cycle has four distinct phases: pre-DNA synthesis, actual DNA synthesis, post-DNA manufacturing, and division (mitosis).
- Mitosis has four subphases: prophase, metaphase, anaphase, and telophase.
- Genetic cells divide through meiosis.
- Meiosis is similar to mitosis, except no DNA replication occurs in telophase; the number of chromosomes in the daughter cell is reduced to half the number of chromosomes in the parent cell.

GENERAL DISCUSSION QUESTIONS

1. How do lipids contribute to the body's ability to maintain homeostasis?
2. What are the differences between DNA and RNA in terms of structure and function?
3. Explain how mitochondria generate energy for cellular activities and why they are called the "powerhouses" of the cell.
4. How do lysosomes protect the cell from potential damage, and what could happen if they malfunction?
5. Discuss the importance of mineral salts in nerve conduction and muscle function.
6. How does the cell membrane regulate the internal environment of the cell?
7. What is the significance of the Golgi apparatus in the synthesis and processing of glycoproteins?
8. How does the structure of the Endoplasmic Reticulum facilitate its role in cellular transport?
9. Compare and contrast the phases of mitosis and meiosis, focusing on their roles in somatic and genetic cells.
10. What are the implications of the Human Genome Project in understanding genetic disorders and developing new treatments?

REVIEW QUESTIONS

1. What is the primary function of carbohydrates in the human cell?
   A. Store genetic information
   B. Provide fuel for cell metabolism
   C. Synthesize proteins
   D. Insulate the body

2. Which of the following organelles is responsible for breaking down large unwanted molecules within the cell?
   A. Ribosomes
   B. Golgi apparatus
   C. Lysosomes
   D. Mitochondria

3. During which phase of the cellular life cycle does DNA synthesis occur?
   A. Prophase
   B. Pre-DNA synthesis
   C. DNA synthesis
   D. Post-DNA synthesis

4. What is the main role of nucleic acids in the cell?
   A. Store energy
   B. Provide structural support
   C. Carry genetic information for replication
   D. Transport molecules across the cell membrane

5. Which organelle is known as the "highway system" of the cell, transporting molecules from one part of the cell to another?
   A. Golgi apparatus
   B. Ribosomes
   C. Endoplasmic reticulum
   D. Centrosomes

6. What is the role of water within the human cell?
   A. Synthesizing proteins
   B. Acting as a transport vehicle for materials
   C. Storing genetic information
   D. Providing insulation for the cell

7. Which of the following processes involves a reduction in chromosome number in the daughter cells?
   A. Mitosis
   B. Meiosis
   C. DNA synthesis
   D. Protein synthesis

8. Which component of RNA distinguishes it from DNA?
   A. Thymine
   B. Uracil
   C. Adenine
   D. Cytosine

9. What percentage of the human body is composed of water?
   A. 50% to 60%
   B. 60% to 70%
   C. 70% to 75%
   D. 80% to 85%

10. Which of the following organelles is primarily involved in energy production within the cell?
    A. Ribosomes
    B. Lysosomes
    C. Mitochondria
    D. Golgi apparatus

6

Molecular and Cellular Radiation Biology

OBJECTIVES

After completing this chapter, the reader will be able to perform the following:

- Define all key terms.
- Explain in what manner ionizing radiation damages living systems.
- List three characteristics of ionizing radiation that determine the extent to which different radiation modalities transfer energy into biologic tissue.
- List the three radiation energy transfer determinants, and explain their concepts.
- Explain why x-rays and gamma rays can also be referred to as a stream of particles called photons.
- Differentiate among the three levels of biologic damage that may occur in living systems as a result of exposure to ionizing radiation and describe how the process of direct and indirect action of ionizing radiation on the molecular structure of living systems occurs.

- Create a diagram to illustrate the various effects of ionizing radiation on a DNA macromolecule, and describe the effects of ionizing radiation on chromosomes, various types of cells, and ultimately the entire human body.
- Explain the target theory.
- List and explain six effects of irradiation on the entire cell that can result from damage to the cell's nucleus.
- Explain the purpose and function of survival curves for mammalian cells.
- List the factors that affect cell radiosensitivity.
- State and describe the law of Bergonié and Tribondeau.
- Describe the effects of ionizing radiation on human blood cells, epithelial tissue, muscle tissue, nervous tissue, and male and female reproductive cells.

CHAPTER OUTLINE

Ionizing Radiation
Radiation Energy Transfer Determinants
    Linear Energy Transfer
    Relative Biologic Effectiveness
    Oxygen Enhancement Ratio
Molecular Effects of Irradiation
    Effects of Irradiation on Somatic and Genetic Cells
    Classification of Ionizing Radiation Interaction
    Direct Action Characteristics
    Radiolysis of Water
    Indirect Action Characteristics
    Specific Effects of Ionizing Radiation on DNA
    Effects of Ionizing Radiation on Chromosomes
    Target Theory
Effects of Irradiation on the Entire Cell

    Instant Death
    Reproductive Death
    Apoptosis
    Mitotic Death
    Mitotic Delay
    Interference With Function
Survival Curves for Mammalian Cells
Cell Radiosensitivity
    Cell Maturity and Specialization
    Oxygen Enhancement Effects
    Law of Bergonié and Tribondeau
    Effects of Ionizing Radiation on Human Cells and Tissues
Summary

KEY TERMS

apoptosis
cell survival curve
chromosome breakage
direct action
free radicals
indirect action

law of Bergonié and Tribondeau
linear energy transfer (LET)
mutation
oxygen enhancement ratio (OER)
point lesion
radiation weighting factor (W_R)

radiolysis
relative biologic effectiveness (RBE)
target theory
wave-particle duality

Radiation biology, also known as Radiobiology, is the branch of biology concerned with the effects of ionizing radiation on living systems. Areas of study included in this discipline are:

- The sequence of events occurring after the absorption of energy from ionizing radiation
- The action of the living system to compensate for the consequences of this energy assimilation
- Injury to the living system that may occur from irradiation

The human body is a complex interconnected living system composed of very large numbers of various types of cells, most of which may be damaged by radiation. Because the potentially harmful effects of ionizing radiation on living systems occur primarily at the cellular level, the preceding chapter placed a strong emphasis on the basics of cell structure, composition, and function. This chapter provides an introduction to those aspects of molecular and cellular radiation biology that are relevant to the subject of radiation protection.

IONIZING RADIATION

Ionizing radiation damages living systems by removing electrons from (ionizing) the atoms comprising the molecular structures of these systems. X-ray and gamma-ray photons can impart energy to orbital electrons in atoms if the photons happen to pass near the electrons. High-energy charged particles such as alpha and beta particles and protons also may ionize atoms by interacting electromagnetically with orbital electrons. The alpha particle, which is composed of two protons and two neutrons and therefore carries an electric charge of +2, strongly attracts the negatively charged electrons as it passes.

Biologic damage, then, begins with the ionization of atoms caused by various types of radiation. Such altered atoms do not bond properly in molecules. If the molecule in question is necessary for the normal function of an organism, then the entire organism may be adversely affected.

RADIATION ENERGY TRANSFER DETERMINANTS

The characteristics of ionizing radiation vary among different types of radiation. Characteristics include:

- Charge
- Mass
- Energy

These attributes determine the extent to which different radiation modalities transfer energy into biologic tissue. To be able to understand how ionizing radiation causes injury and how the effects can vary in biologic tissue, three essential concepts must be studied:

1. Linear energy transfer
2. Relative biologic effectiveness
3. Oxygen enhancement ratio

Linear Energy Transfer

When passing through a medium such as human tissue, ionizing radiation may interact with that medium during its passage, and as a result, lose energy along its path (called a *track*). The average energy deposited per unit length of track is **linear energy transfer (LET)** (Fig. 6.1). This energy average is calculated by dividing the total energy deposited in the medium by the total length of the track. LET is generally described in units of kiloelectron volts (keV) per micron (1 micron [μm] = 10^{-6} m). The rate of transfer of energy from ionizing radiation, used

Path of
electron
E = 350 keV

SI
(IP/cm)

LET
keV/cm

	7	100
	— 1 cm	
	8	200
	— 2 cm	
	9	250
	— 3 cm	
Avg. ~8.3	Avg. ~208	

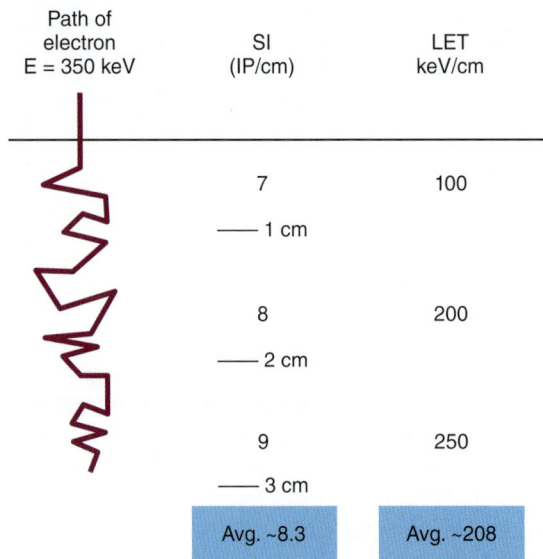

Fig. 6.1 Linear energy transfer. An electron with energy (E) of 350 keV interacts in a tissue-like material. Its actual path is tortuous, changing direction a number of times, as the electron interacts with atoms of the material via excitations and ionizations. As interactions reduce the energy of the electron through excitation and ionization, the electron's energy is transferred to the material. The interactions that take place along the path of the particle may be summarized as specific ionization (SI; ion pairs/cm) or as linear energy transfer (LET; keV/cm) along the straight-line continuation of the particle's trajectory beyond its point of entry. (From Hendee WR, Ritenour ER: *Medical imaging physics*, ed 4, Chicago, 2002, John Wiley & Sons.)

for diagnostic purposes (x-rays), to soft biologic tissue is estimated to be 3 keV/μm, which is considered to be relatively low-LET radiation compared with other types of radiation, which can have values in the megaelectron volt per micron (MeV/μm). Because the amount of ionization produced in an irradiated object is related to the amount of energy it absorbs, and because both chemical and biologic effects in tissue coincide with the degree of ionization experienced by the tissue, the LET value of the radiation involved is an essential factor in assessing potential tissue and organ damage from exposure to that type of ionizing radiation. When LET increases, the chance of a significant biologic response in the radiosensitive DNA macromolecule also increases.

Radiation Categories According to Linear Energy Transfer. Radiation may be divided into two general categories according to its LET (Box 6.1), low or high.

BOX 6.1   General Categories of Linear Energy Transfer Radiation (LET)

Low-LET Radiation	High-LET Radiation
Gamma rays	Alpha particles
X-rays	Ions of heavy nuclei
Electrons	Charged particles released from interactions between neutrons and atoms
	Low-energy neutrons

Low–linear energy transfer radiation. Low-LET radiation is electromagnetic radiation, such as:
- X-rays
- Gamma rays (short-wavelength, high-energy waves emitted by the nuclei of radioactive substances)

Because of a property known as **wave-particle duality**, x-rays and gamma rays, as described in Box 2.1 in Chapter 2 and Appendix E, can also be referred to as streams of moving particles called *photons,* each of which has no mass* and no charge.

Although electromagnetic radiation (EMR) can be quite penetrating, it is sparsely ionizing and interacts randomly along the length of its track. Consequently, EMR photons do not relinquish all their energy quickly. When low-LET radiation interacts with biologic tissue, it causes damage to a cell primarily through an *indirect* action that involves the production of molecules called **free radicals**. These are solitary atoms, for example, a non-molecular hydrogen atom [H]** or most often a combination of atoms such as [OH] that behave as single entities and are chemically reactive as a result of the presence of unpaired valence (outermost) electrons. Also, but much less likely, the low-LET radiation may *directly* induce single-strand breaks in the ladder-like DNA structure. Because low-LET radiation generally causes sub-lethal damage to DNA, repair enzymes can usually reverse the cellular damage.

---

*More precisely the photon has zero rest mass or intrinsic mass. The photon, however, has motional mass associated with its total energy E and this quantity is related to its nonrest mass by Einstein's equation: $E = mc^2$.
**Hydrogen atoms *normally* occur as bound molecular pairs H_2 and not as individual atoms.

High–linear energy transfer radiation. High-LET radiation includes particles that possess substantial: mass and charge.

This type of radiation, unlike low-LET radiation, can produce dense ionization along its path and therefore is much more likely to interact significantly with biologic tissue. Some typical examples of high-LET radiation are:

- Alpha particles
- Ions of heavy nuclei
- Charged particles released from interactions between neutrons and atoms

Low-energy neutrons, which carry no electrical charge, are also a form of high-LET radiation. Since these types of high-LET radiation exhaust their energy rapidly in matter, unless they are of extremely high energies, they cannot travel or penetrate as far as x-ray and gamma-ray photons. Even so, high-LET radiation can be very destructive to biologic matter.

Risk of damage to DNA. Fig. 6.2 demonstrates an electron and an alpha particle passing through the nucleus of a cell in the vicinity of a strand of DNA. The size of the entire area is only approximately 10 nanometers (10 billionths of a meter). The electron is most often a Compton scattered electron, whereas the alpha particle represents one of the particles ejected from the nucleus of an atom after radioactive decay of an element such as radon.

Probability of interaction with DNA. As exhibited in Fig. 6.2, there are many more alpha particle interactions in the small region than electron interactions, the alpha particle is 1000 times the LET of the electron. Each time the particle interacts, it loses some energy and slows down in the cell. When enough interactions have occurred, the particle will essentially be at rest, and interactions beyond this path penetration are unlikely. Because it does not interact as often, the electron, however, can travel significantly farther than the alpha particle. A Compton scattered electron or photoelectron set in motion in a patient exposed to diagnostic x-rays may travel through thousands of cells, having interactions in only some of them and with a low probability that any of these will occur in the DNA. Conversely, an alpha particle, such as the one shown, may travel through only a

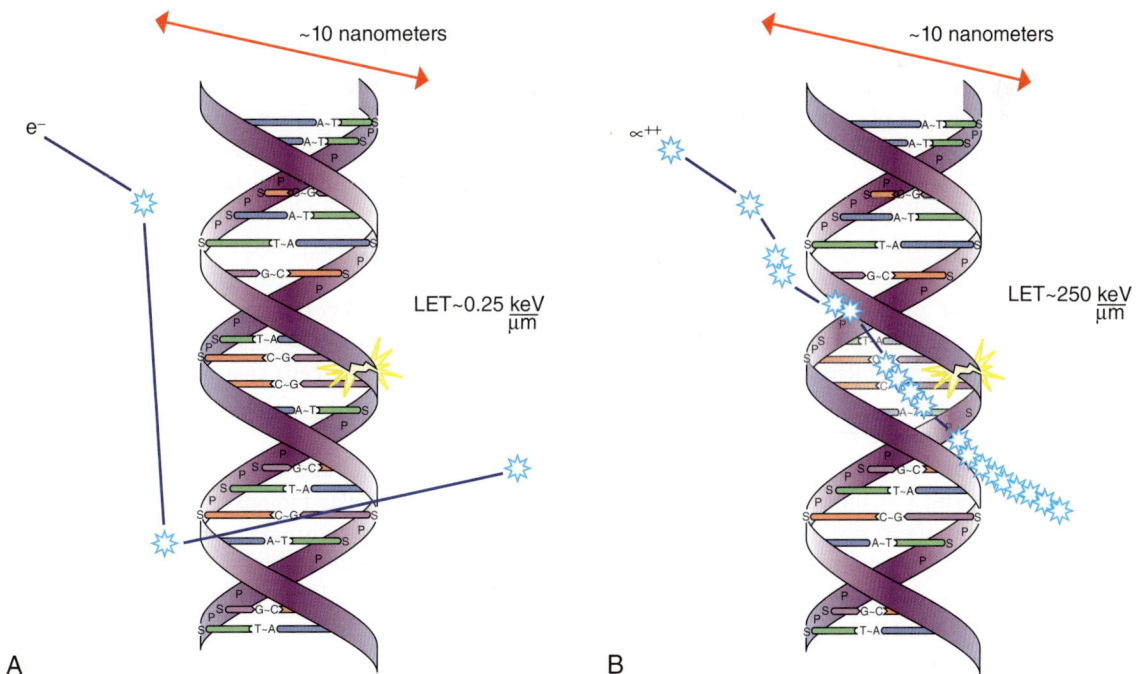

Fig. 6.2 An electron and an alpha particle passing through the nucleus of a cell near a strand of DNA. (A) For an electron, several interactions may occur in the vicinity of a DNA strand and create a risk of damage to the DNA. (B) Because many interactions may occur in the vicinity of a DNA strand, some damage is likely.

few cells, but will have a high probability of interacting with the DNA of a cell it encounters.

High–linear energy transfer radiation and internal contamination. For radiation protection, high-LET radiation is of most significant concern when internal contamination is possible, that is, when a radionuclide has been:

- Implanted
- Ingested
- Injected
- Inhaled

Then, the potential exists for irreparable damage because, with high-LET radiation, multiple-strand breaks in DNA are possible. For example, with a double-strand break in the same rung of the DNA ladder-like structure, complete **chromosome breakage** occurs (see Fig. 6.8A). Repair enzymes are incapable of undoing this damage, and hence cell death will most likely follow.

Relative Biologic Effectiveness

Biologic damage produced by radiation escalates as the LET of radiation increases. Identical doses of radiation of different LETs do not render identical biologic effects. **Relative biologic effectiveness (RBE)** describes the comparative capabilities of radiation with differing LETs to produce a particular biologic reaction. RBE of the type of radiation used is the ratio of the dose of a reference radiation (conventionally 250-kVp x-rays, where kVp is optimal peak kilovoltage) to the dose of radiation of the type in question that is necessary to produce the same biologic reaction in a given experiment. The response is what is produced by a dose of the *test* radiation delivered under the same conditions. Box 6.2 demonstrates the mathematical expression of RBE.

Use of the Relative Biologic Effectiveness Concept for Specific Experiments. The concept of RBE refers to specific experiments with specific cells or animal tissues (e.g., tumor cells in a Petri dish, skin of the left hand of a particular strain of laboratory rat). Because the various types of cells or tissues differ in their biologic response per unit quantity of absorbed dose, the concept of RBE alone is not practical for specifying radiation protection dose levels in humans. To overcome this limitation, a **radiation weighting factor (W_R)** is employed to calculate the equivalent dose (EqD) to

---

BOX 6.2   Mathematical Expression of Relative Biologic Effectiveness (RBE)

$$RBE = \frac{\text{Dose in } Gy_t \text{ from 250 kVp x-rays (reference radiation)}}{\text{Dose in } Gy_t \text{ of test radiation}}$$

Example: A biologic reaction is produced by 2 Gy_t of a test radiation. It takes 10 Gy_t of 250-kVp x-rays to produce the same biologic reaction. What is the RBE of the test radiation?

$$\frac{10}{2} = 5$$

The RBE is 5, which means that the test radiation is five times as effective in producing this biologic reaction as are 250-kVp x-rays.

---

determine the ability of a dose of any kind of ionizing radiation to cause biologic damage. The W_R values are similar to the values of RBE for any particular type of radiation. For example, the W_R for x-radiation is 1, and the RBE for diagnostic x-rays is also 1. The W_R values for different types of ionizing radiation are listed in Table 4.2 in Chapter 4.

Oxygen Enhancement Ratio

The **Oxygen Enhancement Ratio (OER)**, or oxygen effect, refers to the enhancement of the therapeutic or detrimental effect of ionizing radiation due to the presence of oxygen. When tissue is irradiated in an oxygenated state, the tissue is more sensitive to radiation than when it is exposed to radiation under anoxic (without oxygen) or hypoxic (low oxygen) conditions. This is an essential concept in radiation therapy. Cells that are anoxic during irradiation are about three times more resistant than cells that are well oxygenated at the time of irradiation. The OER describes this effect numerically.[1,2]

The OER is the ratio of the radiation dose required to cause a particular biologic response of cells in an oxygen-deprived environment to the radiation dose required to generate an identical response under normal oxygenated conditions. The OER formula is stated in Box 6.3.

In general, x-rays and gamma rays, which are low-LET types of radiation, have an OER of approximately 3.0 when the radiation dose is high. The OER may be less (approximately 2.0) when radiation doses are lower than 2 Gy_t. This surprising result exists because a 2 Gy_t dose is associated with the linear (i.e., straight-line) portion of the linear-quadratic dose–response relationship for cell killing (see Fig. 8.3), whereas higher doses can fall on the curved (i.e., quadratic) portion of the dose–response curve.[3] The term *linear-quadratic* indicates that the equation that best fits the data has conditions that depend on dose (linear dependency) and dose squared (quadratic dependence). Because high-LET radiation, such as alpha particles, produces its biologic effects from direct action—namely, direct ionization and disruption of biomolecules—the presence or absence of oxygen is of little or no consequence to their effects. Therefore the OER of high-LET radiation is approximately equal to 1. For low-LET radiation, a significant fraction of bioeffects are caused by indirect actions in which a *free radical* is formed. Because of their high reactivity, free radicals can dramatically increase the amount of biologic damage. Oxygen, if present in biologic tissues, will react with these chemical entities to produce organic peroxide compounds.* The latter represent non-restorable changes in the chemical composition of the target material. Without oxygen, the damage created by the indirect action of radiation on a biologic molecule may be repaired, but when damage occurs through an oxygen-mediated process, the final result is lasting or fixed. This phenomenon has been called *the oxygen fixation hypothesis*.

MOLECULAR EFFECTS OF IRRADIATION

In living systems, biologic damage stemming from exposure to ionizing radiation is examined on three levels:

- Molecular
- Cellular
- Organic systems

---

*An organic peroxide is any organic (carbon-containing) compound with two oxygen atoms joined together (-O-O-).

Any visible radiation-induced injuries of living systems at the cellular or organic level always begin with damage at the molecular level. Molecular damage results in the formation of structurally changed molecules that may severely impair cellular function.

Effects of Irradiation on Somatic and Genetic Cells

Cells of the human body are highly specialized. Each cell has a predetermined task to perform, and each cell's function is governed and defined by the structures of its constituent molecules. Absorbed energy from ionizing radiation can alter these structures, thereby disturbing the cell's chemical balance and, ultimately, how it operates. When this occurs, the cell no longer performs its normal tasks. If sufficient quantities of somatic cells (i.e., all cells in the body other than female and male germ cells) are affected, entire body processes can be disrupted. Conversely, if radiation damages the germ (reproductive) cells, the damage may be passed on to future generations in the form of genetic mutations.

Classification of Ionizing Radiation Interaction

When ionizing radiation interacts with a cell, ionizations and excitations (the addition of energy to a molecular system that raises it from a ground state to a higher-energy, or excited, state) are produced either in vital biologic macromolecules or in water (H_2O), the medium in which the cellular organelles are suspended. Based on the site interaction, the effect of radiation on the cell is classified as either (Fig. 6.3): a direct or indirect action.

As mentioned previously, in **direct action**, biologic damage occurs as a result of the ionization of atoms on essential molecules produced by an immediate interaction with incident radiation. **Indirect action**, instead, is always a multistage process that first involves the production of free radicals that are usually created by the interaction of the radiation with water (H_2O) molecules. These unstable agents, then, may proceed to interact with cellular molecules. Free radicals are so highly reactive that should they encounter DNA macromolecules, they can cause cell death.

Direct action has some probability of occurring after exposure to any kind of radiation. However, direct action is much more likely to occur after exposure to high-LET radiation such as alpha particles, which produce a vast

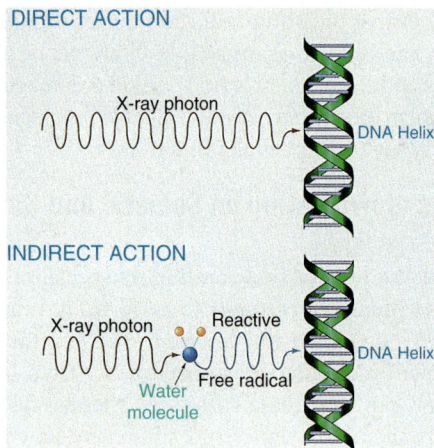

Fig. 6.3 The action of radiation on the cell can be direct or indirect. It is direct when ionizing particles interact with a vital biologic macromolecule such as DNA. The action is indirect when ionizing particles interact with a water molecule, thus resulting in the creation of ions and reactive free radicals that eventually produce toxic substances that can create biologic damage. (From *Radiobiology and radiation protection: Mosby's radiographic instructional series*, St. Louis, 1999, Mosby.)

number of ionizations in a very short distance of travel. This response is in stark contrast to exposure to low-LET radiation, such as x-rays, which are only sparsely ionizing.

Direct Action Characteristics

When ionizing particles interact directly with vital biologic macromolecules such as:

- DNA
- Ribonucleic acid (RNA)
- Proteins
- Enzymes

Damage to these molecules occurs from the absorption of energy through photoelectric and Compton interactions. The ionization, or even the excitation, of the atoms of the biologic macromolecules can result in breakage of the macromolecules' intricate chemical bonds, causing them to become abnormal structures. This change could lead to inappropriate cellular chemical reactions. As an example, when enzyme molecules are damaged by interaction with ionizing particles, essential biochemical processes that depend on the facilitating action of the enzymes may not occur in the cell when needed. Should this occur during the process associated with the synthesis of a particular protein, the protein will not be

manufactured, and if this protein were intended to perform a specific function, its failure to exist would hinder or prevent that function. If other cell operations depend on the suppressed function, these operations will be compromised as well, and consequently, a negative biologic sequence occurs.

Radiolysis of Water

Ionization of Water Molecules. Radiolysis refers to the dissociation of molecules by ionizing radiation. Thus, when x-ray photons interact with water molecules contained within the human body, this can result in their separation into other molecular components. For example, one type of interaction could create an ion pair consisting of a water molecule with a positive charge (HOH^+) and a single electron (e^-). After the original ionization of the water molecule, several other successive reactions are possible. One such outcome is that the positively charged water molecule (HOH^+) may recombine with the electron (e^-) to reform a stable water molecule ($HOH^+ + e^- = H_2O$). If this happens, no damage will occur. Alternatively, the electron (the negative ion) may join with another water molecule to produce a negative water ion ($H_2O + e^- = HOH^-$). This result, however, can have unfavorable consequences.

Production of Free Radicals. The positive water molecule (HOH^+) and the negative water molecule (HOH^-) are fundamentally unstable. Hence, they will soon break apart into smaller molecules. HOH^+ decomposes into a hydrogen ion (H^+) and the neutral oxygen–hydrogen combination called the *hydroxyl radical* (OH^*), whereas HOH^- becomes a hydroxyl ion (OH^-) and a hydrogen radical (H^*). The asterisk symbolizes a free radical. A free radical is a molecular unit that has no net electrical charge but, because of *having an unpaired valence electron*, it is an extremely reactive entity, which typically exists as such for approximately one millisecond before pairing up with another electron, even if to do this it has to break a chemical bond in a vital molecule. In summary, the interaction of radiation with water ultimately results in the formation of an ion pair, H^+ and OH^-, and two free radicals, H^* and OH^* (Fig. 6.4).

Production of Adverse Chemical Reactions and Biologic Damage. Energetic hydrogen and hydroxyl *free radicals* within the human body can initiate undesirable

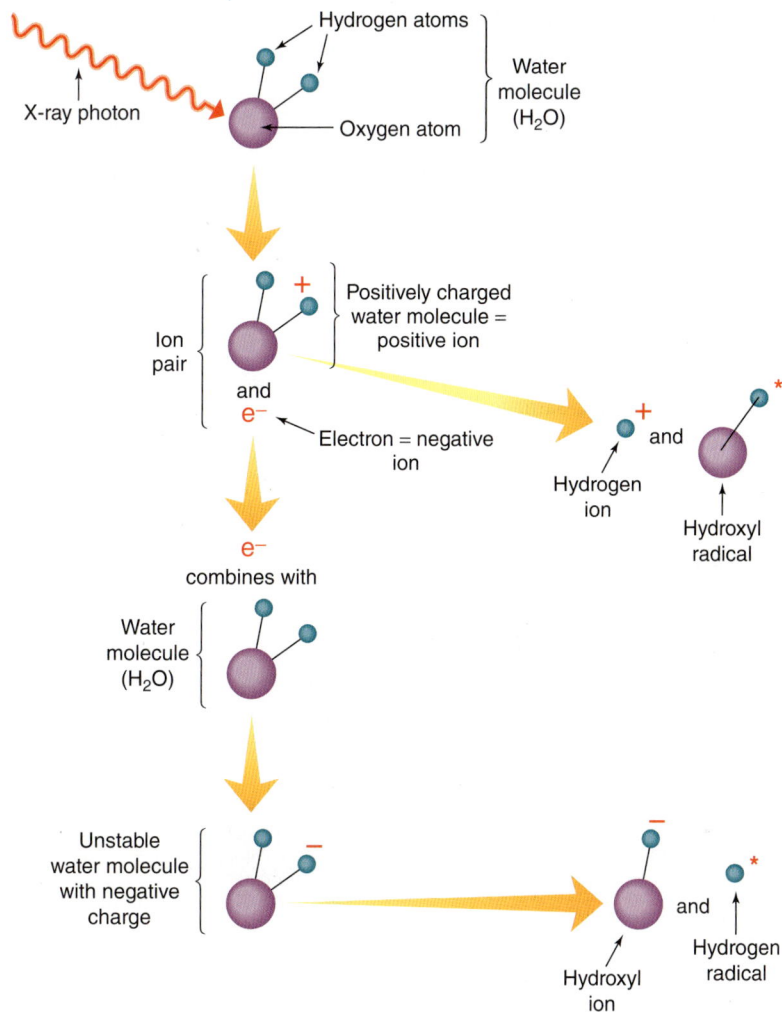

Fig. 6.4 Radiolysis of water. The final result of the interaction of radiation with water is the formation of an ion pair (H+ and OH–) and two free radicals (H* and OH*).

chemical reactions. In the process, the free radicals' excess energy is transferred to some biologic molecules, thereby either breaking these molecules' chemical bonds, or at the very least, causing **point lesions** (i.e., altered areas caused by the fracturing of a single chemical bond) in the molecule. Approximately two-thirds of all radiation-induced damage is believed to be ultimately caused by the hydroxyl free radical (OH*). Also, because free radicals have excess energy and can travel through the cell, they are capable of destructively interacting with other molecules located at some distance from the radicals' place of origin.

Production of Cell-Damaging Substances. Hydrogen and hydroxyl radicals are not the only destructive substances produced during the radiolysis of water. A hydroxyl radical (OH*) can bond with another hydroxyl radical (OH*) and form hydrogen peroxide (OH* + OH* = H_2O_2), a substance that is very poisonous to the cell. Additionally, hydroperoxyl radical (HO_2*) is formed when a hydrogen free radical (H*) combines with molecular oxygen (O_2). The hydroperoxyl radical and hydrogen peroxide are believed to be among the primary substances that produce biologic damage *directly* after the interaction of radiation with water.

Organic Free Radical Formation. Absorption of radiation can cause a healthy organic molecule (for simplicity, known as *RH,* in which *H* stands for hydrogen and *R* can be any organic molecule) to form the free radicals R* (an organic-neutral free radical) and H*. Without oxygen or a force to attract an electron, these radicals usually react with each other to reform the original organic molecule (RH). When oxygen is present, however, R* and H* may react with oxygen molecules (O_2) to form the radicals RO_2* and HO_2*. Hence the original organic molecule (RH) is destroyed and replaced by the radicals RO_2* and HO_2*. These radicals can react with other organic molecules to cause biologic damage. Thus, a small-scale chain reaction of destructive events results when radiation deposits energy within tissue in the *presence of oxygen.*

Indirect Action Characteristics

To summarize, when free radicals previously produced by the interaction of radiation with water molecules act on a molecule such as DNA, the damaging action of ionizing radiation is indirect in the sense that the radiation is not the immediate cause of injury to the macromolecule. The by-products of the radiation, the free radicals, are the direct cause of this damage. Because the human body is 80% water and less than 1% DNA, essentially all effects of low-LET irradiation in living cells result from indirect action.[1] Fig. 6.5 depicts a useful flow chart of the radiobiologic process of indirect action.

Specific Effects of Ionizing Radiation on DNA

Single-Strand Break. If ionizing radiation interacts with a DNA macromolecule, the transferred energy could rupture one of its chemical bonds and possibly sever one of the sugar–phosphate chain side rails, or strands, of the ladder-like molecular structure (single-strand break) (Fig. 6.6). This type of injury to DNA is called a **point lesion.** Such a single alteration along the sequence of nitrogenous bases can result in a gene abnormality. Point lesions commonly occur with low-LET radiation. Repair enzymes, however, are often capable of reversing this damage.

Double-Strand Break. Further exposure of the affected DNA macromolecule to ionizing radiation will likely lead to additional breaks in the sugar–phosphate molecular chain(s). These breaks may also be repaired,

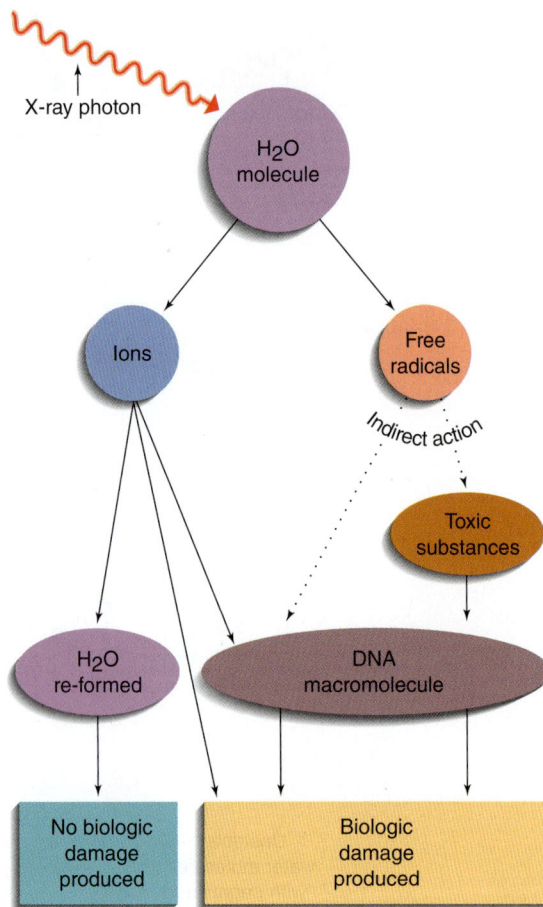

Fig. 6.5 Indirect action of ionizing radiation on biologic molecules. X-ray photons interact directly with a water (H_2O) molecule. The H_2O molecule breaks down into ions and free radicals. The ions can recombine to form a water molecule, thereby creating no biologic damage. The free radicals can migrate to another molecule, such as a DNA molecule located at some distance from the site of the initial ionization, and destructively interact with it by ionizing it or rupturing some chemical bonds. This creates molecular or point lesions in the DNA macromolecule. Alternatively, free radicals can spread biologic damage by combining with other molecules to form toxic substances that also can migrate to distant DNA molecules and destructively interact.

but double-strand breaks (one or more breaks in each of the two sugar–phosphate chains) (Fig. 6.7) are not repaired as easily as single-strand breaks. If a repair does not take place, further separation can occur in the DNA chains, threatening the life of the cell. Double-strand breaks occur more commonly with densely ionizing (high-LET) radiation and often are associated

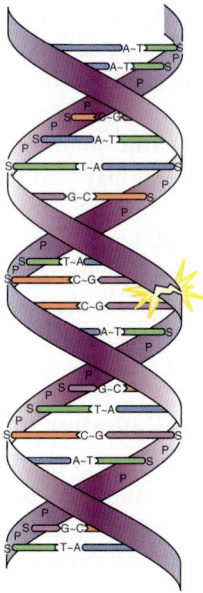

Fig. 6.6 A single-strand break in the ladder-like DNA molecular structure.

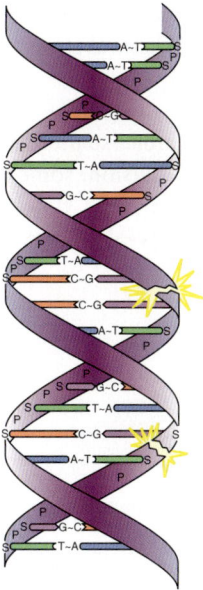

Fig. 6.8 A double-strand break in same rung of the (A) DNA molecular structure causes complete chromosome breakage, (B) resulting in a cleaved or broken chromosome.

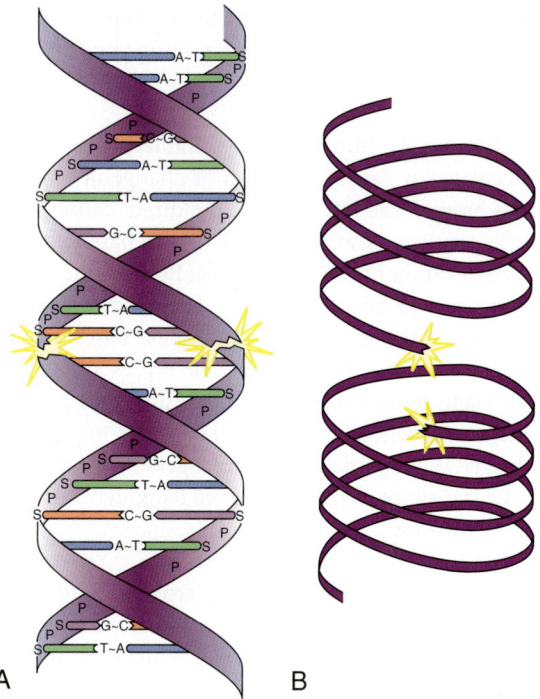

Fig. 6.7 A widely spaced double-strand break in the DNA molecular structure.

with the loss of one or more nitrogenous bases. Thus, when high-LET radiation interacts with DNA molecules, the ionization interactions may be so closely spaced that, by chance, both strands of a DNA chain

are broken. Should both strands be broken at the same nitrogenous base "rung" (Fig. 6.8A) the result will be the same as if both side rails of the ladder were severed at the same step, namely the DNA ladder would be chopped into two pieces. This situation will result in the associated chromosome to be broken. Thus, some types of chromosomal damage that are caused explicitly by high-LET radiation are related to double-strand breaks of DNA. Because the chance of reversing this type of injury is meager, the possibility of a lethal alteration of nitrogenous bases within the genetic sequence is now far more significant.

Chromosome Effect After a Double-Strand Break in the Same Rung of DNA. As mentioned earlier, when two interactions (hits), one on each of the two sugar–phosphate chains, occur within the same rung of the DNA ladder-like configuration (see Fig. 6.8A), the result is a cleaved or broken chromosome (see Fig. 6.8B), with each new portion generally containing an unequal amount of genetic material. If this damaged chromosome divides, each new daughter cell will receive an incorrect amount of genetic material. This defect will culminate in either impaired functioning or death of the newly created daughter cell.

Mutation. Interactions of ionizing radiation with DNA molecules may cause the loss of or change in a nitrogenous base on the DNA chain. The direct consequence of this damage is an alteration of the base sequence (Fig. 6.9) within the DNA molecule. Because the genetic information to be passed on to future generations is contained in the strict sequence of these bases, the loss or change of a base in the DNA chain represents a **mutation**. Damage may not be reversible and may generate acute consequences for the cell, but, more importantly, if the cell remains viable, incorrect genetic information will be transferred to one of the two daughter cells when the cell divides.

Covalent Cross-Links. Covalent cross-linking is the process of chemically joining two or more molecules by a covalent bond, which is the sharing of one or more pairs of electrons between the molecules. Covalent cross-links involving DNA comprise another effect directly initiated by high-LET radiation. With low-LET interactions, however, covalent cross-links are most likely caused by the process of indirect action. After irradiation, some molecules can fragment or change into small, spur-like molecules that become very interactive ("sticky") when exposed to radiation. Such sticky molecules can facilitate cross-linking by

attaching or connecting to other macromolecules or other segments of the same macromolecule chain. Cross-linking can occur in many different patterns. For example, it can form between two places on the same DNA strand. This joining is an *intrastrand cross-link*. Cross-linking may also take place between complementary DNA strands (Fig. 6.10) or between entirely different DNA molecules. These joining's are *interstrand cross-links*. Finally, DNA molecules also may become covalently linked to a protein molecule.[4] These linkages are potentially fatal to the cell if they are not correctly repaired.

Effects of Ionizing Radiation on Chromosomes

Large-scale structural changes in a chromosome produced by ionizing radiation may be as serious for the cell as are radiation-induced changes in DNA. When changes occur in the DNA molecule, the chromosome exhibits the variation. Because DNA modifications are discrete, they do not inevitably result in observable structural chromosome revisions. However, if these distinct effects are numerous enough, such as may be brought about by exposure to very high-LET radiation, then an observable structural chromosome alteration is possible.

Radiation-Induced Chromosome Breaks. After irradiation and during cell division, some radiation-induced chromosome breaks may be viewed microscopically. These changes are revealed during the metaphase

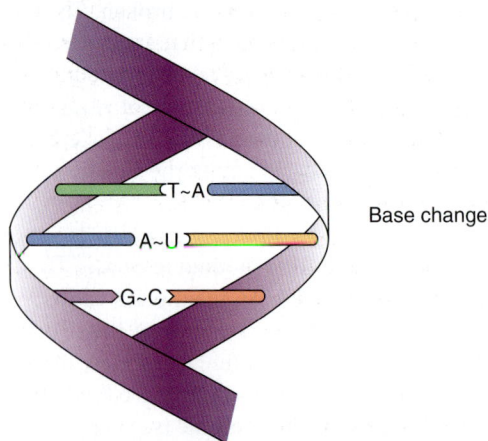

Fig. 6.9 Alteration of the nitrogen base sequence on the DNA chain caused by the action of ionizing radiation directly on a DNA molecule.

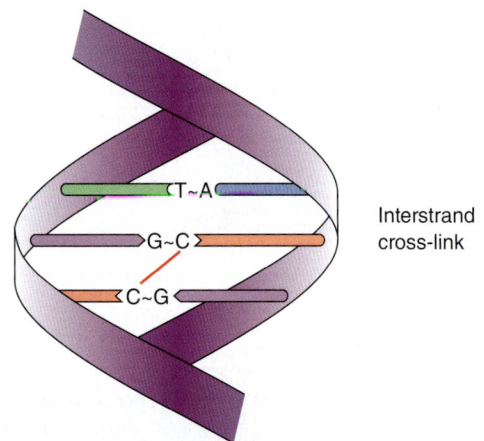

Fig. 6.10 Interstrand covalent crosslink produced by high-LET radiation acting directly on a DNA molecule.

and anaphase stages of the cell division cycle, when the length of the chromosomes is visible. Because the events that precede these phases of cell division are not observable, they can only be assumed to have occurred. What can be seen, however, is the effect of these events—the gross or apparent differences in the structure of the chromosome. Both somatic cells and reproductive cells are subject to chromosome breaks induced by radiation.

Chromosomal Fragments. After chromosome breakage, two or more chromosomal fragments are produced. Each of these fragments contains a fractured extremity. These broken ends are chemically very active and therefore have a strong tendency to adhere, or chemically combine, to another similar end. The fractured fragments can:

- Rejoin in their original configuration
- Fail to rejoin and create an aberration (lesion or anomaly)
- Join to other broken fragments and thereby create new chromosomes that may not appear structurally altered compared with the chromosome before irradiation

Chromosome Anomalies. Two types of chromosome anomalies have been observed at metaphase. They are:

- Chromosome aberrations and
- Chromatid aberrations

Chromosome aberrations result when irradiation occurs early in interphase, before DNA synthesis takes place. In this situation, the break caused by ionizing radiation is in a single strand of chromatin, which is the original chromosome. During the DNA synthesis that follows, the resultant break is replicated when this strand of chromatin lays down an identical strand adjacent to itself (called the *sister chromatid*) if repair is not complete before the start of DNA synthesis. This situation leads to a chromosome aberration in which both chromatids (the arms of the new chromosome) exhibit the break. The break is visible at the next mitosis. Each daughter cell generated will have inherited a damaged chromatid as a consequence of a failure in the repair mechanism. Solitary chromatid aberrations, conversely, result when irradiation of individual chromatids occurs later in interphase, after DNA synthesis has taken place. Then only one chromatid of the X-shaped pair may

undergo a radiation-induced break. Therefore only one daughter cell is affected.

Summary of Structural Changes Caused by Ionizing Radiation. Ionizing radiation interacts randomly with matter, expending energy in the process. Because of this energy transfer, exposure to radiation can lead to the occurrence of a variety of harmful effects in biologic tissue, including the following in cell nuclei:

- A single-strand break in one chromosome
- A break in one chromatid
- A single-strand break in separate chromosomes
- A strand break in separate chromatids
- More than one break in the same chromosome
- More than one break in the same chromatid
- Chromosome stickiness, or clumping together

Consequences to the Cell from Structural Changes Within the Nucleus

1. *Restitution,* the breaks rejoin in their original configuration with no visible damage (Fig. 6.11). In this case, no injury to the cell occurs because the chromatid has been restored to its original condition. The process of healing by restitution is believed to be how 95% of single-chromosome breaks mend.[4]
2. *Deletion,* a part of the chromosome or chromatid is lost at the next cell division, thus creating an aberration known as an *acentric fragment* (Fig. 6.12), which results in a cell mutation.
3. *Broken-end rearrangement,* a grossly misshapen chromosome may be produced. Ring chromatids, dicentric chromosomes, and anaphase bridges are examples of such distorted chromosomes and chromatids (Fig. 6.13). This results in a cell mutation.
4. *Broken-end rearrangement without visible damage to the chromatids,* whereby the chromatid's genetic material has been rearranged, yet the chromatid appears normal. Translocations are examples of such rearrangements (Fig. 6.14). This results in a cell mutation.

Changes such as those outlined in items 2, 3, and 4 inevitably result in mutation because the positions of the genes on the chromatids have been rearranged, thus altering the heritable characteristics of the cell.

Target Theory

The biologic effects of exposure to radiation stem primarily from the ionizations occurring at *sensitive*

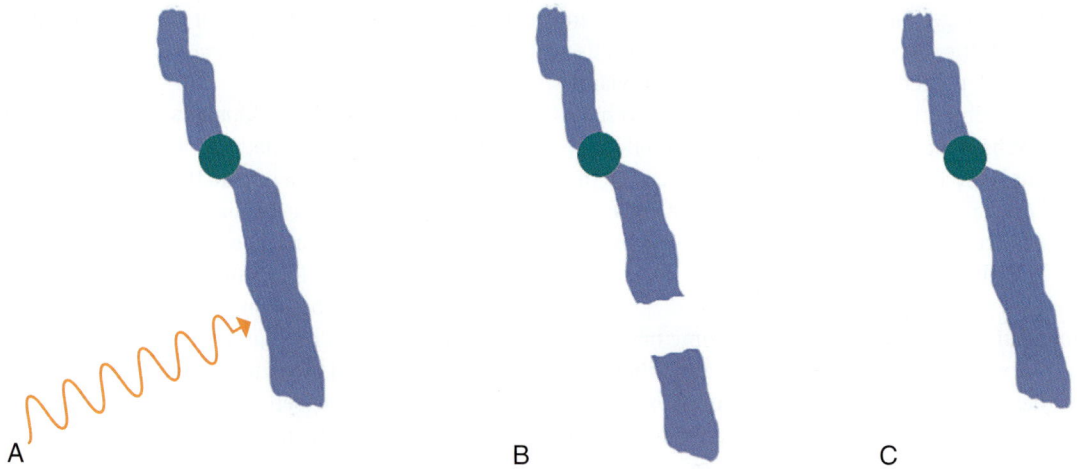

Fig. 6.11 The process of restitution, whereby the breaks rejoin in the original configuration with no visible damage. (A) The chromatid (single-strand chromosome) break occurs because of a photon interaction. (B) The fragment is fully separated from the rest of the chromatid. This same type of damage could occur to a metaphase or X-shaped chromosome if S phase had already occurred. (C) The broken fragment has reattached in its original location through the action of repair enzymes.

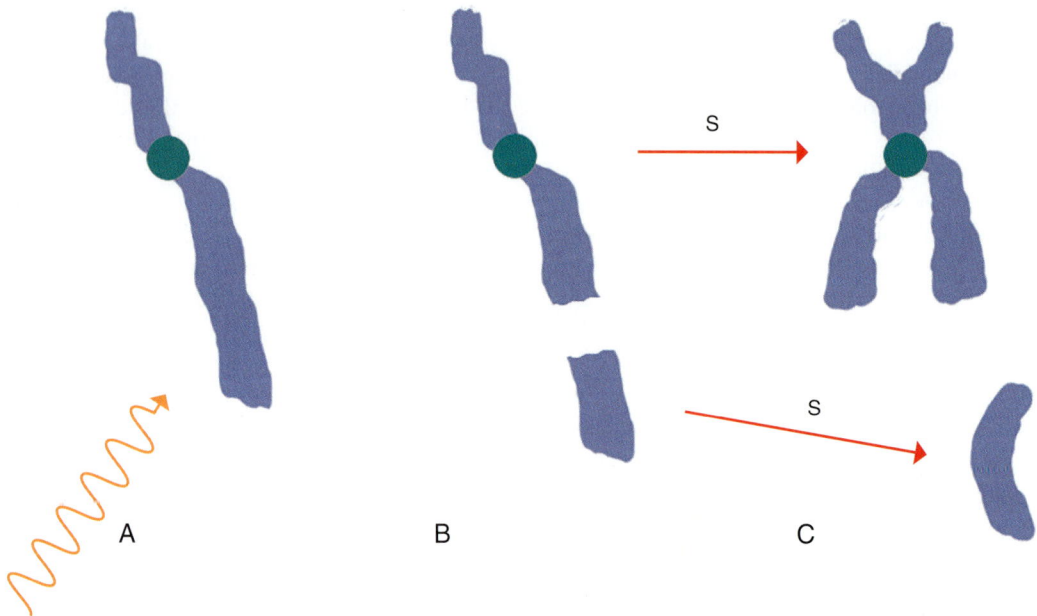

Fig. 6.12 The process of deletion, in which part of a chromosome is lost at the next cell division, thus creating an acentric fragment. (A) The chromatid or single-strand chromosome break results from a photon interaction. (B) The fragment is fully separated from the rest of the chromatid. (C) After the next DNA synthesis phase of the cell cycle (labeled S), the remainder of the single-strand chromosome has been replicated normally, but with fragments missing from the two arms of the metaphase chromosome. The replicated fragment is acentric, a section of genetic material without a centromere.

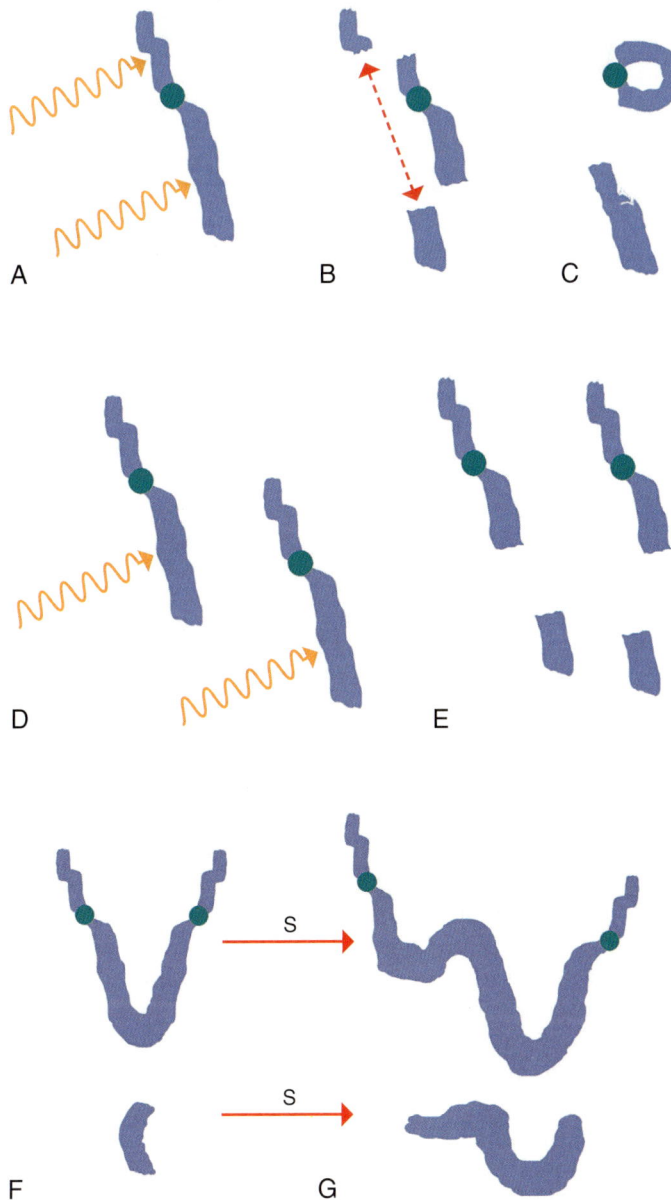

Fig. 6.13 The process of broken-end rearrangement may result in grossly misshapen chromatids. (A) Two chromatid breaks occur in a single chromatid as a result of the interactions of two photons. (B) The fragments from opposite ends unite before the DNA synthesis phase. (C) The ends of the chromatid that are still attached to the centromere also unite and form a "ring" chromatid. (D) Chromatid breaks occur in two different chromatids. (E) The fragments are fully separated from the rest of their respective chromatids. (F) The ends of the chromatids and the ends of the fragments have joined before DNA synthesis, thus forming a dicentric (two centromeres) and an acentric (no centromere) fragment. (G) After DNA synthesis (labeled S), the chromatid is elongated but cannot split in two. The two centromeres are "bridged." This type of chromatid damage leads to reproductive death of the cell (i.e., it cannot replicate or divide into two cells).

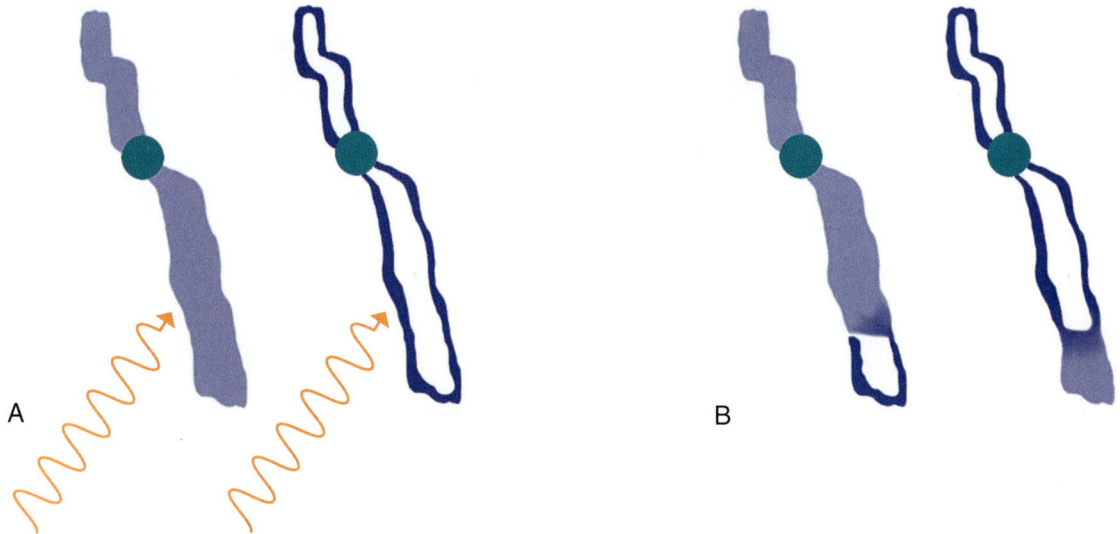

Fig. 6.14 If radiation breaks off parts of two different chromatids that are near each other (A) then the broken parts may reattach to the wrong chromatids (B) resulting in no visible damage. However, this rearrangement of genetic material may drastically alter a cell's function and lead to cell death or failure to replicate. This same type of damage could occur to a chromosome if S phase had already occurred. In this case, the cell may divide, but the genetic material in the daughter cells is compromised and those cells may not function properly.

cellular points secondary to energy transfers from radiation. These affected sites in a cell or, more specifically, on a vital molecule within the cell are known as *targets*. Whether or not such sites are struck by radiation is a random process. From all existing evidence, it appears that producing a serious effect typically requires more than one radiation "hit" on a specific target. The damage from a single hit ordinarily is not conclusive because of repair mechanisms. This concept of radiation damage to specific sensitive locations resulting from discrete and random events is known as **target theory**.

To summarize the importance of target theory, among the many different types of molecules that lie within the cell, a master, or key, molecule that maintains normal cell function, and thereby ensures cell survival, is considered to be present (Fig. 6.15). Because this molecule is unique in any given cell, no similar molecules in the cell are available to replace it; if a critical location on the master molecule is a *target* receiving multiple hits from ionizing radiation, the master molecule may be inactivated. Healthy cell function will then cease, and the cell will die (Fig. 6.16). If, conversely, it receives only a single hit, then the master molecule most likely will still be operational. Experimental data

strongly support this concept and confirm that DNA is the irreplaceable master, or key, molecule that exists as the preeminent vital target. Destruction of other important large-scale molecules that are present in the cell does not typically result in cell death. The reason is that cells have a number of similar molecules to take control and perform necessary functions in the event of the destruction of one or more of the molecules. Consequently, if only a few non-DNA cell molecules are made dysfunctional by radiation exposure, the cell will probably not display any evidence of injury after irradiation.

As radiation passes through the molecular structure of living systems, it does not preferentially seek out master molecules in cells to destroy them; it interacts with these key molecules only by chance. The target theory concept is useful for understanding both cell death and nonfatal cell abnormalities caused by exposure to radiation.

Interactions between ionizing radiation and molecular targets such as DNA occur through both direct and indirect action. However, discerning which of the two types of effects or actions has been at work in any given case of cell death is virtually impossible.

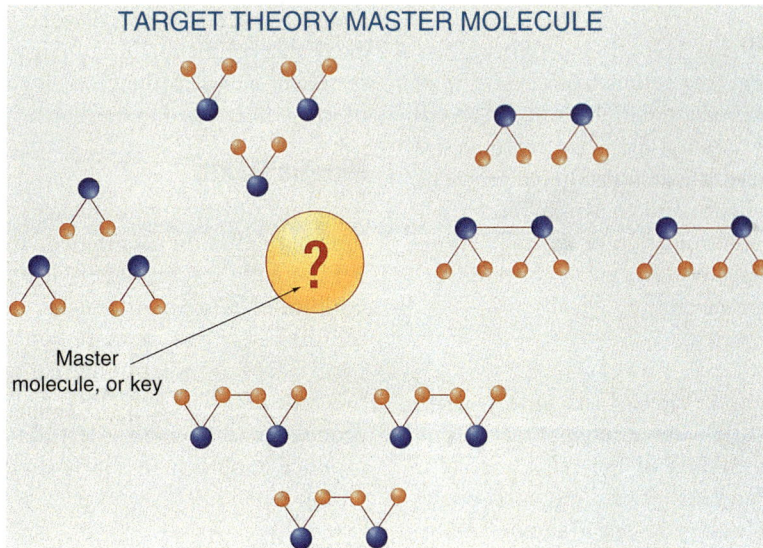

Fig. 6.15 The *yellow circle* depicts a target that represents a potential location for either *direct hits* from external incident radiation or *indirect hits* caused by the formation of very interactive free radicals from incident radiation interactions with the numerous water molecules surrounding the target. (From *Radiobiology and radiation protection: Mosby's radiographic instructional series,* St. Louis, 1999, Mosby.)

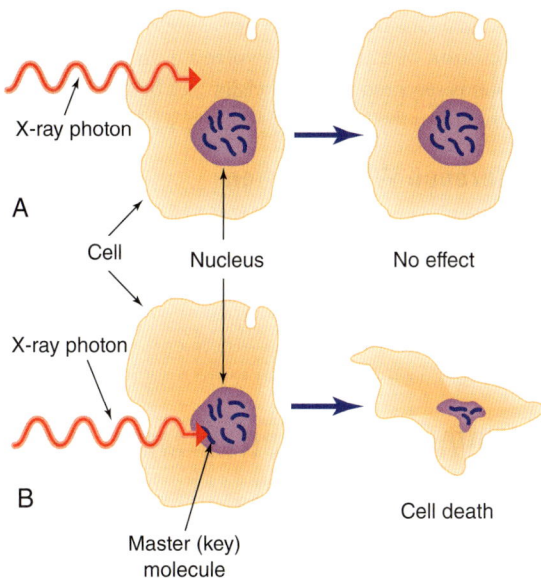

Fig. 6.16 The target theory holds that the cell will die after exposure to ionizing radiation only if the master, or key, molecule (DNA) is inactivated in the process. (A) An x-ray photon passes through the cell without interacting with the master molecule, which is located in the cell's nucleus, no measurable effect results. (B) An x-ray photon enters the nucleus and interacts with and inactivates the master molecule; the cell dies as a result.

EFFECTS OF IRRADIATION ON THE ENTIRE CELL

For the cell as a whole, damage to the cell's nucleus reveals itself in one of the following conditions:
1. Instant death
2. Reproductive death
3. Apoptosis, or programmed cell death (interphase death)
4. Mitotic, or genetic, death
5. Mitotic delay
6. Interference with function

Instant Death

Instant death of large numbers of cells occurs when a volume is irradiated with an x-ray or gamma ray dose of approximately 1000 Gy_t in seconds or a few minutes. This massive influx of energy causes gross disruption of cellular form and structure and severe changes in chemical machinery. As a result of receiving such an enormous dose of ionizing radiation, the cell's DNA macromolecule breaks up and cellular proteins coagulate. Radiation doses high enough to cause this type of damage are vastly more significant than those used for diagnostic examinations or even standard therapeutic treatments.

Reproductive Death

Reproductive death generally results from exposure of cells to doses of ionizing radiation in the range of 1 to 10 Gy_t. Although the cell does not die when reproductive death occurs, it permanently loses its ability to procreate but continues to metabolize and to synthesize nucleic acids and proteins. The termination of the cell's reproductive capabilities does, however, prevent the transmission of damage to future generations of cells.

Apoptosis

A non-mitotic, or non-division, form of cell death that occurs when cells die without attempting division during the interphase portion of the cell life cycle is apoptosis or programmed cell death. Apoptosis occurs spontaneously in both healthy tissue and tumors. Apoptosis can occur in human beings and other vertebrate animals and amphibians, both in the embryo and in the adult. An example of this process is the sequence of events during embryonic development whereby tadpoles lose their tails.

Certain types of *programmed cell death* are integral to the development and maintenance of organisms. Many types of cells are destined to die for the good of the organism. For example, human beings lose webbing between their digits during embryonic development, and throughout life, human skin cells die, are replenished, and maintain the protective outer coating known as *skin*. In apoptosis the cell shrinks and produces tiny membrane-enclosed structures called *blebs*. The cell nucleus breaks up and then the cell itself breaks up, and its fragments are usually ingested by neighboring cells.

Researchers believe that apoptosis may be instigated by radiation under some circumstances. The mechanisms of apoptosis and its relationship with radiosensitivity are areas of active research in radiobiology. It appears that the radiosensitivity of the individual cell governs the dose required to induce apoptosis; the more radiosensitive the cell is, the smaller the dose required to cause apoptotic death during interphase. For example, a few hundred centigray (cGy_t) can initiate apoptosis in sensitive cells such as lymphocytes or spermatogonia, but for less radiosensitive cells, such as those in bone, it seems that apoptosis may require radiation doses of several thousand cGy_t. A special type of radiation therapy seeks to involve activation of the genes that regulate

apoptosis so that its occurrence becomes much more likely after irradiation in a tumor. It should be noted that the phenomenon of apoptosis is considered by many to be integrally related to the "ageing process."

Mitotic Death

Ionizing radiation can adversely affect cell division. Ionizing radiation may impede the mitotic process or permanently inhibit it; cell death follows permanent inhibition. *Mitotic,* or *genetic, death* occurs when a cell dies after one or more divisions. Even relatively small doses of radiation have a possibility of causing this type of cell death. The radiation dose required to produce mitotic death is less than the dose needed to produce apoptosis in slowly dividing cells or nondividing cells.

Mitotic Delay

Exposing a cell to as little as 10 cGy_t of ionizing radiation just before it begins dividing can cause *mitotic delay,* the failure of the cell to start dividing on time. After this delay the cell may resume its normal mitotic function. The underlying cause of this phenomenon is not known. Possible reasons for the delay are as follows:

1. Alteration of a chemical involved in mitosis
2. Proteins required for cell division not being synthesized
3. A change in the rate of DNA synthesis after irradiation

Interference With Function

Permanent or temporary interference with cellular function independent of the cell's ability to divide can also be brought about by exposure to ionizing radiation. If repair enzymes are able to repair the damage, the cell can recover and continue to function properly. Otherwise, the cell will be unable to reproduce or will die.

SURVIVAL CURVES FOR MAMMALIAN CELLS

Cells vary in their radiosensitivity. This fact is particularly important in determining the types of cancer cells that will respond to radiation therapy. A classic method of displaying the sensitivity of a particular type of cell to radiation is the cell survival curve.[5] A cell survival curve is constructed from data obtained by a series of experiments. First, the cells are made to grow "in culture," meaning in a laboratory environment such as a Petri dish. Then the cells are exposed to a specified

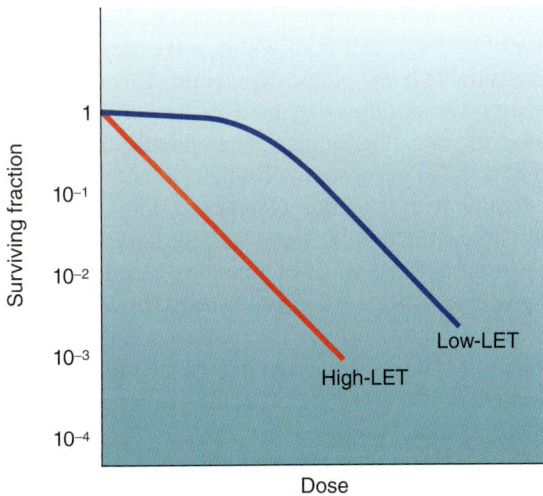

Fig. 6.17 Cell survival curves for the same cell line irradiated with both low- and high-linear energy transfer (LET) radiation. With low-LET radiation, a "shoulder" to the curve at lower doses indicates the cell's ability to repair some damage at low doses. High-LET radiation typically has no shoulder, thus indicating that little or no repair takes place.

dose of radiation. After radiation exposure, the ability of the cells to divide, or form new "colonies" of cells, is measured. The fraction of cells that are able to form new colonies through cell division is then reported as the fraction of cells that have survived irradiation. The process is repeated for a range of radiation doses, and the results are graphed with the logarithm* of the surviving fraction on the vertical axis and the dose on the horizontal axis.

Fig. 6.17 demonstrates two cell survival curves, one for high-LET radiation and one for low-LET radiation. The curve for low-LET radiation exhibits a *shoulder* that displays very little change in survival at low doses, followed by a linear portion in which survival decreases in regular proportions at higher doses. This response indicates that, at low doses, the cell can locate and repair some of the damage. At higher doses the repair mechanism is overwhelmed. For the high-LET curve, no

*In the ordinary decimal counting system, the logarithm (log) of a number N is, by definition, the power to which 10 must be raised to give N (e.g., log 1000 = 3 because 10^3 = 1000). So using logarithm values as one axis of an x–y graph permits a convenient display of very wide-ranging (orders of magnitude) data values.

BOX 6.4 Examples of Radiosensitive and Radioinsensitive Cells

Radiosensitive Cells	Radioinsensitive Cells
Basal cells of the skin	Brain cells
Blood cells such as lympho-	Muscle cells
cytes and erythrocytes	Nerve cells
Intestinal crypt cells	
Reproductive (germ) cells	

survival shoulder exists. If damage occurs, it is usually so extensive that it is irreparable.

CELL RADIOSENSITIVITY

Cell Maturity and Specialization

The human body is composed of different types of cells and tissues, which vary in their degree of radiosensitivity. Immature cells are nonspecialized (undifferentiated) and undergo rapid cell division, whereas more mature cells are specialized in their function (highly differentiated) and divide at a slower rate or do not divide. These factors affect the cells' degree of radiosensitivity. Examples of radiosensitive and radioinsensitive cells are listed in Box 6.4. Because combinations of both immature and mature cells in various ratios form the different body tissues and organs, radiosensitivity varies from one tissue and organ to another.

Oxygen Enhancement Effects

If oxygen is present when a tissue is irradiated, more free radicals will be formed in the tissue; this increases the indirect damage potential of the radiation.

During imaging procedures, fully oxygenated human tissues are exposed to x-radiation or gamma radiation. However, both radiographic and nuclear medicine procedures employ low doses of radiation that are also low LET. Consequently, very few cells are killed by the types of radiation used in these procedures.

In radiation therapy, the presence of oxygen plays a significant role in radiosensitivity and, thereby, treatment efficacy. Cancerous tumors often contain both hypoxic cells, which lack an adequate amount of oxygen, and normally aerated cells. The poorly oxygenated cells severely inhibit the indirect mechanism of radiation interaction with cells and therefore are noticeably radioresistant, particularly to low-LET radiation. However, when oxygen tension in capillaries is increased by high pressure (hyperbaric) oxygenation, hypoxic cells may reoxygenate and become more sensitive to radiation; consequently, the chances of them being destroyed by the indirect action of therapeutic radiation increases. Thus, in the treatment of certain types of cancerous tumors that are known to be significantly oxygen-depleted, hyperbaric oxygen treatments have occasionally been employed in conjunction with standard megavoltage x-ray radiation therapy to enhance the radiation's destruction of tumor cells. Radiosensitization of hypoxic cells has also been accomplished with chemical-enhancing agents, such as misonidazole and variants thereof.[3]

Law of Bergonié and Tribondeau

In 1906, Jean A. Bergonié, a French radiologist, and Louis F. A. Tribondeau, a French physician, observed the effects of ionizing radiation on testicular germ cells of rabbits exposed to x-rays. These researchers established that radiosensitivity was a function of the metabolic state of the cell receiving the exposure. Their findings eventually became known as the **Law of Bergonié and Tribondeau**, stating that the radiosensitivity of cells is directly proportional to their reproductive activity and inversely proportional to their degree of differentiation. Thus the most pronounced radiation effects occur in cells with the least maturity and specialization or differentiation, the greatest reproductive activity, and the longest mitotic phases.[6] Although the law was initially applied only to germ cells, it is true for all types of cells in the human body. Consequently, within the realm of diagnostic imaging, the embryo-fetus, which contains a large number of immature nonspecialized cells, is much more susceptible to radiation damage than is an adult or even a child. All imaging professionals should be ever mindful of this.

Effects of Ionizing Radiation on Human Cells and Tissues

The more mature and specialized in performing functions a cell is, the less sensitive it is to radiation. In the following sections, the radiation response of some of the most critical cell groups is examined in detail.

Blood Cells

Hematologic depression. Ionizing radiation adversely affects blood cells by depressing the number of active cells in the peripheral circulation. A whole-body dose of 0.25 Gy_t delivered within a few days produces a measurable hematologic depression. This dose by far exceeds average doses sustained by the working population of the radiation industry. Therefore the use of blood count tests for purposes of dosimetry is not valid.

Depletion of immature blood cells. Most blood cells are manufactured in the bone marrow. Radiation causes a decrease in the number of immature blood cells (stem or precursor) produced in the bone marrow and hence a reduction, ultimately, in the number of mature blood cells in the bloodstream. The higher the radiation dose received by the bone marrow, the higher will be the resulting cell depletion.

Repopulation after a period of recovery. If the bone marrow cells have not been destroyed by exposure to ionizing radiation, they can repopulate after a period of recovery. The time necessary for recovery depends on the magnitude of the radiation dose received. If a relatively low dose (less than 1 Gy_t) of radiation is received, bone marrow repopulation occurs within weeks after irradiation. Large (1 to 10 Gy_t) to very high (10 or more Gy_t) doses, which severely deplete the number of bone marrow cells, require a more extended recovery period. Very high doses of radiation can cause a permanent decrease in the number of stem cells.

Effects on stem cells of the hematopoietic system. Radiation primarily affects the stem cells of the hematopoietic (blood-forming) system. Erythrocytes, also known as *red blood cells* because of their reddish color due to the presence of hemoglobin*, are the primary carriers of oxygen to the tissues and organs of the body. These transport cells are among the most radiosensitive of human cells. As with all cells, however, that develop from an immature, undifferentiated state to a mature, functional state, the *mature red blood cells*, which do not have a cell nucleus, are much less radiosensitive. Because the population of circulating red blood cells is high and their life span is long, depletion of red blood

---

*Hemoglobin is the main functional component of the red blood cell. It serves as an oxygen-carrying protein. Iron is present within its molecular structure. Because an iron atom has two valence electrons, it can readily bind chemically with a molecule of oxygen. Thus the hemoglobin protein has an affinity for oxygen, which, when achieved, is expressed by the formation of an iron oxide combination. This creates the red color for which the cell is known.

cells is not usually the cause of death in high-dose irradiation (i.e., several Gy_t delivered to the whole body). Death, if it occurs, is typically caused by infection that cannot be overcome by the immune system because of the destruction of *myeloblasts* (an immature cell of bone marrow that is the most basic precursor of granulocyte* white blood cells) and internal hemorrhage resulting from destruction of megakaryoblasts (cells that are the ancestors of platelets**).

Whole-body doses in excess of 5 Gy_t. Humans who receive whole-body doses above 5 Gy_t may die within 30 to 60 days because of effects related to initial depletion of the stem cells of the hematopoietic system. The use of antibiotics or isolation from pathogens in the environment (e.g., placing the patient in a sterile environment, feeding only sterilized food) has been proven to mitigate these effects in animals and humans. Humans, however, recover more slowly than do laboratory animals. The lethal dose in animals is usually specified as LD 50/30 (the dose that produces death in 50% of the subjects within 30 days). The lethal dose in humans is generally stated as LD 50/60 because a human's recovery is slower than that of the laboratory animals, and death may still occur at a later time after a substantial whole-body exposure. Whether survival lasts for 30 days or 60 days, the lethal whole-body dose for humans is generally estimated to be 3.0 to 4.0 Gy_t without treatment and higher if medical intervention is available. Table 6.1 presents an overview of LD 50/30 for various species.

Effects of ionizing radiation on lymphocytes. White blood cells, *leukocytes,* include cells with and without the small grains known as *granules.* Lymphocytes belong to the granule-free category and are of importance in defending the body against foreign substances (antigens) by producing protective proteins (antibodies) to combat disease. Lymphocytes, which survive for only approximately 24 hours, have the shortest life

*Granulocytes, cells that have visible small grains called *granules* inside the cell, are a category of white blood cells that are essential in fighting infections.

**Platelets, also known as *thrombocytes,* are small cell fragments that originate in the bone marrow as pieces broken off from large cells. They continuously circulate within the blood and when they recognize damaged blood vessels, clump together in large numbers at the damaged site, as a result causing a plug or blood clot.

TABLE 6.1 LD 50/30 Values for Various Species

Species	LD 50/30 Gy_t
Human being	3.0–4.0*
Monkey	4.0–4.75
Dog	3.0
Hamster	7.0
Rabbit	7.25
Rat	9.0
Turtle	15.0
Newt	30.0

*Depending on the source of the radiation exposure, LD 50/30 (dose that produces death in 50% of the subjects within 30 days) varies. LD 50/30 may be higher if medical intervention is available. For humans, LD 50/60 may be more realistic because humans are more likely to survive longer than 30 days after an acute whole-body exposure, especially if medical treatment is provided.

span of all blood cells. Lymphocytes are manufactured in the bone marrow and are the most radiosensitive blood cells in the human body. A whole-body radiation dose as low as 0.25 Gy_t is sufficient to noticeably decrease the number of viable lymphocytes present in the circulating blood. When significant numbers of lymphocytes are functionally damaged by radiation exposure, the body loses its natural ability to combat infection and becomes very susceptible to bacterial and viral antigens.

The normal white blood cell count for an adult ranges from 5000 to 10,000/mm³ of blood. At a dose of 0.25 Gy_t or less, blood cell count recovery occurs shortly after irradiation. However, when a higher dose of whole-body radiation (0.5 to 1 Gy_t) is received, the lymphocyte count decreases to zero within a few days. Full recovery generally requires several months after this level of exposure. During that period the body is highly susceptible to antigens.

Effects of ionizing radiation on neutrophils. Neutrophils, another type of white blood cell, but belonging to the granule-containing category, also play an essential role in fighting infection. A whole-body dose of 0.5 Gy_t of ionizing radiation will noticeably reduce the number of neutrophils present in the circulating blood, causing a person to be susceptible to infection. When larger doses of radiation (2 to 5 Gy_t) are received, these cells decrease in actual number to 10% or less within a few weeks of irradiation, with a consequently high potential for severe infection. In this latter situation, it will require several months after the exposure until the number of viable neutrophils present in the blood returns to its original value.

Effects of ionizing radiation on thrombocytes (platelets). Thrombocytes, or platelets, initiate blood clotting and prevent hemorrhage. Thrombocytes have a life span of approximately 30 days. The normal platelet count in the human adult ranges from 150,000 to 350,000/mm³ of blood. A dose of radiation higher than 0.5 Gy_t lessens the number of platelets in the circulating blood, A dose of radiation in the range of 1 to 10 Gy_t, will significantly deplete these cells, and it will take approximately 2 months for them to repopulate. During this period wound clotting will be highly compromised.

Radiation exposure during diagnostic imaging procedures. Neither the blood nor the blood-forming organs of patients should undergo appreciable damage from radiation exposure received during diagnostic imaging procedures. However, numerous studies indicate the inducement of some chromosome aberrations in circulating lymphocytes that have received radiation doses within the diagnostic radiology range. Prime candidates for developing such irregularities are patients either for whom *high-level* fluoroscopy was employed or for whom very long fluoroscopic exposure times occurred (e.g., cardiac catheterization and other specialized invasive procedures).

Monitoring of patients undergoing radiation therapy treatment. A therapeutic dose of ionizing radiation, especially doses delivered to locations that include blood-forming organs, decreases the blood count. Consequently, patients who are undergoing radiation therapy treatment are monitored frequently (in the form of weekly or biweekly complete blood counts, also known as *CBCs*) to determine whether all of their functioning blood constituent counts are adequate.

Occupational radiation exposure monitoring. A periodic blood count is not recommended as a method for monitoring occupational radiation exposure because biologic damage has already occurred when an irregularity is seen in the blood count. In addition, a blood count is a relatively insensitive test that is unable to indicate doses of less than 10 cGy_t accurately. State-of-the-art optically stimulated luminescence (OSL) dosimeters and direct ion storage dosimeters can detect effective radiation doses and therefore may be used to reveal

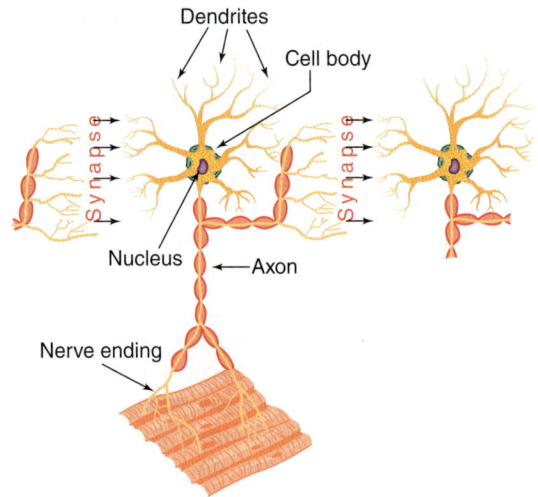

Fig. 6.18 A nerve cell (neuron). Nerve cells relay messages to and from the brain. A message enters a nerve cell through its dendrites, passes through the cell body, and exits the cell through the axon, which transmits the message across a synapse, the communication area leading to the next nerve cell in the chain.

potentially hazardous working conditions before actual harm occurs.

Epithelial Tissue. Epithelial tissue lines and covers body tissue. The cells of these tissues lie close together, with few or no substances between them. Epithelial tissue is devoid of blood vessels, and it regenerates through the process of mitosis. The cells are found in the lining of the intestines, the mucous lining of the respiratory tract, the pulmonary alveoli (tiny air sacs), and the lining of blood and lymphatic vessels. Because the body continually regenerates epithelial tissue, the cells that comprise this tissue are highly radiosensitive.

Muscle Tissue. Muscle tissue contains fibers that affect the movement of an organ or part of the body. Since muscle tissue cells are highly specialized and do not divide, they are relatively insensitive to radiation.

Nervous Tissue. Nervous tissue (conductive tissue) is found in the brain and spinal cord. A nerve cell (neuron) (Fig. 6.18) consists of a cell body, which contains its nucleus, and two kinds of string-like tissue segments, called *processes,* that extend outward from the cell body, namely: *dendrites* (fine tentacle-like extensions that carry impulses toward the cell) and the *axon* (a broad, long, tentacle that carries impulses away from it). Nerve cells relay messages to and from the brain. A message enters the nerve cell through the dendrites. Next, it passes through the cell body and exits the cell through the axon, which transmits the message across a *synapse*, the communicating area leading to the next nerve cell in the chain.

Nerve tissue in the human adult. In the adult, nerve cells are highly specialized. Nerve cells perform specific functions for the body and, similar to muscle cells, do not divide. Nerve cells contain a nucleus. If by exposure to radiation, the nucleus is destroyed, the cell dies and is never restored. If the cell nucleus is damaged, but not destroyed by the radiation, the damaged nerve cell may continue to function but in an impaired fashion. Radiation can also cause temporary or permanent damage in a nerve cell's processes (dendrites and axon). When this occurs, communication with and control of some areas of the body may be disrupted. Whole-body exposure to very high doses of radiation causes severe damage to the entirety of the central nervous system (CNS). A single exposure of radiation above 50 Gy_t of ionizing radiation may lead to death within a few hours or days at the most.

Nerve tissue in the embryo-fetus. Developing nerve cells in the embryo-fetus are more radiosensitive than are the mature nerve cells of the adult. Irradiation of the embryo can lead to CNS anomalies, microcephaly (small head circumference), and intellectual disability. The study of the Japanese atomic bomb survivors provides strong evidence of a "window of maximal sensitivity" extending from 8 to 15 weeks after gestation. This time covers the end of *neuron organogenesis* (a period of development and change of the nerve cells) into the beginning of the fetal period. After this a lower level of elevated risk remains until week 25, at which time the risk is not found to be significantly different from that of young adults. During the window of maximal sensitivity, a 0.1 Sv (10 rem) fetal EqD is associated with as much as a 4% chance of intellectual disability. This level is considered significant compared with risks during a healthy pregnancy. Therefore special consideration is dedicated to the irradiation of the abdomen or pelvis of a pregnant patient, particularly during the period of highest sensitivity. The fetal EqD associated with abdominal fluoroscopy, however, is generally about 0.05 Sv (5 rem). Thus, if the referring physician and radiologist believe that the diagnostic imaging procedure is vital to the medical management of the mother or embryo-fetus, the risk associated with the needed radiation exposure may be justified. For such a situation a genetic study may be recommended afterwards.

Reproductive Cells

Spermatogonia. Human reproductive cells (germ cells) are relatively radiosensitive, although the exact responses of male and female germ cells to ionizing radiation vary since their processes of development from immature to mature status differ. The male testes contain both mature and immature spermatogonia. Because the developed spermatogonia are specialized and do not divide, they are relatively insensitive to low-LET ionizing radiation. The "young" spermatogonia, however, are unspecialized and divide rapidly, and therefore these germ cells are very radiosensitive. A radiation dose of 2 Gy_t may cause temporary sterility for as long as 12 months, and a dose of 5 or 6 Gy_t can cause permanent sterility. Even small doses of ionizing radiation (doses as low as 0.1 Gy_t) could depress the male sperm population. Male reproductive cells that have been exposed to a radiation dose of 0.1 Gy_t or more may cause genetic mutations in future generations. To prevent mutations from being passed on to children, male patients receiving this level of testicular radiation dose should refrain from unprotected sexual relations for a few months after such an exposure. By that time, cells that were irradiated during their most sensitive stages will have matured and disappeared. It is highly unlikely that germ cells of patients undergoing diagnostic imaging procedures would ever receive doses of 0.1 Gy_t, and radiographers working under normal occupational conditions would never receive a gonadal dose of this level.

Ova. The ova, the mature female germ cells, do not divide continuously. After puberty, one of the two ovaries expels a mature ovum approximately every 28 to 36 days (the exact number of days varies among women). During the reproductive life of a woman (from approximately 12 to 50 years old), 400 to 500 mature ova are produced. The radiosensitivity of ova varies considerably throughout the lifetime of the germ cell. Immature ova are very radiosensitive, whereas more mature ova have little radiosensitivity. After irradiation, a mature ovum can still unite with a male germ cell during conception. However, these irradiated cells may contain damaged chromosomes. If fertilization of an egg with damaged chromosomes occurs, genetic damage can be passed on to the child, potentially resulting in congenital abnormalities. In general, whenever chromosomes in male or female germ cells are damaged by exposure to ionizing radiation, mutations can be passed on to succeeding generations. Even low doses of radiation received from diagnostic imaging procedures have a non-zero probability, although incredibly low, of initiating some chromosomal damage.

Significant exposure to ionizing radiation may cause female sterility. The dose necessary to produce sterility depends partly on the age of the patient. Infertility occurs when radiation exposure destroys ova. The ovaries of the female fetus and those of a young child are very radiosensitive since they contain a large number of stem cells (oogonia) and immature cells (oocytes). As the female child matures from birth to puberty, the number of immature cells (oocytes) decreases. Therefore the ovaries become less radiosensitive. This decrease continues up to the age of 30 years; women between the ages of 20 and 30 years exhibit the lowest level of sensitivity. After a woman reaches age 30 years, the *net sensitivity* of the ovaries now increases steadily until menopause because any additional ova that are destroyed are not replenished.[7-9] Thus, since the ovaries of a younger woman are *less sensitive overall* than the ovaries of an older woman, a higher dose of radiation is required to cause sterility in the younger woman.

Temporary sterility usually results from a single radiation dose of 2 Gy_t to the ovaries, but if the radiation dose is fractionated (i.e., given as a combination of smaller doses with time between doses) over several weeks, thus permitting the cells to repair some of the damage, doses as high as 20 Gy_t may be tolerated.[10,11] A single dose of 5 Gy_t generally causes permanent sterility in mature women. Even small doses of low-LET ionizing radiation (doses as low as 0.1 Gy_t) could cause menstrual irregularities, such as delay or suppression of menstruation. Although some evidence suggests that immature ova are capable of repairing radiation damage, women who have received 0.1 Gy_t or more are sometimes advised to postpone attempting conception for 30 days or more to allow the damaged immature ova to be expelled.

SUMMARY

- Linear energy transfer (LET)
  - LET is the average energy deposited per unit length of track by ionizing radiation as it passes through and interacts with a medium along its path.
    - LET is described in units of keV per micron (1 micron [μm] = 10^{-6} m).
  - The LET value of the radiation involved is a significant factor in assessing potential tissue and organ damage from exposure to that type of ionizing radiation.
  - Low-LET radiation (x-rays and gamma rays) doses that are not excessive primarily cause indirect damage to biologic tissues that usually can be reversed by repair enzymes.
  - High-LET radiation (alpha particles, ions of heavy nuclei, and low-energy neutrons) can produce irreparable damage to DNA because of inducing multiple-strand breaks that cannot be undone by repair enzymes.
- Relative biologic effectiveness (RBE)
  - RBE of the type of radiation being used is the ratio of the dose of a reference radiation (conventionally 250-kVp x-rays) to the dose of radiation of the type in question that is necessary to produce the same biologic reaction in a given experiment. The response is what is provided by a dose of test radiation delivered under the same conditions.
  - The concept of RBE is not practical for specifying radiation protection dose levels in humans. Therefore to overcome this limitation, a radiation weighting factor (W_R) is used to calculate the equivalent dose (EqD) to determine the ability of a dose of any type of ionizing radiation to cause biologic damage.
- Oxygen enhancement ratio (OER)
  - OER is a comparative measure used to obtain the amount of cellular injury for a species of ionizing radiation under poorly oxygenated conditions. Specifically, OER is the ratio of the radiation dose required to cause a particular biologic response of cells or organisms in an oxygen-deprived environment to the radiation dose required to generate an identical response under normal oxygenated conditions.
- Radiation-induced biologic damage in living systems is observed on molecular, cellular, and organic systems levels.

- Radiation action on the cell is either direct or indirect, depending on the site of interaction.
  - If sufficient quantities of somatic cells are affected by exposure to ionizing radiation, entire body processes can be disrupted. Conversely, if radiation damages the germ cells, the damage may be passed on to future generations in the form of genetic mutations.
  - Action is direct when biologic damage occurs as a result of the ionization of atoms on essential molecules (e.g., DNA, RNA, proteins, enzymes) produced by straight interaction with the incident radiation.
  - Action is indirect when effects are produced by free radicals created by the interaction of radiation with water molecules; these unstable, highly reactive chemical combinations can cause substantial disruption to vital macromolecules such as DNA and result in cell death.
  - Because the human body is 80% water and less than 1% DNA, virtually all effects of low-LET irradiation in living cells result from indirect action.
  - Point lesions commonly occur with low-LET radiation and are often reversible through the action of repair enzymes.
  - Double-strand breaks of DNA happen more commonly with densely ionizing (high-LET) radiation and often are associated with the loss of one or more nitrogenous bases. The chance of repair from this type of damage is very low; the possibility of a lethal alteration of nitrogenous bases within the genetic sequence is far greater.
  - When two interactions, one on each of the two sugar–phosphate chains, occur within the same rung of the DNA ladder-like configuration, the result is a cleaved or broken chromosome, with each new portion containing an unequal amount of genetic material. If this damaged chromosome divides, each new daughter cell will receive an incorrect amount of genetic material, resulting in either death or impaired functioning of the new daughter cell.
  - Because the genetic information to be passed on to future generations is contained in the strict sequence of nitrogenous bases, the loss or change of a base in the DNA chain represents a mutation.
  - Chromosome aberrations and chromatid aberrations are two types of chromosome anomalies that have been observed at metaphase.

- Consequences to the cell from structural changes within the nucleus can result in restitution, deletion, broken-end rearrangement with or without visible damage to the chromatids.
- Target theory states that when a vital macromolecule or target such as cell DNA is directly or indirectly inactivated by exposure to radiation, the cell will die.
- When a cell nucleus is significantly damaged by exposure to ionizing radiation, the cell can die or experience reproductive death, apoptosis, mitotic death, mitotic delay, or interference with function.
- The cell survival curve is used to display the radiosensitivity of a particular type of cell, which helps determine the types of cancer cells that will respond to radiation therapy.
- The law of Bergonié and Tribondeau states that the most pronounced radiation effects occur in cells with the least maturity and specialization or differentiation, the greatest reproductive activity, and the longest mitotic phases.
  - The embryo-fetus is very susceptible to radiation damage, which can cause central nervous system (CNS) anomalies, microcephaly, and intellectual disability.
  - Lymphocytes are the most radiosensitive blood cells, and when they are damaged the body loses its natural ability to combat infection and becomes more susceptible to bacterial and viral antigens.
  - Because the body continually regenerates epithelial tissue, the cells comprising this tissue are highly radiosensitive.
  - Muscle tissue is relatively insensitive to radiation.
  - Nerve cells in the adult are highly specialized. If the cell nucleus has been damaged but not destroyed by exposure to radiation, the damaged nerve cell may still be able to function but in an impaired fashion. Radiation can cause temporary or permanent damage to a nerve's processes, thus disrupting communication with and control of some body functions.
  - Developing nerve cells in the embryo-fetus are more radiosensitive than are the mature nerve cells of the adult. Studies indicate that the eighth to the fifteenth week after gestation is the time frame of maximal radiosensitivity. A lower but still significant level of risk remains until the 25th week after gestation.
  - Human germ cells are relatively radiosensitive, although the exact responses of male and female germ cells to ionizing radiation differ because

their courses of development from immature to mature status differ. For both males and females, temporary sterilization occurs at 2 Gy_t, and permanent sterilization occurs at 5 to 6 Gy_t.

GENERAL DISCUSSION QUESTIONS

1. How does ionizing radiation damage living systems?
2. What are three characteristics of ionizing radiation that influence energy transfer into biological tissue?
3. What are the three radiation energy transfer determinants?
4. Why can x-rays and gamma rays be referred to as a stream of particles called photons?
5. What are the three levels of biological damage that may occur from ionizing radiation exposure?
6. What is the target theory in relation to ionizing radiation?
7. What are six effects of irradiation on the entire cell resulting from damage to the cell's nucleus?
8. What is the purpose and function of survival curves for mammalian cells?
9. What factors affect cell radiosensitivity?
10. What does the law of Bergonié and Tribondeau state?

REVIEW QUESTIONS

1. What is a primary mechanism by which ionizing radiation causes damage to living cells?
   A. Inducing apoptosis
   B. Ionization of molecules
   C. Increasing cellular respiration
   D. Enhancing protein synthesis
2. Which characteristic of ionizing radiation relates to how much energy is deposited per unit length of tissue?
   A. Relative Biological Effectiveness (RBE)
   B. Linear Energy Transfer (LET)
   C. Oxygen Enhancement Ratio (OER)
   D. Photon energy
3. What is the term for the increased effectiveness of radiation in the presence of oxygen?
   A. Linear Energy Transfer
   B. Relative Biological Effectiveness
   C. Oxygen Enhancement Ratio
   D. Radiation Dose Rate
4. X-rays and gamma rays are often described as streams of particles known as:
   A. Electrons
   B. Neutrons
   C. Protons
   D. Photons
5. Which of the following is NOT a level of biological damage from ionizing radiation?
   A. Cellular damage
   B. Tissue damage
   C. Organismal damage
   D. Molecular repair
6. In target theory, the critical target for ionizing radiation is typically:
   A. The cell membrane
   B. The cytoplasm
   C. The DNA
   D. The mitochondria
7. Which of the following describes the effect of irradiation known as "mitotic death"?
   A. Immediate cell death
   B. Cell division failure due to DNA damage
   C. Programmed cell death
   D. Temporary cell dysfunction
8. What is the primary purpose of survival curves for mammalian cells?
   A. To assess cell differentiation
   B. To evaluate the effectiveness of radiation therapy
   C. To measure cellular respiration rates
   D. To analyze DNA mutations
9. Which factor is NOT known to affect cell radiosensitivity?
   A. Cell type
   B. Oxygen levels
   C. Temperature
   D. Cell cycle stage
10. According to the law of Bergonié and Tribondeau, which type of cells are generally more radiosensitive?
    A. Highly differentiated cells
    B. Slowly dividing cells
    C. Rapidly dividing, less differentiated cells
    D. Mature muscle cells

Early Effects of Radiation Exposure

OBJECTIVES

After completing this chapter, the reader will be able to perform the following:

- Define all key terms.
- Identify factors affecting early tissue reactions and the time frames in which these reactions appear.
- List and describe several possible high-dose consequences of ionizing radiation on living systems.
- Describe acute radiation syndrome (ARS), and list three separate dose-related syndromes that occur as part of this total-body condition.
- Identify and describe the four major response stages of ARS.
- Explain why cells that are exposed to sublethal doses of ionizing radiation recover after irradiation and discuss the cumulative effect that exists after repeated radiation injuries.
- Describe local tissue damage that occurs when any part of the human body receives high radiation exposure.
- List three factors affecting organ and tissue responses to radiation exposure.
- Describe radiation-induced skin damage from a historical perspective.
- Differentiate among the three layers of human skin, and identify other related accessory structures.
- State the single absorbed dose of ionizing radiation that can cause radiation-induced skin erythema within 24 to 48 hours after irradiation, and describe how this dose initially manifests.
- Explain the difference between moderate and large radiation doses with regard to epilation.
- State the energy range of grenz rays, and provide a historical example of their use in treating disease.
- Discuss the concept of orthovoltage radiation therapy treatment, and identify its effects on human skin.
- Discuss the impact on human skin when high-level fluoroscopy is utilized for extended periods during cardiovascular or therapeutic interventional procedures.
- Define cytogenetics, and explain how cytogenetic analysis of chromosomes may be accomplished.
- Explain the process of karyotyping, and identify the phase of cell division in which chromosome damage caused by radiation exposure can be evaluated.
- List two types of chromosomal aberrations that can be caused by exposure to ionizing radiation, and explain what determines the rate of production of these aberrations.

CHAPTER OUTLINE

KEY TERMS

acute radiation syndrome (ARS)
biologic dosimetry
cytogenetics
desquamation
early tissue reactions
epilation
genetic effects

genetic mutations
grenz rays
karyotype
latent period
manifest illness
metaphase
pluripotential stem cell

prodromal stage
radiodermatitis
recovery
somatic effects
somatic tissue reactions

When biologic effects of radiation occur relatively soon after humans receive high doses of ionizing radiation, the biologic responses demonstrated are referred to as early effects. Numerous laboratory animal studies and data from observation of some irradiated human populations provide substantial evidence of the consequences of such responses. Although early tissue reactions are not common in diagnostic imaging, they are discussed in this chapter to provide the reader with a broader and more complete understanding of the impact of high radiation exposure on the human body.

SOMATIC AND GENETIC EFFECTS

The term *somatic* originates from the Greek term "soma" meaning "body." Therefore, somatic effects are effects upon the body that was irradiated. Genetic effects are effects upon future generations due to the irradiation of germ cells in previous generations.

SOMATIC EFFECTS

Depending on the length of time from the moment of irradiation to the first appearance of symptoms of radiation damage, somatic effects are classified as either early or late.

This chapter discusses *early* somatic radiation effects on organ systems. If the consequences include cell killing and are directly related to the dose received, they are somatic tissue reactions. As the radiation dose increases, the severity of early somatic tissue reactions also increases. These results have a threshold, a point at which they begin to appear and below which they are absent (Fig. 7.1). The amount of biologic damage depends on the actual absorbed dose of ionizing radiation.

Early Tissue Reactions

Early tissue reactions vary depending on the duration of time after exposure to ionizing radiation. They may appear within:

* Minutes

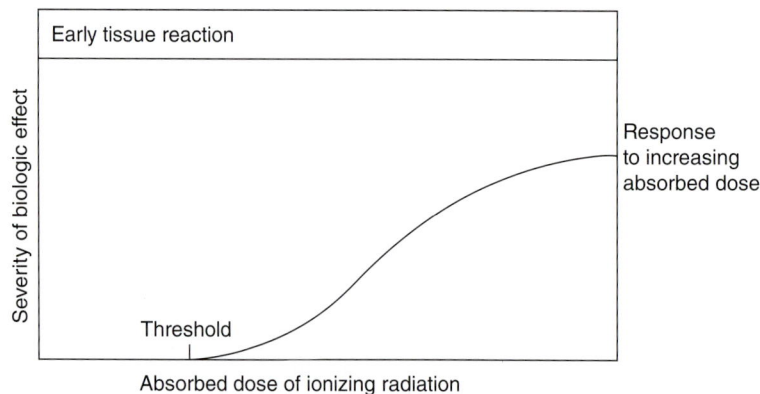

Fig. 7.1 This graph demonstrates the existence of a threshold whereby early tissue reactions of an absorbed dose of ionizing radiation begin and increase in severity as the dose of radiation received increases.

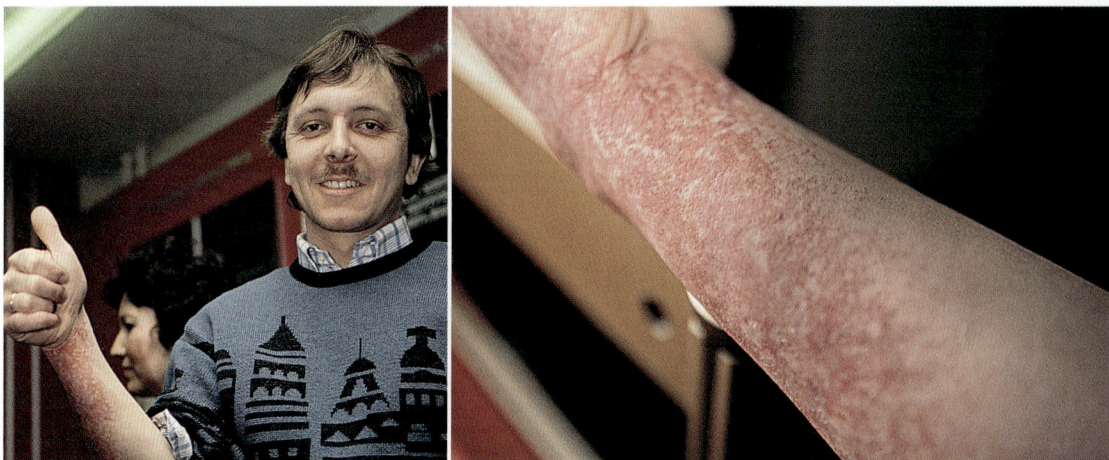

Fig. 7.2 Radiation burns or erythema on the arm of a former worker, who was present at the Chernobyl nuclear power plant during the 1986 radiation accident. (From Ken Graham Photography.)

- Hours
- Days
- Weeks

A substantial dose of ionizing radiation is required to produce biologic changes very soon after irradiation, and the severity of these changes is dose-related. Early tissue reactions are caused by cell death.

Except for specific lengthy high-dose-rate fluoroscopic procedures, diagnostic imaging examinations do not typically impose radiation doses sufficient to cause early tissue reactions. Thus, they are of little concern in this modality. It should be noted, however, that prolonged exposure to x-rays in the diagnostic energy range results in a high radiation dose to the skin, whereas underlying tissues receive a substantially lower dose. Therefore, unacceptably high x-ray exposures in radiology result primarily in skin effects, which are discussed later in this chapter. For completeness of knowledge of radiobiology, radiographers are also expected to understand the consequences of large doses of radiation to the whole body, as would result from exposure to types of radiation other than x-rays.

Possible high radiation dose consequences include:

- Nausea
- Fatigue
- Erythema (diffuse redness over an area of skin after irradiation) (Fig. 7.2)
- Epilation (loss of hair)
- Blood disorders
- Intestinal disorders

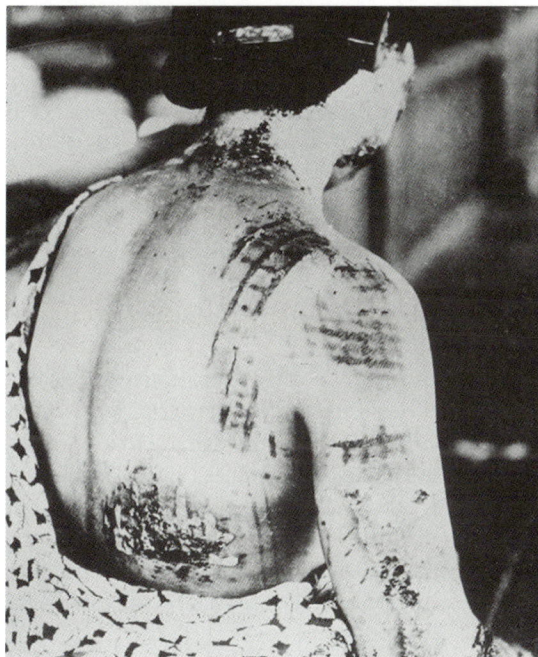

Fig. 7.3 Dry and moist desquamation. The back of this female Japanese atomic bomb survivor demonstrates the pattern of the kimono she was wearing at the time of the bombing. Radiation burns resulting in the shedding of the outer layer of skin is visible. (From PhotoAssist, Inc.)

- Fever
- Dry and moist desquamation (shedding of the outer layer of skin) (Fig. 7.3)
- Depressed sperm count in the male

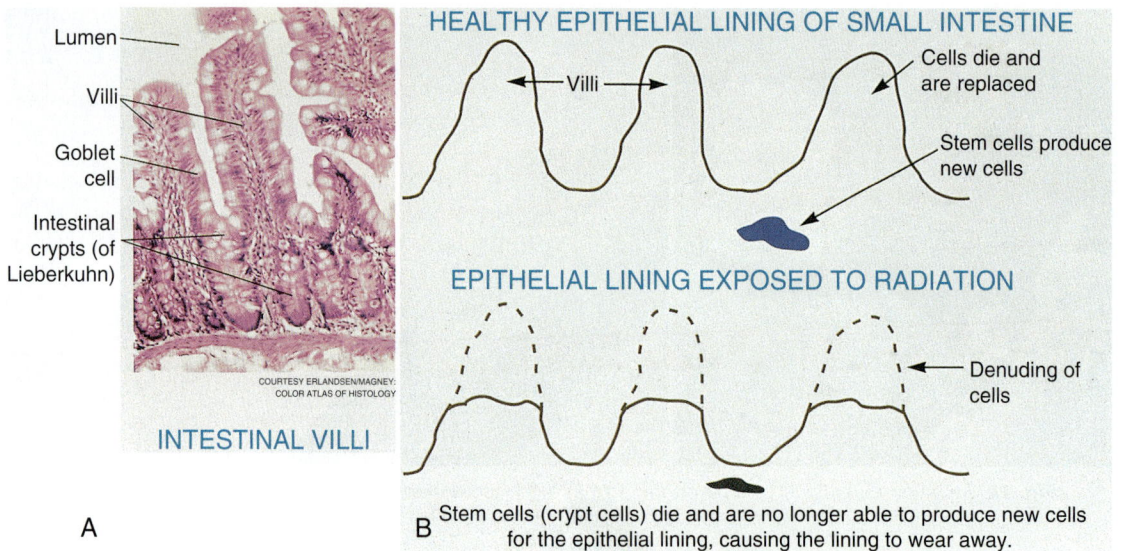

HEALTHY EPITHELIAL LINING OF SMALL INTESTINE

Lumen
Villi
Goblet cell
Intestinal crypts (of Lieberkuhn)

COURTESY ERLANDSEN/MAGNEY:
COLOR ATLAS OF HISTOLOGY

INTESTINAL VILLI

Villi
Cells die and are replaced
Stem cells produce new cells

EPITHELIAL LINING EXPOSED TO RADIATION

Denuding of cells

A

B   Stem cells (crypt cells) die and are no longer able to produce new cells for the epithelial lining, causing the lining to wear away.

Fig. 7.4 (A) Intestinal villi. These are small, finger-like projections that extend into the lumen of the small intestine. Each villus is approximately 0.5–1.6 mm in length. They absorb nutrients from food and move them into the bloodstream. (B) The top drawing depicts the healthy lining of the small intestine. The bottom drawing shows the epithelial lining of the small intestine after it has been exposed to radiation. Stem cells (crypt cells) die and are no longer able to produce new cells for the epithelial lining, thus causing the lining to wear away. (From *Radiobiology and radiation protection: Mosby's radiographic instructional series,* St. Louis, 1999, Mosby.)

- Temporary or permanent sterility in the male and female
- Injury to the central nervous system (at extremely high radiation doses)

The various types of organic damage may be related to the cellular effects discussed in Chapter 6. For example, intestinal disorders are caused by damage to the sensitive epithelial tissue lining the intestines (Fig. 7.4). When the whole body is exposed to a dose of 6 Gy_t of ionizing radiation, many of these manifestations of organic damage occur soon after that and in succession. These early tissue reactions are known as **acute radiation syndrome (ARS)**.

Acute Radiation Syndrome (ARS). ARS, or radiation sickness, occurs in humans after large whole-body doses of ionizing radiation are delivered over a short period (from several hours to a few days). Data from epidemiologic studies of human populations exposed to doses of ionizing radiation sufficient to cause this syndrome have been obtained from:

- Atomic bomb survivors of Hiroshima and Nagasaki
- Marshall Islanders who were inadvertently subjected to high levels of fallout during an atomic bomb test in 1954

- Nuclear radiation accident victims, such as those injured in the 1986 Chernobyl disaster
- Patients who have undergone radiation therapy

Symptoms of acute radiation syndrome. *Syndrome* is the medical term that defines a collection of symptoms. Thus, ARS is a collection of symptoms associated with high-level radiation exposure. Three separate dose-related syndromes or conditions occur as part of the acute radiation syndrome:

- Hematopoietic syndrome
- Gastrointestinal syndrome
- Cerebrovascular syndrome

Hematopoietic syndrome. The hematopoietic form of ARS, or "bone marrow syndrome," occurs when people receive whole-body doses of ionizing radiation ranging from 1 to 10 Gy_t (Fig. 7.5). The hematopoietic system manufactures the corpuscular elements of the blood and is the most radiosensitive vital organ system in humans. Radiation exposure causes the number of red blood cells, white blood cells, and platelets in the circulating blood to decrease. Dose levels that produce this syndrome may also damage cells in other organ systems and cause the affected organ or organ system to fail.

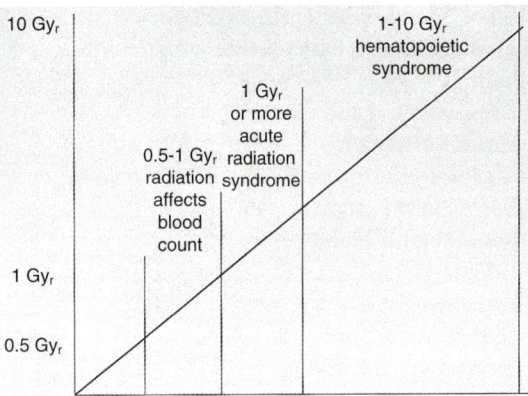

Fig. 7.5 The prodromal (early symptoms) stage of acute radiation syndrome occurs within hours after a whole-body absorbed dose of 1 Gy_t or more is received. Doses ranging from 1 to 10 Gy_t are responsible for causing the hematopoietic form of acute radiation syndrome. (From *Radiobiology and radiation protection: Mosby's radiographic instructional series*, St. Louis, 1999, Mosby.)

For persons with hematopoietic syndrome, survival time shortens as the radiation dose increases. Because bone marrow cells are being destroyed, the body becomes more susceptible to infection (mostly from its intestinal bacteria) and more prone to hemorrhage. When death occurs, it is because of excessive bone marrow destruction causing anemia and little or no resistance to severe infection.

Death may occur 6 to 8 weeks after irradiation in some susceptible human subjects who receive a whole-body dose just exceeding 2 Gy_t. But as the whole-body dose increases from 2 to 10 Gy_t, all irradiated individuals will die and in a shorter period. If the radiation exposure is, however, in the range of 1 to 2 Gy_t, bone marrow cells will eventually repopulate to a level adequate to support life in most individuals. Many of these people recover from 3 weeks to 6 months after irradiation. The irradiated person's general state of health at the time of irradiation strongly influences the possibility of recovery.

Survival probability of patients with hematopoietic syndrome is enhanced by intense supportive care and special hematologic procedures. As an illustration, victims who received doses above 5 Gy_t, such as those of the nuclear power station accident in Chernobyl, benefited from bone marrow transplants from appropriate histocompatible donors. During the surgical procedure, hematopoietic stem cells are transplanted to facilitate bone marrow recovery. This procedure, however, is not an absolute cure for patients with hematopoietic syndrome because many individuals undergoing bone marrow transplants die of burns or other radiation-induced damage they sustained before the transplanted stem cells have had a chance to support recovery.

Gastrointestinal syndrome. In humans, the gastrointestinal (GI) form of ARS appears at a threshold dose of approximately 6 Gy_t and peaks after a dose of 10 Gy_t. Without medical support to sustain life, exposed persons receiving doses of 6 to 10 Gy_t may die 3 to 10 days after being exposed. Even if medical assistance is provided, the exposed person will live only a few days longer. Survival time does not change with dose in this syndrome.

A few hours after the dose required to cause the GI syndrome has been received, the *prodromal*, or beginning, stage occurs. Severe nausea, vomiting, and diarrhea persist for as long as 24 hours. Next is a latent period, which may last for several days. During this time, the outward symptoms disappear. The *manifest illness* stage follows this period of false calm. Again, the human subject experiences:

- Severe nausea
- Vomiting
- Diarrhea
  Other signs and symptoms that may occur include:
- Fever (as in hematopoietic syndrome)
- Fatigue
- Loss of appetite
- Lethargy
- Anemia
- Leukopenia (decrease in the number of white blood cells)
- Hemorrhage (GI tract bleeding because the body loses its blood-clotting ability)
- Infection
- Electrolyte imbalance
- Emaciation

Fatality occurs primarily as a result of catastrophic damage to the epithelial cells that line the GI tract. This results in the death of the exposed person within 3 to 5 days from a combination of infection, fluid loss, and electrolytic imbalance. Although expiration from GI syndrome is primarily from damage to the bowel, it also can be induced by the destruction of the bone marrow.

The small intestine is the most severely affected part of the GI tract. Because epithelial cells function as an essential biologic barrier, their breakdown leaves the body vulnerable to:

- Infection (mostly from intestinal bacteria)
- Dehydration
- Severe diarrhea

Some epithelial cells regenerate in the period before death occurs. However, because of the large number of epithelial cells damaged by the radiation, death may occur before sufficient cell regeneration is accomplished. The workers and firefighters at Chernobyl who did not survive are examples of humans who died as a result of GI syndrome.

Cerebrovascular syndrome. The cerebrovascular form of ARS results when the central nervous system and cardiovascular system receive doses of 50 Gy$_t$ or more ionizing radiation. A dose of this magnitude can cause death within a few hours to 2 or 3 days after exposure. After irradiation, the prodromal stage begins. Signs and symptoms include:

- Excessive nervousness
- Confusion
- Severe nausea
- Vomiting
- Diarrhea
- Loss of vision
- Burning sensation of the skin
- Loss of consciousness

As with the GI syndrome, a latent period, only lasting up to 12 hours, follows. During this time, symptoms lessen or disappear. After the **latent period**, the manifest illness stage occurs. Other severe symptoms now appear, including:

- Disorientation and shock
- Periods of agitation alternating with stupor
- Ataxia (confusion and lack of muscular coordination)
- Edema in the cranial vault
- Loss of equilibrium
- Fatigue
- Lethargy
- Convulsive seizures
- Electrolytic imbalance
- Meningitis
- Prostration
- Respiratory distress
- Vasculitis
- Coma

Injured blood vessels and capillaries permit fluid to leak into the brain, increasing intracranial pressure, and causing tissue damage. The final result of this damage is the failure of the central nervous and cardiovascular systems, which brings death in a matter of minutes. Because the GI and hematopoietic systems are more radiosensitive than the central nervous system, they also fail to function after a dose of this magnitude. However, because death occurs quickly, the consequences of the failure of these two systems are not demonstrated.

An overview of acute radiation lethality is presented in Table 7.1. The radiation dose required to cause a

TABLE 7.1	**Overview of Acute Radiation Lethality**		
Stage	**Dose (Gy$_t$)**	**Average Survival Time**	**Symptoms**
Prodromal	1	Not Applicable	Nausea, vomiting, diarrhea, fatigue, leukopenia
Latent	1–100	Not Applicable	None
Hematopoietic	1–10	6–8 wk (doses over 2 Gy$_t$)	Nausea; vomiting; diarrhea; decrease in number of red blood cells, white blood cells, and platelets in the circulating blood; hemorrhage; infection
Gastrointestinal	6–10	3–10 days	Severe nausea, vomiting, diarrhea, fever, fatigue, loss of appetite, lethargy, anemia, leukopenia, hemorrhage, infection, electrolytic imbalance, and emaciation
Cerebrovascular	50 and above	Several hours to 2–3 days	Same as hematopoietic and gastrointestinal, plus excessive nervousness, confusion, lack of coordination, loss of vision, burning sensation of the skin, loss of consciousness, disorientation, shock, periods of agitation alternating with stupor, edema, loss of equilibrium, meningitis, prostration, respiratory distress, vasculitis, coma

particular syndrome and the average survival time are the most important measures used to quantify human radiation dose lethality. The progression of each syndrome, the length of time required for the consequential chain of events to occur, and the outcome depend on the effective dose received.

Acute radiation syndrome as a consequence of the Chernobyl nuclear power plant accident. The massive explosion that blew apart the unit 4 reactor at the nuclear power station in Chernobyl in the Soviet Union on April 26, 1986, provides an example of humans developing ARS. During the explosion, several tons of burning graphite, uranium dioxide fuel, and other contaminants such as cesium-137, iodine-131, and plutonium-239 were ejected upward into the atmosphere in a 3-mile-high radioactive plume of intense heat. Of 444 people working at the power plant at the time of the explosion, two died instantly, and 29 died within 3 months of the accident as a consequence of thermal trauma and severe injuries caused by whole-body doses of ionizing radiation of approximately 6 Gy_t or more.[1-3]

Without useful physical monitoring devices, biologic criteria such as the occurrence of nausea and excessive vomiting played an essential role in the identification of radiation casualties during the first 2 days after the nuclear disaster. ARS caused the hospitalization of at least 203 people.[3,4] Determining the lapse of time from the exposure of the victims to the onset of nausea and vomiting completed the biologic criteria. Dose assessment was determined from serial measurements of levels of lymphocytes and granulocytes in the blood and quantitative analysis of the frequency of dicentric chromosomes (altered chromosomes with two centromeres) present in blood and hematopoietic cells, originating from bone marrow. The data were compared with doses and effects from earlier radiation mishaps.[2,3] An analysis in which damage to tissues is used to estimate radiation dose is referred to as **biologic dosimetry**.

Acute radiation syndrome as a consequence of the atomic bombing of Hiroshima and Nagasaki. The Japanese atomic bomb survivors of Hiroshima and Nagasaki are examples of a human population affected by ARS as a consequence of war. Follow-up studies of the survivors, who did not rapidly die of this syndrome, demonstrated late tissue reactions (e.g., cataracts) and stochastic effects of ionizing radiation, such as induction of leukemia. The atomic bombing of Japan and the nuclear accident at Chernobyl caused the medical community to recognize the need for a thorough understanding of ARS and the appropriate medical support of persons affected.

Lethal Dose

LD 50/30. The term *LD 50/30* signifies the whole-body dose of radiation that can be lethal to 50% of the exposed population within 30 days. As mentioned previously, the LD 50/30 for adult humans is estimated to be 3.0 to 4.0 Gy_t without medical support (Fig. 7.6). For x-rays and gamma rays, this is equal to an equivalent dose of 3.0 to 4.0 sievert (Sv). Whole-body doses greater than 8 Gy_t will cause the death of the entire population in 30 days without medical support. With intense medical support, some human beings have survived doses as high as 8.5 Gy_t.[5]

LD 10/30, LD 50/60, and LD 100/60. Other measures of lethality also are quoted, such as *LD 10/30, LD 50/60,* and *LD 100/60.* These measures refer to the percentage

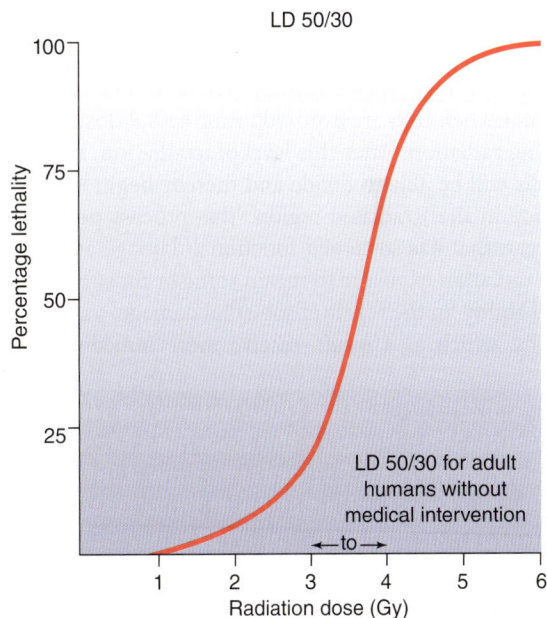

Fig. 7.6 LD 50/30 refers to the whole-body dose of radiation that can be lethal to 50% of the exposed population within 30 days. As can be seen in the graph, no deaths are expected below 1 Gy_t. In this particular graph, which represents the human response to radiation exposure, LD 50/30 is reached at 3.5 Gy_t. This is the point at which half of those exposed to 3.5 Gy_t of ionizing radiation would die. The graph also demonstrates that at a dose of 6 Gy_t, no one is expected to survive. In reality, survival is possible with extensive medical intervention.

of subjects who die after a specified number of days. The values reported in the literature vary widely because most lethal dose data represent an estimate of the role played by radiation in fatalities, while often, other factors (e.g., fire at Chernobyl, physical effects of a large explosion at Hiroshima and Nagasaki, chemical contamination in some nuclear accidents) were present. The medical treatment further complicates the exact specifications of fatal effects that the patient may receive during the prodromal and latent stages before many of the symptoms of ARS appear. When medical treatment is provided promptly, the patient is treated for initial symptoms, and so, answering the question of long-term survival may be delayed. For this reason, LD 50/60 for humans is perhaps the most accurate measure for human survival than any shorter period. Table 7.2 presents estimates of lethal doses, including the treatment provided in the populations studied. Regardless of treatment, whole-body equivalent doses of greater than 12 Gy_t are considered fatal.[6]

Repair and Recovery

Since cells contain a repair mechanism inherent in their biochemistry (repair enzymes), repair and recovery can occur when cells are exposed to sub-lethal doses of ionizing radiation. After this level of irradiation, surviving cells will be able to divide and thereby begin to repopulate in the irradiated region. This process permits an organ that has sustained functional damage as a result of radiation exposure to regain some or most of its useful ability. In the repair of sublethal damage, oxygenated cells, which as a result, receive more nutrients, allow

for a better prospect for recovery than do hypoxic, or poorly oxygenated, cells that consequently receive fewer nutrients. When both cell categories are exposed to a comparable dose of low-LET radiation, the oxygenated cells are more severely damaged, but those that survive can repair themselves and recover from the injury. Even though they are less severely damaged, the hypoxic cells do not repair and recover as efficiently.

Research has shown that repeated radiation injuries have a cumulative effect. Hence a percentage, approximately 10%, of the radiation-induced damage will be irreparable, whereas the remaining 90% may be repaired over time.

Local Tissue Damage

A destructive response in biologic tissue is likely to occur when any part of the human body receives a high radiation dose. Significant cell death usually results, leading to the shrinkage of organs and tissues, a process referred to as *atrophy*. Atrophied organs and tissues can lose their ability to function, or they may recover. If recovery does occur, it may be partial or complete, depending on the types of cells involved and the dose of radiation received. Should this not happen, then necrosis, or death, of the irradiated biologic structure results.

Organ and tissue response to radiation exposure depend on factors such as:
- Radiosensitivity
- Reproductive characteristics
- Growth rate

Some local tissues suffer immediate consequences from high radiation doses. Examples of such tissues include the following:
- Skin
- Male and female reproductive organs
- Bone marrow

Effects on the Skin

From the experiences of early pioneers, radiation accident victims, atomic bomb survivors, and patients who have received radiation therapy or unusually high doses during prolonged fluoroscopy in certain areas, a considerable amount of information is available on radiation-induced skin damage. Recall that many early radiologists and dentists developed radiodermatitis, a significant reddening of the skin caused by excessive exposure to relatively low-energy ionizing radiation that eventually led to cancerous lesions on the hands and

TABLE 7.2 Lethal Dose Values for Healthy Adults Who Receive the Specified Medical Treatment After Exposure to Low–Linear Energy Transfer Radiation at Dose Rates of more than 100 mGy$_a$/min (10 rads/min)		
Effect	**Treatment**	**Dose (Gy$_a$)**
LD 50/60	Minimal	3.2–4.5
LD 50/60	Optimal supportive	4.8–5.4
LD 50/60	Autologous bone marrow transplantation	11

From Fry RJM: Acute radiation effects. In Wagner LK, Fabrikant JI, Fry RJM, editors: *Radiation bioeffects and management: test and syllabus,* Reston, VA, 1991, American College of Radiology.

fingers. In 1898 after personally suffering severe burns, which he ultimately attributed to accumulated radiation exposure, William Herbert Rollins, a Boston dentist, began investigating the potential hazards of radiation exposure. His experimentation led to him becoming the first known determined advocate for radiation protection. Rollins performed experiments on guinea pigs that led to "three important safety practices for radiographers: wear radiopaque glasses; enclose the x-ray tube in protective housing; and irradiate only areas of interest on the patient, covering adjacent areas with radiopaque materials."[7] Unfortunately, at the time Rollins made these insightful recommendations, they were not given much attention. The misfortune of ignoring his suggestions led to continuing radiation-induced injuries. Eventually, however, our pioneers did learn from their transgressions, and these recommendations became universally accepted.

The skin consists of three layers (Fig. 7.7):
- Epidermis, or outer, layer
- Dermis, or middle, layer composed of connective tissue
- Hypodermis, a subcutaneous layer of fat and connective tissue

Accessory structures include hair follicles, sensory receptors, sebaceous glands, and sweat glands. The layers of the skin, as well as the accessory structures, are actively involved in the response of the tissue to radiation exposure.

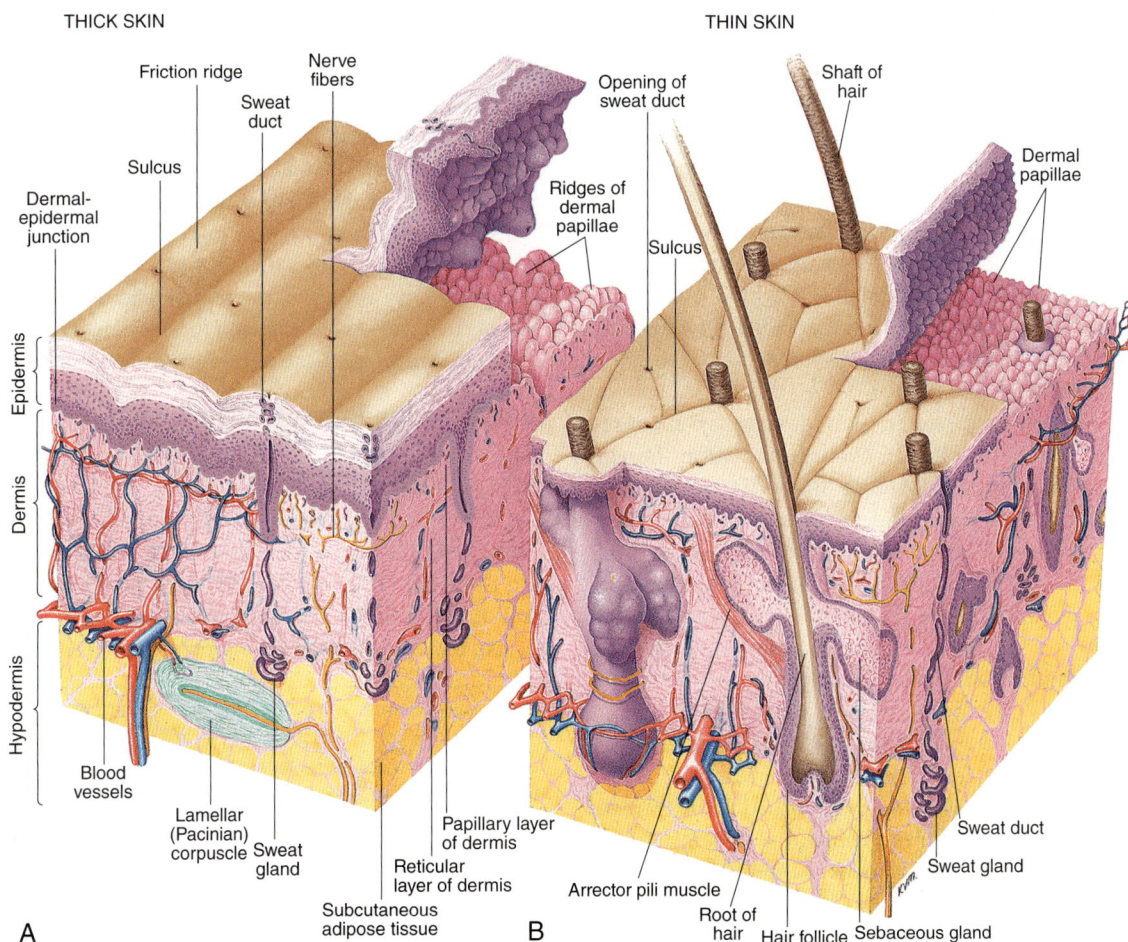

Fig. 7.7 Layers of the skin and accessory structures. (From Patton KT: *Anatomy and physiology*, ed 10, St. Louis, 2019, Elsevier.)

Because the skin functions as an ongoing regenerative protection system, it is relatively radiosensitive. Approximately 2% of the body's surface skin cells are replaced daily by stem cells from an underlying basal layer. The characteristics of these stem cells are responsible for the radiosensitivity of the skin. A single absorbed dose of 2 Gy_t can cause radiation-induced skin erythema within 24 to 48 hours after irradiation. As time progresses, over the next week or two, the erythema becomes much worse, until it reaches its maximal intensity. **Desquamation**, or shedding of the outer layer of skin, occurs at higher radiation doses. Desquamation generally manifests first as moist skin peeling, and then a dry skin flaking may develop (see Fig. 7.3).

Epilation, or hair loss (also called *alopecia*), can be caused by exposure to radiation since hair follicles are growing tissue. Moderate doses of radiation generally produce temporary hair loss, whereas large radiation doses can result in permanent hair loss.

Historically, skin diseases, such as ringworm, were treated and successfully cured by irradiating the affected area with **grenz rays** (x-rays in the energy range of 10 to 20 kVp).[5] These very low-energy photons were adequate to cure the disease. However, if the ringworm was located on the scalp, the local irradiation also caused the hair to fall out, which would typically be followed by regrowth, provided the radiation dose delivered to the patient was not sufficient to cause permanent hair loss.

Significant evidence of skin damage as a consequence of exposure to orthovoltage radiation therapy (x-rays in the range of 200 to 300 kVp), occurred in oncology patients who underwent such treatments in earlier years for deep-seated tumors. When orthovoltage irradiation was utilized for this purpose, the ability of a person's skin to tolerate this exposure actually determined the total amount of treatment radiation the individual could receive. Single-portal orthovoltage radiation treatments caused the patient's skin to obtain a considerably higher radiation dose than the dose received by the tumor because radiation in this energy range was substantially absorbed while traversing the skin and other intervening tissue layers before it reached the tumor. Thus, to deliver a specific dose to the tumor, the superficial, or skin dose, would unavoidably be significantly greater than the tumor dose. Modern radiation therapy treatment utilizes very much higher energy photons (ranging from 6 to 18 megaelectron volt [MeV] produced by linear accelerators*) that minimize skin surface effects and also employ multiple skin entrance locations. The combination of these two activities effectively spares the shallow body tissues from what would now be considered unacceptable exposure levels, while precisely delivering cell-killing doses to solid tumors at any depth and location within the body. High-energy gamma-emitting isotopes such as cobalt 60 (gamma-ray energy of 1.25 MeV) have also historically been utilized to spare skin while successfully treating non-superficial cancers.

The overall goal of any therapeutic treatment is to deposit the radiant energy to an overwhelming extent into an image-guided volume that both encloses the tumor and any microscopic extent of it and also includes a small added margin (this particular volume is called the *planning target volume* or PTV: it allows for uncertainties in planning and treatment delivery) while delivering a substantially lower dose to as much healthy surrounding tissue as possible. This treatment concept is called the therapeutic ratio.

During cardiovascular or other interventional procedures that use high-level fluoroscopy for extended periods, the effects of ionizing radiation on the skin can sometimes be significant. Patient exposure rates have been estimated to range from 100 to 200 mGy_a/min and occasionally even greater. As a result of numerous reported injuries to patients that were associated with the use of high-level fluoroscopy, imposing strict controls on its use is essential.

Effects on the Reproductive System

Some of the early tissue reactions from ionizing radiation have been discussed in Chapter 6.

Human germ cells are relatively radiosensitive. Doses as low as 0.1 Gy_t can depress the male sperm population, and this same dose has the potential to cause **genetic mutations** in future generations. In females, a gonadal dose of 0.1 Gy_t may delay or suppress menstruation.

---

*A linear accelerator is essentially a highly evacuated straight-line cylindrical device that, by virtue of superimposed strong oscillating electrical potentials, accelerates and focuses electrons, injected into it from a heated filament, into a narrow megavoltage energy beam. This beam is then directed by a magnetic field onto a high atomic number target (e.g., tungsten and/or lead). The resulting interactions generate highly energetic x-rays (megavoltage range), which are shaped by thick high atomic number collimators (typically lead or depleted uranium) into a useful beam that can be employed to effectively treat deep-seated tumors while greatly sparing superficial tissues.

Male:

Spermatogonia Spermatocyte Spermatid   Sperm

Female:

Primordial   Mature follicle Corpus luteum   Ovum
follicle

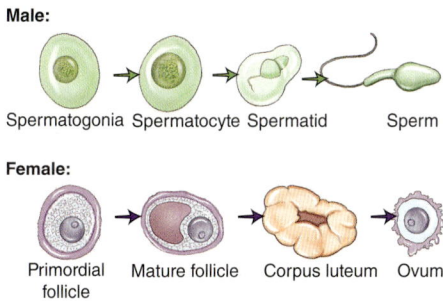

Fig. 7.8 Development of the germ cell from the stem cell phase to the mature cell.

Animal experiments and data from irradiated human populations have provided important information on gonadal response to radiation exposure. Irradiated human populations include:

- Patients who have undergone radiation therapy
- Radiation accident victims
- Volunteer convicts[8,9]

The testes of the male and the ovaries of the female do not respond in the same manner to irradiation because of the differences in the method by which these cells are produced and progress from elementary stem cells to mature cells. The spermatogonia, the stem cells of the testes, continually reproduce. They evolve and become spermatocytes. The latter cells then multiply and develop into spermatids that eventually differentiate and become spermatozoa, or sperm, which are the functionally mature germ cells (Fig. 7.8). The development of the male stem cell into a functionally mature germ cell takes 3 to 5 weeks.[5]

In the female, the oogonia, the ovarian stem cells, multiply to millions of cells only during fetal development, before birth, and then they steadily decline in number throughout life. During the latter part of fetal development, the oogonia become encapsulated by numerous primordial (primary) follicles that grow around them (see Fig. 7.8). The oogonia then become oocytes, which contain follicles that are nests of cells, some of which eventually mature during the reproductive life of a woman. Before these primary oocyte-containing follicles grow into mature follicles, they remain dormant until puberty. Then, just before puberty, the oocytes are reduced in number to only several hundred thousand. Some of the cells of the primary follicles proliferate in response to stimulation by hormones from the pituitary gland, and these cells begin to mature.

At the same time, the ovum contained within each of the follicles undergoes meiosis. As puberty begins, the developed ova, or mature female germ cells*, within the follicles are ejected when the follicles themselves rupture. Usually, only one follicle will fully mature and move toward the surface of the ovary to be expelled, and the others disintegrate. This process occurs at regular time intervals of approximately 28 days. Of the mature ova that are actually enclosed within the follicles, only 400 to 500 are produced, matured, and made available for fertilization during a woman's reproductive life.

Follicles range in size from small to large. Of these, the intermediate-size follicles are the most radiosensitive, and the small follicles are the least radiosensitive. Large, mature follicles possess only a moderate degree of radiosensitivity.[10] During the female menstrual cycle, a mature follicle releases an ovum during the period of ovulation, when a ripe egg is expelled from an ovary into the pelvic cavity. If a waiting male sperm does not fertilize that ovum in the uterus, it will be lost during menstruation and not replaced.

Hematologic Effects

As a brief review, recall that during the 1920s and 1930s, periodic blood counts were the only means of radiation exposure monitoring for radiation workers engaged in radiologic practices. The use of personnel dosimeters for monitoring occupational exposure made the simplistic practice obsolete. When blood counts were used to monitor the effects of radiation exposure among those who worked with radiation, a whole-body radiation dose of 0.25 Gy_t would be required to produce a measurable hematologic depression. Such a dose could cause enough of a decrease in the number of lymphocytes in the blood to render the body vulnerable to infection by foreign invaders. This method, therefore was completely unfounded for modern principles of radiation protection.

Hematopoietic System. The hematopoietic system consists of:

- Bone marrow
- Circulating blood
- Lymphoid organs (lymph nodes, spleen, and thymus gland)

---

*Mature female germ cells or eggs are those that have entered stage M2 of meiosis. The end result of meiosis is the halving of the number of chromosomes and genetic material.

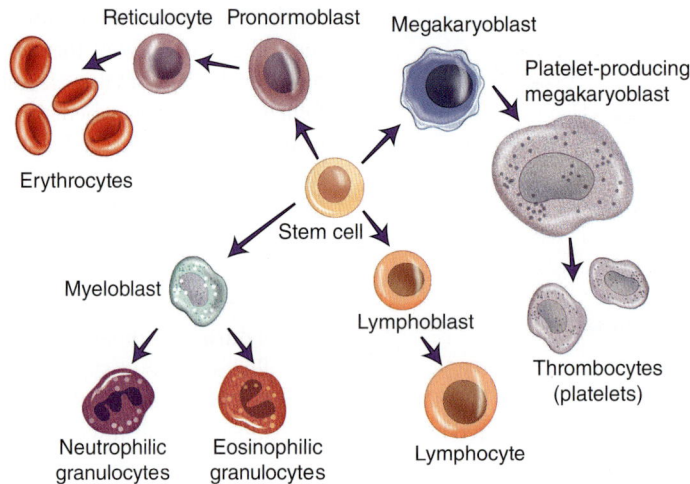

Fig. 7.9 Progressive development of various cells from a single pluripotential stem cell.

Cells of this system develop from a single precursor cell, the **pluripotential stem cell**. The following are other types of cells that originate from this type of primary cell: lymphocytes, granulocytes, thrombocytes or platelets, and erythrocytes. Fig. 7.9 demonstrates the progressive development of these cells from a single pluripotential stem cell. Most of these blood cells are manufactured in bone marrow at different intervals, and when they mature, they enter the blood capillaries and the peripheral circulation. Even though blood cells are continually being produced, the life span of each type of blood cell differs, varying, on average, from only a few hours (e.g., lymphocytes) to almost 120 days (e.g., erythrocytes).

The human body may experience health-related consequences throughout life if there is a decrease in the number of these various cells. Some of these consequences will be increased susceptibility to aggressive infectious organisms, a higher risk of hemorrhage, and anemia.

Radiation doses resulting from diagnostic imaging procedures during which appropriate radiation protection methods have been employed for patients and all personnel result in negligible damage to the blood and the blood-forming organs. However, in this dose range, some chromosomal changes in circulating lymphocytes have been observed.

Cytogenetic Effects

In simple terms, **cytogenetics** may be defined as the study of cell genetics with an emphasis on cell chromosomes. The techniques used to study and observe the chromosomes of each human cell have contributed significantly to advancing genetic analysis and the understanding of the influence of radiation on genetics.

Cytogenetic analysis of chromosomes may be accomplished through the use of a chromosome map called a **karyotype**. This map consists of a photograph or *photomicrograph,* of the human cell nucleus during metaphase, when each chromosome can be individually perceived. The karyotype is constructed by extracting the individual chromosomes and pairing them on the map with their sister chromosomes. These chromosome pairs are usually aligned by size, beginning with the largest pair and ending with the smallest pair (Fig. 7.10)

Metaphase is the phase of cell division in which chromosome damage caused by radiation exposure can be evaluated. *Chromosome aberrations* (deviation from normal development or growth of structures that contain genetic material) and *chromatid aberrations* have been observed at metaphase.

Both low and high radiation doses can cause chromosomal damage that may not be apparent immediately.

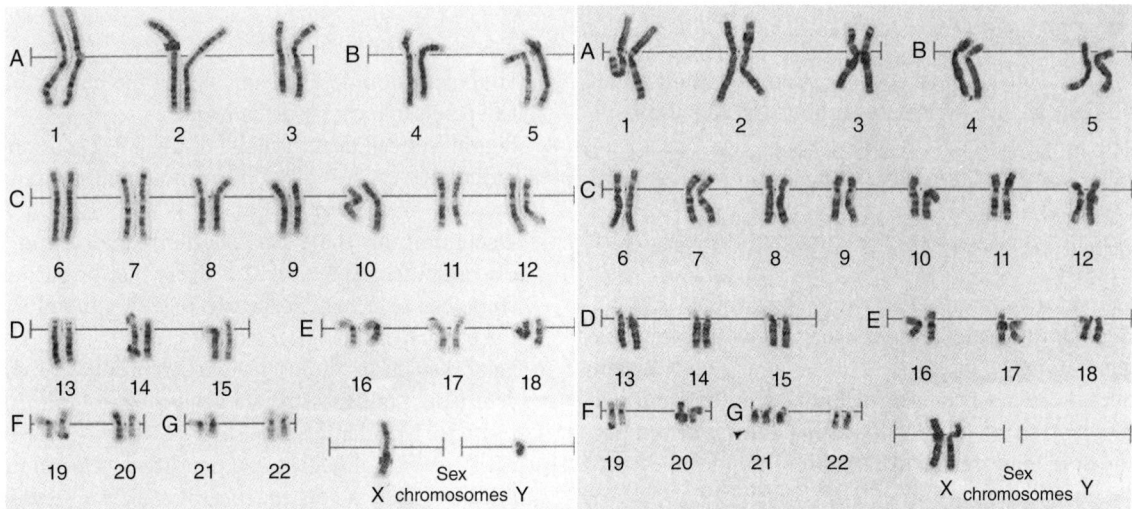

Fig. 7.10 A photomicrograph of the human cell nucleus at metaphase that shows each chromosome individually demonstrated. The karyotype is constructed by cutting out the individual chromosomes and pairing them with their sister chromosomes. These chromosome pairs are usually aligned by size, beginning with the largest pair and ending with the smallest pair. The left karyotype is male, and the right is female. (From Carolyn Caskey Goodner, Identigene, Inc.)

The majority of chromosomal damage results from the process of indirect action of ionizing radiation on vital biologic macromolecules.

Almost every type of chromosome aberration can be caused by exposure to ionizing radiation. However, some aberrations can "only" be produced by radiation exposure.[5] The total radiation dose delivered to a somatic or genetic cell and the duration in which the dose was delivered determine the rate of production of chromosome aberrations.

Attempts have been made to measure chromosome aberrations after diagnostic x-ray imaging procedures, but successful results have not been achieved in these studies. For imaging procedures that involve much higher radiation dose rates, studies demonstrated that radiation-induced chromosome imperfections were observed shortly after the imaging procedure was completed.

Increased frequency of chromosome translocations is an established radiation biomarker and may also suggest increased cancer risk.[11] An occupational epidemiologic study of 146,000 US radiologic technologists began in 1982 and is still in progress. This study is a collaborative effort of the University of Minnesota School of Public Health, the National Cancer Institute, and the American Registry of Radiologic Technologists.[12,13] The purpose of the research is "to determine whether their personal cumulative exposure to diagnostic x-rays was associated with increased frequencies of chromosome translocations"[11] and possible associated cancer risk. Included in the study were mail surveys, telephone interviews, and a collection of 150 blood samples for testing purposes. Results of the blood tests indicated increased chromosome damage as a consequence of cumulative work-related exposure from routine x-ray procedures.[11] For patients, computed tomography (CT) and nuclear medicine procedures can contribute substantially to higher radiation exposure. "Some studies have found increased chromosome abnormalities immediately after radiation exposure from CT scanning"[11,14] or in patients with unusually high numbers of diagnostic procedures.[11,15] These studies, however, have failed to show similar levels for low dose CT versions of the same scan.

SUMMARY

- Biologic effects that occur relatively soon after humans receive high doses of ionizing radiation are generally referred to as *early effects.*
- Early tissue reactions are not common in diagnostic radiology.
- Somatic effects are effects upon the body that was irradiated.
- Genetic effects are effects upon future generations due to the irradiation of germ cells in previous generations.
- Somatic tissue reactions include cell killing and are directly related to the dose of radiation received. As the dose increases, so does the severity of these early tissue reactions.
- Early tissue reactions vary depending on the duration of time after exposure to ionizing radiation. They may appear within minutes, hours, days, or weeks after receiving a high dose of ionizing radiation.
- Possible high radiation dose consequences generally include nausea and fever, extreme fatigue, erythema, epilation, and blood and intestinal disorders. Also, temporary or permanent sterility in the male and female and injury to the central nervous system (at extremely high radiation doses) can occur.
- Acute radiation syndrome (ARS) occurs in humans after large whole-body doses of ionizing radiation delivered over a short period.
  - ARS can manifest as hematopoietic syndrome, gastrointestinal syndrome, and cerebrovascular syndrome.
  - ARS presents in four major response stages: prodromal, latent period, manifest illness, and recovery or death.
- LD (lethal dose) 50/30 signifies the whole-body dose of ionizing radiation that can be lethal to 50% of an exposed population within 30 days.
  - LD 50/30 for adult humans is estimated to be 3 to 4 Gy_t without medical support.
  - When cells are exposed to sub-lethal doses of ionizing radiation, repair and recovery are possible.
  - After receiving a sub-lethal dose of radiation, surviving cells will be able to divide and thereby begin to repopulate in the irradiated region.
  - Approximately 90% of radiation-induced damage may be repaired over time; 10% is irreparable.

- High radiation doses to any part of the human body can result in local tissue damage.
- Significant cell death usually results after substantial radiation exposure, leading to potential atrophy of involved organs and tissues.
- Depending on the types of cells included and the dose of radiation received, recovery may be partial or complete, or it may not occur, resulting in failure of the irradiated biological structure.
- Factors such as radiosensitivity, reproductive characteristics, and growth rate govern organ and tissue response to radiation exposure.
- Many early radiologists and dentists developed radiodermatitis as a consequence of radiation exposure to the skin, which eventually led to the development of cancerous lesions.
  - Human skin consists of three layers and several accessory structures, all of which are actively involved in the response of tissue to radiation exposure.
  - A single absorbed dose of 2 Gy_t can cause radiation-induced skin erythema within 24 to 48 hours after irradiation.
  - High radiation doses to the skin can cause moist skin peeling, and then dry desquamation.
  - Moderate radiation doses to the scalp can cause temporary hair loss, and large radiation doses can result in permanent hair loss.
  - Significant evidence of skin damage as a consequence of exposure to orthovoltage radiation therapy comes from oncology patients who underwent such treatments in earlier years for deep-seated tumors.
  - The use of high-level fluoroscopy for extended periods can result in radiation-induced skin injuries for patients.
- Human germ cells are relatively radiosensitive.
  - In males, a radiation dose to the gonads of 0.1 Gy_t can depress the sperm population and possibly cause genetic mutations in future generations.
  - In females, a gonadal dose of 0.1 Gy_t may delay or suppress menstruation.
- Personnel dosimeters have replaced periodic blood counts as an accurate means to monitor occupational radiation exposure.

- When blood counts were used to monitor the effects of radiation exposure among those who worked with radiation, a whole-body radiation dose of 0.25 Gy_t would be required to produce a measurable hematologic depression.
- The mapping of chromosomes is *karyotyping.*
  - Karyotyping is performed during metaphase, when each chromosome can be individually perceived and radiation-induced chromosome and chromatid aberrations can be observed.
- Chromosomal damage can be caused by both low and high radiation doses.
- Chromosome aberrations have been observed in individuals after completion of some imaging procedures.

GENERAL DISCUSSION QUESTIONS

1. What factors influence early tissue reactions to ionizing radiation, and what are the typical time frames for these reactions to appear?
2. What are some high-dose consequences of ionizing radiation on living systems?
3. What is acute radiation syndrome (ARS), and what are the three dose-related syndromes associated with it?
4. What are the four major response stages of acute radiation syndrome (ARS)?
5. Why do cells exposed to sublethal doses of ionizing radiation recover, and what is the cumulative effect of repeated injuries?
6. What local tissue damage can occur with high radiation exposure in specific parts of the body?
7. What three factors affect organ and tissue responses to radiation exposure?
8. How did historical perspectives shape our understanding of radiation-induced skin damage?
9. What are the three layers of human skin, and what are some related accessory structures?
10. What absorbed dose of ionizing radiation can cause skin erythema within 24 to 48 hours, and how does this dose manifest?

REVIEW QUESTIONS

1. What is one of the primary factors affecting early tissue reactions to ionizing radiation?
   A. Age of the individual
   B. Dose of radiation
   C. Gender
   D. Time of day
2. Which of the following is a potential consequence of high-dose ionizing radiation?
   A. Increased metabolism
   B. Acute radiation syndrome (ARS)
   C. Enhanced tissue regeneration
   D. Improved immune response
3. What are the three dose-related syndromes associated with acute radiation syndrome (ARS)?
   A. Hematopoietic, gastrointestinal, and cerebrovascular
   B. Endocrine, reproductive, and muscular
   C. Dermatological, neurological, and cardiovascular
   D. Musculoskeletal, respiratory, and urinary
4. What is the first stage of acute radiation syndrome (ARS)?
   A. Latent stage
   B. Prodromal stage
   C. Manifest illness stage
   D. Recovery stage
5. Why do cells exposed to sublethal doses of ionizing radiation often recover?
   A. They undergo apoptosis
   B. They have robust repair mechanisms
   C. They become dormant
   D. They divide more rapidly
6. What type of local tissue damage can result from high radiation exposure?
   A. Increased blood flow
   B. Skin burns and necrosis
   C. Enhanced healing
   D. Tissue hypertrophy

7. Which factor does NOT affect organ and tissue responses to radiation exposure?
   A. Radiation dose
   B. Tissue type
   C. Environmental temperature
   D. Rate of exposure
8. What historical practice highlighted the dangers of radiation-induced skin damage?
   A. Use of grenz rays for skin treatment
   B. Early radiology practices
   C. Radiation therapy for cancer
   D. Fluoroscopy in dental exams
9. What are the three layers of human skin?
   A. Epidermis, dermis, and hypodermis
   B. Epidermis, fascia, and muscle
   C. Dermis, subcutaneous, and connective
   D. Epidermis, subcutaneous, and vascular
10. What absorbed dose of ionizing radiation can lead to skin erythema within 24 to 48 hours?
   A. 0.5 Gy
   B. 1 Gy
   C. 2 Gy
   D. 5 Gy

Late Effects of Radiation Exposure

OBJECTIVES

After completing this chapter, the reader will be able to perform the following:

- Define all key terms.
- Explain how scientists use epidemiologic studies to predict the risk of cancer in human populations exposed to low doses of ionizing radiation.
- Explain the purpose of a radiation dose–response curve.
- Draw diagrams demonstrating various dose–response relationships.
- Explain the reason regulatory agencies continue to use the linear dose–response model for establishing radiation protection standards.
- Differentiate between the threshold and nonthreshold relationships.

- List and describe the various late tissue reactions and stochastic effects of ionizing radiation on living systems.
- Describe the concept of risk for radiation-induced malignancies, and explain the models that are used to provide risk estimates.
- Identify ionizing radiation-exposed human populations or groups that prove radiation induces cancer.
- Explain how spontaneous mutations occur.
- Discuss the concept and processes of radiation-induced genetic effects.
- Differentiate between dominant and recessive gene mutations.
- Explain the doubling dose concept, and provide an example of how the number of mutations increases as dose increases.

CHAPTER OUTLINE

Radiation-induced damage at the cellular level may lead to measurable somatic and hereditary damage in the living organism as a whole later in life. These *late effects* are the long-term results of radiation exposure. Some examples of measurable delayed biologic damage are:

- Cataracts
- Leukemia
- Genetic mutations

Cataracts are considered to be a **late tissue reaction** that is nonrandom, whereas leukemia and genetic mutations are viewed as delayed stochastic or random consequences that, if these reactions do appear, they do not do so for extended periods. This chapter focuses on the organic system-level damage from ionizing radiation that occurs months or years after radiation exposure.

EPIDEMIOLOGY

Epidemiology is a "science that deals with the incidence, distribution, and control of disease in a population."[1] Epidemiologic studies consist of observations and statistical analysis of data, such as the incidence of disease within groups of people. The latter studies include the risk of radiation-induced cancer. The incident rates at which these irradiation-related malignancies occur are determined by comparing the natural incidence of cancer occurring in a human population with the prevalence of cancer occurring in an irradiated population. Risk factors are then identified for the general human population.

Epidemiologic studies are of significant value to radiobiologists who use the information from these studies to formulate *dose–response estimates* for predicting the risk of cancer in human populations exposed to low doses of ionizing radiation.

CARCINOGENESIS

Carcinogenesis, also called tumorigenesis, is the formation of a *cancer*. Cancer is the name used for a substantial group of diseases in which healthy cells have been transformed into nonstandard cells that divide uncontrollably. The process leads to an expansive growth of abnormal structures within various locations in the body and the destruction of surrounding body tissues such as bone marrow. The altered or cancer cells readily demonstrate the potential to invade or spread to other parts of the body. Cancer is the most significant late **stochastic effect** caused by exposure to ionizing radiation.

RADIATION DOSE–RESPONSE RELATIONSHIP

Dose–Response Curves

The **radiation dose–response relationship** is demonstrated graphically through a curve (the dose–response [DR] curve) that maps the observed effects of radiation exposure in relation to the dose of radiation received. The "effect" in question may be the incidence of a disease (e.g., cases of cancer per million in a population or fatalities due to cancer per million in a population), or the effect may be its degree of acuteness, such as the severity of cataracts as dose increases. The DR curve is either linear (straight line) or nonlinear (curved to some degree), and it depicts either a threshold dose or a nonthreshold dose (Fig. 8.1).

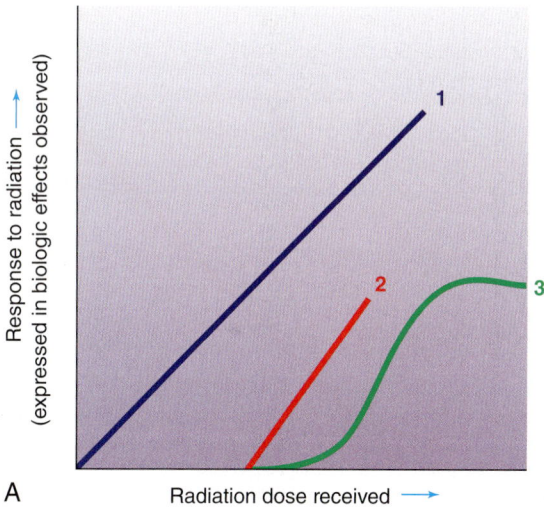

A

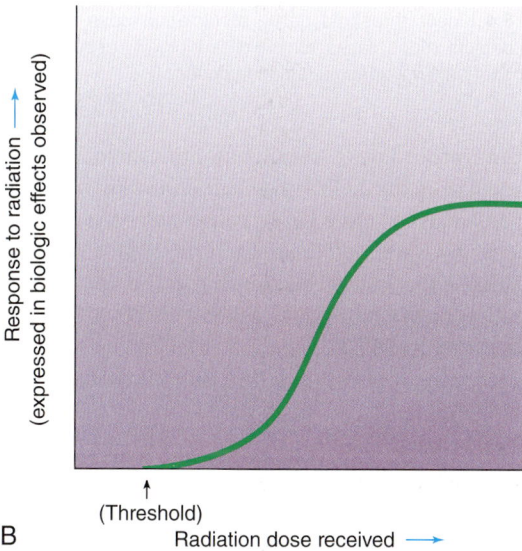

Fig. 8.2 Linear nonthreshold curve of radiation dose–response relationship. The straight-line curve passing through the origin in this graph indicates both that the response to radiation (in terms of biologic effects) is directly proportional to the dose of radiation and that no known level of radiation dose exists below which the chance of sustaining biologic damage is zero. In contrast to a cell-survival curve (Fig. 6.17), as seen in Chapter 6, both the vertical and horizontal axes of a dose–response curve are ordinary linear scales.

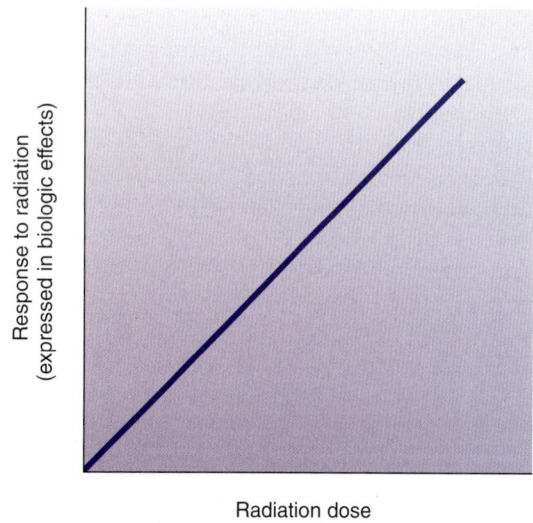

B

Fig. 8.1 (A) 1 represents a linear (straight-line) nonthreshold curve of the radiation dose–response relationship; 2 represents a linear threshold curve of the radiation dose–response relationship; 3 represents a nonlinear threshold curve of the radiation dose–response relationship. (B) Sigmoid (S-shaped, hence nonlinear) threshold curve of radiation dose–response relationship generally employed in radiation therapy to demonstrate high-dose cellular response.

Threshold and Nonthreshold Relationships

The term **threshold** is defined as a point or level at which a response or reaction to an increasing stimulation first occurs. Regarding ionizing radiation, this means that below a certain absorbed radiation dose, no biologic effects are observed. The biologic effects begin to occur only when the threshold dose is reached. A **nonthreshold** relationship indicates that a radiation absorbed dose of any magnitude has the capability of producing a biologic effect. Therefore, if the DR curve is as shown in Fig. 8.2, biologic effect responses will be caused by ionizing radiation in living organisms in a directly proportional manner at any dose above zero. This behavior is referred to as a *linear nonthreshold (LNT) relationship*. LNT proclaims that no radiation dose can be considered absolutely "safe," with the incidence of the biologic effects increasing directly with the magnitude of the absorbed dose.

Risk Models Used to Predict Cancer Risk and Heritable Damage in Human Populations

In a 1980 report, the Committee on the Biological Effects of Ionizing Radiation (BEIR), under the auspices of the National Academy of Sciences, studying atomic bomb survivors concluded that most **stochastic effects** (e.g., cancer) and hereditary effects at low-dose levels from

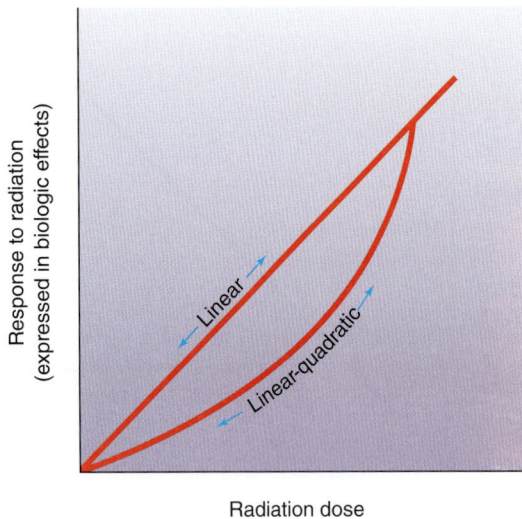

Fig. 8.3 Linear-quadratic nonthreshold dose–response relationship. The curve estimates the risk associated with low-dose levels from low LET radiation.

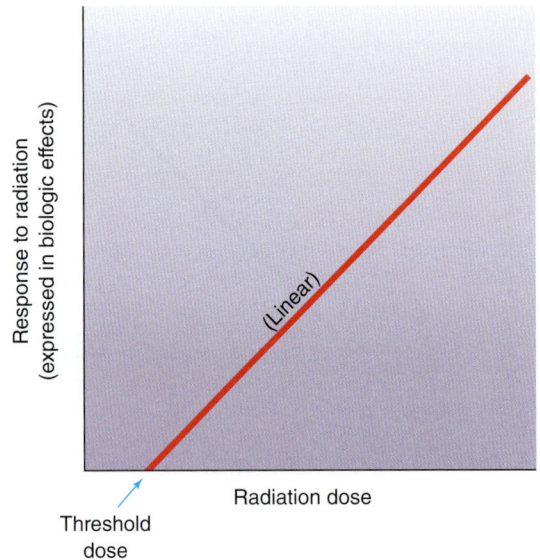

Fig. 8.4 Linear threshold curve of radiation dose–response. This depicts those cases for which a biologic response does not occur below a specific radiation dose.

low LET radiation, such as the type of radiation used in diagnostic radiology, appear to follow a linear-quadratic nonthreshold dose–response curve (LQNT DR) (Fig. 8.3). The term *linear-quadratic* implies that the equation that best fits the data has components that depend on dose to the first power (linear or straight-line behavior) and also on dose squared (quadratic or curved behavior). Since the 1980 report, newer risk models and updated dosimetry techniques have provided a more useful follow-up study of Hiroshima and Nagasaki atomic bomb survivors. In 1990 the BEIR Committee's revised risk estimates indicated that the risk from radiation exposure was about three to four times greater than previously projected. Currently, the committee recommends the use of the **linear nonthreshold curve** of radiation dose–response (LNT DR) for most types of cancers. With the LNT DR curve, if the absorbed dose is doubled, the biologic response probability, and therefore its actual occurrence in a large population sample, is also doubled (see Fig. 8.2).

Risk Models Used to Predict Leukemia, Breast Cancer, and Heritable Damage

Currently, advocates of LNT theorize that because all radiation exposure levels possess the potential to cause biologic damage, radiographers must never fail to employ aggressive radiation safety measures whenever humans are exposed to radiation during diagnostic

imaging procedures. Another nonthreshold risk estimate curve is the **LQNT DR** curve (see Fig. 8.3). This curve displays a *more conservative dose–response outcome for low-level radiation*. The 1990 BEIR Committee considered the LQNT relationship to be an improved reflection of stochastic and genetic effects at low-dose levels from low-LET radiation. The following health concerns are presumed to follow this DR curve:

- Leukemia
- Breast cancer
- Heritable damage

For leukemia, the LQNT hypothesis appears to be supported by an analysis of the leukemia occurrences in Nagasaki and Hiroshima that utilized a more recent reevaluation of the radiation dose distribution in these two cities.[2,3]

Risk Model Used to Predict High-Dose Cellular Response

Acute reactions from significant radiation exposure, such as skin erythema and hematologic depression, may be demonstrated graphically through the use of a radiation *linear threshold dose–response curve* (LT DR) as shown in Fig. 8.4. In this model, a biologic response does not occur below a specific dose level. Laboratory experiments on animals and data from human populations observed after high doses of radiation provided the foundation for this curve. The **sigmoid, or S-shaped (nonlinear), threshold curve** of the radiation dose–response relationship (see Fig. 8.1B) is generally employed in radiation therapy to demonstrate the high-dose cellular response to the radiation absorbed doses within specific tissues, such as skin, the lens of the eye, and various types of blood cells. Different effects require different minimal doses. The tail of the curve indicates that limited recovery occurs at lower radiation doses. At the highest radiation doses, the curve gradually levels off and then veers downward because the affected living specimen or tissue dies before the observable effect appears.

The Rationale for Risk Model Selection

The continued use of the linear dose–response model for radiation protection standards has the potential to exaggerate the seriousness of radiation effects at lower dose levels from low-LET radiation. Regulatory agencies such as the Nuclear Regulatory Commission continue to review scientific literature to determine if the evidence supports changes in the use of this model for setting radiation protection standards. In establishing such standards, the regulatory agencies have chosen to be conservative—that is, to use a model that may overestimate risk at low doses but is not expected to underestimate risk.

SOMATIC EFFECTS

When living organisms that have been exposed to radiation sustain biologic damage, the effects of this exposure are classified as *somatic effects,* from the Greek *sômatikos,* meaning "of the body." The classification of somatic effects may be subdivided into: stochastic effects and tissue reactions.

In stochastic effects, the probability that the effect occurs depends upon the received dose, but the severity of the effect does not. The occurrence of a cancer is an instance of a stochastic or random somatic effect. In tissue reactions, however, both the probability and the severity of the effect depend upon the dose.

A *non-somatic* effect is an effect in the offspring of the individual who was irradiated. An example of a non-somatic effect is the irradiation of an individual's genetic material (sperm or eggs) leading to a genetic malformation in offspring.

> **BOX 8.1   Late Effects of Radiation**
>
> **Late Tissue Reactions**
> Cataract formation
> Fibrosis
> Organ atrophy
> Loss of parenchymal cells
> Reduced fertility
> Sterility
>
> **Teratogenic Effects**
> (i.e., effects of radiation on the embryo-fetus in utero
>   that depend on the fetal stage of development and
>   the radiation dose received)
> Embryonic, fetal, or neonatal death
> Congenital malformations
> Decreased birth weight
> Disturbances in growth and/or development
> Increased stillbirths
> Infant mortality
> Childhood malignancy
> Childhood mortality
>
> **Stochastic Effects**
> Cancer
> Genetic (hereditary) effects

Late Somatic Effects

Late somatic effects are consequences of radiation exposure that appear months or years afterwards. Late effects may be either stochastic or tissue reactions. Stochastic effects, such as the incidence of cancers in a population, typically are not noticeable for many years in the exposed population. Tissue reactions, such as skin effects, may be perceptible sooner in individuals, although months or years may pass before their full expression. Tissue reactions are the result of slowly developing changes to body tissues that may be modified by other factors, such as medical intervention, after the exposure. Stochastic effects, such as the occurrence of cancer, are generally *determined* at the time of irradiation.

Examples of both classes of late effects are listed in Box 8.1.

Risk Estimate for Contracting Cancer From Low-Level Radiation Exposure

Low-level doses are a consideration for patients and personnel exposed to ionizing radiation as a result of diagnostic imaging procedures. The risk estimate for humans contracting cancer from low-level radiation exposure is controversial. No conclusive proof currently exists that low-LET ionizing radiation absorbed doses below 0.1 Gy (10 rads) cause a significant increase in the risk of malignancy. The risk may be negligible or even nonexistent. Sources of such low-level radiation include the following:

- X-rays and radioactive materials used for diagnostic purposes
- Employment-related exposures in medicine and industry
- Natural background exposure

In general, low-level low LET radiation dosage has been defined as an equivalent dose of "0.1 Sv or less delivered over a short time" and as "a larger dose delivered over a longer time—for instance, 0.5 Sv in 10 years."[4] The effective dose of a typical routine two-view chest radiograph is approximately 0.06 mSv (6 mrem) (note: this can be somewhat greater or lesser, depending on the patient's body size) which is far below what is considered a low-level exposure.[5] Numerous laboratory experiments on animals and studies on human populations that have been exposed to *high doses* of ionizing radiation from various causes were conducted to catalog the occurrence and degree of adverse health effects. Using all data available on high radiation exposure, members of the scientific and medical communities have concluded that three categories of harmful health consequences also require study at *low dose levels*:

- Cancer induction
- Damage to the unborn from irradiation in utero
- Genetic effects

Low-Level Effects Summary

Cells that survive the initial irradiation may have incurred some form of damage. Theoretically, radiation damage to just one or a few cells of an individual could produce a stochastic effect such as a malignancy or a hereditary disorder many years after radiation exposure. Tissue reactions such as skin reactions do not usually demonstrate a late onset. Extreme reactions associated with high skin doses may persist for some time but will often occur in weeks or months after the exposure.

Major Types of Late Effects

To summarize, the three major types of late effects are:

- Carcinogenesis
- Cataractogenesis
- Embryologic effects (birth defects)

Of these, carcinogenesis and embryologic effects are considered stochastic events, and cataractogenesis is regarded as a late tissue reaction.

Risk Estimates for Cancer

Exposure to ionizing radiation may cause cancer as a stochastic effect. At high doses, for groups such as the atomic bomb survivors, the risk is measurable in human populations. At low equivalent doses below 0.1 Sv, which includes groups such as occupationally exposed individuals and virtually all patients in diagnostic radiology, this risk is not directly measurable in population studies. Either the risk is overshadowed by other causes (e.g., environmental exposures, genetic predisposition, life-style factors such as smoking) of cancer in humans, or the risk is zero. Current conservative radiation protection philosophy, namely the LNT model, assumes that risk still exists and may be determined by extrapolating from high-dose data, in which risk has been directly observed, down to low doses, in which it has not been observed. Again, this remains a very controversial concept.

Absolute Risk and Relative Risk Models. Risk estimates to predict cancer incidence may be stated in terms of absolute risk or relative risk caused by a specific exposure to ionizing radiation (over and above background exposure). Both models forecast the number of excess cancers or cancers that would not have occurred in the population in question without exposure to ionizing radiation. The **absolute risk** model estimates that a specific number of malignancies will occur as a result of exposure (Fig. 8.5). The **relative risk** model predicts that the number of excess cancers will increase as the natural incidence of cancer increases with advancing age in a population (Fig. 8.6). The risk model is relative in the sense that this model predicts a percentage increase in incidence rather than a specific number of cases. More recent studies of atomic bomb survivors tend to support the relative risk model over the absolute risk model.

Epidemiologic Studies for Determining the Risk of Cancer. Epidemiologic studies suggest that although the radiation doses received by patients in diagnostic radiology imaging could be considered in determining the risk of cancer, the benefit to the patient of the information gained from an imaging procedure greatly exceeds the minimal theoretical risk to the patient for

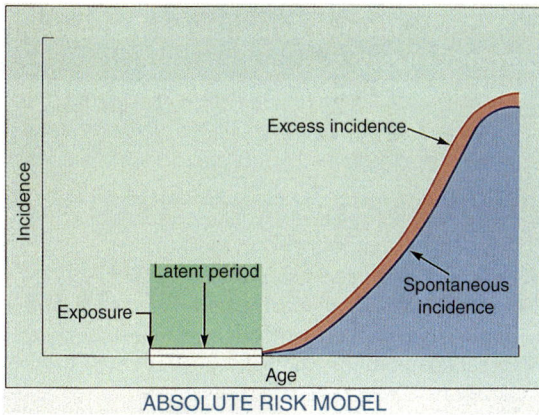

Fig. 8.5 Absolute risk model. This model forecasts that a specific number of malignancies will occur as a result of exposure. (From *Radiobiology and radiation protection: Mosby's radiographic instructional series*, St. Louis, 1999, Mosby.)

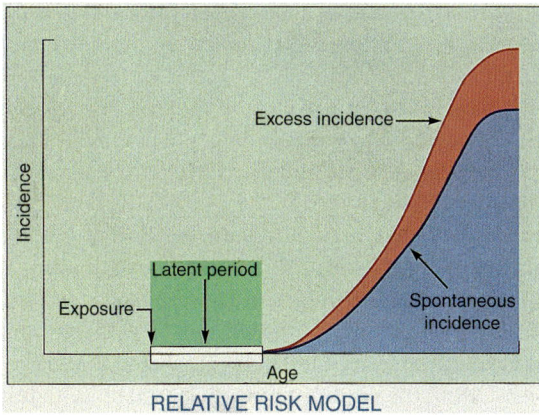

Fig. 8.6 Relative risk model. This model predicts that the number of excess cancers will increase as the natural incidence of cancer increases with advancing age in a population. (From *Radiobiology and radiation protection: Mosby's radiographic instructional series*, St. Louis, 1999, Mosby.)

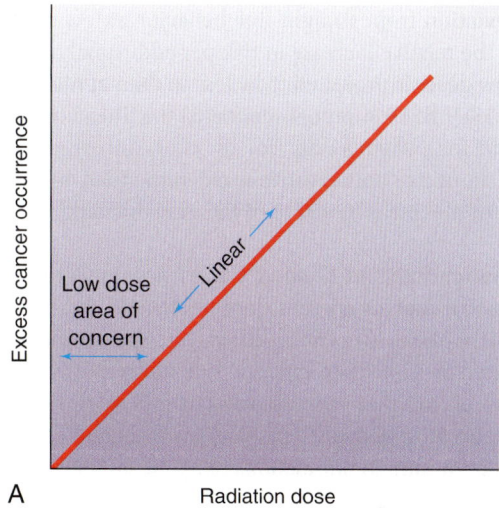

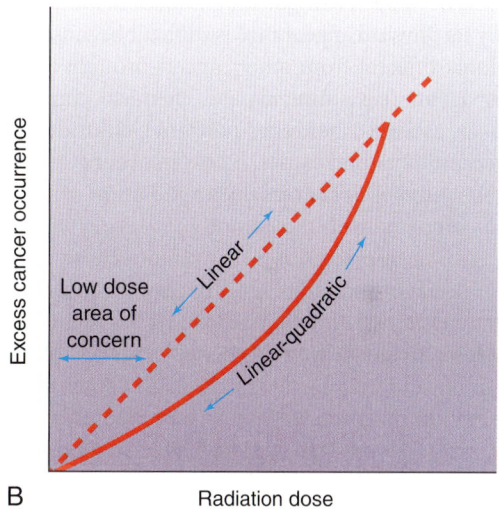

Fig. 8.7 (A) Linear model used to extrapolate the occurrence of cancer from high-dose information to low doses. This model suits current high-dose information satisfactorily but exaggerates the actual risk at low doses and dose rates. (B) Linear-quadratic model used to extrapolate the occurrence of cancer from high-dose information to low doses. This model suits current high-dose information satisfactorily, but risk at low doses may be underestimated.

developing cancer as a late stochastic response to diagnostic radiation exposure. Even at the relatively high doses encountered by the Japanese atomic bomb survivors, the probability of causation of an excess fatal cancer is surprisingly low—approximately 5% per sievert.[6]

Models for Extrapolation of Cancer Risk from High-Dose to Low-Dose Data. Researchers commonly use two models for extrapolation of risk from high-dose to low-dose data, the linear and linear-quadratic models. In the linear model (Fig. 8.7A), the risk per centigray is constant; the occurrence of cancer follows a straight-line or dose-proportional progression throughout the entire dose range. Although this model appears to match the high-dose data, it may substantially overestimate the risk at low doses. The linear-quadratic model (see Fig. 8.7B) includes additional mathematical terms that produce a deviation from straight-line behavior at low doses so that the relative increase in risk per additional centigray at low doses is projected to be less so than at high doses. The 1989 BEIR V report supported the linear-quadratic model for leukemia only. For all other cancers, the BEIR V Committee conservatively recommended the adoption of the linear model to fit the available data.[7]

Radiation-Induced Cancer. Cancer is a random occurrence that does not appear to have a threshold and the severity of the disease is not dose-related (e.g., a patient's leukemia induced by a low-dose exposure is no different from a person's leukemia that was caused by a high-dose exposure).

Laboratory experiments with animals and statistical studies of human populations (e.g., the Japanese atomic bomb survivors) demonstrate that radiation exposure initiates cancer. In humans, this may take 5 or more years to develop. Distinguishing radiation-induced cancer by its physical appearance is difficult because it does not look different from other cancers brought about by other agents (e.g., minerals and chemical compounds such as asbestos, benzene, polyvinyl chlorides, etc.). Cancer from natural causes, however, occurs frequently, and the number of cancers due to radiation exposure is small compared with the *natural incidence of malignancies*, even at received doses many times those encountered in diagnostic radiology. Therefore, cancer caused by low-level radiation is challenging to identify and, therefore, to quantify. In general, evidence of radiation-induced carcinogenesis in humans comes from the observation of irradiated humans and from epidemiologic studies conducted many years after subjects were exposed to *high doses* of ionizing radiation. Examples of these data are listed in Box 8.2. An explanation of each instance follows.

Radium watch-dial painters. During the early years of the last century (the 1920s and 1930s), a radium watch-dial painting industry flourished in some factories in New Jersey. Young, unprotected, and ill-informed young women employed in these factories hand-painted the luminous numerals on watches and clocks with radium-containing paint. The girls used sable brushes to apply the paint. To do the delicate work required, some would place the paint-saturated brush tip on their lips to draw the bristles to a fine point. The girls who followed this procedure, unfortunately, ingested large quantities of radium. Because radium is chemically similar to calcium, the radium was deposited into bone tissue.

> ## BOX 8.2 Human Evidence for Radiation Carcinogenesis
>
> 1. Radium watch-dial painters (1920s and 1930s)
> 2. Uranium miners (early years, and Navajo people of Arizona and New Mexico during the 1950s and 1960s)
> 3. Early medical radiation workers (radiologists, dentists, technologists) (1896 to 1910)
> 4. Japanese atomic bomb survivors (1945)
> 5. Patients with benign postpartum mastitis who were given radiation therapy treatments (mid-1900s)
> 6. Evacuees from the Chernobyl nuclear power station disaster in 1986

Eventually the accumulation of this toxic substance caused:

- Development of osteoporosis (decalcification of bone)
- Osteogenic sarcoma (bone cancer)
- Other malignancies such as carcinoma of the epithelial cells lining the nasopharynx and paranasal sinuses

The bones most frequently affected by ingested radium included the pelvis, femur, and mandible. Doses of 5 Gyt or more are assumed to have caused the malignancies mentioned above. The number of head carcinomas attributed to the radium watch-dial painting industry, although small, is statistically significant. Of 1474 women in the industry, 61 were diagnosed with cancer of the paranasal sinuses and 21 with cancer of the mastoid air cells. Studies also attributed the death of at least 18 of the radium watch-dial painters to radium poisoning or toxicity.

Uranium miners. During the early years of the last century, many people worked in European mines to extract pitchblende, a uranium ore. The most common isotope of Uranium238 U92 is a radioactive element with a very long half-life of 4.5 billion years. Uranium decays sequentially through a series of other heavy radioactive nuclides by emitting alpha, beta, and gamma radiation One of the most important members of its decay family is radium*, which decays to the radioactive gas, radon. Because of its volatile nature, radon was able to seep through tiny gaps in rocks within the mines and created

---

*Radium (atomic number Z = 88, mass number = 226) has an unstable nucleus and decays with a half-life of 1622 years by alpha particle emission to the radioactive element radon (Z = 86, mass number = 222).

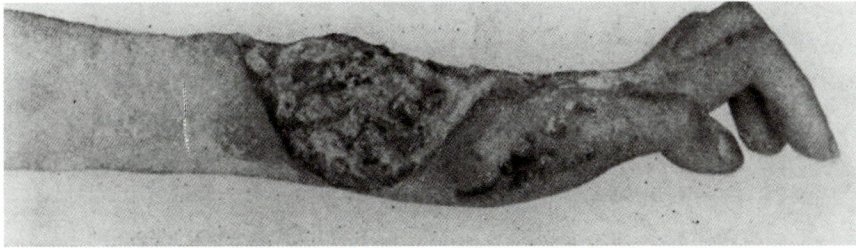

Fig. 8.8 Carcinoma of the distal arm and hand developed after an x-ray burn (in 1904). (From Allen CW: *Radiotherapy and phototherapy including radium and high frequency currents,* New York, 1904, Lea Brothers.)

an ever-present insidious airborne hazard to miners. Consequently, throughout many years of employment, some miners inevitably inhaled significant amounts of radon, leading to approximately 50% of the miners eventually succumbing to lung cancer.

During the 1950s and 1960s, at the height of the Cold War between the United States and the Soviet Union, the US government needed fuel for nuclear weapons and power plants. The Navajo people of Arizona and New Mexico mined uranium to meet this need. Because the government did not regulate working conditions in the mines to ensure safety from exposure—despite awareness of risk—some 15,000 Navajo and other workers in the uranium mines received substantial doses of ionizing radiation by breathing radioactive dust and drinking contaminated water. Researchers have estimated that miners unknowingly received over their employment duration a composite dose as much as 10 Sv (1000 rem) or more.[8] The families of the miners were also affected because the clothing worn by the miners was contaminated by radioactive material.

Early medical radiation workers. Many of the first generation of radiation workers (radiologists, dentists, and technologists) were exposed to large amounts of ionizing radiation without realizing the dangers of this exposure. This exposure resulted in a large number of severe radiation injuries to these individuals. An example was the development of cancerous skin lesions on the hands of radiologists and dentists (Fig. 8.8). When compared with their non-radiologist counterparts, a significant number of these early radiation workers also had a higher incidence of blood disorders such as:

- Aplastic anemia
- Leukemia

Because these workers did not have the benefit of protective devices, which led to some receiving doses estimated at more than 1 Gy/year, the occurrence of these

radiation-induced injuries is very plausible. Today, as a result of educational programs focusing on radiation safety, appropriate usage of protective devices, and safety improvements in imaging equipment, medical imaging technologists should not experience any adverse health effects as a consequence of their occupation. Detailed studies of radiographers and physicians who began their careers in radiology after the 1940s have established that these radiation workers had no increase in adverse health effects as a result of their occupational exposure. This finding is attributed to increased knowledge and use of proper protective measures and improved safety devices.[9]

Incidence of breast cancer in radiation treatment of benign postpartum mastitis. Studies of postpartum patients treated with ionizing radiation for relief of mastitis are another group of individuals in whom the results of radiation exposure to healthy breast tissue via scattered radiation indicate that radiation can cause breast cancer. In a particular study of 531 women who received a mean dose of 247 cGyt, "breast cancer incidence doubled from 3.2% expected to 6.3% actual."[10] Because there is an ongoing concern that mammography performed for either screening or diagnostic purposes could cause the development of breast cancer, epidemiologic studies that provide such statistical information continue to be a high priority.

Japanese atomic bomb survivors

Atomic bomb detonation on Hiroshima and Nagasaki. On August 6, 1945, the United States dropped the first atomic bomb on the Japanese city of Hiroshima, thus marking a pivotal moment in the latter stages of World War II. Three days later, on August 9, 1945, a second bomb was dropped on the city of Nagasaki. Of the 300,000 people living in these two cities at the time of these bombings, approximately 88,000 people were killed,

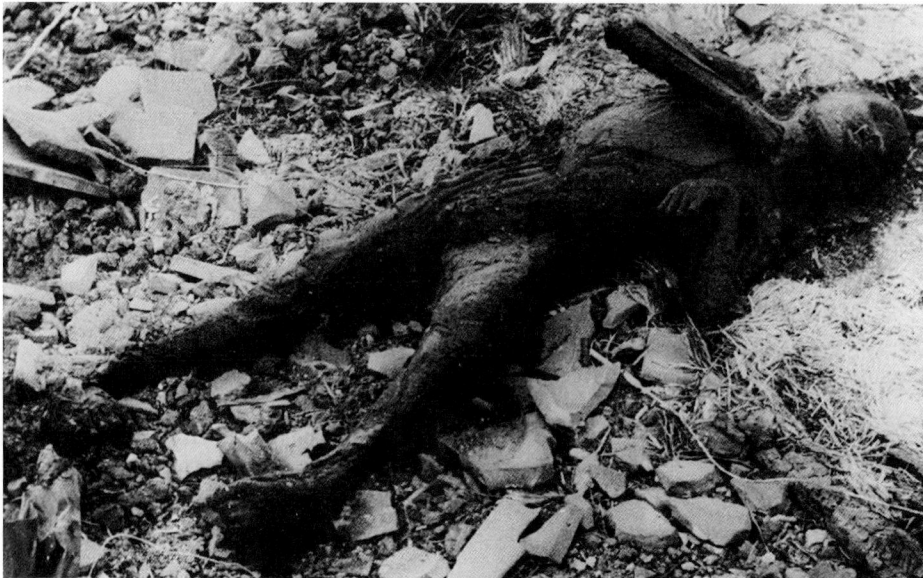

Fig. 8.9 Charred human remains were found in the epicenter of Nagasaki after the detonation of the atomic bomb on August 9, 1945. (From Magnum Photos.)

and at least 70,000 more were injured. Many of those who died were killed by the extreme heat and the shock wave from the blast (Fig. 8.9). Survivors became victims of radiation injuries. These individuals have been observed since that time for signs of stochastic effects of radiation.

Data obtained from epidemiologic studies. Epidemiologic studies of approximately 100,000 Japanese survivors of the atomic bombings at Hiroshima and Nagasaki indicate that ionizing radiation causes leukemia (proliferation of the white blood cells). "Studies of the atomic bomb survivors in both Hiroshima and Nagasaki show a *statistically significant** increase in leukemia incidence in the exposed population compared with the non-exposed population. In the period 1950 to 1956, 117 new cases of leukemia were reported in the Japanese survivors; approximately 64 of these can be attributed to radiation exposure."[1]

---

*Statistical significance indicates (via the value of a numerical probability parameter) whether an observation or result from a study sample is likely due to change or some actual factor of interest such as radiation exposure levels. Therefore, when a finding is deemed *significant*, it means investigators can feel confident to a specific degree (e.g., 95%) that the conclusion is actual and not that the investigators were just fortunate in choosing their investigation sample.

Incidence of leukemia rate of other radiation-induced malignancies. Among the atomic bomb survivors, the number of people living with leukemia has slowly declined since the late 1940s and early 1950s. However, the occurrence rates of other radiation-induced malignancies continued to escalate since the late 1950s and early 1960s. Among these are a variety of solid tumors such as:

- Thyroid cancer
- Breast cancer
- Lung cancer
- Bone cancers

Fig. 8.10 demonstrates the nominal risk of malignancy, as identified by Warren K. Sinclair, from a dose of 0.01 Gyt of uniform whole-body radiation.[11] The graph indicates that leukemia occurs approximately 2 years after the initial exposure, rises to its highest level of incidence between 7 and 10 years, and then declines to almost zero at 30 years. Unlike leukemia, solid tumors have a latent period of approximately 10 years before developing and generally increase in incidence at the same rate that cancer increases as people age. Whether the risk for solid tumors continues to rise beyond 40 years or declines, as with leukemia, is still unknown. Follow-up studies of the atomic bomb survivors may eventually provide the answer.

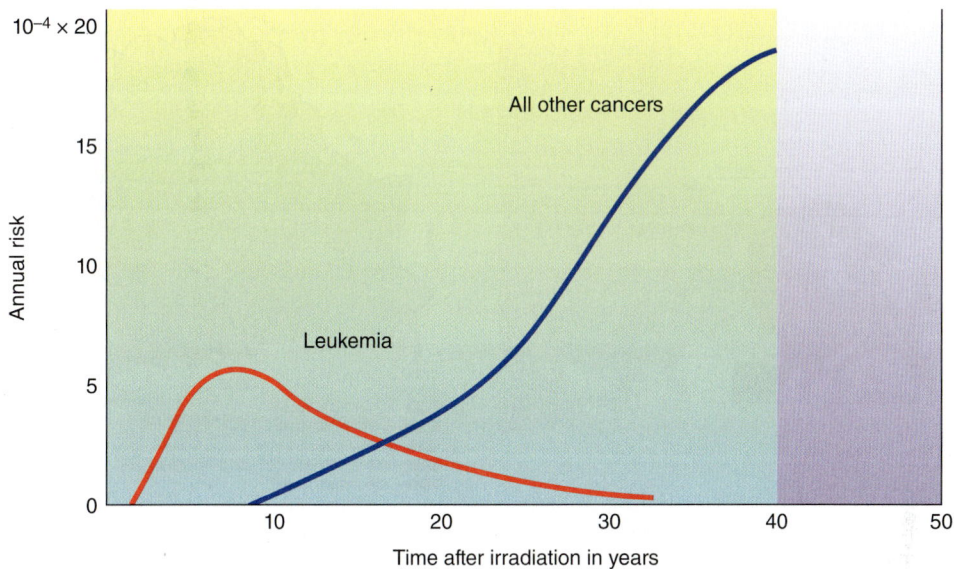

Fig. 8.10 Nominal risk of malignancy from a dose of 0.01 Gyt of uniform whole-body radiation. (From Sinclair WK: Radiation protection recommendations on dose limits: the role of the NCRP and the ICRP and future developments, *J Radiat Oncol Biol Phys* 131:387, 1995.)

Incidence of breast cancer in Japanese women. In general, Japanese women have a lower natural incidence of breast cancer than US and Canadian women.[12] Studies of the female Japanese atomic bomb survivors provide strong evidence that ionizing radiation may induce breast cancer. The incidence of breast cancer in these women rises with radiation dose. Breast cancer follows an LNT curve. Numerous studies of female survivors indicate a relative risk for breast cancer ranging from 4:1 to as high as 10:1.

Effectiveness of ionizing radiation as a cancer-causing agent. Although studies from Hiroshima and Nagasaki confirm that high doses of ionizing radiation will cause cancer, radiation is, in actuality, *not a highly effective cancer-causing agent*. For example, follow-up studies of approximately 82,000 atomic bomb survivors from 1950 to 1978 reveal an excess of only 250 cancer deaths attributed to radiation exposure. Instead of the normally expected 4500 cancer deaths, 4750 occurred. This death rate indicates that of about every 300 atomic bomb survivors, one died of a malignancy attributed to an average whole-body radiation dose of approximately 0.14 Sv.

Radiation dose and radiation-induced leukemia. Epidemiologic data concerning Hiroshima atomic bomb survivors also indicate that a linear relationship exists between radiation dose and radiation-induced leukemia. This means that the chance of contracting leukemia as a result of exposure to radiation is directly proportional to the magnitude of the radiation exposure. Available information for establishing the existence of a threshold dose–response relationship (i.e., whether a harmless dose exists) is incomplete. Hence radiation-induced leukemia is assumed to follow an LNT dose-response relationship compared with leukemia in a population that has not been exposed to ionizing radiation.[13] More recent reevaluations of the quantity and type of radiation that was released in the cities of Hiroshima and Nagasaki provide an improved foundation for radiation dose and damage assessment. Originally, neutron radiation was predominantly credited with the populace irradiation dosage in Hiroshima. However, when more recent studies revealed that the uranium-fueled bomb dropped on Hiroshima provided more gamma radiation exposure and less neutron exposure than previously believed, data on the survivors were updated to reflect this more accurate information. As a result, researchers have established that gamma radiation and neutrons each provided about 50% of the radiation dose inflicted on the population of Hiroshima. Conversely, the inhabitants of Nagasaki, who were exposed to a plutonium bomb, received only 10% of their exposure from neutrons and 90% from gamma radiation. The impact

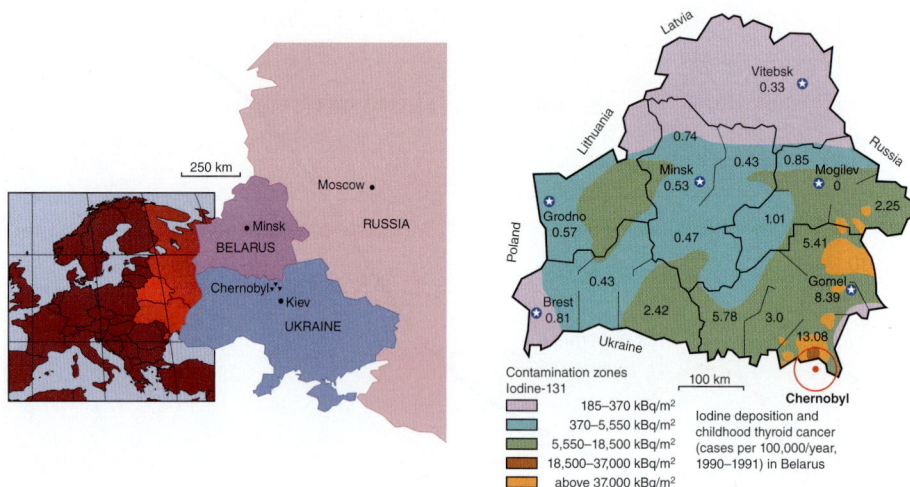

Fig. 8.11 In the first 10 years after the Chernobyl nuclear accident, a dramatic increase in thyroid cancer was seen among children living in the regions of Belarus, Ukraine, and Russia, where the heaviest contamination occurred. Map lines delineate study areas and do not necessarily depict accepted national boundaries. (From Abelin T, Egger M, Ruchti C: Fallout from Chernobyl. Belarus increase was probably caused by Chernobyl, *BMJ* 12:1298, 1994.)

of the nuclear bomb dosimetry revision is a significant increase in cancer risk estimates for both gamma and x-ray irradiation. The BEIR V report provides a summary of the newer estimates.

Conclusions from the Chernobyl nuclear disaster

Need for follow-up studies. The 1986 nuclear power station accident at Chernobyl requires long-term follow-up studies to assess the magnitude and severity of late effects on the exposed population. Detailed observations investigating potential increases in the incidence of leukemia, thyroid problems, breast cancer, and other possible radiation-induced malignancies will continue.

Worldwide effects of the accident. Even today, the possibility of late effects occurring from the Chernobyl power station disaster is still a source of concern worldwide. Because winds carried the radioactive plume in several different directions during the 10 days after the accident, more than 20 countries were affected by fallout, with approximately 400,000 people receiving some degree of radiation exposure. In February 1989, Dr. Richard Wilson, professor of physics at Harvard University in Cambridge, Massachusetts, estimated "that about 20,000 people throughout the world" would develop a radiation-induced malignancy from the Chernobyl accident.[14]

Thyroid cancer from the accident. Iodine-131 (131I) is one of the radioactive materials that became airborne in the radioactive plume. 131I concentrates in the thyroid gland and may produce cancer many years after the initial exposure. Seeking to prevent thyroid cancers, physicians administered potassium iodide (KI) to children in Poland and other countries after the Chernobyl disaster. By acting like a harmless substitute for take-up by the thyroid gland, potassium iodide inhibits the gland's uptake of 131I.

During the first 10 years after the Chernobyl disaster, the incidence of thyroid cancer increased dramatically among children living in the regions of Belarus, Ukraine, and Russia (Fig. 8.11), where the most substantial radioactive iodine contamination occurred. Thyroid cancer has been the "most pronounced health effect" of the radiation accident.[15] As of April 1996, more than 700 cases of thyroid cancer were diagnosed in children residing in these areas. The number of new thyroid cancer cases identified since the Chernobyl incident is significantly higher than anticipated, and by 1998 a total of 1700 cases had been diagnosed.[16] Radiation scientists from the Western and Eastern Hemispheres collaborated to determine the reason for this increase. Some possible explanations for the higher-than-expected number of thyroid cancers are as follows:

1. Chronic iodine deficiency during the years preceding the accident in the children living in the regions contaminated

2. Genetic predisposition to developing thyroid malignancy after radiation exposure in some subgroups of the exposed population[15]

If the first theory is valid, the thyroid glands of these individuals would have preferentially assimilated isotopes of the radioactive material inhaled from a cloud or ingested from contaminated milk supplies. If the second theory is valid, some of the exposed individuals may have a disorder that prevents the mechanism generally used by healthy cells to initiate repair and mend the genetic damage.

Why early studies did not demonstrate a significant increase in the incidence of leukemia after the accident. The fact that radiation causes leukemia, and this disease is assumed to follow an LNT dose–response curve was addressed in the discussion of the Japanese atomic bomb survivors earlier in this chapter. However, early studies of the Chernobyl victims did not demonstrate a significant increase in the incidence of leukemia, possibly because the radioactive iodine and cesium expelled into the environment during the accident may produce damaging health effects in different ways.[17] For example, 131I has a relatively short half-life (about 8 days) and is assimilated by the body and quickly distributed to the thyroid gland, thereby delivering an abrupt, acute dose to that organ. Radioactive cesium, conversely, has a much longer life (e.g., for $55Cs137$, $T_{1/2} = 30$ years), causing whole-body irradiation over a lengthy period through its long-term presence in the environment and food supply lines. This increase possibly escalates the incidence of childhood leukemia. However, it is difficult to detect without very sensitive and reliable monitoring procedures.

Life Span Shortening

Animal Studies. Laboratory experiments on small animals have shown that the life span of small animals that were exposed to nonlethal doses of ionizing radiation was shortened as a consequence of the exposure. When compared with an unexposed control group, the exposed animals died sooner. Radiation was then believed to have accelerated all causes of death. This reduction in the life cycle is known as *nonspecific life span shortening.* It was also believed that radiation accelerated the aging process, thus causing the animals to be more susceptible to several diseases. In actuality, the early demise of the experimental animals usually resulted from the induction of cancer.

Human Studies

American radiologists. In humans, studies of the life span of US radiologists that were conducted by the Radiological Society of North America from 1945 to 1954 indicated that radiologists had a shorter life span than non-radiologist physicians.[13] The process of evaluating the information has been subject to considerable criticism, and the conclusions of the study were considered questionable. Further analysis of the epidemiologic studies showed that the shortening of the life span in both animals and humans was the result of cancer and leukemia and no other "nonspecific" causes or accelerated aging.

American radiologic technologists. Initiated in 1982 and currently still in progress, an extensive study of approximately 146,000 US radiologic technologists (USRT) is continuing to evaluate potential radiation-related adverse health effects resulting from long-term, repeated exposures to low-dose ionizing radiation. These responses include cancer incidence. This occupational epidemiologic study is a collaborative effort among the University of Minnesota, the National Cancer Institute, and the American Registry of Radiologic Technologists (ARRT). The study conducted four major surveys from 1983–2014. The first survey, in 1982, identified current and former radiologic technologists certified for at least two years from 1926–1982. Ultimately, 146,022 technologists enrolled in the study and completed a questionnaire. The surveys provided important information about work practices that were common in the early years before personnel monitoring devices were routinely used.[18,19]

In 1994, the second survey was conducted. Over 90,000 radiologic technologists completed the questionnaire. The third survey, performed in 2004, had over 73,000 participants. As reported in 2004 among the 90,305 technologists who completed the first survey in the mid-1980s, there were 1283 deaths from cancer. A comparison was made between technologists who started working in the 1960s or later and those who began working before 1940. A slightly higher risk of dying from any cancer was found in technologists working before 1940. Technologists, who began working after 1940 did not demonstrate any elevated risk. However, technologists entering the medical radiation industry before 1950 demonstrated a somewhat higher risk of dying from leukemia compared with individuals entering the workforce later. The risk of dying from breast cancer has also been studied in technologists working in the field before 1940, between 1940 and 1950, and in those entering the field in 1960 or later. Technologists who began working before 1940 had the greatest risk of dying of breast cancer, followed by those who worked up to 1950. When the risk of dying of breast cancer in women who began their careers in the 1950s is compared with that in women employed from 1960 or later, the risk is only slightly higher for the women first employed in the 1950s.

The fourth survey, in 2012, had over 58,000 technologists who completed a questionnaire, over 14,000 completed a questionnaire concerning fluoroscopically-guided procedures, and over 6000 completed a questionnaire regarding nuclear medicine procedures. During 2015 and ongoing, the USRT study will focus on the following:

1. Conduct analyses of occupational radiation exposure and risk of specific cancers.
2. Conduct investigations of work history and cancer risk analyses of USRT Cohort members who perform nuclear medicine procedures and fluoroscopically guided procedures.
3. Evaluate the risk of cataracts in the entire USRT Cohort and in technologists who perform nuclear medicine procedures and fluoroscopically guided procedures.
4. Evaluate measures for estimating lifetime exposures to ultraviolet radiation and conduct exposure response analyses of cancer and other serious disease risks concerning estimated lifetime ultraviolet radiation exposure.

Readers interested in obtaining more information about this ongoing study can visit the website at https://radtechstudy.nci.nih.gov/.

Cataractogenesis

The lens of the eye contains transparent fibers that transmit light. The lens focuses light on the retina so that as the image forms, it may be transmitted through the optic nerve (Fig. 8.12B) to the imaging centers in the brain. The probability that a single dose of ionizing radiation of approximately 2 Gyt will induce the formation

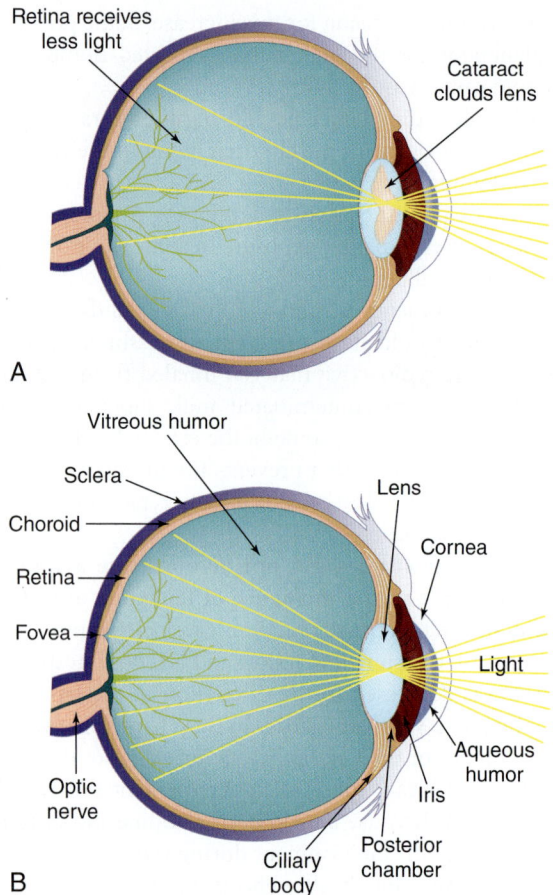

Fig. 8.12 (A) Eye with cataract. (B) Normal eye.

of cataracts (opacity of the eye lens) (see Fig. 8.12A) is high. Cataracts result in partial or complete loss of vision. Laboratory experiments with mice conclude that cataracts may be caused by doses as low as 0.1 Gyt. Highly ionizing neutron radiation (large relative biologic effectiveness [RBE]) is exceptionally efficient in producing cataracts. A neutron dose as low as 0.01 Gyt has been known to cause cataracts in mice. Radiation-induced cataracts in humans follow a threshold nonlinear dose–response relationship. Evidence of human radiation cataractogenesis originates from the observation of small groups of people who accidentally received substantial doses to the eyes. These groups include:

- Japanese atomic bomb survivors.
- Nuclear physicists working with cyclotrons (units that produce beams of high-energy particles such as 150 MeV proton beams) between 1932 and 1960.

- Patients undergoing radiation therapy who received significant exposures to the eyes during treatment.

Recent data indicate that the threshold for cataract induction is lower than previously thought.[20] The threshold for single exposures is now considered to be 0.5 Gy (50 rads).[21] Even with this lower value, the chance of radiographers developing radiation-induced cataracts from general diagnostic imaging procedures is very small. However, in the realm of diagnostic radiology, some very lengthy fluoroscopic procedures can result in significant radiation exposure to the lens of the eye from cumulative scatter radiation. The occupational dose to this sensitive area can be substantially reduced when radiologists and radiographers wear protective eyewear while participating in the examination. In patients, the dose to the lens of the eye can be decreased by also having them wear protective eye shields, provided the use of such shields does not compromise the diagnostic value of the fluoroscopic examination.

Embryologic Effects (Birth Defects)

Stages of Gestation in Humans. All life forms are most vulnerable to radiation during the embryonic stage of development. The period of gestation during which the embryo-fetus is exposed to radiation governs the effects (death or congenital abnormality) of the radiation. Gestation in humans is divided into three stages or periods:

1. Preimplantation, which corresponds to 0 to 9 days after conception
2. **Organogenesis**, which lasts approximately from 10 days postconception to 12 weeks after conception
3. The fetal stage, which extends from the 12th week to term (Fig. 8.13)

Embryonic Cell Radiosensitivity During the First Trimester of Pregnancy. Because embryonic cells begin dividing and differentiating after conception, they are exceptionably radiosensitive and hence may easily be damaged by exposure to ionizing radiation. Thus, the first trimester of pregnancy is the most crucial period concerning harmful consequences from irradiation because the developing central nervous system and related sensory organs of the embryo-fetus contain a large number of stem cells during this period of gestation.

If the embryo receives a high dose of radiation within approximately 2 weeks of fertilization (i.e., before the start of organogenesis), fetal death is the most apparent negative consequence of such an exposure, followed by spontaneous abortion. If this does not occur, the pregnancy will continue to term, either with some adverse effect or without any.[13] Irradiation of the embryo-fetus during the first 12 weeks of development to equivalent doses above 200 mSv (20 rem) frequently may result in fetal death or, at the least, in severe congenital abnormalities.

During the preimplantation stage, the fertilized ovum divides and forms a ball-like structure containing undifferentiated cells. If this structure is irradiated with a dose in the range of 0.05 to 0.15 Gyt, embryonic

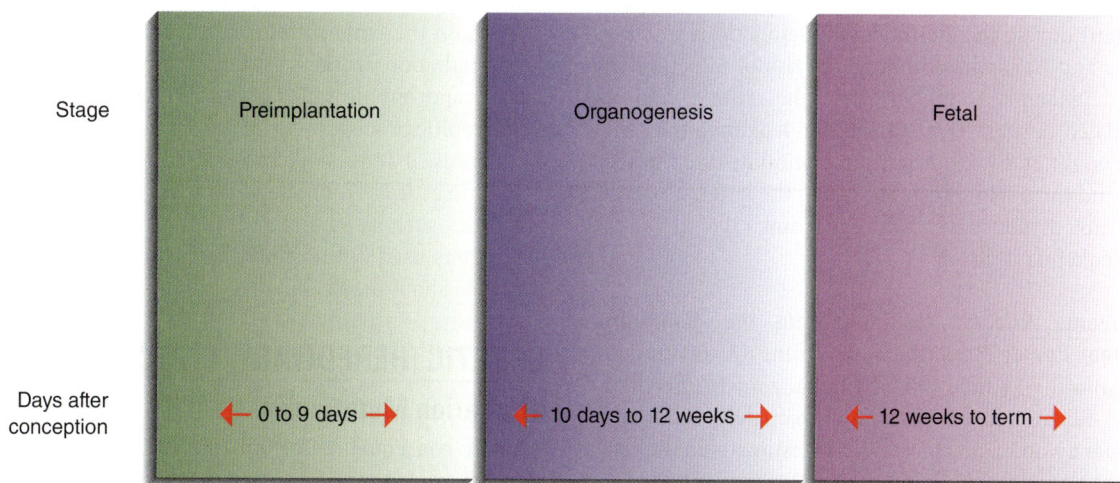

Stage	Preimplantation	Organogenesis	Fetal
Days after conception	← 0 to 9 days →	← 10 days to 12 weeks →	← 12 weeks to term →

Fig. 8.13 Division of gestation in humans. (From Riegh R: *Am J Roentgenol* 89:182, 1963.)

death will occur. Malformations resulting from radiation exposure do not occur at this stage. The developing fetus is most susceptible to radiation-induced congenital abnormalities during organogenesis, which occurs at approximately 10 days and lasts up to 12 weeks after conception. Abnormalities may include:

- Growth inhibition
- Intellectual disability
- Microcephaly
- Genital deformities
- Sensory organ damage

During the late stages of organogenesis, the presence of nonminor abnormalities in the fetus will cause neonatal death (death at birth). Skeletal damage from radiation exposure occurs most frequently during the period from week 3 to week 20 of development. Cancer and functional disorders during childhood are other possible effects of irradiation during the fetal stage (a growth period).

Embryonic Cell Radiosensitivity During the Second and Third Trimesters of Pregnancy. Fetal radiosensitivity decreases as gestation progresses. Hence, during the second and third trimesters of pregnancy when lesser numbers of cells are differentiating, the developing fetus is less susceptible to ionizing radiation exposure. However, even in these later trimesters, congenital abnormalities and functional disorders such as sterility may be caused by radiation exposure.

Much of the evidence for radiation-induced congenital abnormalities in humans comes from more than four decades of follow-up studies of children exposed in utero during the atomic bomb detonations in Hiroshima and Nagasaki. Although the risk of radiation-induced leukemia is higher when the embryo-fetus is irradiated during the first trimester, leukemia may also be brought on by exposure to radiation during the second and third trimesters. Studies of the latter, however, have not demonstrated any significant rates of cancer and leukemia deaths.[22]

Embryonic Effects Resulting from the Chernobyl Nuclear Power Plant Accident. Of the 135,000 evacuees from the 18 mile (30 km) radial zone of the Chernobyl nuclear power plant, approximately 2000 were pregnant women. Each received an estimated quite *sizeable* average total-body equivalent dose of 0.43 Sv (43 rem). No apparent abnormalities were observed in the 300 live babies born by August 1987. However, from 1987 through 1990, the Ministry of Health in Ukraine recorded an increased number of miscarriages, premature births, and stillbirths.[23,24] Also recorded during this period by the ministry was an increase to three times the average rate of deformities and developmental abnormalities in newborns.[23,24]

Review of Fetal Effects by UNSCEAR. Fetal effects such as mortality, malformations, intellectual disability, and childhood cancer were reviewed by the United Nations Scientific Committee on the Effects of Atomic Radiation (UNSCEAR).[25] This group proposed an upper-limit *increased combined radiation risk* for the aforementioned fetal effects of "3 chances per 1000 children (0.3%) for each rem (.01 Sv) of fetal dose."[26] With no radiation exposure, these fetal effects have an estimated *reasonable total risk* of "60 chances per 1000 children (6%)."[26] Thus with radiation exposure, a total risk of 60 per 1000 children plus an additional 3 per 1000 children for each 0.1 Sv (rem) of the fetal equivalent dose was indicated.

Effects of Low-Level Ionizing Radiation on the Embryo-Fetus. The effects of *low-level ionizing radiation* on the embryo-fetus can only be poorly estimated. Documentation of the impact of low-level radiation on the unborn irradiated in utero is insufficient because some types of abnormalities occur in a small percentage (approximately 4%) of all live births in the United States. However, if the exposure occurs during a period of major organogenesis, the abnormality and its occurrence may be more pronounced.

Because the embryo-fetus is extra sensitive to radiation, radiation workers should exercise caution and employ appropriate safety measures when performing radiographic procedures on pregnant patients. For these procedures, if requested, medical physicists can make fetal dose estimates for specific patients based on characteristics such as patient size and the actual technical parameters used in the studies in cases where there are concerns about medical management.

GENETIC (HEREDITARY) EFFECTS

Irradiation Mutations

Biologic consequences of ionizing radiation on future generations are termed **genetic or hereditary effects**. They can occur as a result of radiation-induced damage to the DNA molecule in the sperm or ova of an adult, leading to germ cell alterations, which cause incorrect genetic information to be transmitted to the offspring. Additionally, these effects may manifest as various diseases or malformations. Non-lethal radiation doses received by the germ cells can cause chromosome irregularities that may be transmitted to successive generations.

Natural Mutations

Some modifications in genetic material occur naturally, without a known cause. They are referred to as *spontaneous mutations*. These can be transmitted from one generation to the next and may cause a wide variety of disorders or diseases, including:

- Hemophilia
- Huntington's chorea
- Down syndrome
- Duchenne's muscular dystrophy
- Sickle cell anemia
- Cystic fibrosis
- Hydrocephalus

Hereditary disorders are common in any animal population. In humans, a genetic disorder is present in approximately 10% of all live births in the United States.

Other Agents of Genetic Mutations

There are also additional agents called *mutagens*, which can increase the frequency of mutations. Among these are:

- Viruses
- Multiple specific chemicals

Incapacities of Mutant Genes

Mutant genes cannot correctly govern the cell's normal chemical reactions or adequately control the sequence of amino acids in the formation of specific proteins. These incapacities result in various genetic diseases. For example, sickle cell anemia arises from the defective synthesis of the protein hemoglobin. About 300 amino acids combine to form the hemoglobin molecule. Sickle cell anemia is caused by the omission of only a single vital amino acid.

Dominant or Recessive Point Mutations

Point mutations (genetic mutations at the molecular level) may be either *dominant* (probably expressed in the offspring) or *recessive* (perhaps not expressed for several generations). Radiation is thought to cause primarily recessive mutations. For a recessive mutation to appear in the offspring, both parents must have the same genetic defect. This requires that the defect must be located on the same part of a specific DNA base sequence in each parent. Because this rarely occurs, the effects of recessive mutations are not likely to appear in a population. However, an increase in the number of individuals who receive radiation exposure raises the likelihood that two individuals with the same type of mutation will have children. Therefore, it is essential to limit the radiation exposure of the entire population. Damage from recessive mutations sometimes manifests more subtly and may play a role in many commonly encountered disorders related to metabolism or the immune system.

Ionizing Radiation as a Possible Cause of Genetic (Hereditary) Effects

The most conclusive physical evidence confirming that ionizing radiation causes genetic effects comes from extensive experimentation with fruit flies and mice at high radiation doses. The data on mice have been extrapolated to low doses and then applied to humans. The information obtained from the fruit fly experiments suggests that *genetic effects do not have a threshold dose*. Because this means that even the smallest radiation dose could cause some hereditary damage, there is, according to these data, no such thing as a "100% safe" gonadal radiation dose.

Direct existing data on radiation-induced genetic effects in humans, however, are both contradictory and inconclusive. Some of the data accumulated comes from observation of test groups of children conceived after one or both parents had been exposed to radiation as a result of the atomic bomb detonation in Hiroshima or Nagasaki. As of the third generation of these survivors, no radiation-induced genetic effects are known. However, this does not ensure that they will not be seen in subsequent generations. J. F. Crow, a geneticist who spent many years experimenting with fruit flies, believed that the most frequent mutations in humans are not those leading to obvious hereditary diseases but those causing minor impairments leading to higher embryonic death rates, lower life expectancy, increase in disease, or decreased fertility.[27] The position of the scientific community to date remains unresolved.

In 2001 a UNSCEAR study on the genetic effects of radiation concluded that no radiation-induced inherited diseases had so far been demonstrated in human populations exposed to ionizing radiation. However, some counterexamples have appeared in the scientific literature.[24]

Currently, evidence of radiation-induced hereditary effects has not been detected in persons employed in diagnostic imaging or in patients undergoing radiologic examinations. Even with this information on hand, it is still recommended that irradiation of gonadal tissue should be avoided unless there is a reasonable expectation of medical benefit, e.g., the information obtained from a well-ordered and high-quality diagnostic examination.

Doubling Dose Concept

Animal studies of radiation-induced hereditary changes led to the development of the doubling dose concept, which is a measure of the effectiveness of ionizing radiation in causing mutations. **Doubling dose** is, by definition, the radiation dose that causes the number of spontaneous mutations occurring in a given generation to increase to two times their original occurrence. For example, if 7% of the offspring in each generation are born with mutations in the absence of radiation other than background levels, the

BOX 8.3 Doubling Dose Concept		
Percentage (%) of offspring born in each generation with mutations in the absence of radiation other than background	Estimated radiation dose in sieverts (Sv) received	Percentage (%) of offspring born with mutation after receiving a doubling equivalent dose
7%	1.56 Sv	14%

administration of the doubling dose to all members of the population would eventually increase the number of mutations to 14% (Box 8.3). The radiation doubling dose for humans, as determined from studies of the children of the atomic bomb survivors of Hiroshima and Nagasaki, is estimated to have a mean value of 1.56 Sv (156 rem) based on the hereditary indicators of an unfortunate pregnancy outcome (e.g., stillbirths, significant congenital abnormalities, death during the first postnatal week), childhood mortality, and sex chromosome aneuploidy (possession of an abnormal number of chromosomes).

SUMMARY

- Scientists use the information from epidemiologic studies to formulate dose–response graphical relationships to predict the risk of cancer in human populations exposed to low doses of ionizing radiation.
  - Curves that demonstrate radiation dose–response relationships can be either linear or nonlinear and depict either a threshold or a nonthreshold dose.
  - A linear nonthreshold (LNT) curve is currently used for most types of cancers.
  - Risk of leukemia, breast cancer, and genetic effects associated with low-level radiation is typically estimated with the linear-quadratic nonthreshold (LQNT) curve.
  - Late tissue reactions may be demonstrated graphically through the use of a linear threshold (LT) curve of radiation dose–response.
  - High-dose cellular response may be demonstrated through the use of a sigmoid threshold curve.

- Late effects include carcinogenesis, cataractogenesis, and embryologic (birth) defects.
- Effects that have no threshold, that occur arbitrarily, that have a severity that does not depend on dose, and that occur months or years after exposure are called *stochastic effects*.
- Cancer is the most significant stochastic somatic effect caused by exposure to ionizing radiation.
- Risk estimates are given in terms of absolute risk or relative risk.
  - The absolute risk model estimates that a specific number of malignancies will occur as a result of radiation exposure.
  - The relative risk model predicts that the number of excess cancers rises as the natural incidence of cancer increases with advancing age in a population.
  - Linear and linear-quadratic models are used for extrapolation of risk from high-dose to low-dose data.

- The first trimester of pregnancy is the most critical period for radiation exposure of the embryo-fetus.
  - Radiation-induced congenital abnormalities can occur approximately from 10 days to 12 weeks after conception.
  - Skeletal abnormalities most frequently occur from weeks 3 to 20.
- Radiation exposure even in the second and third trimesters can potentially cause congenital abnormalities, functional disorders, and a predisposition to the development of childhood cancer.
- Genetic effects of ionizing radiation are biologic effects on generations yet unborn.

- Radiation-induced abnormalities are caused by unrepaired damage to DNA molecules in the sperm or ova of an adult.
- There is no 100% safe gonadal radiation dose; even the smallest radiation dose could cause some hereditary damage.
- Doubling dose measures the effectiveness of ionizing radiation in causing mutations; it is the radiation dose that causes the number of spontaneous mutations in a given generation to increase to two times their original occurrence.
- For humans, the doubling dose is estimated to have a mean value of 1.56 Sv.

GENERAL DISCUSSION QUESTIONS

1. How do scientists use epidemiologic studies to assess cancer risk from low doses of ionizing radiation?
2. What is the purpose of a radiation dose–response curve?
3. What are the different types of dose–response relationships, and how can they be represented in diagrams?
4. Why do regulatory agencies prefer the linear dose–response model for radiation protection standards?
5. What is the difference between threshold and nonthreshold relationships in radiation exposure?
6. What are some of the late tissue reactions and stochastic effects associated with ionizing radiation?
7. How is risk for radiation-induced malignancies conceptualized, and what models are used for risk estimation?
8. Can you identify specific populations that have shown increased cancer rates due to ionizing radiation exposure?
9. How do spontaneous mutations occur, and what is their significance?
10. What is the doubling dose concept, and how does it relate to mutation rates?

REVIEW QUESTIONS

1. How do epidemiologic studies help predict cancer risk in populations exposed to low doses of ionizing radiation?
   A. By measuring radiation levels in soil
   B. By comparing cancer rates between exposed and unexposed groups
   C. By analyzing genetic mutations in laboratory settings
   D. By assessing dietary habits in the population
2. What is the primary purpose of a radiation dose–response curve?
   A. To establish safe radiation levels for workers
   B. To illustrate the relationship between radiation dose and biological response
   C. To measure environmental radiation exposure
   D. To determine the effectiveness of radiation therapy
3. Which type of dose–response relationship indicates that even small doses of radiation can increase risk?
   A. Threshold
   B. Nonthreshold
   C. Linear
   D. Biphasic
4. Why do regulatory agencies often use the linear dose–response model for radiation protection?
   A. It is the simplest model available.
   B. It provides a conservative estimate of risk.
   C. It is based on historical data.
   D. It requires fewer resources to implement.
5. What are late tissue reactions to ionizing radiation?
   A. Immediate nausea and vomiting
   B. Long-term effects like cancer and cataracts
   C. Increased metabolic rate
   D. Temporary hair loss

6. Which model is commonly used to estimate the risk of radiation-induced malignancies?
   A. Linear no-threshold model (LNT)
   B. Absolute risk model
   C. Relative risk model
   D. Stochastic risk model

7. Which group of individuals is known to have increased cancer rates due to radiation exposure?
   A. Smokers
   B. Hiroshima and Nagasaki survivors
   C. Athletes
   D. Pregnant women

8. What is the primary cause of spontaneous mutations?
   A. Environmental toxins
   B. Errors during DNA replication
   C. Ionizing radiation
   D. Viral infections

9. What does the doubling dose concept refer to?
   A. The time required to double the radiation exposure
   B. The amount of radiation that doubles the mutation rate
   C. The increase in cancer cases over time
   D. The number of treatments needed to reduce cancer risk

10. Which type of genetic mutation is characterized by a single altered gene that can manifest in the phenotype?
   A. Chromosomal aberration
   B. Recessive mutation
   C. Dominant mutation
   D. Spontaneous mutation

Dose Limits for Exposure to Ionizing Radiation

OBJECTIVES

After completing this chapter, the reader will be able to perform the following:

- Define all key terms.
- List and describe the function of the four major organizations that share the responsibility for evaluating the relationship between radiation equivalent dose and induced biologic effects and five US regulatory agencies responsible for enforcing established radiation effective dose limiting standards.
- Explain the function of the radiation safety committee (RSC) in a medical facility, and describe the role of the radiation safety officer (RSO) by listing the various responsibilities the RSO must fulfill.
- Explain the purpose of the Radiation Control for Health and Safety Act of 1968 and the Consumer-Patient Health and Safety Act of 1981.
- List the important provisions of the code of standards for diagnostic x-ray equipment that began on August 1, 1974.
- Explain the ALARA concept.
- Discuss the current radiation protection philosophy.
- Identify radiation-induced responses that warrant serious concern for radiation protection.
- Explain the concept of risk as it relates to the medical imaging industry.
- Describe the effective dose limit and the effective dose limiting system.
- Identify the risk from exposure to ionizing radiation at low absorbed doses.
- Discuss the current National Council on Radiation Protection and Measurements recommendations.

- Calculate the cumulative effective dose (CumEfD) for the whole body of a radiation worker.
- Discuss the significance of radiation effective dose action limits in health care facilities.
- Explain the concept of radiation hormesis.
- State the following in terms of International System (SI) units:
  - Annual occupational effective dose limit and CumEfD limit for whole-body radiation exposure excluding medical and natural background exposure, which are based on stochastic effects
  - Annual occupational equivalent dose limits for tissues and organs such as the lens of the eye, skin, hands, and feet, which are based on tissue reactions
  - Annual effective dose limits for continuous (or frequent) exposure and for infrequent exposure of the general public from human-made sources other than medical and natural background, which are based on stochastic effects
  - Annual equivalent dose limits for tissues and organs such as the lens of the eye, skin, hands, and feet of members of the general public, which are based on tissue reactions
  - Annual effective dose limit for an occupationally exposed student under the age of 18 years (excluding medical and natural background radiation exposure)
  - Occupational monthly equivalent dose limit to the embryo-fetus (excluding medical and natural background radiation) once the pregnancy is known

CHAPTER OUTLINE

KEY TERMS

action limits
agreement states
ALARA Concept
annual occupational effective
  dose limit
cumulative effective dose
  (CumEfD) limit
effective dose (EfD)
effective dose (EfD) limiting
  system

effective dose limit (EDL)
equivalent dose (EqD)
**International Commission on
  Radiological Protection
  (ICRP)**
lifetime effective dose
**National Council on Radiation
  Protection and Measurements
  (NCRP)**
Negligible individual dose (NID)

**Nuclear Regulatory Commission
  (NRC)**
radiation hormesis
radiation-induced malignancy
radiation safety committee (RSC)
radiation safety officer (RSO)
stochastic effects
tissue reactions
tissue weighting factors (W$_t$)

Exposure of the general public, patients, and radiation workers to ionizing radiation must be limited
to minimize the risk of harmful biologic effects. To
this end, scientists have developed occupational and

nonoccupational **effective dose (EfD)** limits and **equivalent dose (EqD)** limits for tissues and organs such as
the lens of the eye, skin, hands, and feet. An **effective
dose (EfD) limiting system** (i.e., a set of numeric dose

limits that are based on calculations of the various risks of cancer and genetic [hereditary] effects to tissues or organs exposed to radiation) has been incorporated into Title 10 of the Code of Federal Regulations, Part 20, a document prepared and distributed by the US Office of the Federal Register. The rules and regulations of the Nuclear Regulatory Commission (NRC) and fundamental radiation protection standards governing occupational radiation exposure are included in this document.

BASIS OF EFFECTIVE DOSE LIMITING SYSTEM

The concept of radiation exposure and the associated risk of radiation-induced malignancy is the basis of the effective dose limiting system. Information contained in Reports 184 and 116 of the National Council on Radiation Protection and Measurement (NCRP) and Publication No. 60 of the International Commission on Radiological Protection (ICRP) serves as a resource for the revised recommendations. Future radiation protection standards are expected to continue to be based on *risk*.

Because medical imaging professionals share the responsibility for patient safety from radiation exposure and themselves are subject to such exposure in the performance of their duties, they must be familiar with previous, existing, and new guidelines. By staying informed, imaging professionals will be more conscious of beneficial radiation safety practices. A radiographer can obtain the required knowledge by becoming familiar with the functions and recommendations of the various advisory groups and regulatory agencies discussed in this chapter (Fig. 9.1).

RADIATION PROTECTION STANDARDS ORGANIZATIONS

The following discussion examines the four major organizations responsible for evaluating the relationship between radiation EqD and induced biologic effects. These organizations are also extensively occupied with formulating risk estimates of somatic and genetic effects of irradiation. They are respectively entitled:

1. International Commission on Radiological Protection (ICRP)
2. National Council on Radiation Protection and Measurements (NCRP)

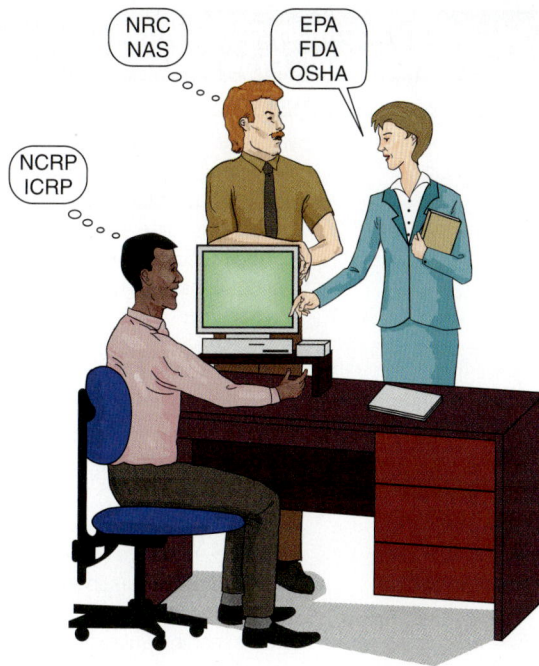

Fig. 9.1 The various advisory groups and regulatory agencies, usually referred to by abbreviations and acronyms, may be extremely confusing.

3. United Nations Scientific Committee on the Effects of Atomic Radiation (UNSCEAR)
4. National Academy of Sciences/National Research Council Committee on the Biological Effects of Ionizing Radiation (NAS/NRC-BEIR)

A brief operational summary of these radiation standards organizations is presented in Table 9.1.

International Commission on Radiological Protection

The International Commission on Radiological Protection (ICRP) is considered the international authority on the safe use of sources of ionizing radiation. The ICRP is composed of a main commission with 12 active members, a chairman, and 4 standing committees, which include committees on radiation effects, radiation exposure, protection in medicine, and the application of ICRP recommendations.[1] Since its inception in 1928, the ICRP has been the leading international organization responsible for providing clear and consistent radiation protection guidance through its recommendations for occupational dose limits and public dose limits.

TABLE 9.1   Summary of Radiation Protection Standards Organizations

Organization	Function
International Commission on Radiological Protection (ICRP)	Evaluates information on biologic effects of radiation and provides radiation protection guidance through general recommendations on occupational and public dose limits
National Council on Radiation Protection and Measurements (NCRP)	Reviews regulations formulated by the ICRP and decides ways to include those recommendations in US radiation protection criteria
United Nations Scientific Committee on the Effects of Atomic Radiation (UNSCEAR)	Evaluate human and environmental ionizing radiation exposure and derive radiation risk assessments from epidemiologic data and research conclusions; provide information to organizations such as the ICRP for evaluation
National Academy of Sciences/National Research Council Committee on the Biological Effects of Ionizing Radiation (NAS/NRC-BEIR)	Reviews studies of biologic effects of ionizing radiation and risk assessment and provides the information to organizations such as the ICRP for evaluation

BOX 9.1   Objectives of the National Council on Radiation Protection and Measurements

Objectives 4 to 7 are identified in the charter of the council (Public Law 88-376) as follows:
"To:

4. Collect, analyze, develop, and disseminate in the public interest information and recommendations about (a) protection against radiation (b) radiation measurements, quantities, and units, particularly those concerned with radiation protection.
5. Provide a means by which organizations concerned with the scientific and related aspects of radiation protection and of radiation quantities, units, and measurements may cooperate for the effective utilization of their combined resources, and to stimulate the work of such organizations.
6. Develop basic concepts about radiation quantities, units, and measurements, about the application of these concepts, and about radiation protection.
7. Cooperate with the International Commission on Radiological Protection, the International Commission on Radiation Units and Measurements, and other national and international organizations, government and private, concerned with radiation quantities, units, and measurements and with radiation protection."

From National Council on Radiation Protection and Measurements (NCRP): *Limitation of exposure to ionizing radiation, Report No. 116,* Bethesda, MD, 1993, NCRP. Reprinted with permission from the National Council on Radiation Protection and Measurements, http://NCRPonline.org.

Initially, these recommendations were published as reports in selected scholarly journals. Since 1959, the ICRP has had a series of publications, and from 1977 onward, the scientific journal *Annals of the ICRP* has published ICRP information. The ICRP only makes recommendations; it does not function as an enforcement agency. Recommendations are also supplied by scientific articles published in scholarly journals and by organizations such as UNSCEAR and NAS/NRC-BEIR, which are discussed later in this chapter. Each nation must develop and enforce its specific regulations.

National Council on Radiation Protection and Measurements

In the United States, a nongovernmental, nonprofit, private corporation known as the **National Council on Radiation Protection and Measurements (NCRP),** chartered by Congress in 1964, reviews the recommendations formulated by the ICRP. The NCRP determines how ICRP recommendations are incorporated into US radiation protection criteria. The council implements this task by assembling general relevant guidelines and publishing them in the form of various NCRP reports which can be purchased from NCRP Publications in Bethesda, Maryland. A listing of current NCRP reports available for purchase at cost may be found at www.ncrp.com.

Because the NCRP is not an enforcement agency, the enactment of its recommendations lies with federal and state agencies that have the power to enforce such standards after they have been established. The NCRP's objectives are listed and described in Box 9.1. Governmental enforcement organizations (e.g., the NRC, the EPA, and all state governments) use the recommendations of the NCRP as the scientific basis for their radiation protection activities.[2] Nongovernmental groups desiring to improve their radiation safety practices and their promotion and disbursement of pertinent radiation protection materials refer to this public service organization for guidance.

United Nations Scientific Committee on the Effects of Atomic Radiation (UNSCEAR)

UNSCEAR, established in 1955, is another group that plays a prominent role in the formulation of radiation protection guidelines. This group evaluates human and environmental ionizing radiation exposures from a variety of sources, including:

- Radioactive materials
- Radiation-producing machines
- Radiation accidents

UNSCEAR uses epidemiologic data (e.g., information from follow-up studies of Japanese atomic bomb survivors), data acquired from the Radiation Effects Research Foundation (a group run by the government of Japan primarily to study the survivors), and research conclusions to derive radiation risk assessments for radiation-induced cancer and genetic (hereditary) effects.

National Academy of Sciences/National Research Council Committee on the Biological Effects of Ionizing Radiation (NAS/NRC-BEIR)

NAS/NRC-BEIR is another advisory group that reviews studies of the biologic effects of ionizing radiation and risk assessment. This group formulated the 1990 BEIR V Report, *Health Effects of Exposure to Low Levels of Ionizing Radiation*. BEIR V supersedes four earlier BEIR reports that listed studies of biologic effects and the associated risk of groups of people who were either routinely or accidentally exposed to ionizing radiation. Such groups include:

- Early radiation workers
- Atomic bomb victims of Hiroshima and Nagasaki
- Evacuees from the Chernobyl nuclear power station disaster

As previously noted, recommendations for EfD limits and EqD limits are made by the ICRP, NCRP, UNSCEAR, and NAS/NRC-BEIR. Based on these recommendations, limits on radiation exposure are established by congressional acts or state mandates. National and state agencies are charged with the responsibility of enforcing standards after they have been established.

US REGULATORY AGENCIES

After radiation protection standards have been determined, responsible agencies must enforce them for the protection of the general public, patients, and occupationally exposed personnel.

Regulatory agencies include the following:
1. Nuclear Regulatory Commission (NRC)
2. Agreement states
3. Environmental Protection Agency (EPA)
4. US Food and Drug Administration (FDA)
5. Occupational Safety and Health Administration (OSHA)

A summary of the US regulatory agencies is presented in Table 9.2.

TABLE 9.2 Summary of US Regulatory Agencies

Agency	Function
Nuclear Regulatory Commission (NRC)	Oversees the nuclear energy industry, enforces radiation protection standards, publishes its rules and regulations in Title 10 of the US Code of Federal Regulations, and enters into written agreements with state governments that permit the state to license and regulate the use of radioisotopes and certain other material within that state
Agreement states	Enforce radiation protection regulations through their respective health departments
Environmental Protection Agency (EPA)	Facilitates the development and enforcement of regulations pertaining to the control of radiation in the environment
US Food and Drug Administration (FDA)	Conducts an ongoing product radiation control program, regulating the design and manufacture of electronic products, including x-ray equipment
Occupational Safety and Health Administration (OSHA)	Functions as a monitoring agency in places of employment, predominantly in industry

Nuclear Regulatory Commission

The **Nuclear Regulatory Commission (NRC)**, formerly known as the *Atomic Energy Commission,* is a federal agency that has the authority to control the possession, use, and production of atomic energy in the interest of national security. This agency also has the power to enforce radiation protection standards. However, the NRC does not regulate or inspect x-ray imaging facilities. The primary function of the NRC is to oversee the nuclear energy industry. This agency supervises the:

- Design and working mechanics of nuclear power stations
- Production of nuclear fuel
- Handling of expended fuel
- Supervision of hazardous radioactive waste material

Additionally, the NRC controls the manufacture and use of radioactive isotopes formed in nuclear reactors (also known as *by-product* materials) and used in:

- Research
- Industry
- Nuclear medicine imaging procedures
- Therapeutic treatments

Users of such radioactive materials must be formally licensed by the NRC and will receive periodically unannounced inspections by NRC staff to determine whether these users comply with the provisions of their licenses. Failure to pass these inspections can result in significant fines and even license suspension. Until 2008, the NRC did not regulate the use of radioactive substances that either are naturally occurring, like radium, or are produced outside of a reactor by high-energy particle accelerators, such as cyclotrons. These materials are designated as *NARM* ("naturally occurring and/or accelerator produced materials"). Two common examples of cyclotron-produced radioisotopes are:

- Thallium-201 (201Tl) used in nuclear medicine for heart stress tests
- Palladium-103 (103Pd) used for therapeutic prostate seed implants

NARM materials were formerly solely regulated by state bureaus of radiation protection. In 2008, the NRC expanded its definition of by-product substances to include NARM materials. This meant that all facilities in *nonagreement* states (i.e., those states that have decided to maintain their own self-designed independent radiation protection program for radioactive materials), must be in full compliance with NRC regulations and additionally would have to amend their NRC radioactive materials license to include all NARM materials that they are currently using.

The NRC writes rules and regulations. The US Office of the Federal Register prepares and distributes these rules in Title 10 of the US Code of Federal Regulations. Radiation protection standards governing occupational radiation exposure may be found in Part 20 of Title 10, abbreviated 10 CFR 20.

Agreement States

The NRC has the authority to enter into written contracts with state governments. These agreements permit the contracting state to undertake the responsibility of licensing and regulating the use of radioisotopes and certain other radioactive materials within that state.

Most states in the United States have entered into such "agreements" with the NRC, thereby also assuming responsibility for enforcing radiation protection regulations through their respective health departments. These states are known as **agreement states**. In *nonagreement states*, both the state and the NRC jointly inspect and enforce radiation protection regulations by sending agents at different times to health care facilities. Hospitals are evaluated to determine whether they comply with existing radiation safety regulations. Individual states may also legislate regulations regarding radiation safety to be above and beyond those mandated by the NRC. Inspection of nuclear reactors and assurance of adherence to federal radiation safety regulations in the agreement or nonagreement states fall solely under the jurisdiction of the NRC.

Environmental Protection Agency (EPA)

The EPA, established in 1970 through the reorganization plan of US President Richard M. Nixon, was created to bring several departments under one organization that would be responsible for protecting the health of humans and for safeguarding the natural environment from industrial practices and harmful waste disposal.

The EPA, as part of its general overseer responsibilities, also facilitates the development and enforcement of regulations pertaining to the *control of radiation in the environment.* Specifically, it:

- Directs relevant federal agencies
- Oversees the general area of environmental monitoring
- Has oversight authority for specific areas such as determining the action level for radon

US Food and Drug Administration (FDA)

Under Public Law 90-602, the Radiation Control for Health and Safety Act of 1968, the FDA conducts an ongoing product radiation control program, regulating the design and manufacturing of electronic products, including diagnostic x-ray equipment.

A more detailed explanation of the Radiation Control for Health and Safety Act of 1968 is discussed later in this chapter.

To determine the level of compliance with standards in a given radiology facility, the FDA conducts on-site inspections of x-ray equipment, particularly mammography units. Compliance with FDA standards ensures the protection of occupationally and nonoccupationally exposed persons from faulty manufacturing.

Occupational Safety and Health Administration (OSHA)

OSHA functions as a monitoring agency in places of employment, predominantly in industry. OSHA regulates occupational exposure to radiation through Part 1910 of Title 29 of the US Code of Federal Regulations (29 CFR 1910). The agency is responsible for regulations concerning an employee's "right to know" about hazards that may be present in the workplace. A series of statutes passed by the individual states requires that employees be made aware of these potential risks in the workplace. The act covers:

- Hazardous substances
- Infectious agents
- Ionizing radiation
- Nonionizing radiation (e.g., ultraviolet, microwaves, etc.)

The act requires employers to evaluate their workplaces for harmful agents and to provide training and written information to their employees. OSHA also regulates training programs in the workplace.

RADIATION SAFETY PROGRAM

Requirement

Facilities providing imaging services *shall have* an active and detailed radiation safety program to ensure adequate safety of patients and radiation workers. The implementation of an effective program begins with the administrative personnel of the facility. Individuals in executive positions must provide the resources necessary for creating and maintaining this program. They can:

- Delegate operational funds in the budget
- Oversee the development of policies and procedures
- Provide the equipment needed for starting and continuing the program

Radiation Safety Committee and Radiation Safety Officer

The NRC mandates that a **radiation safety committee (RSC)** be established for the facility. This committee imparts guidance for the program and facilitates its ongoing operation. A **radiation safety officer (RSO)** should also be selected to:

- Oversee the program's daily operation
- Provide for formal review of the program each year

An RSO is usually a medical physicist, health physicist, radiologist, or other individual qualified through adequate training and experience. This person is designated by a health care facility and approved by the NRC and the state.

Responsibilities of the Radiation Safety Officer. The RSO is responsible for developing an appropriate radiation safety program for the facility that follows internationally accepted guidelines for radiation protection. This individual is also charged with ensuring that the facility's operational radiation practices are such that all persons, especially those who are or could be pregnant, are adequately protected from unnecessary exposure. To fulfill this responsibility, the management of the facility must grant the RSO the authority necessary to implement and enforce the policies of the radiation safety program.

The RSO must also review and maintain radiation-monitoring records for all personnel and be available to provide counseling for individuals (e.g., those who receive monitor readings above allowable limits).

Required Training and Experience for a Radiation Safety Officer. The necessary training and experience for an RSO is described in Part 35.50 and Part 35.900 of Title 10 of the Code of Federal Regulations. The NRC publishes regulatory guides to accompany its rules. Although legally health care facilities do not need to comply with the guide, they frequently choose to do so to facilitate the chances of a successful outcome of an NRC inspection or approval of license changes. The guide is the NRC's interpretation of how to implement its own rules.

> **BOX 9.2   Allowable Pathways for a Nominated Radiation Safety Officer to Meet Training and Experience Requirements as Described in 10 CFR 35.50 and 10 CFR 35.900**
>
> 1. Certification by one of the professional boards approved by the Nuclear Regulatory Commission (NRC)
> 2. Didactic and work experience as described in detail in the regulations
> 3. Identification as an authorized user, authorized medical physicist, or authorized health physicist on the license, with experience in the types of uses for which the individual has radiation safety officer (RSO) responsibilities

> **BOX 9.3   Duties That 10 CFR 35.24 Requires the Licensee to Freely Provide the Radiation Safety Officer to Perform**
>
> 1. Identify radiation safety problems.
> 2. Initiate, recommend, or provide corrective action.
> 3. Stop unsafe operations involving by-product material.
> 4. Verify implementation of corrective actions.

Three pathways exist for obtaining the training and experience required for the RSO position (identified in Box 9.2).

Authority of the Radiation Safety Officer. 10 CFR 35.24 requires that the licensee provide the RSO:

- Sufficient authority
- Organizational freedom
- Management prerogative to perform specific duties

These tasks are identified in Box 9.3. The licensee must establish, in writing, the authority, functions, and responsibilities of the RSO. Because the RSO is responsible for the day-to-day supervision of the facility's radiation safety program, this individual must have independent authority to stop operations that are considered unsafe. Also, the RSO must be given adequate time and resources and have a sufficient commitment from management to ensure that radioactive materials are used in a safe manner. The NRC requires the name of the RSO on the facility's radioactive materials license to ensure that licensee management has identified a responsible, qualified person who can directly interact with the NRC during inspections and also concerning any inquiries regarding the facility's safety program. Usually, the RSO is a full-time employee of the licensed facility; however, the NRC has authorized individuals who are not employed by the licensee (e.g., a consultant) to fill the role of an RSO or to provide support to the facility's RSO. Training for this role is included in 10 CFR 35. A list of these requirements can be found in Appendix H.

RADIATION CONTROL FOR HEALTH AND SAFETY ACT OF 1968

In 1968, the US Congress passed the Radiation Control for Health and Safety Act (Public Law 90-602) to protect the public from the hazards of unnecessary radiation exposure resulting from electronic products such as microwave ovens and picture tube color televisions. Diagnostic x-ray equipment also was included. The act permitted the formation of the Center for Devices and Radiological Health (CDRH). The CDRH falls under the jurisdiction of the FDA. Essentially, it is responsible for conducting an ongoing electronic product radiation control program including establishing standards for the manufacture, installation, assembly, and maintenance of machines for radiologic procedures. Further responsibilities include:

- Assessing the biologic effects of ionizing radiation
- Evaluating radiation emissions from electronic products in general
- Conducting research to reduce radiation exposure

Code of Standards for Diagnostic X-ray Equipment

The code of standards for diagnostic x-ray equipment (Public Law 90-602) went into effect on August 1, 1974. This code applies to complete systems and major components manufactured after that date. Some relevant provisions of the standards for diagnostic x-ray equipment are listed in Box 9.4.

Public Law 90-602 does not regulate the diagnostic x-ray user. It is strictly an equipment performance standard.

ALARA CONCEPT

In 1954, the National Committee on Radiation Protection (later known as the *National Council on Radiation*

*Mathematically, reproducibility is specified by the *coefficient of variation C*, which is by definition equal to the standard deviation (SD), of at least five successive output measurements employing the same technique factors divided by the average, or mean value, of those measurements. The regulation requires that *C* must not exceed 0.05.

SD is an indicator of how measurements for a group, e.g., grades in a class exam, are dispersed from the average value. A low standard deviation means that most of the measured values are close to the average. A high standard deviation means that the values range much farther away from the average value.

Protection and Measurements) put forth the principle that radiation exposures should be kept "as low as reasonably achievable" (ALARA) with consideration for economic and societal factors. According to NCRP

Report No. 160, "The protection from radiation exposure is as low as reasonably achievable when the expenditure of further resources would be unwarranted by the reduction in exposure that would be achieved."[3]

The **ALARA concept** is accepted by all regulatory agencies. In 1987, the NCRP described it as "the continuation of good radiation protection programs and practices which traditionally have been effective in keeping the average and individual exposures for monitored workers well below the limit."[4] It may also be referred to as *optimization* per ICRP Publication No. 37 and Publication No. 55. Medical imaging personnel and radiologists share the responsibility to keep occupational and nonoccupational dose limits ALARA.

In practice this translates into EfDs and EqDs well below maximum allowable levels. This goal can be simply achieved through the employment of proper safety procedures performed by qualified personnel. Such methods should be clearly explained in a facility's radiation safety program. To define ALARA, health care facilities typically adopt *investigation levels*, defined as level I and level II. In the United States, these levels are traditionally one-tenth to three-tenths of the applicable regulatory limits.

Model for the ALARA Concept

The ALARA concept adopts an extremely conservative model concerning the relationship between ionizing radiation and potential risk. The relationship is the linear nonthreshold model discussed in Chapter 8 (reproduced in Fig. 9.2). The central principle of radiation protection is that in the interest of safety, the risk of injury should be overestimated rather than underestimated.

FOOD AND DRUG ADMINISTRATION WHITE PAPER

The US FDA supports the premise that "each patient should get the right imaging examination, at the right time, with the right radiation dose."[5] This declaration is clearly stated in the FDA document known as *the White Paper,* published in February 2010, in which they announced "the launch of a cooperative *Initiative to Reduce Unnecessary Radiation Exposure from Medical Imaging.*"[5] Working in conjunction with its partners, the FDA intends to take action to:

1. "Promote safe use of medical imaging devices"[5]

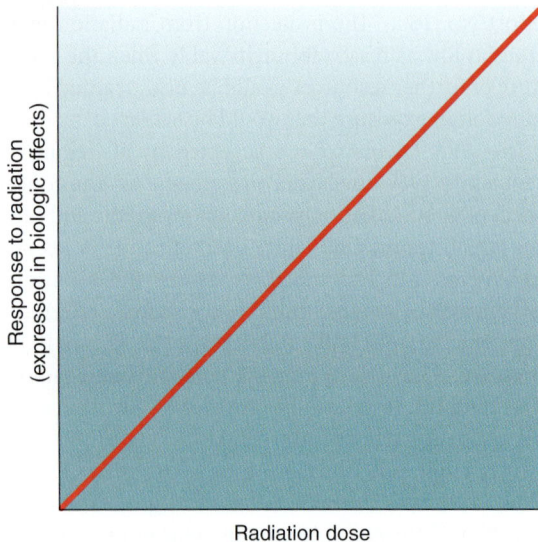

Fig. 9.2 Dose–response curve. Hypothetical linear (straight-line) nonthreshold curve for radiation dose–response relationship. The straight-line curve passing through the origin in this graph indicates both that the response to radiation (in terms of biologic effects) is directly proportional to the dose of radiation and that no known level of radiation dose exists below which absolutely no chance of sustaining biologic damage is evident.

2. "Support informed clinical decision"[5]
3. "Increase patient awareness"[5]

By coordinating these efforts, the FDA will be able to "optimize patient exposure to radiation from certain types of medical exams, and thereby reduce related risks while maximizing the benefits of these studies."[5]

CONSUMER-PATIENT RADIATION HEALTH AND SAFETY ACT OF 1981

The Consumer-Patient Radiation Health and Safety Act of 1981 (Title IX of Public Law 97-35) (see Appendix I) provides federal legislation requiring the establishment of minimum standards for the accreditation of educational programs for persons who perform radiologic procedures and the certification of such persons. The purpose of this federal act, under the directorship of the Secretary of Health and Human Services, is to ensure that regular medical and dental radiologic practices adhere to rigorous safety provisions. Individual states are encouraged to enact similar statutes and administer certification and accreditation programs based on the

---

BOX 9.5   Recent Changes in the Terminology Used to Describe Radiation Effects for the Purpose of Radiation Protection Guidelines

Approximate Year of Adoption	Terminology
1977–1991	stochastic vs. nonstochastic[6]
1991–2012	stochastic vs. deterministic[7]
2012–present	stochastic vs. tissue reactions (early or late)[8,9]

standards established therein. Because no legal penalty exists for noncompliance, many states, unfortunately, have not responded with appropriate legislation.

RADIATION-INDUCED RESPONSES OF CONCERN IN RADIATION PROTECTION

Categories for Radiation-Induced Responses

At present, the two main categories of radiation-induced responses of serious concern for humans are:
1. Tissue reactions
2. Stochastic (probabilistic) effects

Changes in Terminology From the 1970s to the Present

The ICRP and the NCRP update radiation protection terminology to recognize current scientific principles used to describe radiation effects. This progression in terminology is summarized in Box 9.5.[6–9]

Tissue Reactions. In the preceding chapters, tissue reactions were described as biologic somatic effects of ionizing radiation that can be directly related to the dose received. These reactions exhibit a threshold dose below which the response does not typically occur and above which the severity of the biologic damage increases as the dose increases. For example, if a specific dose of radiation is required to cause a skin burn, a higher dose of radiation will cause the skin burn to be more severe. When radiation-induced biologic damage escalates, it does so because greater numbers of cells interact with the increased number of x-ray photons that are present at higher radiation exposures. In general, tissue reactions *typically* occur only after large doses of radiation. However, tissue reactions could also result from long-term individual low doses of radiation sustained over several years. In either instance, the cumulative amounts of such radiation doses are usually much higher than those typically encountered by a patient in diagnostic radiology.*

Early and late tissue reactions. Tissue effects may be early, such as:

- Diffuse redness over an area of skin after irradiation (erythema)
- A decrease in the white blood cell count (leukopenia)
- Epilation, or loss of hair

As was discussed in Chapter 7, other, and much more severe, early consequences of radiation sickness can also arise, such as:

- Hematopoietic syndrome
- Gastrointestinal syndrome
- Cerebrovascular syndrome

Recall that these effects usually occur within a few hours or days after very high-level radiation exposure to a significant portion of the body. Some late tissue reactions due to high-level radiation exposure, though, occur months or more afterward. They include:

- Cataract formation
- Fibrosis
- Organ atrophy
- Loss of parenchymal cells
- Reduced fertility
- Sterility caused by a decrease in reproductive cells

Early tissue reactions such as erythema and late tissue reactions such as cataract formation have a high probability of occurring when entrance radiation doses exceed 2 Gyt.

For tissue reactions caused by high doses, their frequency of occurrence is not linear with respect to dose but instead follows a nonlinear threshold curve that is sigmoidal (S-shaped) with a threshold (see Fig. 8.1B).

Stochastic Effects. Since stochastic effects are non-threshold, randomly occurring biologic somatic changes, their chances of occurrence increase with each radiation exposure. Examples of stochastic effects are:

- Cancer
- Genetic alterations

Stochastic responses may be demonstrated with the use of both the linear (see Fig. 8.2) and the linear-quadratic dose–response curves (see Fig. 8.3). Because a stochastic event is an all-or-none, random effect, ionizing radiation will normally induce some cancers within a large general population, but determining beforehand which members of that population will develop cancer is not possible. Injury may result from exposure to a single cell or from damage in a sensitive substructure, such as a gene. The assumption is that no minimal safe dose exists. The frequency of an occurrence in a population increases in proportion to the magnitude of the absorbed dose of ionizing radiation delivered to the entire population. Therefore, the net effect on the population group depends not only on the number of individuals irradiated but also on the mean dose that each individual receives.

A summary of both early and late tissue reactions and stochastic (probabilistic) effects is presented in Box 9.6.

BOX 9.6   Summary of Serious Radiation-Induced Responses of Concern

Tissue Reactions	Stochastic (Probabilistic)
Early Reactions	**Effects**
Erythema (diffuse redness over an area of skin after irradiation)	Cancer
Blood changes (decrease of lymphocytes and platelets)	**Genetic (Hereditary) Effects**
Epilation (loss of hair)	Mutagenesis (irradiation
Acute radiation syndrome	of DNA of somatic
Hematopoietic syndrome	cells leading to abnor-
Gastrointestinal syndrome	malities in new cells
Cerebrovascular syndrome	as they divide in that
	individual)
Late Reactions	
Cataract formation	
Fibrosis	
Organ atrophy	
Loss of parenchymal cells	
Reduced fertility	
Sterility	

---

*A significant exception to this is high-dose-rate fluoroscopic procedures. For these studies, entrance dose rates as great as 200 mGy_a/min are possible. A fluoroscopic exposure of 15 minutes at this level would result in a patient entrance dose of approximately 3 Gy_a.[10]

Effective Dose (EfD) Limiting System

|
ASSESSES
|

Radiation exposure
and
associated risk of biologic effects

|
FOR
|

Radiation workers
and
the general public

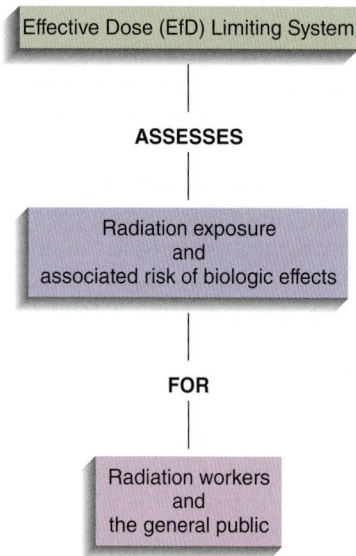

Fig. 9.3 Effective dose (EfD) limiting system.

CURRENT RADIATION PROTECTION PHILOSOPHY

Both genetic and somatic responses to ionizing radiation were considered in developing the present EfD limiting recommendations. The current radiation protection philosophy is based on the assumption that a linear non-threshold relationship exists between radiation dose and biologic response. Thus, even the most minuscule dose of radiation has a nonzero possibility of causing some harm. The current philosophy also acknowledges that ionizing radiation possesses a beneficial potential. This philosophy proposes that, when employed, the potential benefits of exposing the patient to ionizing radiation must far outweigh any potential risk.

Effective Dose Limiting System

The EfD limiting system is the current method for controlling the risk of biologic damage to radiation workers and the general public from radiation exposure (Fig. 9.3). The **effective dose limit (EDL)** is the upper-boundary dose of ionizing radiation that results in a negligible risk of:

- Bodily injury
- Hereditary damage

EDLs may be specified for whole-body exposure, partial-body exposure, and exposure of individual organs.

Separate limits are set for occupationally exposed individuals and the general public. The sum of both the external and internal whole-body exposures is considered when effective dose limits are established. Their values are such as minimizing the risk to humans in terms of early and late tissue reactions and stochastic effects. Natural background and medical exposure are not included.

Upper boundary safe radiation exposure limits for occupationally exposed persons are associated with risks that are similar to those encountered by employees in other industries that are generally considered to be reasonably safe. These industries include:

- Manufacturing
- Trade
- Civil Service

Quantitative values for radiation risks are derived from the complete injury that may be caused by radiation exposure. Because many conflicting views continue to exist on assessing the risk of cancer from low-level radiation exposure, the trend has been to create more rigorous radiation protection standards.

Occupational Risk

The potential for terminal cancer, shortening of life span because of the induction of cancer, hereditary imperfections triggered by reproductive cell mutations, other abnormalities, and overall poorer quality of life are collectively taken into account in formulating occupational risk standards.

As mentioned previously, the risk to a radiographer from radiation exposure may be equated with occupational risk in generally safe industries. That risk is estimated to be a 2.5% chance of a fatal accident over an entire career. The lifetime fatal risk in hazardous occupations, however, is many times greater. A few examples of such occupations include:

- Logging
- Deep-sea fishing
- Iron and steel workers

To ensure that the hazard to radiation workers is no greater than the threat to the general public, the NCRP proposes that radiation protection programs for radiation workers be designed to prevent individual workers from obtaining a total external plus internal cumulative EfD in excess of their age in years times 10 mSv.[4] Consider the following situation: A worker at age 40 years has been employed at a nuclear power plant for 10 years.

He had previously been employed as a radiation worker in another industry, during which he received a cumulative EfD of 100 mSv (10 rem). Therefore, the radiation protection program for his current position should have ensured that he has not accumulated a total EfD greater than 300 mSv (30 rem) during his 10 years of employment.

The Vulnerability of the Embryo-fetus to Radiation Exposure

The fact that the embryo-fetus in utero is particularly sensitive to radiation exposure has already been established. Epidemiologic studies of atomic bomb survivors exposed in utero provided conclusive evidence of a dose-dependent increase in the incidence of severe intellectual disability for fetal doses higher than approximately 0.4 Sv. The most significant risk for radiation-induced intellectual disability occurred when the embryo-fetus was exposed 8 to 15 weeks after conception.

BASIS FOR THE EFFECTIVE DOSE LIMITING SYSTEM

Concept Underlying Radiation Protection

The essential concept underlying radiation protection is that any organ in the human body is vulnerable to damage from exposure to ionizing radiation. Even though some organs are known to be more sensitive to radiation than others, every organ is considered to be at some risk due to the assumed random nature of somatic or hereditary radiation-induced effects.

The EfD limiting system includes, for the determination of EqD for tissues and organs, all radiation-vulnerable human organs that can contribute to potential risk, rather than only those human organs considered critical. In earlier recommendations such as NCRP Report No. 39 (released in 1971), only vital organs such as the gonads, blood-forming organs, and lung tissue were identified.[11]

Tissue Weighting Factor

Although this factor was previously discussed, a brief description follows to reinforce a greater understanding of its importance as it relates to the EfD limiting system. The EfD limiting system is an attempt to equate the various risks of cancer and genetic effects on the tissues or organs that were exposed to radiation. Because

---

BOX 9.7   Organ or Tissue Weighting Factors for Calculating Effective Dose

0.01	0.12
Bone surface	Red bone marrow
Skin	Colon
	Lung
0.05	**Stomach**
Bladder	
Breast	**0.20**
Liver	Gonads
Esophagus	
Thyroid	
Remainder*,†	

*The remainder takes into account the following additional tissues and organs: adrenals, brain, small intestine, large intestine, kidney, muscle, pancreas, spleen, thymus, and uterus.
†In extraordinary circumstances in which one of the remainder tissues or organs receives an equivalent dose in excess of the highest dose in any of the 12 organs for which a weighting factor (WT) is specified, a WT of 0.025 should be applied to that tissue or organ and a WT of 0.025 to the average dose in the other remainder tissues or organs.
From National Council on Radiation Protection and Measurements (NCRP): *Limitation of exposure to ionizing radiation, Report No. 116,* Bethesda, MD, 1993, NCRP. Reprinted with permission from the National Council on Radiation Protection and Measurements, http://NCRPonline.org.

---

various tissues and organs do not have the same degree of sensitivity to these effects, the system employed must compensate for the differences in risk from one organ to another. Therefore a **tissue weighting factor (W_T)** is used. This factor "indicates the ratio of the risk of stochastic effects attributable to irradiation of a given organ or tissue (T) to the total risk when the whole body is uniformly irradiated."[12] Organ or Wt factors recommended by the ICRP in Report No. 60, released in 1991, and adopted by the NCRP in Report No. 116, published in 1993, are reproduced in Box 9.7.

CURRENT NATIONAL COUNCIL ON RADIATION PROTECTION AND MEASUREMENTS RECOMMENDATIONS

National Council on Radiation Protection and Measurements Reports

The NCRP periodically reiterates and updates its position on radiation protection standards and publishes recommendations on these standards in the form of reports. Recommendations contained in NCRP Report No. 184 now supersede those contained in NCRP Reports No. 116, No. 91, and No. 39. A summary of some critical issues and changes follows.

NCRP Report No. 184, *Medical radiation exposure of patients in the United States,* November 2019, is an update to NCRP Report No. 160, *Ionizing radiation exposure of the population of the United States* (2009). This new Report revises medical radiation exposure information with data collected between 2006 and 2016. The 2009 report (No. 116) revealed a dramatic increase in medical radiation exposure over the previous 25 years: medical exposure comprised nearly half of all radiation exposure to the US population, primarily due to an increase in computed tomography (CT) scanning and cardiac nuclear medicine procedures. A decade has passed since the publication of NCRP Report No. 160, and changes in technology, the emergence of campaigns for dose reduction and optimization, indications for specific examinations, and reimbursement appear to have favorably affected medical radiation exposure and dose to the US population. There has been *a substantial reduction in radiation doses to the US population* since NCRP Report No. 160 was published in 2009. The annual nontherapeutic medical radiation dose to the US population in 2006 was 2.92 mSv and decreased to 2.16 mSv in 2016 (Fig. 9.4).

Cumulative Effective Dose (Cumefd) Limit.

A radiation worker's **lifetime effective dose** must be limited to this individual's age in years times 10 mSv. This is known as the **cumulative effective dose (CumEfD) limit** and it pertains to the whole body. Adhering to this limit ensures that the lifetime risk for these workers remains acceptable. CumEfD limits, however, do not include:

- Radiation exposure from natural background radiation
- Exposure acquired as a consequence of a worker's undergoing medical imaging procedures

The limits do include the possibility of both:

- Internal exposure
- External exposure

The CumEfD is, therefore the sum or total of both the internal and external EqDs.

Medical imaging personnel seldom receive EqDs that are a significant fraction of the **annual occupational effective dose limit**. A radiation safety program that is well structured and properly maintained will ensure that individual occupational exposure will not remotely approach 50 mSv (5000 mrem) in any given year.

International Commission on Radiological Protection Recommendation for Downward Revision of the Annual Effective Dose Limit.

In 1991, the ICRP recommended that the annual EfD limit for occupationally exposed persons be reduced from 50 mSv to 20 mSv as a result of information obtained regarding the Japanese atomic bomb survivors in whom the risk of radiation from the atomic bomb detonations was estimated to be approximately three to four times greater (more damaging) than previously estimated.[13] Although the NCRP has not changed from the 50 mSv limit, in the future it could very well *recommend* a lower limit on the annual occupational EfD because of the:

1. Revised risk estimates derived from the more recent reevaluations of dosimetric studies on the atomic bomb survivors of Hiroshima and Nagasaki[11]
2. Appearance, as a result of longer follow-up time, of increased numbers of solid tumors in the survivor population
3. In the United States, lowering the current limits is the responsibility of the NRC, individual states, and the FDA.

Limits for Nonoccupationally Exposed Individuals.

In addition to limits for occupationally exposed individuals, the NCRP recommends EDLs for nonoccupationally exposed individuals who are not undergoing medical imaging procedures. The NCRP-recommended annual EDL is 1 mSv (100 mrem) for continuous or frequent exposures from artificial sources other than medical irradiation and natural background and a limit of 5 mSv annually for infrequent exposure.[4] These nonoccupational values established for individual members of the general public are designed to restrict their chances of harm from annual cumulative exposure "to reasonable *levels of risk* compared with risks from other common sources, i.e., about 10^{-4} to 10^{-6} annually."[4] The 5 mSv annual limit for *infrequent exposure* is made because "annual exposures in excess of the 1 mSv recommendation, usually to a small number of people, need not be regarded as especially significant to the group as a whole provided it does not often occur to the same groups and that the average exposure to individuals in these groups does not exceed an average annual EfD of about 1 mSv."[4]

NCRP Report No. 184:

MEDICAL RADIATION EXPOSURE OF PATIENTS IN THE UNITED STATES

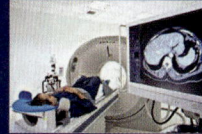

National Council on Radiation Protection and Measurements

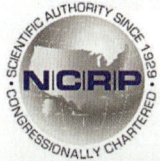

NCRP Report No. 184, *Medical Radiation Exposure of Patients in the United States,* is an update to NCRP Report No. 160, *Ionizing Radiation Exposure of the Population of the United States* (2009). This new Report updates medical radiation exposure information with data collected between 2006 and 2016.

> **There has been a substantial reduction in medical radiation doses to the U.S. population since NCRP Report No. 160 was published in 2009.**

The 2009 report revealed a dramatic increase in medical radiation exposure over the previous 25 years; medical exposure was essentially half of all radiation exposure to the U.S. population, primarily due to an increase in computed tomography (CT) scanning and cardiac nuclear medicine.

A decade has passed since the publication of NCRP Report No. 160, and changes in technology, emergence of campaigns for dose reduction and optimization, indications for specific examinations, and reimbursement appear to have affected medical radiation exposure and dose to the U.S. population.

NCRP Report No. 184 includes a historical introduction, background content listing, information about relevant dose metrics, a discussion of International Commission on Radiological Protection (ICRP) tissue weighting factors and computational phantoms, and modality-specific medical radiation exposure and dose information.

The audience for this Report is primarily federal and state agencies responsible for the health and well-being of individuals exposed to ionizing radiation and those agencies with responsibility for ensuring radiation protection safety in medicine. NCRP Report No. 184 includes useful information for health physicists, medical physicists, physicians and other medical professionals, radiation safety officers, managers, workers, members of the public, and the media.

Purchase a copy of NCRP Report No. 184:
Medical Radiation Exposure of Patients in the United States
https://ncrponline.org/shop/reports/report-no-184/

Fig. 9.4 US medical radiation doses are decreasing. EUS refers to effective dose for data pertaining to US averages. (With permission of the National Council on Radiation Protection and Measurements (NCRP): Medical radiation exposure of patients in the United States, report no. 184, Bethesda, MD, 2019, NCRP, http://NCRPonline.org.)

NCRP Report No. 184:

MEDICAL RADIATION EXPOSURE OF PATIENTS IN THE UNITED STATES

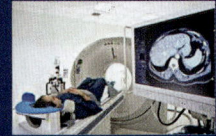

National Council on Radiation Protection and Measurements

U.S. Medical Radiation Doses Are Decreasing

There has been a **15-20% reduction in non-therapeutic medical radiation dose** to the U.S. population in the decade between 2006 and 2016.

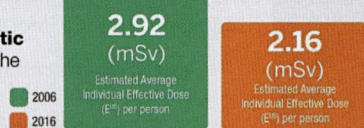

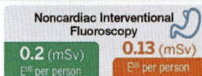

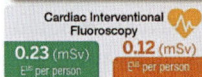

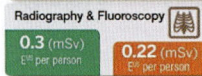

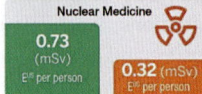

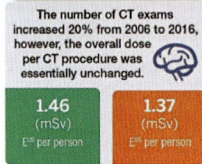

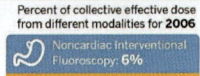

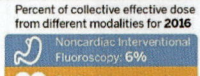

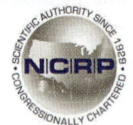

■ 2006
■ 2016

2.92 (mSv)
Estimated Average Individual Effective Dose (E^{US}) per person

2.16 (mSv)
Estimated Average Individual Effective Dose (E^{US}) per person

Noncardiac Interventional Fluoroscopy
0.2 (mSv) E^{US} per person   **0.13** (mSv) E^{US} per person

Cardiac Interventional Fluoroscopy
0.23 (mSv) E^{US} per person   **0.12** (mSv) E^{US} per person

Radiography & Fluoroscopy
0.3 (mSv) E^{US} per person   **0.22** (mSv) E^{US} per person

Nuclear Medicine
0.73 (mSv) E^{US} per person   **0.32** (mSv) E^{US} per person

The number of CT exams increased 20% from 2006 to 2016, however, the overall dose per CT procedure was essentially unchanged.
1.46 (mSv) E^{US} per person   **1.37** (mSv) E^{US} per person

Percent of collective effective dose from different modalities for **2006**
Noncardiac Interventional Fluoroscopy: 6%
Cardiac Interventional Fluoroscopy: 8%
Radiography & Fluoroscopy: 11%
Nuclear Medicine: 25%
Computed Tomography: 50%

Percent of collective effective dose from different modalities for **2016**
Noncardiac Interventional Fluoroscopy: 6%
Cardiac Interventional Fluoroscopy: 6%
Radiography & Fluoroscopy: 10%
Nuclear Medicine: 15%
Computed Tomography: 63%

Note: When current data are compared with NCRP Report 160 utilizing ICRP weighting factors from ICRP Publication 60, the results are the same except for Nuclear Medicine (0.41 mSv), Computed Tomography (1.45 mSv) and total dose (2.33 mSv). For more detail, please see Figure 14.2 in the report.

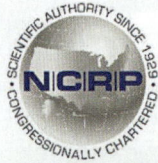

Purchase a copy of NCRP Report No. 184:
Medical Radiation Exposure of Patients in the United States
https://ncrponline.org/shop/reports/report-no-184/

Fig. 9.4, cont'd

Limits for Pregnant Radiation Workers. To limit radiation exposure for pregnant radiation workers and the unborn during potentially sensitive periods of gestation, the NCRP "recommends" a monthly EqD limit not exceeding 0.5 mSv (50 mrem) per month to the embryo-fetus and a maximum during the entire pregnancy not to exceed 5.0 mSv (500 mrem) after declaration of the pregnancy. Notably, the recommended monthly limit is more stringent. Nevertheless, both limits are proposed to reflect that not all pregnant workers are monitored monthly and that personnel dosimetry does not result in exact measures of EqD, just approximations based on the personnel dosimeter readings. This 9-month EqD value excludes both medical and natural background radiation. The value is designed to significantly restrict the total lifetime risk of leukemia and other malignancies to persons exposed in utero.[4] The occurrence of tissue reactions is expected to be statistically negligible if the EqD remains at or below the recommended limit.

Limits for Education and Training Purposes. For education and training purposes, the same dose limits apply to students of radiography as to individuals under 18 years of age. The limit for any education and training exposures of individuals under the age of 18 years is an EfD of 1 mSv (100 mrem) annually. Occasional exposure for the purpose of education and training is permitted, provided special care is taken to ensure that the annual EfD limit of 1 mSv is not exceeded.

Limits for Tissues and Organs Exposed Selectively or Together With Other Organs. Annual occupational dose limits for tissue reactions, for tissues and organs exposed selectively, or together with other organs have been set to prevent excessive doses to those organs and tissues. They include 150 mSv for the crystalline lens of the eyes and 500 mSv for localized areas of the skin, the hands, and the feet.[4] Even though the established annual dose limit for localized areas of skin provides adequate protection for that organ against stochastic effects, it will be necessary to specify an additional limit to prevent tissue reactions.

Negligible Individual Dose. An annual **negligible individual dose (NID)** of 0.01 mSv/year (1 mrem/year) per source or practice has been determined to be a dose of negligible risk. This means that at this EfD level, a reduction of individual exposure is unnecessary.

ACTION LIMITS

Health care institutions work to ensure that personnel dose limits do not approach EfD limits. Radiologic technologists' personnel dosimeter readings should be significantly below a tenth of the maximum EfD limits, even for those technologists who receive the most exposure. Hospitals typically establish internal **action limits**. These limits are typically 1/10th of the annual dose limit. The purpose of action limits is to trigger an investigation when these limits are exceeded that could uncover the reason for any abnormal exposure. A frequent cause for an excessive reading is due to a personnel dosimeter remaining in an x-ray room while exposures are subsequently made because the dosimeter had unknowingly fallen off the uniform of a technologist, or was forgotten on a lead apron. Also, sometimes work habits, such as where the technologist usually stands during interventional radiography, can lead to personnel readings that exceed the action limit. The RSO may then initiate corrective action. In general, the RSO must be an active participant along with the imaging department manager in an ongoing program that is designed to prevent all occupationally exposed personnel from receiving the maximum allowed exposures.

RADIATION HORMESIS

The concept of **radiation hormesis** is that there exists a beneficial result in groups of individuals from continuing exposure to small amounts of radiation. This theory fundamentally contradicts the perception that repeated low doses of radiation will generate an accumulation of mutations that inevitably will result in transforming a normal cell into one that continues to divide without end, ultimately leading to cancer.

In Report No. 5 of the National Academy of Science on the BEIR V, conclusions regarding the adverse effects on the health of low levels of ionizing radiation are based on extrapolations from radiation EqDs greater than 0.5 Sv. Such radiation levels are more than a factor of 100 times greater than ordinary background radiation levels (3.3 mSv/year). BEIR V espouses the very conservative linear "no threshold" view of the Japanese atomic bomb lifetime survival study (LSS) data. However, studies from the Radiation Effects Research Council in Hiroshima have demonstrated an apparent threshold dosage in the atomic bomb LSS data that is approximately in the range of 0.2 to 0.5 Sv. This equivalent dose range is of the same order as the amount of natural radiation that average US residents receive *in their lifetimes*. What is curious is that the LSS data seems to indicate that Japanese atomic bomb survivors with moderate radiation EqD totals of 5 mSv to 50 mSv (0.5 rem to 5 rem), the equivalent of 1.5 to 15 years of natural radiation, have a reduced cancer death rate compared with a normally exposed control population. Additional recent reanalysis of the atomic bomb survivor data have shown that effects on survivors are more consistent with a threshold model than the LNT model.[14] All of this contradicts the predictions of the BEIR V report and, if fully substantiated, casts doubt on the BEIR V conclusion that any amount of radiation is potentially harmful. The reverse could be true, at least for very moderate amounts of radiation exposure! More specifically, in seven Western states with background radiation levels higher than other states by approximately 1 mSv (100 mrem) per year, residents experience about 15% fewer cancer deaths per 1000 individuals than the US average. There is also much evidence from animal studies that support the view that low doses of radiation reduce the chances of both cancer and nonmalignant disease occurrence.[15]

A study was conducted in China from 1972 to 1975 of two stable populations of approximately 70,000 persons, each of whose annual background radiation levels differed by about 2 mSv. This study disclosed a cancer rate in the more exposed population of only about 50% of that of the other group. Annex B of the UNSCEAR 1994 Report, discusses the beneficial aspects of low-dose radiation.[16] All of these suggest a potential *radiation hormesis effect,* which is a positive consequence of radiation for populations continuously exposed to moderately higher levels of radiation than ordinary background levels. During human evolution over millions of years, advantageous genetic mutations caused by radiation exposure may have occurred, resembling those that allow lower animals today to demonstrate radiation hormesis. Therefore, to assume a definite risk from minimal amounts of radiation exposure (two, three, or four times normal background levels) may be entirely incorrect.

In earlier chapters, it has been stated that the risk from low-level, low-LET radiation exposure is mainly a long indirect process involving the production of highly reactive free radicals. These chemical agents have the capacity to damage cellular DNA. However, the human body has an elaborate system of antioxidants that can neutralize many of these reactants. When the immune system is subjected over a period of time to low doses of radiation, it initiates adaptive protection responses[17] that can lessen potential DNA damage and consequently the malignant transformation of cells. However, until the radiation hormesis theory is sufficiently proven, the medical radiation industry will continue to adhere to a rigid principle of ALARA and the no-threshold concept for radiation protection purposes.

OCCUPATIONAL AND NONOCCUPATIONAL DOSE LIMITS

Effective Dose Limits for Radiation Workers and the Population as a Whole

For the protection of radiation workers and the population as a whole, EfD limits have been established as guidelines (Table 9.3). All medical imaging personnel should be familiar with current NCRP recommendations. For this group, the most critical item is the 50 mSv/year (5 rem/year) whole-body occupational dose limit. This annual upper boundary is designed to limit the stochastic (probabilistic) effects of radiation. It takes into account the EqD in all radiation-sensitive organs found in the body.

Special Limits for Selected Areas

Because the tissue weighting factors (see Box 9.7) used for calculating EfD are so small for some organs, an organ that is associated with a low weighting factor may receive an unreasonably large dose. In contrast, the EfD for the whole person remains within the total allowable limit. Therefore, special limits are set for the crystalline lens of the eye and localized areas of the skin, hands, and feet to prevent unwanted tissue reactions. These special limits are given in Table 9.3 for both occupational personnel and the general public.

At present, the ICRP and most governmental regulatory agencies in other countries limit exposure of the lens of the eye for occupational personnel to less than 20 mSv (2 rem) per year. In the United States, the NCRP is continuing to study the matter but is unlikely to change its guidance in the near future.[18] Although this NCRP value of 150 mSv (15 rem) suggests a large discrepancy with the whole-body permitted dose equivalent, the NCRP, in addition to its special limit for the lens of the eye, maintains a cumulative lifetime limit of 10 mSv (1 rem) times the worker's age, which indicates a de facto lower limit to the lens.

TABLE 9.3 Summary of the National Council on Radiation Protection and Measurements (NCRP) Recommendations*† (NCRP Report No. 116)

	Equivalent Dose Limits
A. Occupational exposures‡	
1. Effective dose limits	
a. Annual	50 mSv (5 rem)
b. Cumulative	10 mSv (1 rem) × age in years
2. Equivalent dose annual limits for tissues and organs	
a. Lens of eye	150 mSv (15,000 mrem)
b. Localized areas of the skin, hands, and feet	500 mSv (50,000 mrem)
B. Guidance for emergency occupational exposure‡ (see Section 14, NCRP No. 116)	
C. Public exposures (annual)	
1. Effective dose limit, continuous or frequent exposure‡	1 mSv (100 mrem)
2. Effective dose limit, infrequent exposure‡	5 mSv (500 mrem)
3. Equivalent dose limits for tissues and organs‡	
a. Lens of eye	15 mSv
b. Localized areas of the skin, hands, and feet	50 mSv
4. Remedial action for natural sources	
a. Effective dose (excluding radon)	>5 mSv (>500 mrem)
b. Exposure to radon and its decay products§	>26 (J/s)m^{-3}¶
D. Education and training exposures (annual)‡	
1. Effective dose limit	1 mSv (100 mrem)
2. Equivalent dose limit for tissues and organs	
a. Lens of eye	15 mSv
b. Localized areas of the skin, hands, and feet	50 mSv
E. Embryo and fetus exposures‡	
1. Equivalent dose limit	
a. Monthly	0.5 mSv
b. Entire gestation	5.0 mSv (500 mrem)
F. Negligible individual dose (annual)‡	0.01 mSv (1 mrem)

*Excluding medical exposures.

†See Tables 4.2 and 13.1 in NCRP Report No. 116 for recommendations on radiation weighting factors and tissue weighting factors, respectively.

‡Sum of external and internal exposures, excluding doses from natural sources.

§WLM stands for working level month and refers to a cumulative exposure for a working month (170 hours). As applied to radon and its daughter products, 1 WLM represents the cumulative exposure experienced in a 170-hour period resulting from a radon concentration of 100 pCi/L. The occupational limit for miners is 4 WLM per year, which results in an equivalent dose of approximately 0.15 Sv per year.

¶A measure of the rate of release of energy (joules per second) by radon and its decay products per unit volume of air (cubic meters).

SUMMARY

- Effective Dose Limiting System.
  - Adherence to occupational and nonoccupational effective dose (EfD) limits helps prevent harmful biologic effects of radiation exposure.
  - The concept of cellular damage by radiation exposure and the associated risk of radiation-induced malignancy is the basis of the EfD limiting system.

- The sum of both external and internal whole-body doses is taken into consideration when establishing the cumulative effective dose (CumEfD) limit.
- Accounting for tissue weighting factors is essential because various tissues and organs do not have the same degree of radiation sensitivity.
- Different biologic threats posed by different types of ionizing radiation must be taken into

consideration even when the dose in gray from each is the same.

- Radiation hormesis is the hypothesis that a positive effect exists for specific populations that are continuously exposed to moderately higher levels of radiation.

- Major organizations and their functions involved in regulating radiation doses include the following:
  - The United Nations Scientific Committee on the Effects of Atomic Radiation (UNSCEAR) and the National Academy of Sciences/National Research Council Committee on the Biological Effects of Ionizing Radiation (NAS/NRC-BEIR) supply information to the International Commission on Radiological Protection (ICRP).
  - The ICRP makes recommendations on occupational and public dose limits.
  - The National Council on Radiation Protection and Measurements (NCRP) reviews ICRP recommendations and may or may not adopt them into recommendations for US radiation protection policy.
  - The Nuclear Regulatory Commission (NRC) is the watchdog of the nuclear energy industry; it controls the manufacture and use of radioactive substances.
  - The Environmental Protection Agency (EPA) develops and enforces regulations pertaining to the control of environmental radiation.
  - The US Food and Drug Administration (FDA) regulates the design and manufacture of products used in the radiation industry.
  - The Occupational Safety and Health Administration (OSHA) monitors the workplace and regulates occupational exposure to radiation.

- Individual health care facilities that medically use radiation must establish a radiation safety committee (RSC) and designate a radiation safety officer (RSO).
- The RSO is responsible for developing a radiation safety program for the health care facility; maintains personnel radiation-monitoring records provides counseling and takes corrective actions in all radiation safety situations.
- The ALARA concept (optimization) states that radiation exposure should be kept "as low as reasonably achievable."
- Acute radiation-induced responses in exposed humans may be classified as either tissue reactions or stochastic effects.
  - Tissue reactions are those biologic somatic effects of ionizing radiation that exhibit a threshold dose below which the effect does not typically occur and above which the severity of the biologic damage increases as the dose increases.
  - Stochastic effects are nonthreshold, randomly occurring biologic somatic changes in which the chance of occurrence of the effect rather than the severity of the effect is proportional to the dose of ionizing radiation.
- EfD limits for occupationally exposed personnel include the following:
  - The NCRP has established an annual occupational EfD limit of 50 mSv and a lifetime EfD that does not exceed 10 mSv (1 rem) times the occupationally exposed person's age in years.
  - Internal action limits are established by health care facilities to trigger an investigation when the limits are exceeded to uncover the reasons for any unusually high exposures received by individual staff members.

GENERAL DISCUSSION QUESTIONS

1. What are the four major organizations responsible for evaluating the relationship between radiation dose and biological effects?
2. What is the function of the Radiation Safety Committee (RSC) in a medical facility?
3. What are the responsibilities of a Radiation Safety Officer (RSO)?
4. What was the purpose of the Radiation Control for Health and Safety Act of 1968?
5. What does the ALARA concept stand for, and why is it important?

6. What are radiation-induced responses that warrant serious concern for radiation protection?
7. How does the concept of risk relate to the medical imaging industry?
8. What is the effective dose limit, and why is it important?
9. What are the current recommendations from the National Council on Radiation Protection and Measurements (NCRP)?
10. What is the concept of radiation hormesis?

REVIEW QUESTIONS

1. Which organization provides recommendations on radiation protection practices?
   A. National Institute of Standards and Technology (NIST)
   B. International Commission on Radiological Protection (ICRP)
   C. Food and Drug Administration (FDA)
   D. Environmental Protection Agency (EPA)

2. What is the primary role of the Radiation Safety Committee (RSC) in a medical facility?
   A. To manage patient care
   B. To oversee the radiation safety program
   C. To conduct medical imaging procedures
   D. To regulate employee work hours

3. What is one of the responsibilities of a Radiation Safety Officer (RSO)?
   A. Performing diagnostic imaging
   B. Monitoring radiation exposure levels
   C. Managing hospital finances
   D. Scheduling patient appointments

4. What was the purpose of the Consumer-Patient Radiation Health and Safety Act of 1981?
   A. To reduce the cost of medical imaging
   B. To establish standards for radiation-emitting products
   C. To ensure radiation safety in patient care
   D. To eliminate the use of ionizing radiation in medicine

5. What is the ALARA concept in radiation safety?
   A. A standard for equipment calibration
   B. A principle for minimizing radiation exposure
   C. A method for patient diagnosis
   D. A guideline for medical billing

6. Which of the following is a serious concern for radiation protection?
   A. Increased patient throughput
   B. Radiation-induced cancer
   C. Enhanced imaging technology
   D. Improved staff training

7. What is the effective dose limit for radiation workers primarily designed to protect against?
   A. Immediate radiation burns
   B. Long-term health effects
   C. Equipment malfunction
   D. Operational costs

8. What does the concept of radiation hormesis suggest?
   A. All radiation exposure is harmful.
   B. Low doses of radiation may have beneficial effects.
   C. High doses of radiation are always lethal.
   D. Radiation exposure should be completely avoided.

9. Which agency is responsible for enforcing radiation safety standards in the United States?
   A. Federal Communications Commission (FCC)
   B. Occupational Safety and Health Administration (OSHA)
   C. Nuclear Regulatory Commission (NRC)
   D. National Aeronautics and Space Administration (NASA)

10. What is the purpose of the Code of Standards for Diagnostic X-Ray Equipment established in 1974?
    A. To regulate the cost of imaging services
    B. To set safety standards for x-ray equipment
    C. To eliminate unnecessary medical imaging
    D. To improve patient comfort during procedures

10

Equipment Design for Radiation Protection

OBJECTIVES

After completing this chapter, the reader will be able to perform the following:

- Define all key terms.
- Explain the requirements and purposes for a diagnostic-type protective tube housing, x-ray control panel, radiographic examination table, and source-to-image distance indicator.
- Describe the light-localizing variable-aperture rectangular collimator and explain how this apparatus functions as an x-ray beam limitation device for fixed and mobile radiographic equipment.
- Explain the importance of luminance of the collimator light source, state the requirements for good coincidence between the radiographic beam and the localizing light beam, and explain the function of the collimator's positive beam limitation (PBL) feature.
- Explain the function of x-ray beam filtration in diagnostic radiology, list two types of filtration used to filter the beam adequately, describe half-value layer (HVL), and provide examples of HVLs required for selected peak kilovoltages.
- Explain the function of a compensating filter in radiography, and list two types of such filters.

- Explain the significance of exposure reproducibility and exposure linearity.
- Discuss the concept of automatic exposure control and identify its radiation safety benefits.
- Explain how radiographic grids increase patient dose.
- State the minimum source-skin distance (SSD) that must be used for mobile radiography to ensure patient safety, and the reason for this minimum SSD requirement.
- Explain the process of digital radiography and computed radiography, and discuss why care must be taken to ensure that patients undergoing digital imaging procedures are not overexposed.
- Explain how patient exposure may be reduced during routine fluoroscopic procedures, C-arm fluoroscopic procedures, digital fluoroscopic procedures, interventional and high-dose (high-level control [HLC]) fluoroscopy interventional procedures.
- Discuss the use of fluoroscopic equipment by nonradiologist physicians who perform interventional procedures and identify the responsibilities of the radiographer during such procedures.

CHAPTER OUTLINE

KEY TERMS

automatic exposure control (AEC) and phototiming
brightness
computed radiography (CR)
control panel, or console
cumulative timer
diagnostic-type protective tube housing
digital fluoroscopy (DF)
digital radiography (DR)
digital subtraction angiography (DSA)

entrance skin irradiation rates
exposure linearity
exposure reproducibility
filtration
half-value layer (HVL)
high-level control fluoroscopy (HLCF)
image intensifier (II)
image matrix
light-localizing variable-aperture rectangular collimator
off-focus radiation

positive beam limitation (PBL)
primary protective barrier
pulsed progressive systems
radiographic examination table
radiographic grid
roadmapping
scattered radiation
source-to-image receptor distance (SID)
source-to-skin distance (SSD)
useful, or primary, beam
x-ray beam limitation device

State-of-the-art diagnostic radiographic and fluoroscopic equipment incorporates features that radiologists and technologists can use to optimize the quality of the image while at the same time reducing radiation exposure to patients. This chapter provides an overview of equipment components and accessories and methods that imaging professionals can use to minimize radiation exposure of patients.

RADIATION SAFETY FEATURES OF RADIOGRAPHIC EQUIPMENT, DEVICES, AND ACCESSORIES

All necessary measures must be taken to ensure that radiographic equipment operates safely. Every diagnostic imaging system must have a protective tube housing and a correctly functioning control panel, or console. The radiographic examination table and other devices and accessories also are required to be constructed to reduce the patient's radiation dose.

Diagnostic-Type Protective Tube Housing and Functions

A diagnostic-type protective tube housing (Fig. 10.1) is required to safeguard the patient and imaging personnel from off-focus, or leakage, radiation by restricting the emission of x-rays to the area of the useful, or primary, beam (those x-rays emitted through the x-ray port, or tube window). The housing enclosing the x-ray tube must be constructed with lead lining to reduce radiation leakage through any portion of the housing away from the useful beam. Leakage radiation is measured at a distance of 1 meter from the x-ray source, and must not exceed an air kerma rate of 0.88 mGy/hr (or exposure rate of 100 mR/hr) when the tube is operated at its highest voltage at the highest current that allows continuous operation. The protective tube housing also serves as a shield against the high voltage entering the x-ray tube, thereby preventing electric shock while also facilitating the cooling of the x-ray tube. Because the x-ray tube and housing assembly are relatively heavy, the overall structure is robustly built to provide

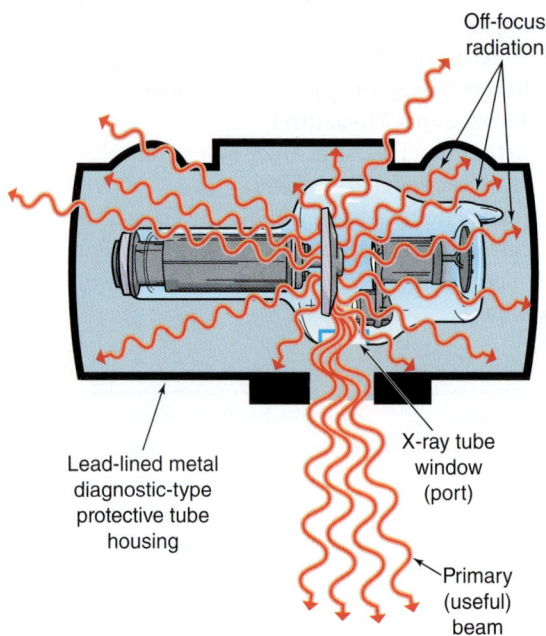

Fig. **10.1** A lead-lined metal diagnostic-type protective tube housing protects patients and imaging personnel from off-focus, or leakage, radiation by restricting x-ray emission to the area of the primary (useful) beam.

needed mechanical support and minimize the potential for damage of the x-ray tube if rough handling occurs.

Control Panel, or Console

The **control panel, or console**, is the place where technical exposure factors such as milliamperes (mA), peak kilovoltage (kVp), and exposure duration (mS) are selected and visually displayed. For the radiation safety of the radiographer, it must be located behind a properly shielded barrier that also has a radiation-absorbent window, which permits continuous observation of the patient during any procedure. It is mandatory that the control panel fully display the conditions of exposure and provide a positive indication when the x-ray tube is energized.[1] It is also required that the exposure hand control be mechanically affixed to the console such that it cannot be activated while the operator is in an unshielded location. For some state-of-the-art operating consoles, digital controls for kVp and mAs are available on a *touch* screen. Generally, when an x-ray exposure begins, a tone is emitted, and a radiation sign illuminates. When the exposure terminates, the sound stops and the "x-ray on" light goes out.

Radiographic Examination Table

The **radiographic examination table** must be strong enough to adequately support patients whose weight can be up to 400 pounds. Frequently, this piece of equipment has a free-moving tabletop that allows easy movement of the patient during an imaging procedure. The thickness of the tabletop must be uniform, and for under-table x-ray tubes as used in fluoroscopy, the patient support surface should be as radiolucent as possible, thereby reducing excessive x-ray tube emission. A carbon fiber material is commonly used in the tabletop to meet this requirement.

Source-to-Image Receptor Distance Indicator

When imaging a patient, radiographers must have a means to accurately measure the distance from the anode focal spot to the image receptor to ensure that the quality control recommended* **source-to-image receptor distance (SID)** is maintained. To meet this need, radiographic equipment comes with an indicator that will perform this function. Previously, a simple device such as a tape measure was attached to the collimator or tube housing so that the radiographer could manually measure the SID. Current radiographic systems are equipped with lasers to automatically accomplish this task. SID accuracy is essential. "Distance and centering indicators must be accurate to within 2% and 1% of the SID, respectively."[1]

X-Ray Beam Limitation Device for Fixed and Mobile Radiographic Equipment

The primary x-ray beam *shall be* adequately collimated so that it is no larger than the size of the image receptor being used for the examination. With modern equipment, this is accomplished by providing the unit with a **light-localizing variable-aperture rectangular collimator** to automatically

---

*For most ordinary x-ray imaging examinations, a standard distance of 100 to 120 cm (40 to 48 inches) is now used in many radiography facilities. For chest radiography of patients who can assume an upright position, a 180-cm (72-inch) distance is traditional. However, an SID as great as 300 cm (120 inches), is sometimes employed. Multiple benefits of increased SID include: reduced magnification distortion of the anatomical parts; an increase in the amount of accurately resolved detail or spatial resolution because as the distance between the source and the image receptor increase, the diverging x-rays become more perpendicular to the object imaged; and an approximate 10% reduction in radiation dose to the patient.[2]

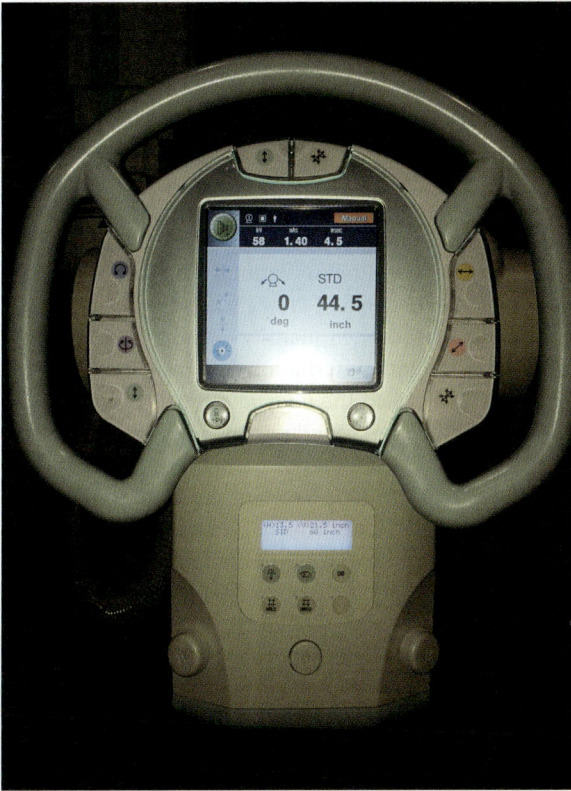

Fig. 10.2 Light-localizing variable-aperture rectangular collimator.

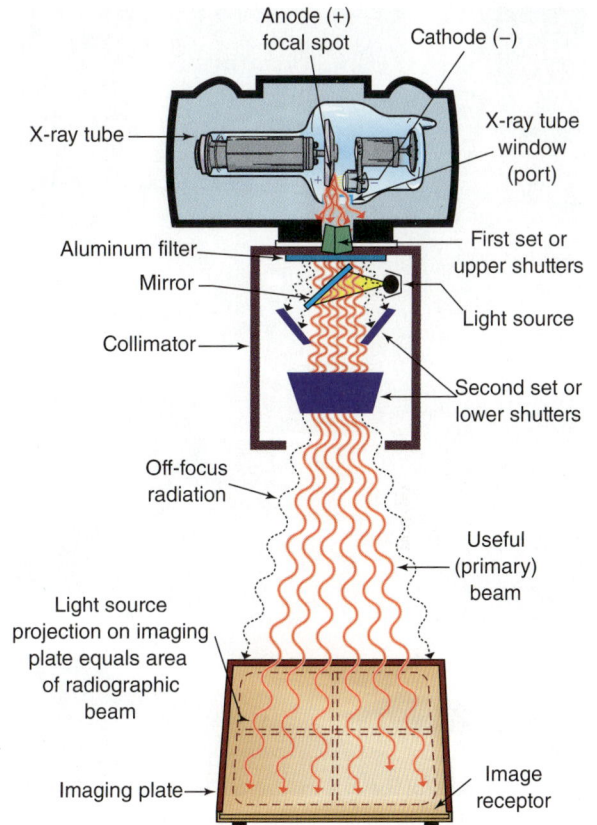

Fig. 10.3 Diagram of a typical collimator demonstrating a radiographic beam-defining system: 1, anode focal spot; 2, x-ray tube window; 3, first set of shutters, or upper shutters; 4, aluminum filter; 5, mirror; 6, light source; 7, second set of shutters, or lower shutters. The metal shutters collimate the radiographic beam so that it is no larger than the image receptor.

or manually adjust the x-ray beam to a specific size and shape (either rectangular or square) (Fig. 10.2). Therefore the collimator serves as the **x-ray beam limitation device** that approximates the size of the anatomical area or part to be included in the radiation field.

Scattered radiation can be defined as all the nonuseful-image-forming radiation that arises from the interaction of an x-ray beam with the atoms of a patient or any other object in the path of the beam. Restricting or *collimating* the size of the x-ray field to include only a slight margin around the anatomic structures of clinical interest reduces the amount of scatter radiation reaching the image receptor. Subject contrast in the radiographic image is thereby much improved because less muddling of the image occurs.

Light-Localizing Variable-Aperture Rectangular Collimators

Construction. The light-localizing variable-aperture rectangular collimator is used in multipurpose x-ray units. It is box-shaped and contains the radiographic beam–defining system (Fig. 10.3). This system consists of:

- Two sets of adjustable lead shutters mounted within the device at different levels
- A light source to illuminate the x-ray field and permit it to be centered over the area of clinical interest
- A mirror to deflect the light beam toward the patient to be imaged

The first set of shutters, the upper shutters or initial collimation, are mounted as close as possible to the tube window to substantially limit the amount of x-rays emitted from parts of the tube other than the focal spot and exiting at various angles from the x-ray tube window. This **off-focus radiation** can never be entirely eliminated because the shutters cannot be physically placed immediately beneath the actual focal spot of the x-ray tube. However, by situating them as close as possible to the tube window, this off-focus radiation can be reduced

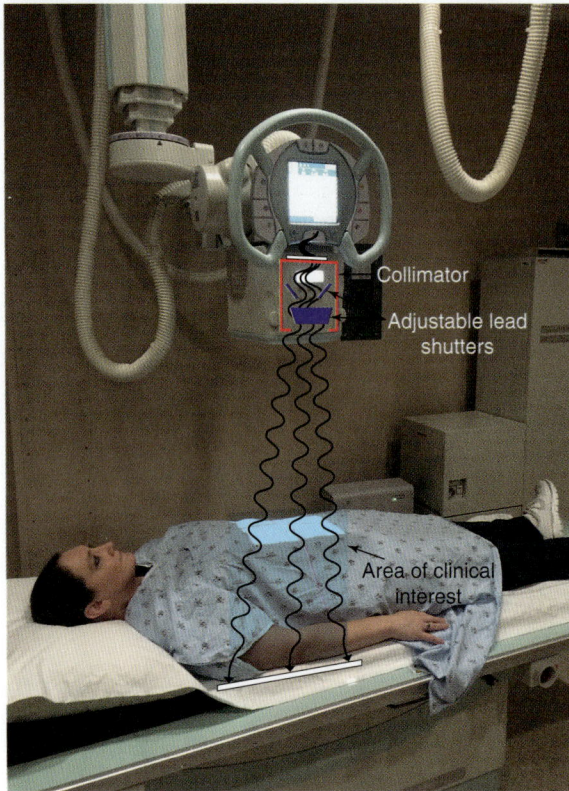

Fig. 10.4 Collimator containing the radiographic beam-defining system, which establishes the parameters (margins) of the beam. Adjustable lead shutters limit the cross-sectional area of the beam and confine it to the area of clinical interest.

significantly, thereby decreasing the patient's exposure and some potential exposure to the radiographer.

The second set of collimator shutters, the lower shutters, are mounted below the level of the light source and mirror and function to further confine the radiographic beam to the area of clinical interest (see Figs. 10.3 and 10.4). This set of shutters consists of two pairs of lead plates oriented at right angles to each other. Each set may be adjusted independently so that the radiographer can select an appropriate size radiation field.

Skin sparing. To minimize skin exposure to electrons produced by photon interaction with the collimator, the patient's skin surface should be at least 15 cm below the collimator for fixed radiographic equipment. Some collimator housings contain "spacer bars," which project down from the housing to prevent the collimators from being closer than 15 cm to the patient. Portable, or mobile, radiographic units are required to maintain a source-to-skin distance of at least 30 cm.

Luminance. Luminance is a technical term referring to the **brightness** of a surface. Specifically, luminance quantifies the intensity of a light source (i.e., the amount of light per unit area coming from its surface). Luminance is determined by measuring the concentration of light over a particular field of view. The primary unit is the *candela per square meter*, known more simply as the *nit*. One candela corresponds to 3.8 million billion photons per second being emitted from a light source through a specific field of view (FOV) or solid angle.*

There is also another quantity associated with brightness. The Systeme International (SI)-derived unit of *luminous flux*, called the *lumen*, is equal to the amount of light emitted per second passing into a solid angle of one steradian from a uniform source of one candela. One lumen corresponds to about the same brilliance as a normal birthday candle has at a distance of one foot. In the English system of units, a related unit is the *foot-candle*, which corresponds to one lumen *per square foot*.

According to standard regulation criteria, luminance must be high enough so that a calibrated light meter reading taken at a distance of 100 cm will in the English system of units be equal to at least *15 foot-candles* when averaged over the four quadrants of a 25 × 25-cm field size.

Example: What is the corresponding "luminance" in SI units associated with an instrument reading of 15 foot-candles?

Solution: One foot-candle is approximately one lumen *per square foot*. The SI unit of luminance is the candela *per square meter*. Therefore a conversion between square feet and square meters has to be done. That conversion is 10.76 square feet to 1 square meter. Consequently, a reading of 15 foot-candles corresponds to a collimator light source with a luminance of approximately 161 (15 × 10.76) candela per square meter or 161 *nit*.

The luminance of the collimator light source must be sufficient to permit the localizing light beam to outline the desired margins of the radiographic beam adequately on the patient's anatomy. Because the light field and the x-ray field are designed to coincide, if the light field were not sufficiently bright, a radiographer could incorrectly position the x-ray field on a patient or, at the

---

*A measure of the size of the FOV (as seen through a camera lens) from some particular point that a given object covers. It is a gauge of how much of an object is perceived by an observer looking from that point. The dimensionless unit of solid angle is the steradian, with 4π steradians covering or encompassing a full sphere field of view.

very least, have difficulty accurately centering the x-ray beam. With insufficient light intensity, an x-ray unit will fail some state inspections.

If the luminance of the collimator light source is sufficient, the localizing light beam will be able to satisfactorily outline the margins of the radiographic beam on the area of clinical interest on patients of all skin pigmentations.

Coincidence between the radiographic beam and the localizing light beam. When a light-localizing variable-aperture rectangular collimator is used, good coincidence (i.e., very similar physical size and overlapping alignment) between the x-ray beam and the localizing light beam is essential to eliminate collimator cutoff of the body structures that need to be imaged. The standard of acceptance is that the sum of the cross-table and along-the-table alignment differences between the x-ray and light beams must not exceed 2% of the SID. This condition is also imposed on the relative "sizing" differences between the x-ray and light beams. These two coincidence requirements are respectively known as:

- Alignment
- Congruence

As an example, 100 cm (or 40-inches in nonmetric units) is a commonly used SID in radiography. For this, the maximum allowable total difference in length and width alignments of the projected light field with the radiographic beam at the level of the image receptor must be no more than 2% of 100 cm, which equals 2 cm ($\approx$ 0.8 inch). Acceptable congruence at a 100-cm (40-inch) SID requires that the sum of the dimensions of the x-ray field should also differ from the length and width span of the light field by no more than 2 cm ($\approx$ 0.8 inches).

The SID used in radiography depends on the individual type of radiographic projection. For example, a 180-cm (or a 72-inch) SID is typically used for routine upright chest x-ray examinations performed on ambulatory patients. In some imaging departments, the use of 120-cm (or 48-inch) SID for many projections has become standard instead of using 100-cm (or 40-inch) SID because increasing the SID causes less geometric divergence of the x-ray beam as it traverses the thickness of the patient's body. The increased SID will improve the sharpness, or spatial resolution, of the radiographic image and decrease the patient's dose.[1-4]

Positive beam limitation. Between 1974 and 1994, the federal government of the United States required all new fixed x-ray installations to be equipped with automatic collimation, or **positive beam limitation (PBL)** devices. The purpose of this mechanism is to restrict the size and shape of the x-ray beam so it does not exceed the size of the selected image receptor. PBL apparatus consists of electronic sensors in an image receptor holder, which, when activated, send signals to the collimator housing that mechanically adjust the collimators so that the x-ray field dimensions match the size of the image receptor. If special conditions require the radiographer to have complete control of the system, the PBL can be overridden by a turn of a key located on the collimator. A warning light is then automatically lit to alert the radiographer that the PBL system is no longer activated. Since 1994 new radiographic installations surprisingly are no longer required by federal law to include automatic collimation. However, many manufactures of new x-ray equipment continue to include the PBL feature in the interest of radiation safety.

In summary, the PBL system illustrates an essential principle of patient protection during radiographic procedures. Even without PBL, the radiographer must always ensure that x-ray beam collimation is satisfactory by adjusting it so that it is no larger than the image receptor (Fig. 10.5). State requirements, however, for agreement, both in alignment and congruence, of a PBL's system's setting with the actual dimensions of the radiographic beam vary from 2% to 3% of the SID.

Filtration

Purpose and Effects of Radiographic Beam Filtration. **Filtration** of the radiographic beam results in the absorption of most of the lower-energy photons (long wavelength, or soft x-rays) from the heterogeneous beam (Fig. 10.6). This increases the mean energy, or "quality," of the x-ray beam and is commonly referred to as "hardening" the beam. The remaining photons will be of higher mean energy and therefore less likely to be absorbed via the photoelectric interaction in body tissue. On the other hand, if adequate filtration were not present, very low-energy photons (20 keV or lower) would enter the patient and be almost totally absorbed in the body, thus markedly increasing the patient's radiation dose, especially near or at the surface, but contributing nothing to the imaging process. To reduce absorbed dose to the patient, in general radiography, the low-energy photons therefore should be removed from the radiographic beam through proper filtration. The filter material used for this includes elements that are both inherent to and added to the x-ray tube.

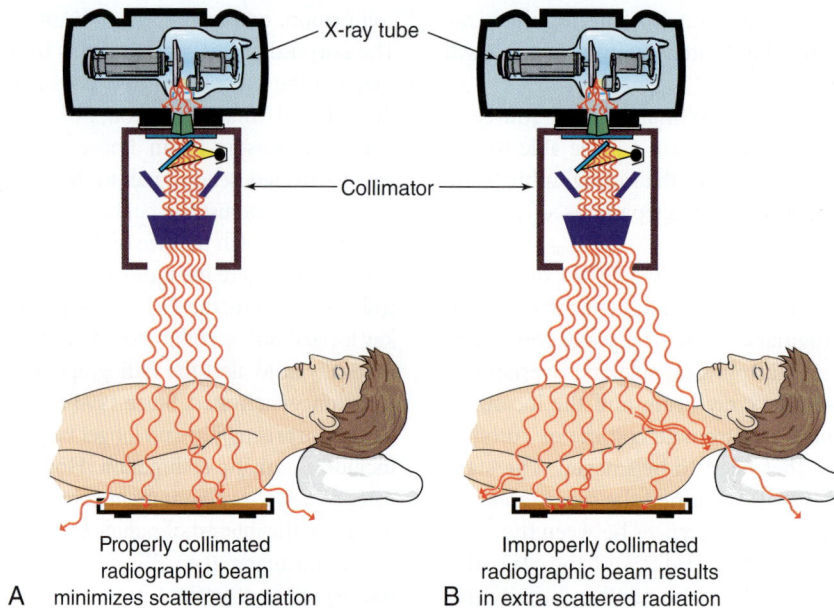

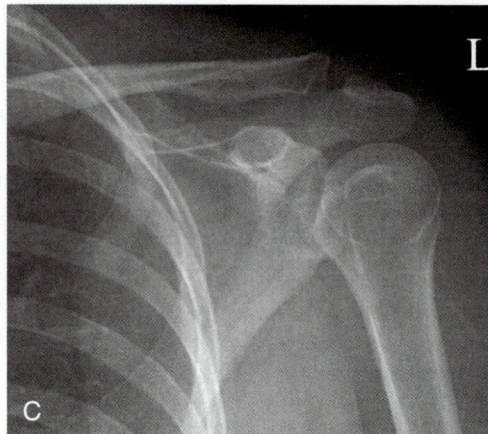

Fig. 10.5 Collimate the radiographic beam so that it is no larger than the image receptor. Limiting the beam to the area of clinical interest decreases the amount of tissue irradiated and minimizes patient exposure by reducing the amount of scattered and absorbed radiation. (A) Good collimation. (B) Poor collimation. (C) Anteroposterior radiograph of the shoulder demonstrating good collimation. (C, From Lampignano J, Kendrick LE: *Textbook of radiographic positioning and related anatomy*, ed 11, St. Louis, 2025, Elsevier.)

Types of Filtration. The following two types of filtration are available:

- Inherent filtration
- Added filtration

Inherent, or intrinsic, filtration, which is always present, includes the:

- Glass envelope encasing the x-ray tube
- Insulating oil surrounding the tube
- Glass window in the tube housing

This intrinsic material provides the same amount of filtration as a 0.5-mm thickness of aluminum. The light-localizing collimator mirror delivers an additional

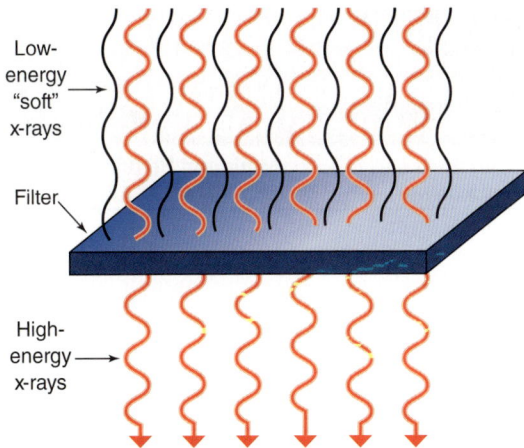

Fig. 10.6 Filtration removes low-energy photons (long-wavelength or "soft" x-rays) from the beam by absorbing them and permits higher-energy photons to pass through. This reduces the amount of radiation that the patient receives.

Added filtration typically consists of:

Thin sheets of aluminum (or the equivalent) of a millimeter to submillimeter thickness

This extra filtration is generally located outside the glass window of the tube housing above the collimator shutters. It is readily accessible to service personnel and may be changed as the x-ray tube ages.

Requirement for Total Filtration. The inherent filtration and added filtration jointly combine to equal the required amount necessary to filter the useful beam adequately (Box 10.1).

The kVp of a given x-ray unit determines the amount of attenuation required. Total filtration of 2.5 mm aluminum equivalent for fixed x-ray units operating above 70 kVp is the regulatory standard (Fig. 10.7).[5] Therefore the manufacturer needs only to place an additional 1

attenuation of almost 1 mm aluminum equivalent. Therefore there is always a minimum of about 1.5 millimeters of equivalent aluminum filtration imposed on the x-ray beam before it exits from the collimator.

BOX 10.1 Total Filtration

Total filtration = Inherent filtration plus added filtration

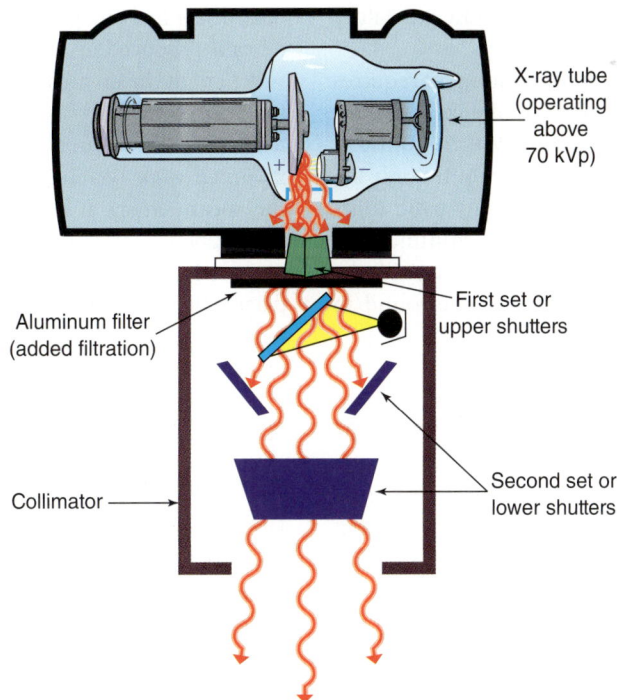

Fig. 10.7 A minimum of 2.5 mm aluminum equivalent total filtration is required for fixed radiographic units operating at above 70 kVp.

BOX 10.2 Summary of Required Minimum Total Filtration

Stationary (Fixed) Radiographic Equipment

Tube Potential Minimum Total Filtration Required (kVp)	Minimum Total Filtration Required (Specified in mm Al Eq)*
Above 70	2.5
50–70	1.5
Below 50	0.5

Mobile Diagnostic Units and Fluoroscopic Equipment

Mobile diagnostic units and fluoroscopic equipment require a minimum of 2.5 mm Al Eq total permanent filtration.

Al Eq, Aluminum equivalent.
*Modified from National Council on Radiation Protection and Measurements (NCRP): *Medical x-ray, electron beam, and gamma-ray protection for energies up to 50 MeV (equipment design, performance, and use)*, Report No. 102, Bethesda, MD, 1989, NCRP.

TABLE 10.1 Half-Value Layer Required by the Radiation Control for Health and Safety Act of 1968 and Detailed by the Bureau of Radiological Health* in 1980

Peak Kilovoltage	Minimum Required HVL in Millimeters of Aluminum
30	0.3
40	0.4
50	1.2
60	1.3
70	1.5
80	2.3
90	2.5
100	2.7
110	3.0
120	3.2

HVL, Half-value layer.
*The Bureau of Radiological Health changed its name to the Center for Devices and Radiological Health in 1982.

mm aluminum equivalent filter between the tube housing and collimator to meet the minimum regulatory requirement.

Stationary (fixed) radiographic equipment requires a total filtration of 1.5 mm aluminum equivalent for x-ray units operating at 50 to 70 kVp. In contrast, fixed units operating at below 50 kVp require only 0.5 mm aluminum equivalent.[5] Mobile diagnostic units and fluoroscopic equipment require a minimum of 2.5 mm aluminum equivalent. A summary of the required minimum total filtration may be found in Box 10.2.

Filtration for General Diagnostic Radiology. In general diagnostic radiology, aluminum (Z = 13) is the metal most widely selected as a filter material because it effectively removes very low-energy (soft) x-rays from a polyenergetic (heterogeneous) x-ray beam without severely decreasing the x-ray beam intensity. In addition, aluminum is:

- Lightweight
- Sturdy
- Relatively inexpensive
- Readily available

In compliance with the Radiation Control for Health and Safety Act of 1968, a diagnostic x-ray beam must always be adequately filtered. This means that a sufficient quantity of low-energy photons has been removed from a beam produced at a given kVp. The **half-value layer (HVL)** of the beam must be measured to verify this. HVL is defined *as the thickness of a designated absorber required to decrease the intensity of the primary beam by 50% of its initial value*. A radiological physicist should obtain this measurement at least once a year and also after an x-ray tube is replaced or repairs have been made on the diagnostic x-ray tube housing or collimation system. For diagnostic x-ray beams, the HVL is expressed in millimeters of aluminum. Because it is a measure of beam quality, or effective energy of the x-ray beam, a certain minimal HVL is required at a given kVp. Examples of required HVLs for selected kVp values are listed in Table 10.1.

Compensating Filters

Dose reduction and uniform radiographic imaging of body parts that vary considerably in thickness or tissue composition may be accomplished by use of *compensating filters* constructed of:

- Aluminum
- Lead-acrylic
- Other suitable materials

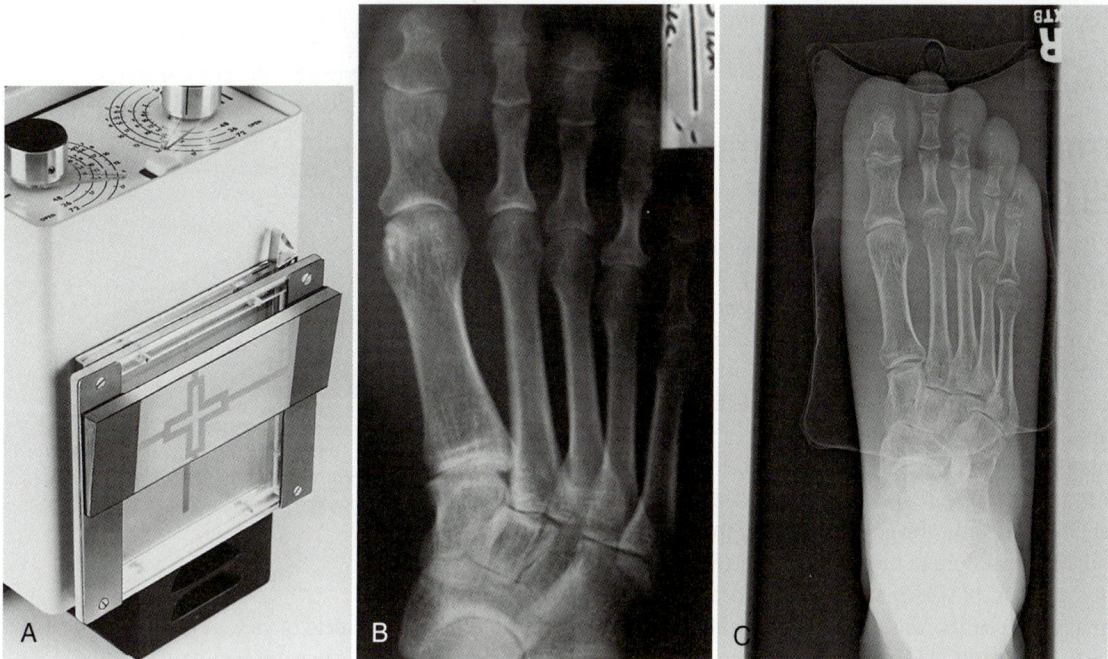

Fig. 10.8 (A) Wedged-shaped lead-acrylic compensating filter used to provide uniform density for (B) a dorsoplantar projection of the foot without a compensating filter. (C) A dorsoplantar projection of the foot with a wedge-shaped lead-acrylic compensating filter.

These devices are shaped so as to partially attenuate x-rays that are directed toward the thinner, or less dense, anatomic areas while permitting more x-radiation to strike the thicker, or denser, areas to be imaged. For example, the *wedge filter* (Fig. 10.8) is used to provide uniform density when the foot is undergoing radiography in the dorsoplantar projection. For this examination, the wedge is attached to the lower rim of the collimator and positioned with its thickest part toward the toes and thinnest part toward the heel.

The *trough*, or *bilateral, wedge filter*, which is used in some dedicated chest radiographic units, is another example of a compensating filter. This filter is thin in the center to permit adequate x-ray penetration of the mediastinum and thick laterally to reduce exposure of the aerated lungs. With this device, a radiographic image with a uniform average density is obtained. Some modern digital systems correct for such nonuniformities of exposure with digital image processing rather than by using a physical filter.

Required Radiation Exposure Characteristics

Exposure Reproducibility. Exposure reproducibility has been previously defined as consistency in radiation output intensity for identical generator settings from one single exposure to subsequent exposures. This means that the x-ray unit must be able to duplicate certain radiographic exposures for any given combination of kVp, mA, and time settings. A variance of 5% or less is acceptable. Reproducibility may be verified by using the same technical exposure factors to make a series of repeated radiation exposures and then, observing with a calibrated ion chamber, how radiation intensity typically varies.

Exposure Linearity. Exposure linearity, also previously described, refers to a *consistency* in output radiation intensity at any selected kVp when generator settings are changed from one milliamperage and time combination (mAs = mA × exposure time) to another. *Linearity (L)* has been mathematically defined as the ratio of the difference in mSv/mAs or mR/mAs values between two successive generator stations to the sum of those mSv/mAs or mR/mAs values. It must be less than 0.1 (i.e., L cannot exceed 10%).

AUTOMATIC EXPOSURE CONTROL (AEC) AND PHOTOTIMING

The **Automatic Exposure Control (AEC)** system (also often referred to as "**phototiming**") of a radiographic unit is essentially an *x-ray exposure termination device* that ends the radiation when a predetermined amount of radiation is received by an arrangement of sensors. Once correctly calibrated*, it is available as an exposure feature that supplements and/or replaces the usage of a manual technique chart.

Automatic exposure systems are designed to produce an acceptable diagnostic image while limiting the total amount of radiation exposure to the patient. When activated, technical factors such as kVp and mA and focal spot size are normally selected by the radiographer, whereas *duration is controlled by the AEC*. However, there are other AEC systems, for example, predominantly used in fluoroscopy systems, which will also automatically set extra exposure factors, such as the x-ray tube current and voltage.

For safety considerations, all radiographic automatic exposure systems have a mandatory, and always engaged, *backup timer* feature. This allows the device to terminate the radiation appropriately while still protecting the patient from excessive overexposure if a problem occurs. Backup time is typically set to 150% to 200% of the expected exposure time.

Differences in automatic exposure systems lie in the type of device used to convert radiation into electricity or, more precisely, electrical signal. Two types of detection systems have historically been used: photomultipliers** and ionization chambers. *Phototiming* specifically refers to the use of photomultiplier tubes, and although today these are only present in older systems, the terminology is still frequently used. The standard type of AEC system utilizes ionization chambers. Regardless of the kind of automatic exposure system employed, almost all systems have a set of three radiation-measuring detectors, arranged in some particular manner to monitor the intensity distribution of

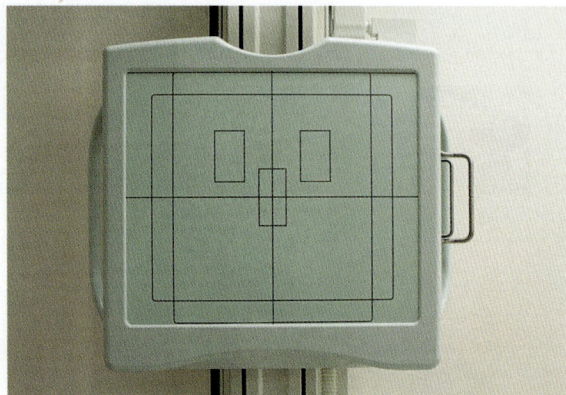

Fig. 10.9 Automatic exposure control (AEC) system with upright bucky unit. The location of three AEC detector chambers are outlined on the face of the device. (From Johnston JN: *Essentials of radiographic physics and imaging*, ed 4, St. Louis, 2026, Elsevier.)

radiation over the field of view. A common spatial separation in detectors is shown if Fig. 10.9.

Radiographic Grids

A **radiographic grid** (Fig. 10.10) is a device made of parallel radiopaque strips alternately separated with low-attenuation strips of a material such as aluminum or plastic.

When x-rays pass through an object, some of the photons are scattered away from their original path as a result of coherent and Compton scattering processes. Radiographic quality is highest when these scattered photons are not recorded on the image. If scattered photons are recorded, a diffused additional darkening of the image occurs, which detracts from the viewer's ability to distinguish among the different structures of the object being imaged. Ideally, only those photons that have passed through matter with no deviation from their original geometric path should be recorded.

To minimize the influence of scattered photons, a grid is inserted between the patient and the image receptor. It is designed to act as a sieve to block the passage of photons that have been scattered beyond some maximum angle from their original path (Fig. 10.11). This significantly improves:

---

*Annual calibrations by a qualified medical physicist employing standard phantoms of varying thicknesses to test both reproducibility and accuracy are regulatory required.

**A photomultiplier is an analog, vacuum tube device that converts x-ray photon energy into electrical signals. It has been largely supplanted by solid-state devices and ionization chambers, both of which are more durable and have much longer useful lifetimes.

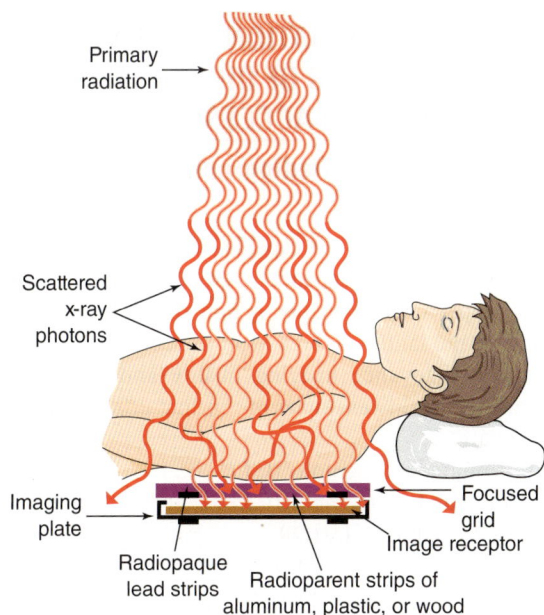

Primary radiation

Scattered x-ray photons

Imaging plate

Focused grid
Image receptor

Radiopaque lead strips

Radioparent strips of aluminum, plastic, or wood

Fig. 10.10 Radiographic grids remove scattered x-ray photons that emerge from the patient being imaged before this scattered radiation reaches the image receptor and decreases radiographic quality.

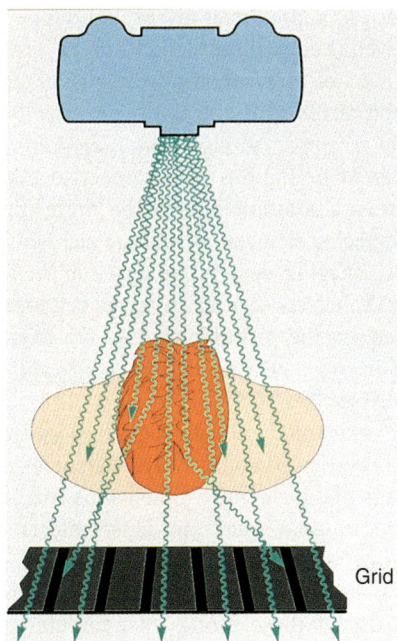

Grid

Fig. 10.11 The radiographic grid acts as a sieve to block the passage of photons that have been scattered at some angle from their original path. (From *Radiobiology and radiation protection: Mosby's radiographic instructional series*, St. Louis, 1999, Elsevier.)

- Radiographic contrast
- Visibility of detail

Generally, this device is used when the thickness of the body part to be irradiated is 10 cm (about 4 inches) or greater. Although the use of a grid increases a patient's dose, the benefit obtained in terms of the improved quality of the completed image, making available a greater quantity of diagnostic information, is a fair compromise. Because several different types of grids are available, care must be taken to ensure that the correct type and the optimal grid ratio are used for a particular examination, or a repeat examination may be necessary, which would additionally increase patient dose. In newer **digital radiography (DR)** equipment, an electronic grid is employed. This electronic grid is actually *a software application*. The electronic grid is used in the same manner as the physical grid; however, exposure factors do not need to be increased.

Grid Ratio and Patient Dose. As previously noted, grids are made of parallel radiopaque lead strips alternately separated by low-attenuation strips of aluminum, or plastic fiber. Therefore because some amount of the image receptor is covered with lead, more mAs must be used to compensate for the decrease in signal from the image receptor. Thus, patient dose increases whenever a grid is inserted. Grid ratio is defined as the height of the lead strips divided by the distance between each strip. Grids with higher ratios (e.g., 10:1) contain more lead. Therefore patient dose increases as grid ratio increases. High-ratio grids, however, reduce scatter radiation more effectively than do low-ratio grids, so there is a trade-off between patient dose and improvement of image quality. Grid ratios higher than 12:1 are not normally used.

Effect of Source-Skin Distance on Patient Entrance Exposure. For all types of x-ray units when the **source-skin distance (SSD)** is small, because of the relatively greater rate of spreading out of the x-ray beam at close distances from the x-ray source than at larger distances, the patient's entrance exposure is significantly larger than the exit exposure. However, by increasing the SSD, the relative spatial divergence of the x-ray beam over the thickness of the patient will be decreased even when a grid is not employed. The radiographer thereby maintains a more uniform distribution of exposure throughout the patient.

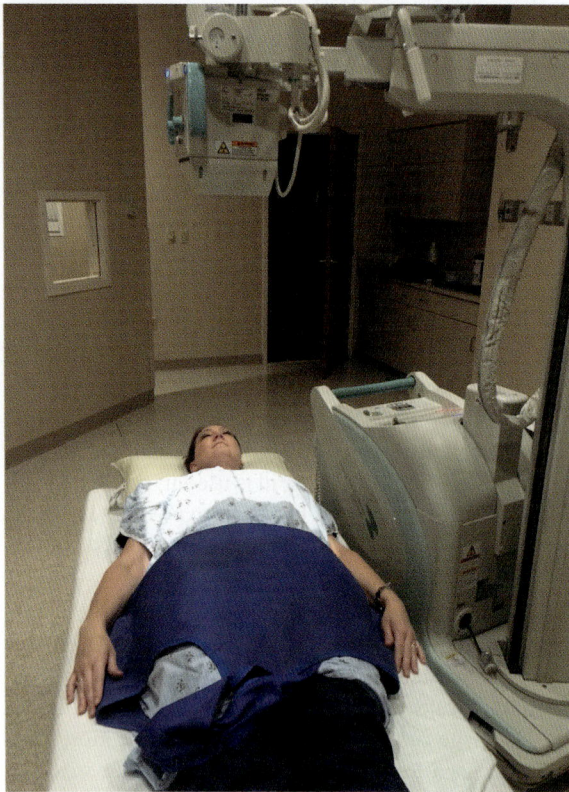

Fig. 10.12 Mobile radiographic examinations require a minimal source-skin distance of 30 cm (12 inches). The 30 cm distance limits the effects of inverse square fall-off of radiation intensity with distance.

Mobile, or Portable, Radiographic Units

Mobile (portable) units should be used to perform radiographic procedures only on patients who cannot be transported to a fixed radiographic installation (an x-ray room). Mobile units are not designed to replace specially designated imaging rooms and require special precautions to ensure both patient and radiographer safety. When operating a mobile unit, the radiographer, while wearing a lead apron, must stand at a distance of 6 feet away from the patient and also use an SSD of *at least* 30 cm (12 inches) (Fig. 10.12). The 30 cm (12 inch) distance limits the effects of the inverse square fall-off of radiation intensity with distance. This fall-off is more pronounced the shorter the SSD. In practice, much longer distances (e.g., 100 cm [40 inches] from the x-ray source to image receptor or even 120 cm [48 inches]) are generally used.

GENERAL INFORMATION AND RADIATION SAFETY FEATURES OF DIGITAL IMAGING EQUIPMENT AND ACCESSORIES

Digital Processed Radiography Imaging Modes

Modern computers are capable of rapidly processing vast amounts of independent groups of information. This property, in particular, is now the backbone in all imaging modalities, as well as in the continuing efforts to further advance imaging quality and detail. The primary modality examples of this that utilize beams of x-rays are:

- Computed tomography (CT)
- Computed radiography (CR)
- Digital radiography (DR)
- Digital fluoroscopy (DF)
- Digital mammography (DM)

Digital Imaging Overview

All nonanalog or digital images have many similar properties regardless of the engineering technology with which they are acquired, simply because they are all numerical approximations of nondigital (analog) signals. Even though these signals may be produced by vast numbers of x-ray photons, the overall strength of the signal is recorded as one number at each location on the image receptor. All el*ectronic* radiography devices have inherent limitations with respect to both spatial and contrast resolution due to the finite dimensions of their detector elements or picture elements (pixels). All digital imaging devices are also subject to certain artifacts (i.e., effects seen in an image system that were introduced by the technology used in acquiring the image or images) such as *aliasing, moiré patterns, and contouring* (see Box 10.3).

These unwanted effects occur because digital images are produced collectively by an array or matrix of elements that have finite dimensions and are always subject to random quantum noise effects (mottle), which grow in importance as the matrix elements become finer.

With any of these modes of computer-processed radiography, the latent (unprocessed) image formed by x-ray photons on a radiation detector is an electronic image.[6] Because this anatomic information is

BOX 10.3 Image Aliasing, Morié Patterns, and Contouring Defects

In computer graphics, *aliasing* is an image distortion that shows up most simply as the jagged, or saw-toothed, appearance of curved or diagonal lines.

Moiré patterns occur when an object that is being imaged contains many fine, repetitive details. As a result, strange-looking wavy patterns are overlayed on the image. This is shown in the figure below.

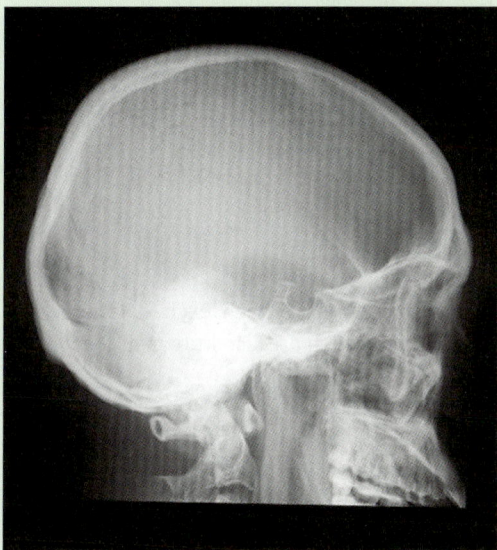

(From Carter CE, Vealé BL: *Digital radiography and PACS*, ed 3, Philadelphia, 2019, Elsevier.)

Contouring artifacts usually show up as patterns of small blocks in an otherwise smooth image. An example of this are adjacent groups of rectangular or block-like images of different intensity or brightness superimposed on what is really a clear smooth sky. These blocks become very much more noticeable as the image is viewed on larger devices or monitors.

are composed of numerical data that can be easily manipulated by a computer.[7]

The numeric values of the digital image are aligned in a fixed number of rows and columns (an array) that form many individual miniature square boxes, each of which corresponds to a particular place in the image. These individual boxes collectively constitute the **image matrix**. Each miniature square box in this matrix is a *picture element*, or *pixel*. The pixels collectively produce a two-dimensional representation of the information contained in a volume of tissue.[8] The size of the pixels determines the sharpness of the image. The resolution is finer when pixels are smaller. One example of a standard matrix size is 512 pixels high by 512 pixels wide, or simply 512 × 512. A range of other matrix sizes are also used, such as 1024 × 1024. For the same field of view (FOV), the latter corresponds to four times as many elements distributed over the same area. The pixels are therefore smaller, which leads to improved patient image detail. It should be noted that such resolution increases, however, are associated with very substantial increases in the quantity of data to be computer processed.

Digital image receptors used in DR convert the energy of x-rays into electrical signals. The image receptor is divided into small detector elements that make up the pixels of the digital image. There are various types of these image receptors. Some use a *scintillator*, such as amorphous silicon,* to convert the x-ray energy into visible light. The visible light is then transformed into electrical signals by an assortment of transistors or an array of charge-couple devices (CCDs), such as those found in video cameras. Other systems use a *photoconductor*, such as amorphous selenium,* to convert the x-ray energy directly into electrical signals that are then read by an ordered grouping (matrix) of transistors. In these systems, the number and size of small transistors or CCDs determine the number and size of pixels in the digital image. Advances in materials technology have resulted in pixel sizes as small as 50 micrometers, which approaches the resolution of screen-film imaging systems (Fig. 10.13).

subsequently collected by a computer and shown on its display, it is called a *digital image*.[7] The familiar radiographic densities then appear as levels of brightness associated with shades of gray. The shades of gray that are displayed on a computer screen constitute the contrast in the image. The number of different shades of gray that can be stored in memory and subsequently displayed is known as the *grayscale*. All digital images

---

*Amorphous refers to a noncrystalline grouping of silicon atoms ($_{14}Si^{28}$) or selenium atoms ($_{34}Se^{79}$) in which, rather than in a regular geometric pattern, the silicone atoms or the selenium atoms are distributed in a continuous random fashion.

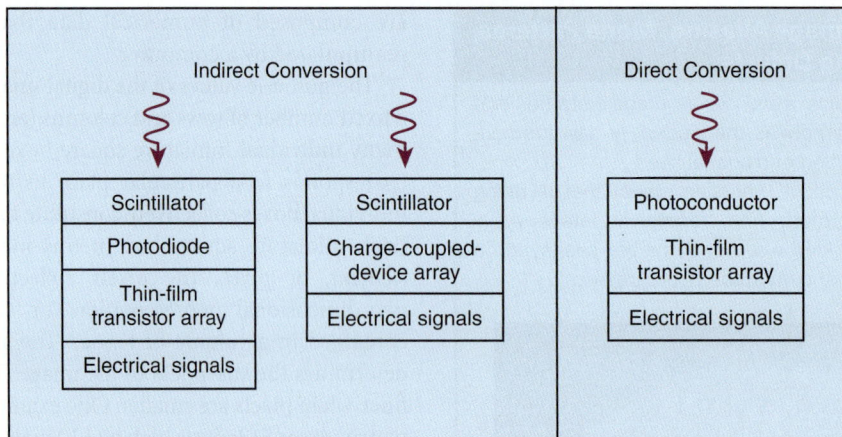

Fig. 10.13 Some large area detectors provide indirect conversion of x-ray energy to electrical charge through intermediate steps involving photodiodes or charge-coupled devices. Other area detectors provide direct conversion of x-ray energy to electrical charge through the use of a photoconductor. (From Hendee WR, Ritenour ER: *Medical imaging physics*, ed 4, Chicago, 2002, John Wiley & Sons.)

Digital images can quickly be accessed via a PACS* network at multiple workstations at the same time, thus allowing image viewing to be very convenient for physicians providing patient care. Patient information and reports can be included in the patient's imaging file, along with records from other imaging modalities.[9]

Computed Radiography (CR)

Computed radiography (CR) is the descriptive term for those x-ray systems that generate images using the process of *photostimulable luminescence* (PSL). In this technique, the energy of the conventional diagnostic x-ray beams passing through a patient is not projected onto x-ray film within a cassette but rather is deposited onto a modified crystalline material known as a photostimulable phosphor (PSP).** The absorbed energy produces a latent (undeveloped) image composed of PSP molecules with electrons that have been excited (energy raised) into fixed states, which are also known as local potential energy traps.

The number and locations of these trapped excited electrons is a molecular photo of the originally projected x-ray energy. The electrons are released from their traps by gaining added energy from absorbing external light of a specific wavelength (photostimulation). These electrons subsequently lose their excess energy by the release of the photostimulable light (PSL) they absorbed. An image-reading unit employing a helium-neon laser is used to scan the light, which then can be measured and enumerated to create a digital image. A computer stores the digital image for visual display on a monitor. If desired, the image can be printed on a laser film when a hard copy is needed. While the digital image is displayed on a monitor, the radiographer, by manipulating the computer mouse (Fig. 10.14) or scrolling a touch screen cursor, can adjust the image to the correct:

- Size
- Brightness
- Contrast

After adjustments have been completed, the image or images are sent through a PACS system for review by a radiologist. In CR, the receptor can be erased with white light and reused to acquire another projection.

CR was useful as an interim step in converting older imaging equipment to digital techniques, since the

---

*PACS refers to a *picture archiving and communication system* imaging technology which provides throughout an authorized and secure computer network both economical storage and convenient remote access to images from multiple modalities. The universal format for PACS image storage and transfer is called *dicom* (Digital Imaging and Communications in Medicine.)

**Europium-activated barium fluorohalide (BaFX:Eu) is the most commonly employed phosphor in which "*X*" represents a combination of a bromide (e.g., potassium bromide KBr) and an iodide (e.g., sodium iodide NaI), typically 85% and 15%, respectively.[1]

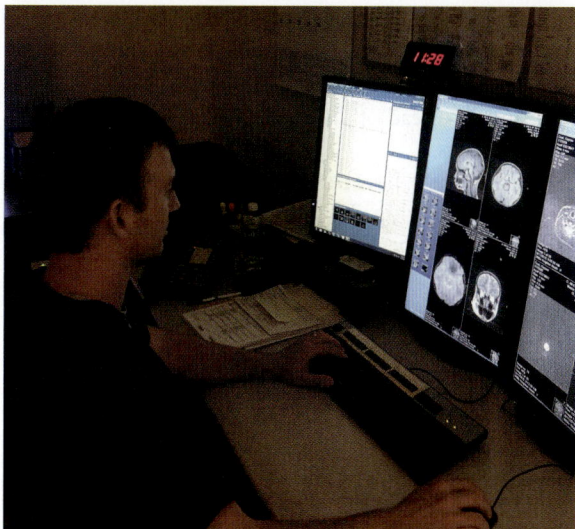

Fig. 10.14 The radiographer at the monitor uses the mouse to adjust the computed radiography image of the body part to the proper size, density, and contrast before electronically sending the image for reading.

CR plate or cassette could be substituted for the film-screen cassette in older equipment with no further modifications. However, the speed of image acquisition and dose efficiency considerations indicate that there will be an eventual conversion of all equipment to DR in the future.

Kilovoltage. The kVp controls the penetrating ability of the x-ray beam as it passes through human anatomy and also affects radiographic contrast in the image. The size of the part or area of the body to be imaged and the type of subject contrast desired in the completed image determine kVp selection.[2] In CR imaging, unlike film-screen imaging, it has been found that with respect to kilovoltage, there is a substantial amount of flexibility available for selection of the degree of desired subject contrast. Regulatory standards require that technique charts indicating optimal kVp values for all CR projections must be available in the x-ray room near the operating console for radiographers.

X-ray Beam Collimation. For the computer to form a CR image correctly, the body area or part being irradiated must be accurately positioned in or near the center of the CR image receptor. In practical application, only one projection per image is obtained on a CR imaging plate.

Use of Radiographic Grids. The CR imaging plate can absorb low-energy scattered photons; therefore, it is sensitive to scatter radiation both before and after it is sensitized by exposure to a radiographic beam.[3] Because of this increased sensitivity, a radiographic grid should be used more frequently. For chest radiography, Carlton and Adler advocated the use of a grid for optimum images when chest measurements exceed 24 to 26 cm.[3] Some CR imaging manufacturers recommended the use of a grid for particular radiographic projections that require relatively high-kVp settings. Grid selection depends on several factors: the size of the anatomic features to be imaged, kVp selected, amount of scatter removal preferred, and grid frequency (lines per centimeter or inch).[3]

It is customary and, for the best image quality, necessary to use a grid for anatomy sections more than 10 cm thick or for techniques that exceed 70 kVp. This need remains true with both CR and DR. In general, the problem a radiographer faces with CR is that the mAs required and, consequently, the patient dose received usually are higher than for non-CR. The addition of a grid will only further increase that dose. Many quality assurance teams, however, realize that CR, because of its wider exposure latitude, reduces the need for grid use on the pediatric population. As a result, satisfactory nongrid pediatric protocols have been developed and implemented.

Digital Radiography (DR)

DR systems, unlike CR, use as image receptors active-matrix flat panels consisting of a detection layer deposited over an array of thin-film transistors and photodiodes. Current state-of-the-art digital sensors are more sensitive or responsive to diagnostic energy x-rays than radiographic film, and thus much less radiation (up to 70% less) is often only required to produce a digital image.

Digital Rradiography Systems Advantages and Disadvantages. DR systems offer several advantages over CR. Some of these include:

- Lower doses—the PSP plates used in CR have a lower efficiency of detection compared to DR detectors. Thus, a higher radiation dose with CR is needed to obtain adequate image quality.
- Greater ease of use and faster patient throughput.
- *Immediate* imaging results: CR requires the cassette be removed from the x-ray machine and then

placed into a reader. This is a labor-intensive step that requires the technologist to leave the patient and workstation with each imaging procedure, even if for a short time.

- Additional image manipulation.
- Much less overall maintenance (e.g., avoidance of CR cassette testing, cleaning, and storage space requirements).

There are, however, several disadvantages of DR relative to CR, namely[10]:

- DR is much more costly
- CR is compatible with a wide range of preinstalled traditional systems
- Multiple cassette sizes with CR allow for greater flexibility than the single detector size of DR
- The CR PSP imaging plates are subject to mechanical damage and also to chemical oxidation but can be replaced without great expense. DR receptors, while well protected from mechanical damage, do not last forever; they experience gradual aging processes, and their replacement cost is high.

An additional prospective disadvantage of DR relative to CR is that most DR systems either do not allow the user to change the grid to accommodate the imaging task or have a preinstalled grid that is not easily accessible. These conditions can result in the use of grids for pediatric imaging, thereby unnecessarily increasing a child's radiation dose. Because of this, DR facilities need to collaborate with their radiation safety officer (RSO) and physics group more than ever before to ensure the highest-quality low-radiation dose imaging for the smallest patients. During acceptance testing of a new DR system, a technologist should inquire whether or not grids are removable from the digital imaging equipment.

Repeat Rates in Digital Imaging

Because image contrast and overall light intensity may be manipulated after image acquisition, digital imaging eliminates the need for almost all repeat images required as a result of improper technique selection (Fig. 10.15). However, repeat rates for reasons of poor positioning are not lowered. Since, for DR, the image receptor is part of the imaging equipment and does not need to be removed for processing, the technologist can simply view the image on a monitor at the control panel. This raises a concern regarding the number of repeats required due to mispositioning. There is no *direct*

"penalty" to a technologist for repeating images because of poor technique, so the examination and resultant radiation exposure could potentially be delivered multiple times, instead of just once, without the knowledge of supervisors.

Early reports have indicated an increase in repeat rates in DR imaging. The increase is fundamentally due to the ease of repeating an image. It appears that technologists are in many cases seeking to obtain the perfect image, without the consideration of increased exposure to the patient.

Digital imaging systems, both DR and CR, separate the process of acquisition from the display and thereby permit a relatively large degree of viewing manipulation of the raw images by the radiographer and/or the radiologist upon examination. Since digital devices also typically have wide exposure latitude,* this can result in a wide range of received patient doses, from very low to extremely high.

An "appropriate" patient exposure is the lowest value that is needed to provide a resultant image of sufficient quality for a radiologist to confidently make an accurate differential diagnosis. However, except for extreme overexposure or underexposure, both DR and CR images can be *manipulated*, because of the separation between acquisition and display, to exhibit satisfactory contrast resolution sensitivity. This is predominately due to the ability of digital detector systems to adjust or rescale the received projection data to a useful grayscale viewing scope or range. Thus, it may be so, in many situations, that the patient has needlessly received a larger radiation exposure often without the knowledge of anyone involved in the diagnostic reading of the case. In some exceptional situations, an overexposure factor of three or more might happen. In general, it has quite often been discovered that a phenomenon known as *"dose creep"* occurs due to the lack of negative impact observed when the patient's anatomy is overexposed but the display still exhibits quality images.

To remedy potential overexposure and thereby adhere to as low as reasonably achievable (ALARA) practices, either each image taken by a digital system

---

*Exposure latitude refers to how much an image receptor can be overexposed or underexposed and still be able to yield a useful image.

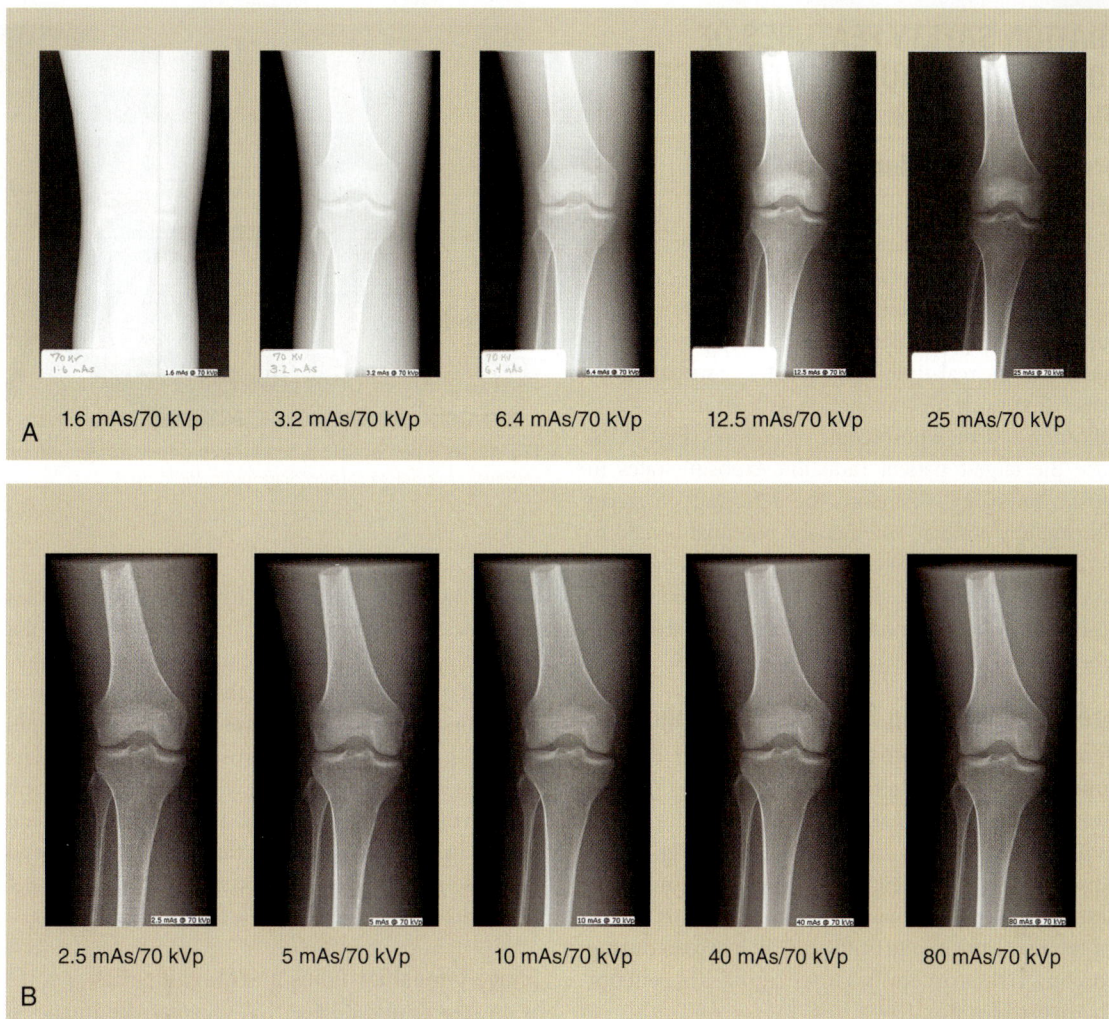

Fig. 10.15 (A) The images obtained with a screen-film image receptor system illustrate how changing technical exposure factors greatly affects film image quality. (B) Computed radiography (CR) images obtained through the same technique ranges as those used for (A) have much less effect on image quality because "CR image contrast is constant, regardless of radiation exposure." (From Betsy Shields, Presbyterian hospital, Charlotte, North Carolina. In Bushong SC, editor: *Radiologic science for technologists: physics, biology and protection*, ed 13, St. Louis, 2026, Elsevier.)

could be monitored by an independent quality control technologist at a separate monitor, which might be quite tedious, or a quality control exposure counting system could be devised whereby for each technologist the number of images per examination is compared with the quantity ordered.

Alternatively, there is, however, a safety feature installed with most digital detector systems: an *exposure index (EI) indicator*, derived from data collected with anthropomorphic phantoms, that supplies the relative speed and sensitivity of the *digital receptor* to incident x-rays. The EI value *ideally* provides a guide to the technologist regarding the proper radiographic techniques to select that will yield an optimal image for a specific examination in terms of both acceptable image quality and patient radiation dose. Usually, during commissioning of a new digital system, a table of appropriate EIs will be determined for that system.

RADIATION SAFETY FEATURES OF FLUOROSCOPIC EQUIPMENT, DEVICES, AND ACCESSORIES

Fluoroscopic Procedures and Patient Irradiation Rates

Fluoroscopy is a continuous irradiation process that demonstrates dynamic motion of or through selected anatomic structures (e.g., a stomach filled with barium sulfate and air during an upper gastrointestinal series) by generating and displaying real-time imaging of those structures on a monitor that works in conjunction with an image signal amplification system. Fluoroscopic procedures (Fig. 10.16) produce the largest patient radiation exposure rates in diagnostic radiology. Therefore the referring physician should carefully evaluate whether the potential benefit to the patient, in terms of information gained, outweighs any adverse somatic or genetic effects of the examination. If the fluoroscopic procedure is necessary, every reasonable effort must be taken to minimize patient exposure time.

Fluoroscopic Imaging Systems: Non-digital

Brightness of the Fluoroscopic Image and Patient Absorbed Dose. Non-digital fluoroscopy (Fig. 10.17) involves the use of a signal amplification device called an *image intensifier (II) tube* (depicted in Fig. 10.18 and discussed in great detail in the next section). This apparatus markedly increases the brightness or intensity of the real-time image produced on a screen during fluoroscopy. II fluoroscopy has three significant benefits, which are listed in Box 10.4.

The x-ray **image intensifier (II)** converts the pattern of x-rays transmitted through the patient into a corresponding and amplified visible light pattern. With an II the overall illumination of the raw fluoroscopic image is increased to roughly 10,000 times that of the image obtained by non-II fluoroscopic systems* while operating

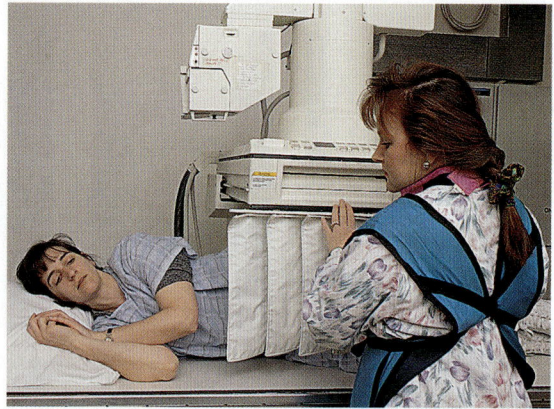

Fig. 10.16 Fluoroscopic procedures produce the largest patient radiation exposure rate in diagnostic radiology.

under the same conditions. This very large increase in brightness has dramatically improved the radiologist's perception of the fluoroscopic image and at the same time enabled a decrease in patient absorbed dose. Image intensification fluoroscopy requires much smaller milliamperage than does pre-II fluoroscopy (approximately 1 to 1.5 mA and even less can now be used for many procedures, whereas 3 to 5 mA and more was usually required before image intensification fluoroscopy). The resultant decrease in exposure rate, for *similar examination durations*, yields a sizable dose reduction for the patient.

Image Intensifier Tubes and Magnification. An II tube is an "electronic device that receives the image-forming x-ray beam and converts it into a visible-light picture of high intensity."[1] A simple diagram of this tube with components labeled is shown in Fig. 10.18. Magnification, or multifield, features are present in the vast majority of II systems. They are also found in **digital fluoroscopy (DF)** units (see the discussion on DF presented later in this chapter). Multifield image intensification tubes vary in size, but the 30/25/20 cm (12/10/8 inch) diameter tri-field model is typical for general-purpose fluoroscopic units. However, other sizes and magnification modes are also available.* When

---

*A pre-image intensification fluoroscopic system consisted of the fluoroscopic tube, mounted beneath the radiographic table, producing x-rays that passed through the tabletop and the patient before striking a zinc-cadmium sulfide (ZnCdS) screen. The latter then phosphoresced, producing an image of the anatomy of interest. Unfortunately, this image was very dim, and to be adequately discerned by the radiologist, a photographic dark-room situation always had to be created.

---

*Many current II systems are available with four selectable viewing modes or magnifications: for example, 20 cm, 17 cm, 15 cm, 12 cm: 12", 9", 6", 4" are other available selections.

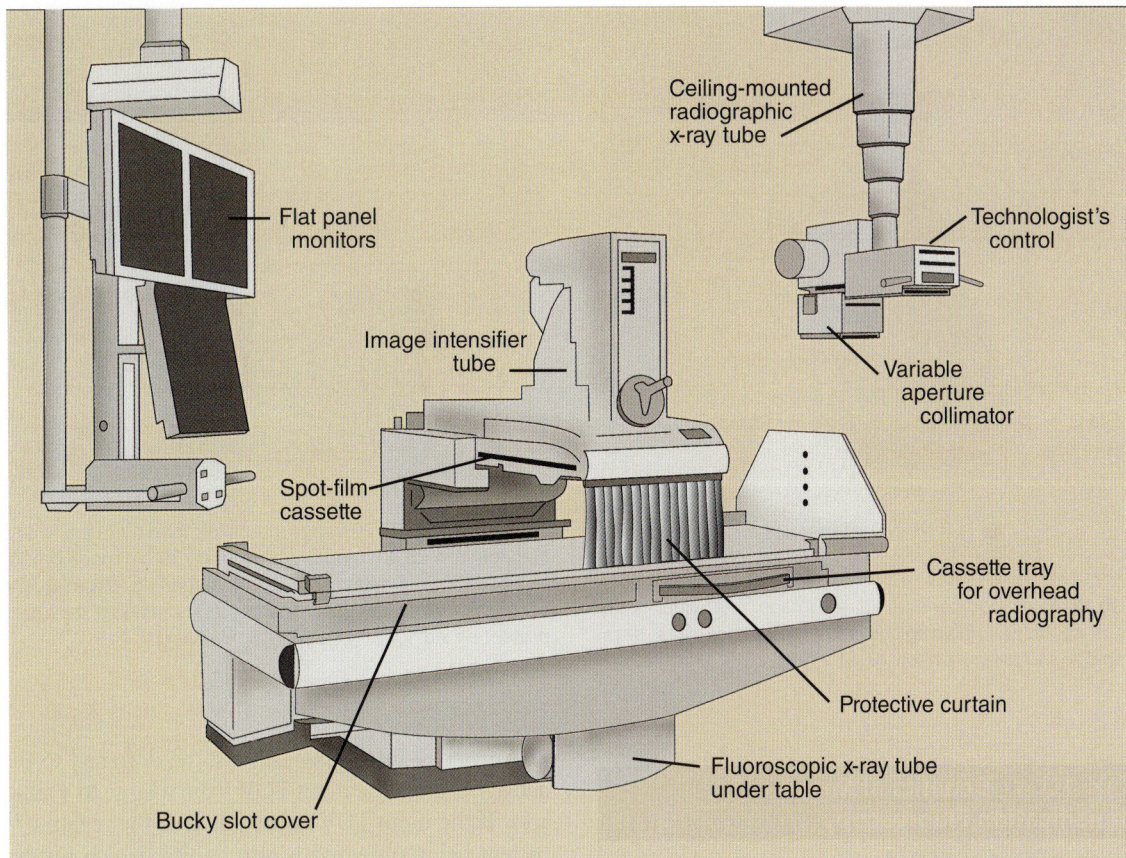

Fig. 10.17 Image intensification fluoroscopy unit. The x-ray tube used in this unit is mounted beneath the unit's radiographic table, which supports the patient. The image intensifier and other image detection devices are then drawn forward and placed over the patient on the table to perform the examination. Other fluoroscopic equipment arrangements are possible. (From Bushong SC: *Radiologic science for technologists: physics, biology and protection*, ed 10, St. Louis, 2013, Elsevier.)

the normal viewing mode of 30 cm (12 inches) is used, photoelectrons emitted from the entire surface of a convex shaped cesium iodide (CsI) phosphor (i.e., the input surface when the x-ray photons passing through the patient first strike the II assembly) are accelerated and converge on a focal point from which they subsequently spread out again and advance to the surface of a zinc-cadmium sulfide output phosphor as shown in Fig. 10.18.

If magnification in the fluoroscopic image is desired, the viewing mode can be changed to the smaller 25 cm mode (10 inches) or even less (e.g., 20 cm or 8 inches in many new systems). With this selection, the voltage on the electrostatic focusing lenses is increased, thereby

causing the focal point of the electrons to move closer to the input phosphor surface or a greater distance away from the output phosphor.[1] As a result, only photoelectrons from the central 25 cm, or 20 cm, diameter portion of the input phosphor, instead of its entire surface area, actually reach the output phosphor of the image intensifier. This added distance from the focal point localization of the photoelectrons to the output phosphor surface, however, *creates a larger image but with a decreased FOV* (Fig. 10.19).

In magnification mode, the quality of the enlarged image, *if there are no other changes*, as viewed on a monitor, is somewhat degraded. This reduction in image clarity occurs because of the decrease in *minification gain*

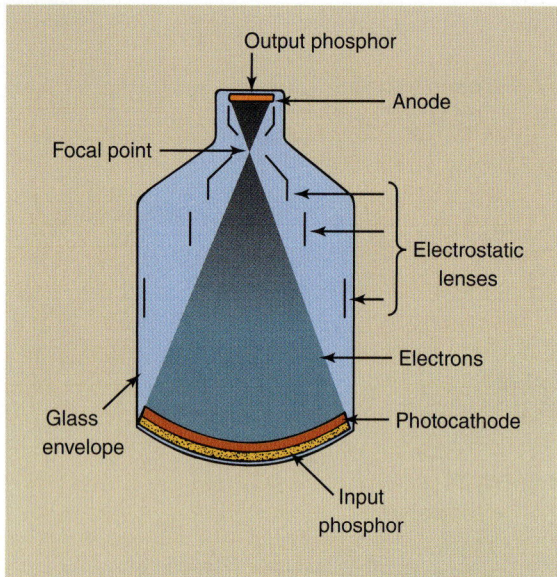

Fig. 10.18 Basic components of an image intensifier tube. (From Bushong SC: *Radiologic science for technologists: physics, biology and protection*, ed 10, St. Louis, 2013, Elsevier.)

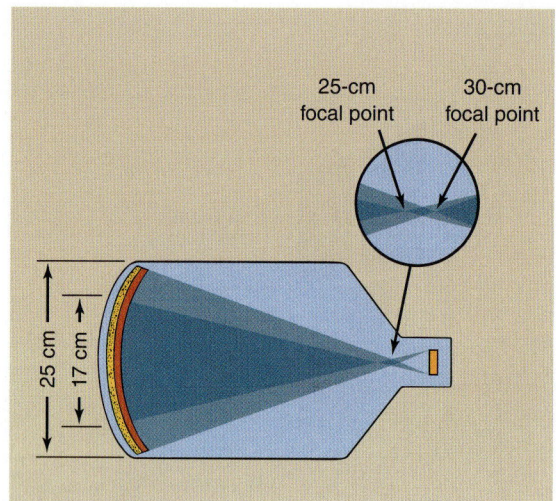

Fig. 10.19 A 30/25/20 image intensifier tube produces a magnified image in 25 cm mode, whereas the 20 cm mode produces an image that is even more highly magnified. (From Bushong SC: *Radiologic science for technologists: physics, biology and protection*, ed 10, St. Louis, 2013, Elsevier.)

BOX 10.4 Benefits of Image Intensification Fluoroscopy

- Increased image brightness
- Saving of time for the radiologist
- Patient dose reduction

(i.e., an increase in brightness) when fewer photoelectrons are available to strike the output phosphor on the image intensifier. Therefore the resultant image is dimmer. Because it is necessary and desirable to maintain a constant level of light intensity on the view monitor, fluoroscopic mA increases automatically to counter this illuminance loss. The overall quality of the image will now be enhanced relative to the larger-diameter modes because a greater number of x-ray photons are being used to form the magnified image. This image will have a more even appearance (less noise), and it will be possible to distinguish among similar tissues more readily because of improved contrast. However, the increase in tube mA necessarily raises the dose to the patient. Thus, magnification modes are only used when diagnostically needed.

An **image intensifier** can also be designed to *interactively* change the input FOV from a large to a smaller area. If the input FOV is halved, then the region of the patient being observed is also halved, which results in two-fold *magnification of the image.*

Pulsed Fluoroscopy. Pulsed, or intermittent, fluoroscopy involves manual or automatic periodic activation of the fluoroscope x-ray tube by the fluoroscopist, rather than continuous activation. This practice:

- Significantly decreases patient dose, especially in long procedures
- Helps extend the life of the tube

In pulsed mode the system software automatically turns the radiation beam on and off at an operator-selected repetition rate. The most common rates are 30, 15, and 7.5 pulses per second, with each radiation pulse lasting no more than 10 milliseconds. Shorter pulse durations lessen the effects of any patient motion thereby improving the sharpness of the image but decrease the signal-to-noise ratio because of the smaller number of x-rays involved. A 30 p/s rate would typically be used for imaging studies involving very rapid anatomic or process motion (e.g., interventional catheter procedures) to achieve acceptable temporal resolution.

Barium swallow studies, on the other hand, could make use of 7.5 p/s. Many systems include a *last image hold feature* that allows the fluoroscopist to momentarily halt the radiation and review the most recent image before giving the patient another pulse of radiation. Frequently utilizing the last image hold feature during long procedures will noticeably reduce patient absorbed dose.

Limiting Fluoroscopic Field Size. The radiologist must limit the size of the fluoroscopic field to include only the area of clinical interest. This involves visually moving the shutters placed between the x-ray tube and the patient to define the desired field of view. When fluoroscopic field size is limited, patient *integral dose* (i.e., volumetric dose) decreases substantially. For lengthy examinations, however, it is possible to spread out the patient entrance irradiation area and thereby minimize the possibility for skin effects while maintaining the same anatomic field of view. This spreading out is accomplished by moving or rotating the patient so that the radiation enters at multiple portions of the patient surface instead of just the same limited region during the procedure.

The selected primary beam length and width must always be confined within the image receptor boundary. Regardless of the distance from the x-ray source to the image receptor, the useful beam should not extend outside the image receptor. Ideally, visible borders ought to appear on the image monitor. If this is not so, a patient could receive a substantial radiation dose in certain procedures to sensitive areas adjacent to the study area. Thus, this conformity (alignment and congruence) between the x-ray field and the input phosphor of the II is an essential item of regulatory concern.

Radiation Delivery Factors

Selection of technique exposure factors for adult patients. During *manual* fluoroscopic procedures, the fluoroscopist must select technical exposure factors that will minimize patient dose. Increasing the kVp and filtration reduces the patient exposure and dose rate. Most fluoroscopic examinations employ a range of 75 to 110 kVp for adult patients, depending on the body area being examined. This kVp range produces the correct level of fluoroscopic image brightness. Lower kVp increases patient dose because a less penetrating x-ray beam necessitates the use of a higher milliamperage to obtain adequate image intensity. The operator can further limit excessive entrance irradiation of the patient by ensuring

that the x-ray **SSD** is not less than 38 cm (15 inches) for stationary (fixed) fluoroscopes and not less than 30 cm (12 inches) for mobile fluoroscopes (C-arms). A 30-cm (12-inch) minimal distance is required, but an increased distance to 38 cm (15 inches) is preferred for all current systems. In addition, positioning the II input phosphor surface as close as is practical to the patient will further reduce the patient's entrance exposure and dose rate.

Selection of technique factors for children. Quality radiation safety practices with fluoroscopic procedures for children necessitates *a decrease in kVp by as much as 25%.* The kVp chosen should depend on anatomic part thickness, just as it does in radiography. In addition to decreasing kVp, maintaining SSD and minimizing the height of the II entrance surface above the patient will further limit excessive entrance irradiation of the pediatric patient.

Filtration. The function of a filter in fluoroscopy, as in radiographic procedures, is to reduce the patient's skin absorbed dose from soft x-rays. Adequate layers of aluminum equivalent material placed within the collimator assembly in the path of the useful beam remove the more harmful lower-energy photons from the beam by absorbing them. A minimum of 2.5 mm total aluminum equivalent filtration must be permanently installed in the path of the useful beam of the fluoroscopic unit. With current systems, a total aluminum equivalent filtration of at least 3.0 mm or markedly higher is typical. Although increases in filtration cause a loss of fluoroscopic image brightness, using higher kVps can somewhat compensate. As in radiography, the minimum permanent filtration of the x-ray beam is federally mandated, and therefore the HVL of the beam must be measured to confirm agreement with regulatory standards. In *routine* fluoroscopy, an x-ray beam HVL of 3 to 4.5 mm aluminum is considered acceptable when kVp ranges from 80 to 100.

Cumulative Timing Device. A **cumulative timer** must be provided and used with each fluoroscopic unit. This resettable device measures the collective x-ray beam-on time and sounds an audible alarm or, in some cases, temporarily interrupts the radiation until it is reset after the fluoroscope has been activated for 5 minutes. It also serves to alert the fluoroscopist to the amount of time the patient has been receiving x-ray exposure. Activating the fluoroscope for shorter periods will not only cause the patient to receive less radiation exposure but also the fluoroscopist and the radiographer. Total fluoroscopic beam-on time should be documented for every fluoroscopic procedure.

Entrance Irradiation Rate Limitations. Current federal standards limit **entrance skin irradiation rates*** of general-purpose intensified fluoroscopic units with maximum technique factors engaged to a maximum of 88 mGya per minute entrance absorbed dose rate (or 10 R/min entrance exposure rate), as measured at the tabletop using an average phantom, with the II entrance surface at a prescribed 30 cm (12 inches) above the tabletop. This limit for conventional fluoroscopic systems has been imposed to provide protection against patients accidentally receiving skin-damaging entrance dose levels in short periods. Fluoroscopic units equipped with *high-level control (HLC)*, however, may produce a skin entrance dose rate as great as 176 mGya per minute (20 R/min entrance exposure rate). Because certain lengthy fluoroscopic procedures can result in the largest patient doses in *diagnostic x-ray* imaging, sometimes reaching the level of therapeutic doses with potential physical damage to the patient, a concerted effort must be made to keep fluoroscopic exposure rates and cumulative exposure times within established limits.

Primary Protective Barrier. A **primary protective barrier** (i.e., shielding in the direct line of the transmitted patient irradiation) of 2 mm lead equivalent is required by regulatory guidelines for a fluoroscopic unit. The II assembly or a digital detector is designed to provide this barrier to direct radiation. The assembly must be physically joined with the x-ray tube and interlocked so that the fluoroscopic x-ray tube cannot be activated when the II or other detection system is in a parked, unaligned, and unconnected position.

Fluoroscopic Exposure Control Switch. According to state and federal regulations, the fluoroscopic exposure control switch (e.g., the foot pedal) must be of the *dead-man type*, meaning that only continuous pressure applied by the operator can keep the switch activated and the fluoroscopic tube emitting x-radiation. This clearly implies that the exposure automatically terminates if the person operating the switch becomes incapacitated (e.g., has a medical emergency) or, for any reason, removes his or her foot from the pedal.

Mobile Fluoroscopic Systems

Radiation Safety Features of Mobile C-arm Fluoroscopy. A mobile C-arm fluoroscopic unit is a portable x-ray unit that has a C-shaped multiorientable gantry arm. An x-ray tube is attached to one end of its curved arm and an II attached to the other end. C-arm fluoroscopes (Fig. 10.20) are frequently used in the operating room for orthopedic procedures (e.g., pinning of

---

*One must be precise in the terminology used for entrance or tabletop fluoroscopy radiation levels, for example, there is the term, *entrance or tabletop exposure rate*, which has been and still is specified by regulatory agencies and medical physicists in R/min, and on the other hand there is the usage of mGy_a/min which is correctly described as *entrance or tabletop absorbed dose rate* and sometimes even as *exposure dose rate*. Fluoroscopic dose rate and exposure rate are not the same. There is a numerical conversion factor existing between them, called the rads (cGy) per roentgen factor "*f*," which is about 0.88. The f factor reflects the fact that not all incident or entrance x-ray photons interact with and deliver energy to surface tissue atoms. Thus, an *entrance exposure rate* of 10 R/min in reality corresponds to an *entrance absorbed dose rate* of about 8.8 cGy_a/min or 88 mGy_a/min.

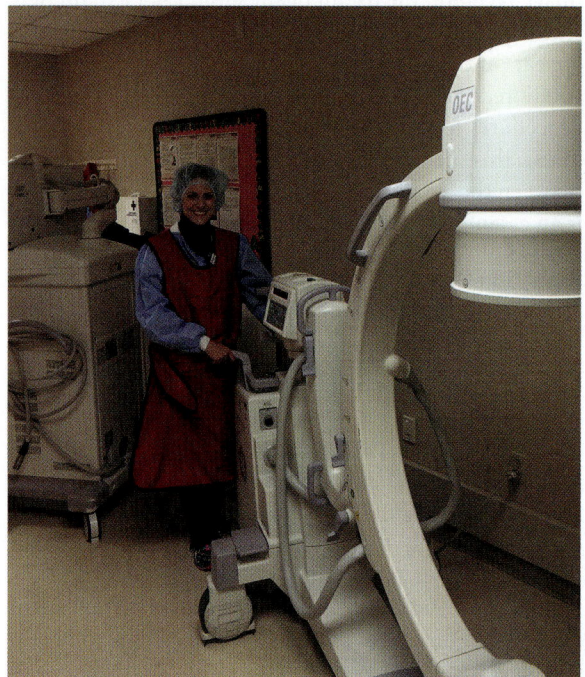

Fig. 10.20 C-arm fluoroscope and monitor.

a fractured hip). They are also employed quite commonly for:

- Cardiac imaging
- Interventional procedures

The use of C-arm fluoroscopy in interventional procedures carries the potential for a relatively large patient radiation dose. C-arm fluoroscope operators, if standing close to the patient, could also receive a significant increase in occupational exposure from patient scatter radiation during such cases. For these reasons, equipment operators, including attending physicians, must have appropriate education and training to ensure that they will be able to follow guidelines for safe C-arm operation and also meet radiation safety protocols essential to patient and personnel safety. A necessary component of this is the wearing of wrap-around lead aprons and thyroid shields by all involved personnel throughout each procedure.

Mobile fluoroscopic units are required to have a minimal source-to-end of collimator assembly distance of 30 cm (12 inches). Some type of spacer or collimator extension is customarily installed to prevent any part of the patient from coming closer than 30 cm (12 inches) to the tube target. During C-arm fluoroscopy procedures, the patient-II distance should be as short as possible (Fig. 10.21). This reduces patient entrance dose. For further dose-reduction purposes it is preferable to position the C-arm so that the x-ray tube is under the patient. With the x-ray tube in this position, scatter radiation is attenuated (Fig. 10.22) toward personnel above the knee level. However, when the x-ray tube is positioned over the patient, scatter radiation is not attenuated by the table, and therefore it is more intense, and radiation exposure of personnel increases correspondingly.

RADIATION SAFETY FEATURES OF DIGITAL FLUOROSCOPIC EQUIPMENT

Digital Fluoroscopy (DF)

Pulsed Progressive Systems. Various methods are used to obtain digital images in fluoroscopic equipment. The electrical signal from the video camera attached to the output phosphor may be digitized. In newer equipment, the analog TV camera may be replaced by a digital device such as a CCD camera or other digital detector. In whatever manner the digital image is acquired, the use of digital technology offers the possibility of several methods of dose reduction. One such method utilizes a brief high-intensity pulse of radiation to create an entire image on the output phosphor. The lines composing the image are progressively scanned (i.e., from left to right followed by right to left and so on, usually referred to as *raster scanning*, from top to bottom) to provide the image that appears on a monitor during a brief period (one-sixtieth of a second). The x-ray beam is deactivated while the image

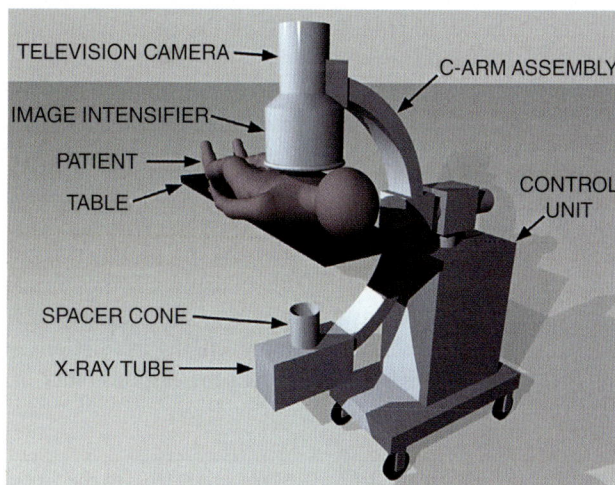

Fig. 10.21 To reduce the patient's entrance dose during C-arm fluoroscopy, the patient–image intensifier distance should be as short as possible. (Courtesy Mark Rzeszotarski.)

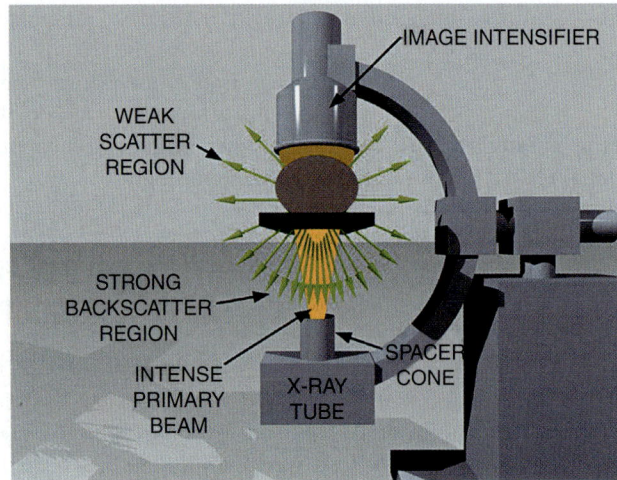

Fig. 10.22 To reduce scatter radiation during C-arm fluoroscopy, position the C-arm so that the x-ray tube is under the patient whenever possible. (Courtesy Mark Rzeszotarski.)

is being scanned, thereby decreasing patient dose, and then pulsed back on for the next image. These systems are known as **pulsed progressive systems** and are commonly used to lower patient dose.

Last Image Hold. Another dose-reduction technique that is particularly effective in DF systems is the *last image hold* feature. For this feature, the image formed when the x-ray tube was last energized remains on the monitor so that no further radiation exposure is needed to regenerate it. In a digital system, using embedded processing software, this retained image could also be composed of several frames of information that have been added together to reduce the effect of quantum or random noise that would be particularly apparent in a single frame.

Digital Subtraction Angiography (DSA) and Interventional Systems

Interventional Procedures. Digital techniques have had a major impact on interventional fluoroscopy. The goal in interventional procedures is to locate high-contrast, small objects such as catheters, stents,* or electrical leads for electronic implants. Not only are these devices in the

millimeter-size range, but they are also moved within the patient as part of the procedure to implant the devices or to inject liquids such as glues,** steroids, or anesthetics. Contrast material is sometimes injected to improve the visibility of the devices or the leading edge of catheters. The visualization of high-contrast, small objects with a digital imaging system requires that the pixel elements reveal very small regions of the patient. In addition, images must be updated at a reasonable rate to reveal the location of objects in the patient as the objects are moved. In the latest DF systems, the II has been replaced by a "flat-panel" detector that is similar to those used in DR. A flat-panel digital detector for fluoroscopy meets the same technical requirements as previously described (direct or indirect conversion of x-ray energy to stored electronic values) but is also capable of recording images rapidly, as many images or "frames" as are required per second to be perceived as motion and presented in a live digital video format. The advent of these techniques has allowed the performance of more complicated procedures that are sometimes associated with much longer exposure times for patients. Some of the data related to these lengthy irradiations are provided in Chapter 2. It is still the responsibility of the imaging team to make

---

*A stent is a tubular support that can be placed inside a blood vessel, canal, or duct to create a pathway or relieve an obstruction.

**Injection of glues or glue embolization is an interventional technique that uses a chemical called n-butyl cyanoacrylate, which is usually shortened to NBCA, to block problematic arteries.

sure that acceptable risk versus benefit principles are applied. While the radiation risk may be increased compared to other imaging techniques, the benefit of repair of life-threatening conditions must also be considered.

Digital Subtraction Angiography. One of the most significant advances in digital imaging in vascular and interventional fluoroscopy over the past 50 years has been **digital subtraction angiography (DSA)**. In vascular fluoroscopy, the objective is the visualization of blood vessels. This may be necessary to complete an interventional procedure, or it may be used to reveal vascular problems such as occlusion (blockage), stenosis (narrowing), or aneurysms (abnormal bulging). It usually includes the injection of contrast material to enhance vascular appearance. DSA implies the performance of arithmetic operations on the pixel values of digital images. Since the individual images or frames of the digital video are available as a matrix of signal (voltage) values that are stored in a computer, pairs of images may be *subtracted*. In image subtraction, the digital values recorded for each corresponding pixel of an image pair are subtracted from each other. This process produces a resultant image *that "only" consists of features that have changed between the initial two images.*

In DSA, a "mask" image (simply a reference image of the same area before the contrast is administered) is obtained prior to the injection of contrast material. Subsequent images may be subtracted from the initial mask so that the main difference between pairs of images (the movement of contrast material) is emphasized. Therefore the contrast material that lines the vessels of interest enhances the appearance of the vessels, revealing features such as narrowing, or stenosis. Interventional procedures may use this information to guide the insertion of stents to open occluded blood vessels. For complex interventional procedures, this increased vascular contrast allows visualization of small vessels surrounding arteriovenous malformations.* Additional clarity may be obtained by remasking (redefining the image from which subsequent images are subtracted) when catheters approach the malformation.

Roadmapping. In situations where the vasculature is complex or overlying structures provide a confusing background, the location of the catheter may be difficult to determine visually. More contrast material could be injected to improve visibility, but the image would still be cluttered, and there are limits to the amount of contrast material that can safely be injected into the patient so as to avoid potential kidney damage. A technique known as **roadmapping** is useful in this situation. If the patient is not moving and the FOV is not altered, a static image of the vasculature may be obtained through subtraction, pre- and postcontrast injection, as in standard DSA. This static image may be preserved as a lower-contrast "ghost" image or as a reversed-contrast lighter image. In either case, it serves the function of a stationary map over which the outline of the catheter can be shown as it advances to the position where it is needed. Fig. 10.23 illustrates a roadmap procedure used for a catheter approaching an aneurism.

RADIATION SAFETY FOR HIGH-LEVEL CONTROL INTERVENTIONAL PROCEDURES

Justification for Use of High-Level Control Interventional Procedures

As mentioned previously, interventional procedures are invasive actions performed by a physician with the aid of fluoroscopic imaging. The interventional physician, usually a radiologist or a cardiologist, inserts catheters into vessels or directly into patient tissues for the purpose of:

- Drainage
- Biopsy
- Alteration of vascular occlusions (obstructions) or malformations

For these procedures, **high-level control fluoroscopy (HLCF)** is often employed. HLCF is an operating mode for state-of-the-art fluoroscopic equipment in which entrance radiation levels are substantially higher than those normally employed in routine procedures. The higher entrance exposure rate or entrance dose rates allows the examination of smaller and lower-contrast objects that are not ordinarily discerned during standard fluoroscopy. HLCF therefore is used for those interventional procedures in which visualization of fine catheters or other not easily seen structures is crucial. An audible signal constantly reminds personnel that the HLC is engaged. *It is strongly recommended that pulsed mode and frequent last image hold be the standard methods of operation when HLCF is being used.*

---

*An abnormal tangle of blood vessels connecting arteries and veins, which disrupts normal blood flow and oxygen circulation.

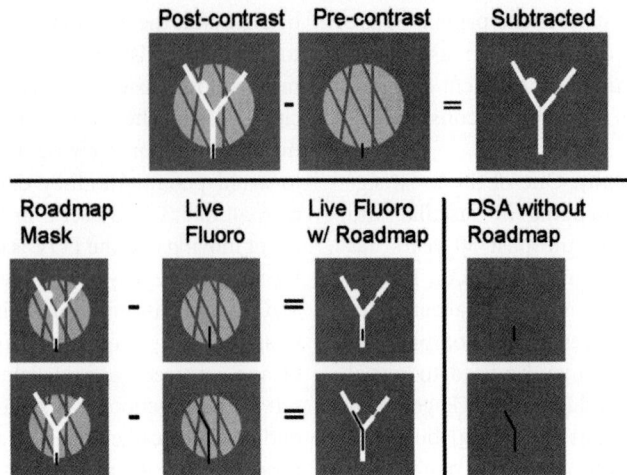

Fig. 10.23 Roadmapping: First, the digital subtraction angiography (DSA) of the vascular structure is performed. The postcontrast frame associated with maximum vessel opacification becomes the roadmap mask; subsequent digital fluoroscopic (*Fluoro*) images are subtracted from the roadmap mask. The result in live fluoroscopic images of the inserted catheter or wire overlaid on a static image of the vasculature (with distracting underlying tissue removed). (From Pooley RA, McKinney JM, Miller DA: The AAPM/RSNA physics tutorial for residents: digital fluoroscopy, *Radiographics* 21(2):521–534, 2001).

Public Health Advisory About the Dangers of Overexposure of Patients and Exposure Rate Limits

Many of the fluoroscopically guided therapeutic interventional procedures have the potential for substantial patient exposure. On September 30, 1974, the US Food and Drug Administration (FDA) issued a public health advisory to alert health care workers to the probability and dangers of overexposure of patients through the use of high-level fluoroscopy. The FDA x-ray equipment standards, *issued in 1994*, limited the *tabletop exposure rate* of fluoroscopic equipment for routine procedures to a maximum of 10 R/min unless an HLC was present, in which case routine fluoroscopy maximum tabletop exposure rates were set at 5 R/min when the system was not in HLC mode and *unlimited when it was in HCL mode.*[11] The authors of these 1994 standards believed that the unrestricted high-level capability was necessary for certain vital situations involving therapeutic interventional procedures in which the potential risks to the patient of much increased radiation exposure would be subordinate to a successful medical outcome of an intervention. As a safeguard, however, HCL was required to have *manual continuous positive pressure on a special high-level foot pedal*, accompanied by a steady audible signal to remind personnel that the high-level fluoroscopic mode was in

use. In this operational mode, patient entrance exposure rates have been estimated to range from 20 to 120 R/min (176 to 1056 mGya/min entrance or skin dose rates). When the rule was issued, total patient irradiation was limited by the heat-loading capabilities of the x-ray tube. Amazingly, the thinking or belief at that time was that the tube would reach its heat limit before any detectable patient early tissue reactions could occur. By the early 1990s, however, advances in x-ray tube heat dissipation technology and the increased frequency of vascular interventional procedures that require long fluoroscopic times (Box 10.5) had created a situation in which very serious skin reactions had been reported in some patients. Radiogenic skin injuries such as *erythema* (diffuse reddening) and *desquamation* (sloughing off of skin cells) are early tissue reactions in which the severity of the disorder increases with radiation dose. As the data in Table 10.2 demonstrate, a half-hour of total high-level beam-on time at one location on a patient's skin is sufficient to produce erythema. In this case, the skin injury does not usually appear for approximately 10 days. Because manifestations of skin injury are delayed, a radiologist would not typically be the first person to observe the onset of the symptoms. Therefore patient monitoring, radiation dosimetry, and accurate record-keeping are essential for the future medical management of adverse reactions. The FDA has

BOX 10.5   Procedures Involving Extended Fluoroscopic Time

- Percutaneous transluminal angioplasty
- Radiofrequency cardiac catheter ablation
- Vascular embolization
- Stent and filter placement
- Thrombolytic and fibrinolytic procedures
- Percutaneous transhepatic cholangiography
- Endoscopic retrograde cholangiopancreatography
- Transjugular intrahepatic portosystemic shunt
- Percutaneous nephrostomy
- Biliary drainage
- Urinary or biliary stone removal

From the US Food and Drug Administration (FDA): *Public health advisory: avoidance of serious x-ray-induced skin injuries to patients during fluoroscopically guided procedures*, Rockville, MD, 1994, FDA.

recommended that a notation be placed in the patient's record if a skin dose in the range of 1 to 2 Gyt is received. The location of the area of the patient's skin that received the absorbed dose should also be noted using:

- A diagram
- Annotated photograph
- Narrative description

Since 2000, however, alarmed state regulatory agencies have imposed a restriction on high-level radiation

entrance rates. With the II at a distance of 30 cm ($\approx$ 12 inches) above the tabletop, the maximum *continuous* fluoroscopic entrance exposure rate permitted is 20 R/min (176 mGya/min entrance dose rate). This is not true, though, for pulsed mode for which the instantaneous exposure rates values can be very much higher.

Use of Fluoroscopic Equipment by Nonradiologist Physicians.
Fluoroscopic devices are capable of subjecting the patient, the physician, and other personnel close to the fluoroscopic equipment to substantial amounts of direct and/or indirect ionizing radiation. These devices include:

- C-arm fluoroscopes
- Fluoroscopes on stationary equipment with HCL mode used for interventional procedures
- Biplane (dual x-ray tubes) interventional fluoroscopic systems*

Ongoing education and training in the safe use of fluoroscopic equipment should be mandatory for nonradiologist physicians and equipment operators. Many institutions have therefore established through their

---

*Biplane x-ray fluoroscopy systems consist of a double c-arm independent configuration with each c-arm having its own x-ray source and corresponding detector panel. The two c-arms are in the mechanical arrangement that allows them to generate multiple oblique dual-angle projections.

TABLE 10.2   Radiation-Induced Skin Injuries

Effect	Typical Threshold Absorbed Dose (Gyt)[†]	HOURS OF FLUOROSCOPIC "ON TIME" TO REACH THRESHOLD*		Time to Onset of Effect[‡]
		Usual Fluoroscopic Dose Rate of 0.02 Gya/min	High-Level Dose Rate of 0.2 Gya/min	
Early transient erythema	2	1.7	0.17	Hours
Temporary epilation	3	2.5	0.25	3 weeks
Main erythema	6	5.0	0.50	10 days
Permanent epilation	7	5.8	0.58	3 weeks
Dry desquamation	10	8.3	0.83	4 weeks
Dermal atrophy	11	9.2	0.92	0.14 weeks
Telangiectasias	12	10.0	1.00	0.52 weeks
Moist desquamation	15	12.5	1.25	4 weeks
Late erythema	15	12.5	1.25	6–10 weeks
Dermal necrosis	18	15.0	1.50	0.10 weeks
Secondary ulceration	20	16.7	1.67	0.6 weeks

*Time required to deliver the typical threshold dose at the specified dose rate.
[†]The unit for absorbed dose is the gray (Gyt) in the International System of Units.
[‡]Time after single irradiation to observation of effect.
Modified from Wagner LK, Eifel PJ, Geise RA: Potential biological effects following high x-ray dose interventional procedures, *J Vasc Interv Radiol* 5:71, 1994.

RSOs radiation safety accreditation programs that must be taken and passed before nonradiologist physicians are permitted to use such devices.

Some of the causes of elevated radiation exposures to personnel during interventional procedures include:

- Operation of the fluoroscopic tube for long periods in continuous mode in place of pulsed mode
- Failure to use the protective curtain or floating shields on the stationary fluoroscopic equipment's II as a means of protection

Monitoring and documenting procedural fluoroscopic time are essential. The responsibility for this documentation has generally belonged to the radiographer assisting with the procedure. With newer systems, the computer software automatically produces a record of both accumulated continuous and pulsed radiation time, as well as estimates of delivered dose and dose area product. In addition, if a physician loses track of how long a procedure is taking and how much radiation is being delivered to a localized area of the patient's body, it becomes the radiographer's ethical responsibility to call this to the physician's attention in the interest of the safety of all concerned. In the event of a critical situation in which there is markedly excessive fluoroscopic irradiation time, the radiographer is responsible for notifying an appropriate supervisor, who should then implement the imaging facility's relevant established protocol.

The National Cancer Institute and the Society of Interventional Radiology have conjointly designed guidelines to assist physicians in developing strategies that will enable them to fulfill their interventional clinical objectives while controlling patient radiation dose and minimizing exposure to occupationally exposed personnel. These strategies are listed in Box 10.6.

BOX 10.6   Strategies to Manage Radiation Dose to Patients, Operators, and Staff During Interventional Fluoroscopy

Immediate	Long-Term
Optimize Dose to Patient	
Use proper radiologic technique:	Include medical physicist in decisions:
• Maximize distance between x-ray tube and patient	• Machine selection and maintenance
• Minimize distance between patient and image receptor	Incorporate dose-reduction technologies and dose-measurement devices in equipment
• Limit use of electronic magnification	Establish a facility quality improvement program that includes an appropriate x-ray equipment quality assurance program, overseen by a medical physicist, which includes equipment evaluation/inspection at appropriate intervals
Control fluoroscopic time:	
• Limit use to necessary evaluation of moving structures	
• Employ last image hold function to review findings	
Control images:	
• Limit acquisition to essential diagnostic and documentation purposes	
Reduce dose:	
• Reduce field size (collimate) and minimize field overlap	
• Use pulsed fluoroscopy and low frame rate	
Minimize Dose to Operators and Staff	
Keep hands out of the beam	Improve ergonomics of operations and staff:
Use movable shields	• Train operators and staff in ergonomically good positioning for use of fluoroscopy equipment; periodically assess their practice
Maintain awareness of body position relative to the x-ray beam:	
• Horizontal x-ray beam: operator and staff should stand on the side of the image receptor	• Identify and provide the ergonomically best personal protective gear for operators and staff
• Vertical x-ray beam: the image receptor should be above the table	• Urge manufacturers to develop ergonomically improved personal protective gear
Wear adequate protection:	• Recommend research to improve ergonomics for personal protective gear
• Protective, well-fitted lead apron	
• Leaded glasses	

From the National Cancer Institute, Division of Cancer Epidemiology and Genetics, Radiation Epidemiology: *Branch: interventional fluoroscopy: reducing radiation risks for patients and staff*, NIH Publication No. 05-5286, Rockville, MD, 2005, National Institutes of Health.

SUMMARY

- A diagnostic-type tube housing protects the patient and imaging personnel from off-focus, or leakage, radiation by restricting the emission of the x-rays to the area of the useful, or primary, beam.
- Leakage radiation from the tube housing measured at 1 m from the x-ray source must not exceed 0.88 mGya/h (100 mR/h) when the tube is operated at its highest kilovoltage at the highest current (mA) that allows continuous operation.
- The control panel, or console, must be located behind a suitable protective barrier that has a radiation-absorbent window that permits satisfactory observation of the patient during any procedure. This panel must indicate the conditions of exposure and provide indication when the x-ray tube is energized.[1]
- The radiographic examination tabletop must be of uniform thickness, and for under-table tubes as used in fluoroscopy, the patient support surface also should be as radiolucent as possible, which will lead to reducing the patient's radiation dose.
- Radiographic equipment must have an source-to-image receptor distance (SID) indicator.
- X-ray beam limitation devices must be used to confine the useful beam before it enters the anatomic area of clinical interest.
- The patient's skin surface should always be at least 15 cm below the collimator to minimize exposure to the epidermis.
- Good coincidence between the x-ray beam and the light-localizing beam of the collimator is necessary; both alignment and length and width dimensions of the two beams must correspond to within 2% of the SID.
- Exposure to the patient's skin may be reduced through proper filtration of the radiographic beam.
- Compensating filters are used in radiography to provide uniform imaging of body parts when considerable variation in thickness or tissue composition exists.
- Diagnostic x-ray units must have consistent exposure reproducibility, that is, the ability to duplicate specific radiographic exposures for any given combination of kVp, mA, and time.
- Exposure linearity is essential. When a change is made from one mA station to a neighboring mA station, the most that linearity can vary is 10%.

- Radiographic grids increase patient dose in radiography. Their use for the examination of thicker body parts is a fair compromise because they remove scattered radiation emanating from the patient that would otherwise degrade the completed image.
- Because of increased sensitivity of photostimulable phosphor to scatter radiation before and after exposure to a radiographic beam, a grid may be used more frequently during computed radiography (CR) imaging. The use of a grid does increase patient dose but significantly improves radiographic contrast and visibility of detail.
- To limit the effects of inverse fall-off of radiation intensity with distance during a mobile radiographic examination, an x-ray source-skin distance (SSD) of at least 30 cm (12 inches) must be used.
- With digital radiography, the image receptor is divided into small detector elements that make up the two-dimensional picture elements, or pixels, of the image.
- Radiographers must always strive to select correct technical exposure factors from the beginning to avoid overexposing patients when digital images are obtained.
- The digital image ultimately acquired in both CR and digital radiography (DR) can be displayed on a monitor for viewing and evaluation and can also be printed if a hard copy is desired.
- Fluoroscopic procedures produce the largest patient radiation rates levels in diagnostic radiology. Therefore multiple safety guidelines should always be adhered to.
- During C-arm fluoroscopic procedures, the patient-image intensifier distance should be as short as possible.
- During digital fluoroscopy, the use of pulsed progressive systems with last image hold and roadmapping will significantly lower patient dose.
- High-level control fluoroscopy (HLCF) is often engaged in interventional procedures and produces entrance radiation rate levels that are substantially higher than those allowed for routine fluoroscopic procedures.
- If skin dose is received in the range of 1 to 2 Gyt, the Food and Drug Administration (FDA) requires that a notation be placed in the patient's record.

GENERAL DISCUSSION QUESTIONS

1. What are the requirements and purposes of a diagnostic-type protective tube housing in radiographic equipment?
2. How does the light-localizing variable-aperture rectangular collimator function as an x-ray beam limitation device?
3. Why is the luminance of the collimator light source important, and what is the function of the positive beam limitation (PBL) feature?
4. What is the function of x-ray beam filtration, and what are two types of filtration used in diagnostic radiology?
5. What is a compensating filter in radiography, and can you list two types?
6. What is meant by exposure reproducibility and exposure linearity in radiography?
7. What is automatic exposure control (AEC), and what are its radiation safety benefits?
8. How do radiographic grids increase patient dose?
9. What is the minimum source-skin distance (SSD) required for mobile radiography, and why is this requirement important?
10. What precautions must be taken to prevent overexposure in digital imaging procedures?

REVIEW QUESTIONS

1. What is the primary purpose of diagnostic-type protective tube housing?
   A. To improve image quality
   B. To shield against leakage radiation
   C. To enhance patient comfort
   D. To increase x-ray production
2. How does a light-localizing variable-aperture rectangular collimator function?
   A. It focuses the x-ray beam on the patient.
   B. It limits the size of the x-ray beam to the area of interest.
   C. It increases the intensity of the x-ray beam.
   D. It reduces the exposure time during imaging.
3. What is the significance of the luminance of the collimator light source?
   A. It determines the radiation dose.
   B. It affects the visibility of the light beam for alignment.
   C. It impacts the overall weight of the collimator.
   D. It enhances the x-ray beam quality.
4. Which type of filtration is commonly used to filter the x-ray beam in diagnostic radiology?
   A. Lead filtration
   B. Glass filtration
   C. Aluminum filtration
   D. Plastic filtration
5. What is the function of a compensating filter in radiography?
   A. To increase the radiation dose
   B. To even out the radiation dose across the image receptor
   C. To reduce the exposure time
   D. To enhance the quality of x-ray images

6. What does automatic exposure control (AEC) do in radiographic imaging?
   A. Automatically adjusts the tube voltage
   B. Maintains consistent image brightness by adjusting exposure time
   C. Limits the patient dose to zero
   D. Increases the exposure time for low-density areas
7. How do radiographic grids affect patient dose?
   A. They decrease the patient dose significantly.
   B. They have no effect on patient dose.
   C. They increase the required radiation dose to achieve quality images.
   D. They eliminate the need for exposure adjustments.
8. What is the minimum source-skin distance (SSD) for mobile radiography?
   A. 6 inches (15 cm)
   B. 12 inches (30 cm)
   C. 18 inches (45 cm)
   D. 24 inches (60 cm)
9. What is a critical consideration when performing digital radiography?
   A. Ensuring the x-ray tube is always vertical
   B. Monitoring exposure to avoid overexposure
   C. Using higher kVp settings at all times
   D. Reducing the number of images taken
10. What role do radiographers play during interventional procedures performed by nonradiologist physicians?
   A. They are responsible for diagnosing patient conditions.
   B. They assist with patient positioning only.
   C. They ensure radiation safety and monitor exposure levels.
   D. They manage the financial aspects of the procedure.

Management of Patient Radiation Dose

OBJECTIVES

After completing this chapter, the reader will be able to perform the following:

- Define all key terms.
- Explain the meaning of a holistic approach to patient care and recognize the need for effective communication between imaging department personnel and the patient.
- Discuss how to minimize or eliminate voluntary motion and how involuntary motion can be compensated for during a diagnostic radiographic procedure.
- Discuss shielding concepts and identify anatomic areas of the body that should be protected with specific area shielding.
- Explain current patient gonadal shielding and fetal shielding practices in diagnostic radiology and discuss the rationale for such practices with modern digital x-ray equipment.
- Discuss the need to use appropriate radiographic technical exposure factors for all radiologic procedures and show how these factors may be adjusted to reduce patient dose.
- Explain how a radiographer can achieve a balance in radiographic exposure factors to ensure the presence of adequate information in the completed image while minimizing patient dose.
- Clarify how adequate immobilization and correct image postprocessing techniques reduce radiographic exposure for the patient.
- Compare the use of an air gap technique for specific examinations with the use of a mid-ratio grid (8:1).
- Describe the benefits of repeat analysis programs.
- List six nonessential radiologic examinations and explain why each is considered unnecessary.
- List four ways to indicate the amount of radiation received by a patient from diagnostic imaging procedures and provide details for each.
- Discuss the concept of fluoroscopically guided positioning and clarify why this is an unacceptable practice.
- Define the term *genetically significant dose (GSD)*.
- Describe special precautions employed in radiography to protect the pregnant or potentially pregnant patient during an x-ray examination.
- Discuss the protocol to be followed when irradiation of an unknown pregnancy occurs and explain how the absorbed dose to the patient's embryo-fetus is determined.
- Explain the reason children require special radiation protection when they undergo conventional diagnostic imaging procedures.
- Pledge to Image Gently and Image Wisely.
- Explain the use of Dual Energy X-Ray Absorptiometry (DEXA, or DXA scan) for determining bone loss by measuring bone mineral density (BMD) and compare the radiation exposure of the patient and radiographer with that of conventional x-ray imaging and computed tomography.

CHAPTER OUTLINE

Effective Communication
  Verbal Messages and Body Language
  Importance of Patient Instructions
  Appropriate Communication for Procedures That
    Will Cause Pain or Discomfort

Repeat Radiographic Exposures Resulting from
  Poor Communication
Immobilization
  Need for Patient Immobilization
  Types of Patient Motion

KEY TERMS

air gap technique
Alliance for Radiation Safety in
   Pediatric Imaging
bone marrow dose
dual-energy x-ray absorptiometry
   (DEXA, or DXA scan)
effective communication

entrance skin exposure (ESE)
fluoroscopically guided
   positioning (FGP)
genetically significant dose (GSD)
gonadal dose
Image Gently Campaign
Image Wisely Campaign

repeat image
scattered radiation
skin dose
thermoluminescent dosimeters
   (TLDs)

During a diagnostic x-ray procedure, a holistic approach to patient care is essential. A holistic approach means considering for treatment the whole person rather than just the area of interest. Holistic patient care begins with effective communication between the radiographer and the patient. **Effective communication** is "an interaction that produces a satisfying result through an exchange of

information"[1] and can be accomplished through verbal messages, body language, and clear and concise instructions. This type of dialog alleviates the patient's uneasiness and increases the likelihood of full cooperation and successful completion of the procedure. To provide appropriate care for all patients, the radiographer should develop easily understandable communication skills.

Radiographers must limit the patient's exposure to ionizing radiation by:

- Employing appropriate radiation reduction techniques
- Using protective devices, accurate positioning of the body or body part, and techniques that minimize radiation exposure

Patient exposure can be substantially reduced by:

- Use of proper body or body part immobilization and other motion reduction techniques
- Proper x-ray beam limitation devices
- Adequate filtration of the x-ray beam
- Use of specific area shielding
- Selection of suitable technical exposure factors used in conjunction with computer-generated digital images
- Use of appropriate digital image processing
- Elimination of repeat radiographic exposures

This chapter provides an expansive overview of methods and techniques that radiographers can use to minimize the patient's exposure to radiation during radiologic examinations.

EFFECTIVE COMMUNICATION

Verbal Messages and Body Language

When verbal messages and gentle body language, or nonverbal messages, are understood as intended, communication between the radiographer and the patient is effective. Good communication:

- Encourages reduction in anxiety and emotional stress
- Enhances the professional image of the radiographer as a person who cares about the patient's well-being
- Increases the chance for successful completion of the x-ray examination, thereby reducing the potential of repeat exposures resulting from poor communication

Everyone within the imaging department should always behave as a compassionate professional. Words and actions must demonstrate understanding and respect for human dignity and individuality.

Importance of Patient Instructions

Each encounter with a patient during a diagnostic x-ray procedure should begin with clear and concise instructions (Fig. 11.1). When health care professionals do not thoroughly explain procedures, patients fear the unknown and become anxious, especially during lengthy examinations. To alleviate the problem, the radiographer must take adequate time to explain the procedure in simple terms that the patient can understand. Patients

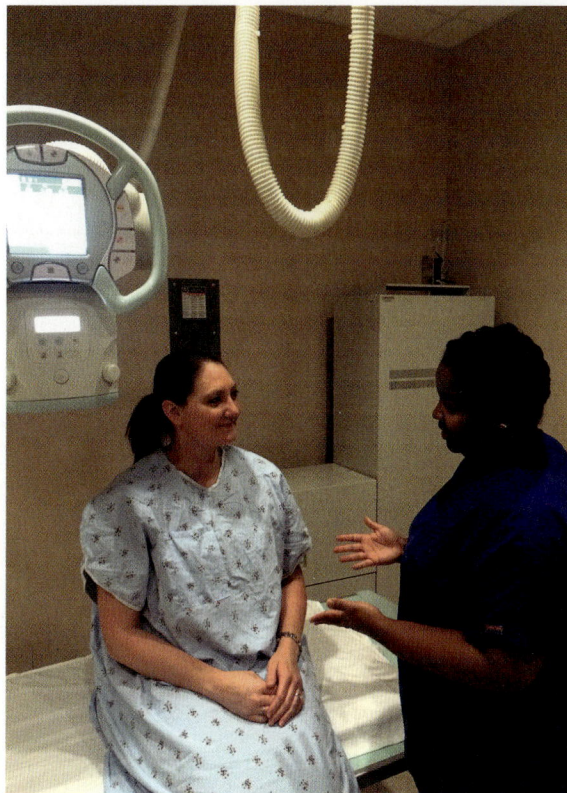

Fig. 11.1 Clear, concise instructions promote effective communication between the radiographer and the patient.

should also be given the opportunity to ask questions. The radiographer must listen attentively to these questions and answer them truthfully in an appropriate tone of voice and in accordance with ethical guidelines. This creates a sense of trust between the patient and the radiographer and encourages any further discourse.

Appropriate Communication for Procedures That Will Cause Pain or Discomfort

If the radiographic procedure will cause pain, discomfort, or any strange sensations, the patient must be fully informed before the procedure begins (Fig. 11.2). However, to prevent the patient from imagining more pain or discomfort than the procedure will cause, the radiographer should try not to overemphasize this aspect of the examination.

Repeat Radiographic Exposures Resulting from Poor Communication

Repeat radiographic exposures can sometimes be attributed to poor communication between the

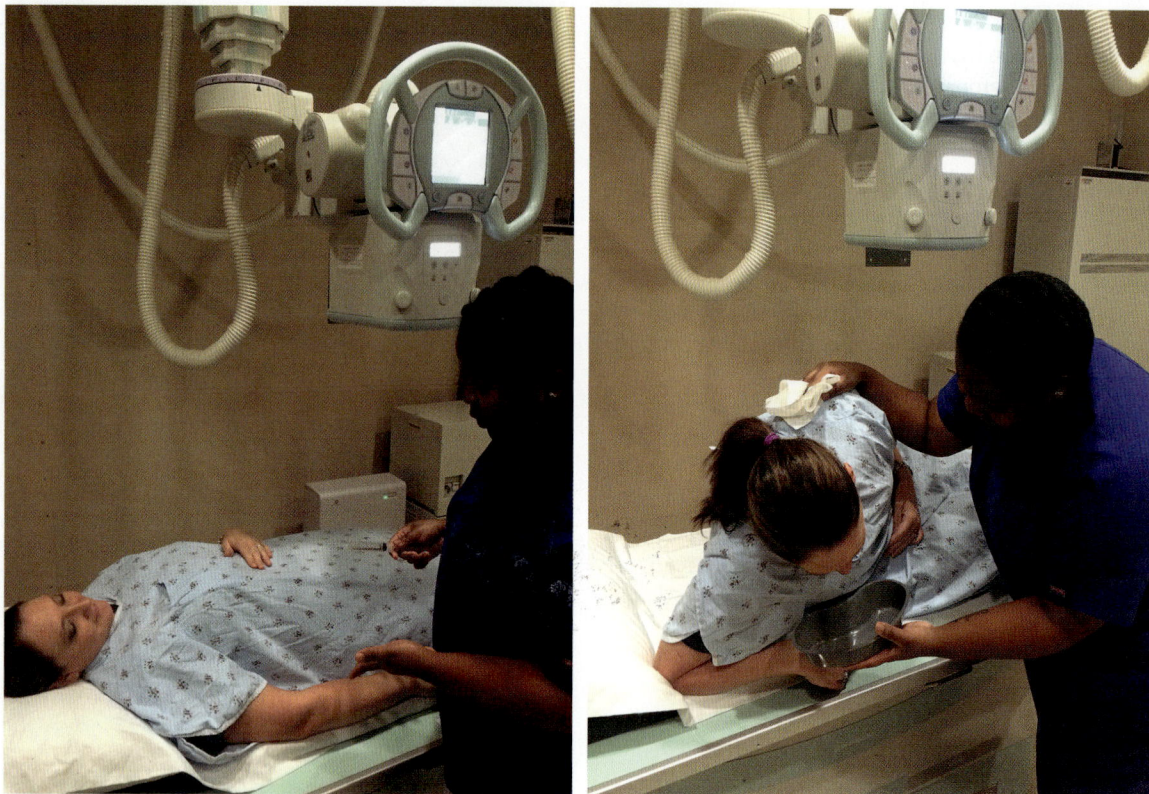

Fig. 11.2 Before the procedure begins, inform the patient of any pain, discomfort, or strange sensations that they might experience during the procedure.

radiographer and the patient. Inadequate or misinterpreted instructions may prevent the patient from being able to cooperate as needed. For example, during an interventional radiographic examination that creates some uncomfortable warmth, patients could move suddenly because they are surprised or want to inform the technologist or physician that something seems to be wrong. Such physical movement usually results in a repeat period of exposure. Effective communication between the radiographer and patient can prevent this problem from occurring.

IMMOBILIZATION

Need for Patient Immobilization

If a patient moves during a radiographic exposure, the radiographic image will be blurred. Because blurred images have little or no diagnostic value, a repeat examination is necessary, even though it results in additional radiation exposure for the patient. Proper body or body part immobilization and the use of motion reduction techniques can eliminate or at least minimize any patient motion.

Types of Patient Motion

Patient motion may be classified as:
- Voluntary
- Involuntary

Voluntary motion would, under normal circumstances, be expected to be controlled by the patient. Inability to exercise such control may be attributed to:
- The patient's advanced age
- Breathing problems or irregularities
- Increased anxiety
- Physical discomfort
- Fear of the examination
- Fear of unfavorable prognosis
- Mental instability

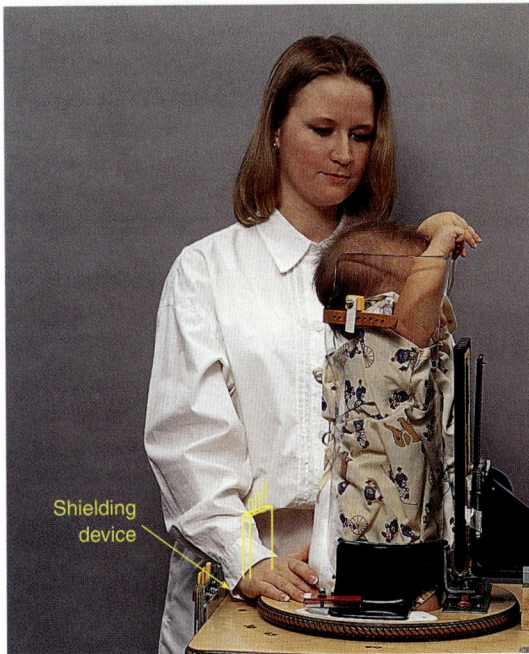

Fig. 11.3 Adequate immobilization during radiographic examinations eliminates or at least minimizes voluntary motion. This restraint has a shield *(left)* that may be adjusted to protect the child's reproductive organs from radiation exposure when that area of the body is not of clinical interest.

To eliminate voluntary motion during radiography, the radiographer must gain the cooperation of the patient or adequately immobilize that individual during the radiographic exposure (Fig. 11.3). Various suitable restraining devices are available to immobilize the whole body or the individual body part to be imaged. These aids should be used whenever necessary. *Involuntary motion*, caused by muscle groups such as those associated with the digestive organs or the heart, cannot be willfully controlled. Other clinical manifestations also cause involuntary motion. These include:

- Chills
- Tremors such as those experienced by patients with Parkinson's disease
- Muscle spasms
- Pain
- Active withdrawal

Decreasing the exposure time with an appropriate increase in milliamperes (mA) to maintain sufficient milliampere-seconds (mAs) for useful radiographic brightness (the amount of luminance of an image on a display monitor) and using very-high-speed imaging receptors can, to a high degree, compensate for involuntary motion.

PROTECTIVE SHIELDING

Need for Protective Shielding

The potential for radiation exposure to the radiosensitive body organs and tissues of a patient requires the use of precise patient positioning and, in many cases, personal shielding (i.e., a device made of lead or lead-impregnated materials that will adequately attenuate ionizing radiation) to reduce or eliminate a radiation dose that could otherwise result in biologic damage. Areas of the body that should be shielded from the useful beam whenever possible are the:

- Lens of the eye
- Breasts
- Thyroid gland

Gonadal Shielding

After some decades of experience with modern digital x-ray equipment and as a result of improvements in dosimetry estimates of the efficacy of shielding with modern equipment and techniques, professional and scientific societies are modifying shielding practices in diagnostic radiology.

In April of 2019, the American Association of Physicists in Medicine (AAPM) issued a position statement regarding the use of patient gonadal shielding and fetal shielding (Policy PP32-A). The statement indicated that patient gonadal shielding and fetal shielding during diagnostic imaging procedures should be discontinued as routine practice (AAPM, 2019). The statement is based on research indicating that patient shielding may jeopardize the benefits of the radiologic examination. Specifically, when a lead shield is placed incorrectly within the collimated x-ray beam and automatic exposure control is used, the lead shield may obscure anatomic information or interfere with the automatic exposure control system. Furthermore, these effects may compromise the diagnostic efficacy of the examination or increase the patient's radiation dose because of the attenuation characteristics of the shield. Because of these risks and the statistically seen minimal to nonexistent benefit associated with fetal and gonadal shielding, AAPM now recommends that the use of shielding should be discontinued.[2] Since the AAPM statement,

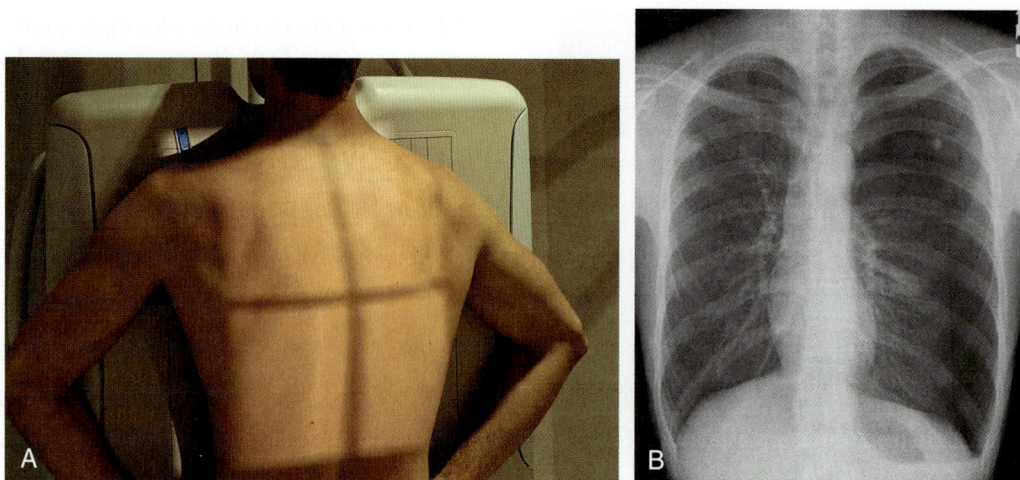

Fig. 11.4 (A) Adequate and precise collimation of the radiographic beam must always be the first step in gonadal protection. (B) When the gonads are not in the area of clinical interest, precise collimation of the radiographic beam reduces gonadal exposure. (From Lampignano J, Kendrick LE: *Bontrager's textbook of radiographic positioning and related anatomy*, ed 10, St. Louis, 2021, Elsevier.)

many organizations have supported the position statement, including thre NCRP, ACR, ASRT, and ARRT.

Adequate collimation of the radiographic beam, to include only the anatomy of interest (Fig. 11.4), must always be the first step in gonadal protection.

CARES Committee. Subsequent to ther publication of their AAPM position statement, and as a response to radiologic technologists' and radiologic science educators, the AAPM has formed the CARES (Communicating Advances in Radiation Education for Shielding) Committee. This group includes members from more than 14 professional organizations worldwide, representing medical and health physicists, radiologic technologists, and organizations that oversee educational programs for radiologic technologists, radiologists, and state regulators. CARES' purpose is for all stakeholders to educate the profession regarding the AAPM gonadal shielding position statement. It is of the utmost importance that the shield is not to any degree located within the collimated area of exposure because if AEC is used, it will not allow the exposure to terminate because it attempts to penetrate the lead shield.

Specific Area Shielding

Radiosensitive organs and tissues may be selectively guarded against the primary beam during a diagnostic radiographic examination. Shields for the lens of the eye are the contact type and are positioned directly on the patient.[3] They can reduce or eliminate exposure to that highly sensitive area.

TECHNICAL EXPOSURE FACTORS
Appropriate Selection

The selection of *scientifically correct* technical exposure factors for each x-ray examination is essential to ensure a useful diagnostic image with minimal patient dose. A high-quality image has sufficient brightness to display anatomic structures, an appropriate level of subject contrast to differentiate among such structures, the maximum amount of spatial resolution,* and a minimal amount of distortion. Limiting the amount of quantum noise, or mottle,** caused when too few x-rays reach the image receptor, is a concern.[4] The appropriate technical factors are determined by considerations such as those listed in Box 11.1.

---

*Spatial resolution is the recorded detail in the radiographic image.

**Quantum noise, or mottle, is a blotchy radiographic image that results when an insufficient quantity of x-ray photons reaches the image receptor.

BOX 11.1   Technical Exposure Factor Considerations

- Mass per unit volume of tissue of the area of clinical interest
- Effective atomic numbers and electron densities of the tissues involved
- Type of image receptor
- Source-to-image receptor distance (SID)
- Type and quantity of filtration employed
- Type of x-ray generator used
- Balance of radiographic brightness required

Use of Standardized Technique Charts

When a properly calibrated AEC system is not employed to obtain a uniform selection of x-ray exposure factors, well-managed imaging departments make use of standardized technique charts that have been established for each x-ray unit. As was discussed in the previous chapter, a digital image receptor is capable of responding to a large variation in x-ray exposures, after which a modern computer processing system can produce acceptable images, even when significant overexposure has occurred. This raises an important radiation safety issue in that unnecessarily high radiation exposure levels could result in medical images of acceptable image quality such that patient overexposure may not be noticed. Because of this, the standardization of technique charts has become even more critical. Radiology departments cannot rely on vendors and other agencies to set technical standards. Establishing and validating protocols with the aid of their quality assurance team helps radiology departments ensure consistency in the diagnostic quality of their digital examinations and minimizes the potential for exposure technique selection errors.[4]

The radiographer is responsible for consulting an available standardized technique chart before making each radiographic exposure to ensure an acceptable diagnostic image is acquired using exposure factors that yield minimal patient dose. Neglecting to use such technique charts necessitates estimating the technical exposure factors, which may result in:

- Poor-quality images
- Repeat examinations
- Additional and unnecessary exposure to the patient

Systematizing exposure techniques, however, does not mean that radiographers use the same protocol for all patients in all situations. Exposure techniques must be adjusted for patients' specific conditions and history. Proper and consistent use, however, of applicable exposure technique charts, adequate peak kilovoltage (kVp), and a well-calibrated AEC are all essential to producing quality diagnostic images consistently while minimizing patient radiation exposure.[4]

Use of High-kVp and Low-mAs Exposure Factors to Reduce Dose to the Patient

Technique factors that minimize the radiation dose to the patient should be selected whenever possible. The use of higher kVp permits lower mAs settings, which reduces patient entrance dose (Fig. 11.5A, B). In digital imaging, the amount of exposure (related to the mAs setting) reaching the digital image does not directly affect the amount of brightness produced, because of computer processing. Adequate penetration of the anatomic part, which is kVp dependent, is needed to create the differences in x-ray intensities exiting the part relative to adjacent structures to produce the desired level of contrast. As long as the part is adequately penetrated, increasing kVp by 15% with a corresponding decrease in mAs reduces patient exposure significantly while yielding satisfactory image quality. The radiographer must always seek to achieve a balance in technical radiographic exposure factors to:

- Ensure the presence of adequate information in the acquired image
- Minimize patient dose (see Fig. 11.5C)

POSTPROCESSING OF THE RADIOGRAPHIC IMAGE

When digital images are acquired, correct image postprocessing is essential to produce a high-quality diagnostic image. For this, any artifacts produced by the image receptor, software, or patient-related problems must be controlled. Artifacts are unwanted densities in the image that are not part of the patient's anatomy and may negatively affect the ability of a radiologist to interpret the image correctly. Failure to eliminate these defects, or at least to reduce them significantly, can result in an unacceptable digital image and can, therefore, necessitate a repeat examination, thus increasing patient dose.

High kVp, low mAs

Low kVp, high mAs

X-ray tube

High-energy, penetrating x-ray beam

Low-energy, x-ray beam

Small absorbed dose

Large absorbed dose

A

B

75 kVp
16 mAs   Good chest radiograph

100 kVp
4.5 mAs   Good chest radiograph*

*Reduces patient exposure by 70%

C

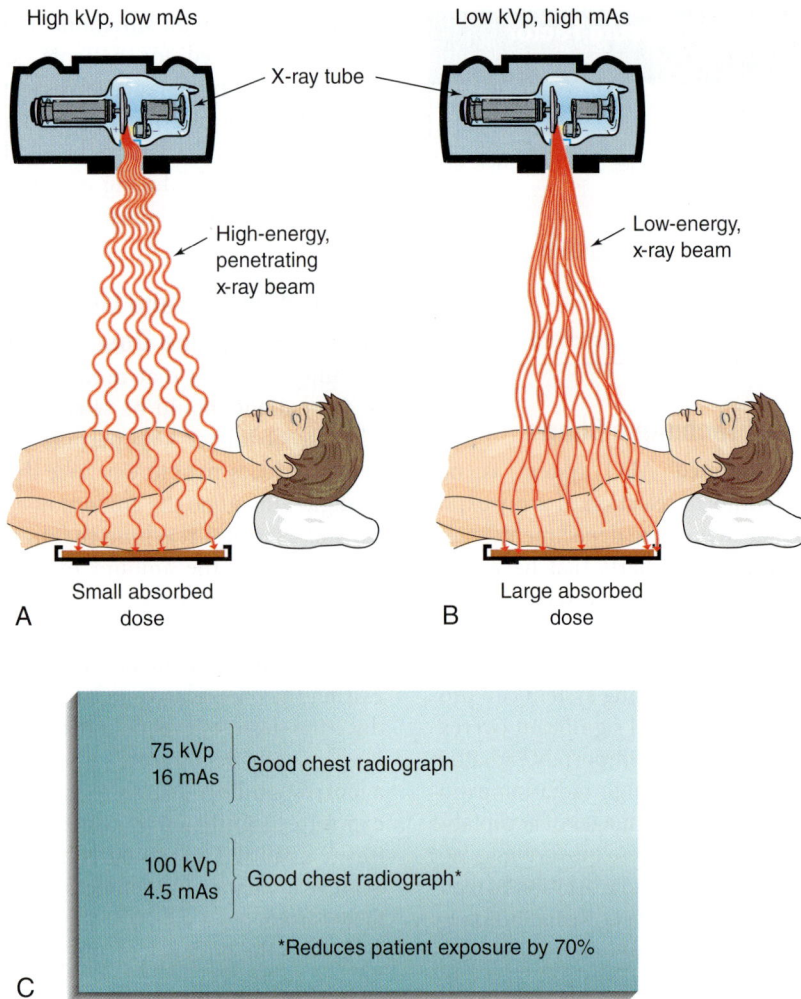

Fig. 11.5 The use of higher kilovoltage (kVp) and lower milliamperage and exposure time in seconds (mAs) reduces patient dose. (A) The use of high kVp and low mAs results in a high-energy, penetrating x-ray beam and a small patient-absorbed dose. (B) The use of low kVp and high mAs results in a low-energy x-ray beam of greater intensity, the majority of which the patient will easily absorb. (C) Example of a higher kVp, lower mAs technique resulting in a 70% reduction in patient exposure without significantly compromising radiographic quality.

Quality Control Program

To ensure quality control in the acquiring and processing of digital images, it is indispensable that every imaging department establishes a *quality control program* that includes regular monitoring and maintenance of all processing and image display equipment in the facility. Such a program will promote quality assurance by decreasing the likelihood of producing suboptimal-quality images, repeat exposures, unnecessary absorbed patient dose, and incorrect x-ray projections.

Radiographers are the operators of sophisticated imaging equipment and therefore are the individuals who may first recognize any equipment malfunction. Problems that occur in digital imaging (either computed radiography [CR] or digital radiography [DR]) tend, unfortunately, to be *systematic*, which can affect the quality of every image and the degree of radiation exposure of every patient until these problems are identified and corrected. Mandated full acceptance testing of new equipment, regular calibration and performance evaluation of existing equipment, and proactive and consistent image review quality control can prevent these systematic errors.[4] QC programs documentation should include step-by-step procedures for performance, monitoring, and continuing quality control.[3–8]

AIR GAP TECHNIQUE

Reduction of Scattered Radiation

The air gap technique is an alternative procedure to use in place of a radiographic grid for reducing scattered radiation during specific examinations (e.g., cross-table lateral projection of the cervical spine, areas of chest radiography). This technique works by using an increased object-to-image receptor distance (OID). Less scatter radiation at the detector decreases image blurring and thereby improves radiographic image contrast. If magnification is not desired, a corresponding increase in source-to-image receptor distance (SID) may be made.

To perform the air gap technique, the image receptor is placed 10 to 15 cm (4 to 6 inches) from the patient, and the x-ray tube is positioned approximately 300 to 366 cm (10 to 12 feet) away from the image receptor. The scattered x-rays from the patient are disseminated in many directions at acute angles to the primary beam when the radiographic exposure is made. Because of the increased distance between the anatomic structures being imaged and the image receptor, a higher percentage of the scattered x-rays produced is less likely to strike the image receptor (Fig. 11.6). This air gap method effectively provides an adequate grid-type scatter cleanup effect. In general, the use of an air gap technique requires the selection of technical exposure factors that are comparable to those used with an 8:1 ratio grid. Therefore when a patient dose is compared with a non-grid technique, it is higher, but when compared with the patient dose resulting from the use of a mid-ratio grid (8:1), the dose from an air gap technique is about the same.

High-Peak Kilovoltage Radiography

In high-kVp radiography that employs kVp settings of 90 or above, air gap techniques are, for the most part, not as effective. Still, some facilities that perform chest radiography by using kVp settings of 120 to 140 do successfully use air gap techniques. In general, when x-rays are scattered through greater angles, such as occurs for images produced at less than 90 kVp, air gap techniques are more successful.

REPEAT IMAGES

Consequences of Repeat Images

A repeat image is an image that must be performed more than once because of human or mechanical error during the production of the initial image. This additional imaging, unfortunately, increases patient dose. If the patient's gonads were included in the imaged area, then the gonads would have received a double dose of radiation. Occasionally, an additional image is permissible when it is recommended by the radiologist to obtain additional diagnostic information. However, repeat exposures resulting from carelessness or poor judgment on the part of the radiographer must be eliminated. The radiographer should, from the beginning of the examination:

- Correctly position the patient
- Select the appropriate technical radiographic exposure factors that will ensure the production of optimal-quality images

Increase in Repeat Rates

Repeat rates for previously film-based radiology departments were documented to be in the range of 10% to 15%, and their leading cause was attributed to the use of incorrect technical factors. With the advent of digital imaging, it was expected that repeat rates would decrease to zero because digital equipment imaging systems can correct errors related to technical factors. A series of research studies, however, have reported repeat rates in many digital departments at approximately 5%, and some, unfortunately, at the same rate as for the earlier film-screen systems' departments. Some studies have even demonstrated repeat rates as high as 17%. Digital imaging significantly changed the cause of repeated images, shifting from exposure-related to *positioning errors*. The unexpected increase in repeat rates has in many instances been ultimately attributed to the trifling ease of retaking an exposure in direct DR. Since there is no imaging receptor to be further processed as in CR and film-screen radiography, the image can be repeated quickly with a modification in the patient's positioning. Some radiographers often strive for a perfect image, even when the initial image would be deemed acceptable.[9] Repeating an exposure to improve an already

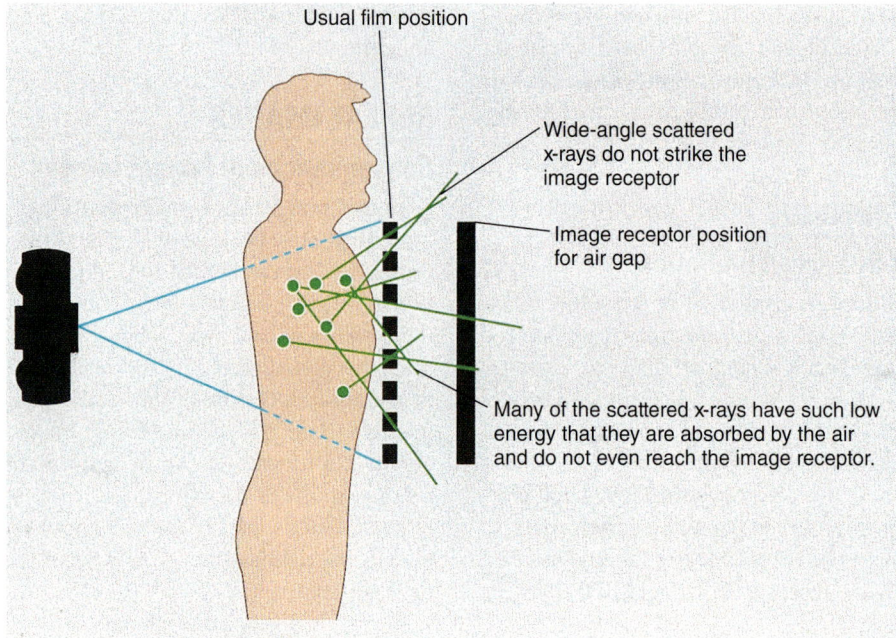

Fig. 11.6 The air gap technique. (From *Radiobiology and radiation protection: Mosby's radiographic instructional series*, St. Louis, 1999, Elsevier).

acceptable image is unnecessary and will only increase patient radiation dose needlessly.

The Benefit of a Repeat Analysis Program

Health care facilities can gain significantly by implementing and maintaining a *repeat analysis program*. Repeat analysis is particularly critical in CR and DR. In these modalities repeating exposures because of improper technique is not usually necessary. In digital imaging, overexposed or underexposed images can be adjusted by computer to *appear technically acceptable*. Consequently, it is essential for the delivery of nonexcessive patient exposures that a qualified medical physicist makes exposure measurements for the techniques employed at the site to ensure that they are within acceptable ranges. With CR or DR, it is necessary to develop a policy whereby the digital files that correspond to retaken images can be recovered for analysis, since this would not happen automatically. Analysis of a department's repeat rate:

- Provides valuable information for process improvement
- Helps minimize patient exposure
- Improves the overall performance of the department[4]
- Some categories for unacceptable images are listed in Box 11.2.

> **BOX 11.2   Reasons for Unacceptable Images**
>
> - Patient mispositioning
> - Incorrect centering of the radiographic beam
> - Patient motion during the radiographic exposure
> - Incorrect collimation of the radiographic beam
> - Presence of external foreign bodies
> - Postprocessing artifacts

CONCERN ABOUT RISK OF EXPOSURE DURING DIAGNOSTIC IMAGING PROCEDURES

Benefit Versus Risk

As a result of increased numbers of people in the United States being required to and subsequently undergoing diagnostic imaging procedures each year, concern about the *collective risk* of radiation exposure from these procedures continues to grow. Imaging personnel must, therefore, always strive to employ techniques that produce high-quality images with the lowest radiation exposure.

Since the responsibility for ordering a radiologic examination lies with the referring physician, in making

BOX 11.3   Unnecessary Radiologic Procedures

- A chest x-ray examination automatically scheduled on admission to the hospital. This examination should not be performed without clinical indications of chest disease or another important concern that justifies exposing the patient to ionizing radiation. This includes presurgical patients. A panel of physicians appointed by the US Food and Drug Administration (FDA)[10] concluded that a chest x-ray examination is not necessary for every presurgical patient. Patients admitted for treatment of pulmonary problems or diseases, however, may benefit from a preadmission chest x-ray examination.
- A chest x-ray examination as part of a preemployment physical. Very little information about previous illness or injury can be gained through this examination, and it is unlikely to be useful to the employer.
- Lumbar spine examinations as part of a preemployment physical. As with the preemployment chest x-ray examination, this examination provides minimal data about previous illness or injury that would be useful to an employer.
- Chest x-ray examination or other unjustified x-ray examination as part of a routine health checkup.

Radiologic procedures should not be performed unless a patient exhibits symptoms that merit radiologic investigations.
- Chest x-ray examination for mass screening for tuberculosis (TB). Such examinations are of negligible value for most people. Testing for TB may be done with more efficient procedures. However, some x-ray screening may still be acceptable for high-risk groups such as members of the medical and paramedical community, people working in such fields as education and food preparation, and selected groups of workers such as miners and workers dealing with material such as asbestos, beryllium, glass, and silica.[3]
- Whole-body computed tomography (CT) screening. Patients may elect to undergo this type of CT procedure without an order from a referring physician. They can simply locate a facility that offers this service to the general public. Currently, the disease detection rate does not justify the relatively high radiation dose received by the patient from this procedure. Until there is evidence of a significant disease detection rate, whole-body CT screening should not be done.[3]

the decision to order the examination, the physician must determine whether the benefit to the patient, in terms of medical information gained, sufficiently justifies subjecting the patient to whatever degree of risk is produced by the absorbed radiation resulting from the procedure.

Nonessential Radiologic Examinations

Some traditional radiographic examinations are very often casually performed in the *absence of definite medical indications*. This practice unnecessarily exposes the patient to radiation even though there is virtually no useful medical information gained from the procedure. Examples of nonessential radiologic examinations are described in Box 11.3.

Specifying the Amount of Radiation Received by a Patient During a Diagnostic Imaging Procedure

In general, the amount of radiation received by a patient from diagnostic imaging procedures may be presented in three ways:

1. Entrance skin exposure (ESE) (includes skin and glandular)
2. Bone marrow dose
3. Gonadal dose

Although each type of specification has significance in estimating the risk to the patient, ESE is the most frequently reported because it is the simplest to determine.

Skin Dose. Skin dose is used in radiation safety terminology to refer to the dose to the *epidermis*, the most superficial layers of the skin. The thickness of the epidermis varies from one anatomic area to another. It is more substantial in areas such as the palms of the hands and soles of the feet. The primary function of the epidermis is to protect underlying tissues and structures.

Entrance skin exposure (ESE) may be converted to patient skin dose by using well-documented multiplication factors. These will be explicitly discussed and illustrated in several examples. When actual patient measurements are not available, reasonably accurate estimates can still be made, which is why ESE is so widely used in assessing the amount of radiation received by a patient.

Thermoluminescent dosimeters (TLDs) are the sensing devices most often used to determine skin dose directly. A small, relatively thin pack of TLDs is secured to the patient's skin in the middle of the clinical area of interest and exposed during a radiographic procedure. Because lithium fluoride (LiF), the sensing material in the TLD, responds similar to human tissue when exposed to ionizing radiation, an accurate determination of surface dose can be made (see Table 2.5 for a list of permissible skin entrance exposures for various radiographic examinations). In fluoroscopy, the amount of radiation that a patient receives at the entrance surface of the skin is usually estimated by measuring the radiation exposure rate at the tabletop* and then multiplying by the fluoroscopy time. The placement of thermoluminescent dosimeters at the tabletop can be used to verify that estimate.

Gonadal Dose

Difference in gonadal dose received by male and female patients. Since genetic effects may result from exposure to ionizing radiation, protection of the reproductive organs is of particular concern in diagnostic radiology (see Table 2.5 for a list of typical gonadal doses from various radiographic examinations). For several examinations identified in Table 2.5, differences in dose received exist between male and female patients. Protection of the ovaries in the female patient by overlying tissue accounts for these differences. As a consequence of their anatomic location, the female reproductive organs receive about three times more exposure during a given radiographic procedure involving the pelvic region than do the male reproductive organs. In diagnostic radiology, the relatively low **gonadal dose** for a single human is by itself considered statistically unimportant. However, should that low gonadal dose value be applied to each member of a large population group, then that dose value may become far more genetically significant.

Genetically significant dose. The concept of **genetically significant dose (GSD)** is used to assess the overall impact of a gonadal dose on a populace. GSD is defined as the equivalent dose (EqD) to the reproductive organs that, if received by every human in a large population

group, would be expected to bring about an identical gross genetic injury to that total population, as does the sum of the actual doses received by exposed individual members of the population. In other words, if 5000 individual inhabitants of a population group of 500,000 each were to receive 0.05 Sv (5 rem) of gonadal radiation EqD and the other 495,000 inhabitants were not to receive any EqD, the gross genetic effect would be identical to the effect that would occur if all 500,000 individual inhabitants each were to receive 0.0005 Sv (0.05 rem) of gonadal radiation. The concept of GSD implies, therefore, that the genetic consequences of substantial absorbed doses of gonadal radiation received by a small number of individuals becomes significantly less when averaged over an entire population rather than applied to just a few of its members.

Additional genetically significant dose considerations. For a population group, the GSD considers that some people receive radiation to their reproductive organs during a given year, whereas others do not. Also, it accounts for the fact that radiation exposure in members of the population who cannot bear children (e.g., those beyond reproductive years) has no genetic impact. Hence the GSD is the average annual gonadal EqD to members of the population who *are of childbearing age*. It includes the number of children who may be expected to be conceived by members of the exposed population in a given year. According to the US Public Health Service, the estimated GSD for the population of the United States is approximately 0.20 millisievert (20 mrem).

Bone Marrow Dose. In humans, bone marrow is of great importance because it contains large numbers of stem, or precursor, blood cells that could be either depleted or, worse, even eliminated by substantial exposure to ionizing radiation. Because irradiation of bone marrow may be responsible for inducing leukemia, the dose to this organ becomes very significant.[3] **Bone marrow dose** may also be described in terms of the *mean marrow dose*, which is defined as "the average radiation dose to the entire active bone marrow."[3] For example, if in the course of performing a specific radiographic procedure, 25% of the active bone marrow were in the useful beam and received an average absorbed dose of 0.8 mGy_t, the mean marrow dose would be 0.2 mGy_t. Because multiple bony areas span the entire body, the radiation dose absorbed by the organ that is called "bone marrow" cannot be measured accurately by a direct method; it can

---

*The entrance exposure rate is obtained from ionization chamber measurements with the chamber situated just beneath a patient equivalent phantom slightly offset from the tabletop as part of routine medical physicist equipment surveys.

only be estimated. In diagnostic radiology, the bone marrow dose is one of the values that has been used to provide an approximation of patient-absorbed doses even though hematologic effects are generally negligible for doses associated with this modality.

Table 2.5 provides typical bone marrow doses for various radiographic examinations performed on human adults. The levels indicated in Table 2.5 are usually less for children because the active bone marrow is more evenly spread out, and significantly lower technical radiographic exposure factors are used. Although each dose listed in Table 2.5 results from fragmentary exposure of the human body, it is averaged over the whole body.

Fluoroscopically Guided Positioning

Fluoroscopic guided positioning (FGP) is the practice of using fluoroscopy to determine the exact location of the central ray before taking a radiographic exposure.[11] Some radiologic technologists (RTs) believe that the use of FGP results in less dose to the patient than does a repeat radiograph. However, the ASRT adopted the following positioning statement:

The ASRT recognizes that the routine use of fluoroscopy to ensure proper positioning before making an exposure is an unethical practice that increases patient dose unnecessarily and should never be used in place of appropriate skills required of a competent radiologic technologist.[12]

Even though the ASRT does not condone FGP, some imaging facilities continue to allow RTs to use fluoroscopy as a positioning aid because they believe that it:
- Is faster than having a repeat exposure
- Reduces the number of repeat exposures
- Provides less radiation exposure to the patient

The Standard of Ethics as published by the American Registry of Radiologic Technologists (ARRT) serves as a guide for practicing technologists in maintaining a high level of ethical conduct and in providing for the protection, safety, and comfort of patients.[13] Blind positioning, or positioning using the radiographer's skill and the anatomic landmarks on the patient, without a repeat exposure, provides the patient with the lowest dose. However, some technologists argue that the chance of repeating the image is reduced when using FGP. This argument *does not hold true* according to the current repeat rates of 7% to 8%.[14] For example, if a technologist has a repeat

rate of 10%, it would not be ethical to overexpose 90% of the patients with FGP to lower the repeat rate. Thus, the usage of FGP by technologists is a practice that should be avoided. It is prohibited by many state regulatory agencies. Where FGP is permitted, the repeat rate depends on the:
- Technologists' skills in the operation of the fluoroscopic equipment
- Communication between the technologist and the patient
- Patients' cooperation
- Patients' condition

Therefore the chance of a repeat during an FGP examination is still present, and ultimately it is the technologist's professional responsibility to reduce the amount of radiation exposure to all patients, not just those who may need to have a repeat examination.

Studies indicate that patient ESE increases with the use of FGP when a repeat exposure is needed.[15] Blind positioning provides the lowest patient ESE.

The current scientific consensus is that all dose levels of ionizing radiation have a non zero potential for producing detrimental effects (the linear non-threshold concept previously discussed). At the same time, however, procedures in radiology, such as fluoroscopy and other imaging modalities, are providing vital information to physicians for diagnosis or treatment of disease. Thus, risk versus benefit must always be considered.

Exposure of patients to medical x-rays is commanding increasing attention in society for two reasons:
1. The frequency of x-ray examinations, including many repetitive studies in short periods, among all age groups, is expanding annually. This increase indicates that physicians are relying more and more on radiologic examinations to assist them in patient care and diagnosis.
2. Concern among public health officials is growing regarding the risk of late effects associated with these multiple medical x-ray exposures.[3]

A review of the literature emphasized the following guidelines:
- No diagnostic procedure using ionizing radiation should be conducted unless its benefit outweighs its risk.
- Exposures should be kept ALARA, with the procedure optimized to reduce radiation hazards.
- The ESE dose level specified in regulations must not be exceeded.

- To maintain ALARA and follow the ASRT position statement and the ARRT code of ethics, *technologists must not use FGP positioning of patients.*

PROTECTING THE PREGNANT OR POTENTIALLY PREGNANT PATIENT

Position of the American College of Radiology on Abdominal Radiologic Examinations of Female Patients

Because much evidence suggests that the developing embryo-fetus is very radiation-sensitive, special care is taken in radiography to prevent unnecessary exposure of the abdominal area of pregnant women. Unfortunately, many women are not aware that they are pregnant during the earliest stage of pregnancy, and this means that exposure to the abdominal area of potentially pregnant (i.e., fertile) women are a concern.[16,17] When the referring physician does not consider radiologic procedures urgent, they may be regarded as elective examinations. They can be booked at an appropriate time to meet patients' needs and safety requirements. However, the official position of the ACR, the primary professional organization of radiologists in the United States, is as follows:

> *"Abdominal radiological examinations that have been requested after full consideration of the clinical status of a patient, including the possibility of pregnancy, need not be postponed or selectively scheduled."[15]*

Although elective scheduling is not always attempted in departments with high workloads, it is the policy of some facilities that women of childbearing years should be made aware of the NCRP recommendations and given a choice as to when they want to have a non-urgent abdominal examination. The NCRP recommendation states that abdominal examinations should be performed during the first few days after the onset of menses to minimize the possibility of irradiating an embryo.[17,18]

Determining the Possibility of Pregnancy

Whenever a female patient of childbearing age is to have an x-ray examination, it is essential that beforehand the radiographer carefully question the patient regarding

any possibility of pregnancy. Part of this questioning involves asking the patient for the date of her last menstrual period (LMP). If the patient is to receive substantial pelvic irradiation and there is doubt about her pregnancy status, then, provided there are no overriding medical concerns, it is strongly recommended that the result of a pregnancy test be obtained before the pelvis is irradiated.

Irradiation During an Unknown Pregnancy

Even with precautionary steps, it is likely that a radiographer will encounter many occasions when a patient who was confident that she could not be pregnant later discovered that she was pregnant at the time of her x-ray examination. This revelation is usually communicated to the imaging department by the patient's obstetrician and is accompanied by a request for the amount of radiation dose that the patient's embryo-fetus received from the x-ray study. The following discussion attempts to illustrate in a simplified manner how the radiography team can appropriately respond to such queries by presenting several case examples.

The first step in the process is to list the specifics of the x-ray examination in as much detail as possible. A useful form can be developed to assist in this process (Fig. 11.7). The information that is needed to fill out this form is listed in Box 11.4.

The following question sometimes arises if a pregnant patient is inadvertently irradiated. Should a therapeutic abortion be performed to prevent the birth of an infant because of radiation exposure during pregnancy? Studies of groups such as the atomic bomb survivors of Hiroshima have shown that damage to the newborn is unlikely for doses below 0.2 Gy. Because essentially, all diagnostic medical procedures result in fetal exposures of less than 0.01 Gy (1 cGy), the risk of abnormality is minimal. The position of the NCRP is stated in Box 11.5.[17]

Procedure to Follow and Responsibility for Absorbed Equivalent Dose Determination to the Patient's Embryo-Fetus

When the details of the x-ray examination have been collected and listed on an appropriate summary form, they must be conveyed to the radiation safety officer or to the medical physicist providing x-ray quality assurance services. It is then that individual's task to determine

Facility: _____

Imaging Department

REQUEST FOR PATIENT RADIATION DOSE
PATIENT X-RAY EXAM RECORD

Patient's name: _____ X-ray study #: _____
Date of birth: _____ Exam date: _____
Date of last menstrual period: _____
Referring physician: _____
Physician requesting radiation dose: _____
Radiologist: _____ Radiographer: _____
Examination: _____ X-ray room unit: _____

RADIOGRAPHIC

Projection	Patient thickness	Film	kVp	mAs	SID	Number of images	Gonadal shield

FLUOROSCOPIC

Anatomic location	kVp (mean)	mA (mean)	Fluoro time	Exam description

SPOT FILMS

Anatomic location	kVp	mA	Time (msec)	Number of spots	Special details

Fig. 11.7 Request for patient radiation dose form.

the absorbed EqD to the patient's embryo-fetus. The calculation process makes use of actual measurements of radiation output on the individual x-ray unit or units and incorporating that with the examination data list supplied by the radiographer. It also uses published absorbed dose data tables. What eventually is obtained and presented by the medical physicist, radiologist, or radiation safety officer to the patient's physician is a *calculated estimate* of the approximate EqD to the embryo-fetus due to the x-ray examination.

Sample Case to Estimate Approximate Equivalent Dose to the Embryo-Fetus

Several typical cases (somewhat simplified) are presented to illustrate one of the methods that may be used to obtain this calculated estimate. Here, it is not the purpose to provide an advanced presentation, but instead, to offer a basic method that makes use of fundamental principles and demonstrates the importance of the radiographer's input in the process. The most significant factor is the correction to the measured radiation output at a given kVp due to the patient's anatomical thickness and the distance from the image receptor to the tabletop. The product of the radiation output dose rate at the patient's radiation entrance surface (mGy_a/mAs) at

the kVp selected and the mAs used for the x-ray projection considered yields the ESE_d for that projection, a quantity that needs to be obtained for each x-ray exposure given to the patient. The most common measurements of milligray per mAs are at a distance of 100 cm from the x-ray tube target. These values as a function of kVp and mAs are usually tabulated during each annual survey of the x-ray unit by a qualified medical physicist. For a patient with thickness T in centimeters and a *typical distance of 8 cm from the image receptor to the tabletop*, the radiation output at the patient's entrance surface for selected mAs is determined as shown in Fig. 11.8, which illustrates all the geometric quantities of interest.

Since the skin surface is closer to the x-ray tube target, the milligray per mAs value will be greater than it is at 100 cm. How much greater is determined from the inverse square law and given by Equation 11.1 below:

$$(mGy_a/mAs) \text{ at skin surface}$$
$$= (mGy_a/mAs) \text{ at } 100 \text{ cm} \times (100/[92-25])^2$$

As an example, assume the following values:

$$(mGy_a/mAs) \text{ at } 100 \text{ cm} = 0.06$$
$$T = 25 \text{ cm}$$

Then:

$$(mGy_a/mAs) \text{ at skin surface} = 0.06 \times (100/67)^2$$
$$= 0.06 \times (100/2.23)$$
$$= 0.13 \text{ mGy}_a/mAs$$

The patient's ESE_d for an x-ray exposure is now given by Equation 11.2 and obtained as shown:

$$ESE_d = (mGy_a/mAs) \text{ at skin surface} \times mAs \text{ used}$$

Example:

$$mAs \text{ used} = 30$$
$$(mGy_a/mAs)_s = 0.13$$
$$ESE_d = 0.13 \times 30$$
$$= 3.9 \text{ mGy}$$

After the ESE_d has been determined for each x-ray exposure, it is necessary to obtain conversion factors that will yield a value for the uterine absorbed dose attributable to each exposure. In 1977, the NCRP published Report No. 54, *Medical Radiation Exposure of Pregnant*

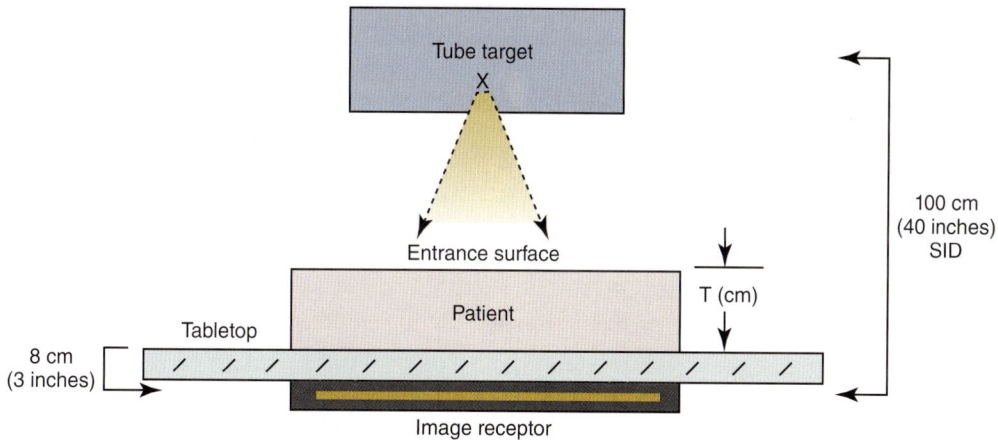

Fig. 11.8 As the diagram shows, the distance from the tube target to the tabletop is 100 cm (40 inches) minus 8 cm (3 inches). The distance from the tube target to the top of the patient in centimeters is therefore equal to 100−8−T where the patient's thickness, T, is specified in centimeters. To convert this value to inches just divide by 2.54.

and Potentially Pregnant Women. Table 4 in this report has been a valuable resource for helping establish the uterine dose. Although other useful and more recent data tables exist, this table has been reproduced here as Table 11.1 to illustrate a simple method for fetal dose estimation. To use the table, it is necessary to know for each x-ray projection the ESE_d, the anatomic location, the beam quality (half-value layer [HVL]), and the image receptor size.

Sample Case to Obtain an Approximate Estimate of the Fetal Equivalent Dose

Two typical x-ray examinations will be considered, and an approximate estimate of the fetal EqD resulting from each study obtained. These are presented in detail in boxes labeled as Case 11.1 and Case 11.2.

Irradiating a Known Pregnant Patient

If the physician believes it is in the best interest of a pregnant or potentially pregnant patient to undergo a radiologic examination, the examination should be performed and extra efforts made to minimize the dose of radiation the patient receives to her lower abdomen and pelvic regions. This can be accomplished by consciously selecting the smallest technical exposure factors that will still yield a diagnostically acceptable image for the examination and by precisely collimating the radiographic beam to include only the anatomic area of interest. When the patient's lower abdomen and pelvic

regions do not have to be included in the area to be irradiated, they should be protected with a lead apron or other suitable protective shield so that a developing embryo- fetus does not receive unnecessary radiation exposure from external scatter and the edges of the selected radiation field (Fig. 11.9).

PEDIATRIC CONSIDERATIONS DURING RADIOGRAPHIC IMAGING

Vulnerability of Children to Radiation Exposure

Children are much more vulnerable to the late effects of radiation than are adults. Hence, children require special consideration when they undergo diagnostic x-ray studies. Some of these considerations are described in the following sections. Because children have a greater life expectancy, they may easily survive long enough to develop late effects like leukemia or another radiogenic malignancy such as lung or thyroid cancer. According to studies published in 1978, the risk of radiation-induced leukemia in children after a substantial dose of ionizing radiation is approximately two times that of adults.[19] For low doses such as those generally encountered in conventional diagnostic radiology, data are still inconclusive. With this concern in mind, radiographers must take every precaution to minimize exposure in all pediatric patients.

TABLE 11.1   Embryo (Uterine) Doses for Selected X-Ray Projections (mcGy/R)*,†

Anatomy or Study	Projection	SID (Inches)	Image Receptor Size (Inches)‡	BEAM QUALITY (HVL MM ALUMINUM)					
				1.5	2.0	2.5	3.0	3.5	4.0
Pelvis, lumbopelvic	AP	40	17 × 14	142	212	283	353	421	486
	LAT	40	14 × 17	13	25	39	56	75	97
Abdominal§	AP	40	14 × 17	133	199	265	330	392	451
	PA	40	14 × 17	56	90	130	174	222	273
	LAT	40	14 × 17	13	23	37	53	71	91
Lumbar spine	AP	40	14 × 17	128	189	250	309	366	419
	LAT	40	14 × 17	9	17	27	39	53	69
Hip	AP (1)	40	10 × 12	105	153	200	244	285	324
	AP (2)	40	17 × 14	136	203	269	333	395	454
Full spine (chiropractic)	AP	40	14 × 36	154	231	308	384	457	527
Urethrogram	AP	40	10 × 12	135	200	265	327	386	441
Upper GI	AP	40	14 × 17	9.5	16	25	34	45	56
Femur (one side)	AP	40	7 × 17	1.6	3.0	4.8	6.9	9.4	12
Cholecystography	PA	40	10 × 12	0.7	1.5	2.6	4.1	6.0	8.3
Chest	AP	72	14 × 17	0.3	0.7	1.3	2.0	3.1	4.3
	PA	72	14 × 17	0.3	0.6	1.2	2.0	3.0	4.5
	LAT	72	14 × 17	0.1	0.3	0.5	0.8	1.2	1.8
Ribs, barium swallow	AP	40	14 × 17	0.1	0.3	0.5	0.9	1.4	2.0
	PA	40	14 × 17	0.1	0.3	0.5	0.9	1.5	2.2
	LAT	40	14 × 17	0.03	0.08	0.2	0.3	0.4	0.6
Thoracic spine	AP	40	14 × 17	0.2	0.4	0.8	1.4	4.1	3.0
	LAT	40	14 × 17	0.04	0.1	0.2	0.4	0.5	0.8
Skull, cervical spine, scapula, shoulder, humerus	—	40	—	<0.01	<0.01	<0.01	<0.01	<0.01	<0.01

AP, Anteroposterior; *GI*, gastrointestinal; *HVL*, half-value layer; *LAT*, lateral; *PA*, posteroanterior; *SID*, source-to–image receptor distance.

*Average dose to the uterus in millicentigray per roentgen entrance skin exposure (free-in-air) (ESE$_d$). The latter value in roentgens is essentially equal, in these energy ranges, to 10 mGy ESE$_d$ or 1 cGy ESE$_d$.

†Adapted from NCRP report No. 54 Rosenstein (1976).

‡Field size is collimated to the image receptor.

§Includes retrograde pyelogram; kidney, ureter, and bladder (KUB); barium enema, lumbosacral spine, intravenous pyelogram (IVP); renal arteriogram.

Data modified from National Council on Radiation Protection and Measurements (NCRP): *Medical exposure of pregnant and potentially pregnant women*, Report No. 54, Washington, DC, 1977, NCRP.

Children Require Smaller Radiation Doses Than Do Adults

In general, smaller doses of ionizing radiation are sufficient to obtain useful images in pediatric imaging procedures than are necessary for adult imaging procedures. For example, an entrance exposure dose below 5 millicGy (mcGy, previously millirads: mrads) results from an AP projection of an infant's chest,[20] whereas the same projection or a PA projection of an adult's chest yields entrance exposure doses that can range from 10 to 25 mcGy.

CASE 11.1   Obstruction Series

X-ray projection details:

Although a 180 cm (72 inch) source-to-image receptor distance (SID) would normally be used for a posteroanterior (PA) upright chest projection, for purposes if simplifying the calculation, the SID will be kept at 100 cm (40 inch) the same for all projections in this series.

PA chest projection

(1) 80 kVp, 10 mAs, 100 cm SID, large CR image receptor, 25-cm patient thickness Erect anteroposterior (AP) abdomen

(1) 75 kVp, 32 mAs, 100 cm SID, large CR image receptor, 20-cm patient thickness Supine abdomen

(1) 70 kVp, 50 mAs, 100 cm SID, large CR image receptor, 20-cm patient thickness

Calculation:

The first step is to obtain the value of mGy$_a$/mAs for each projection. To determine this value, a reference value $(mGy_a/mas)_{100-cm}$ is needed for the x-ray unit involved and the kVp used. To comply with state rules and regulations, a medical physicist measures these values yearly for each x-ray tube. If the measured reference mGy$_a$/mAs values for the three projections are 0.01, 0.04, and 004, respectively, then substituting these numbers into Equation 11.1 along with the corresponding SIDs and patient thicknesses yields: $(mGy_a/mAs)_s$ PA chest = 0.02 $(mGy_a/mAs)_s$ erect AP abdomen = 0.08, and supine abdomen = 0.08, respectively. From Equation 11.2 the entrance skin exposure does (ESE$_d$) value is then given by:

$$ESE_d \text{ PA chest} : 0.02 \times 10 \times 0.2 \, mGy = 0.02 \, cGy$$
$$ESE_d \text{ erect AP abdomen} : 0.08 \times 32 = 2.5 \, mGy = 0.26 \, cGy$$
$$ESE_d \text{supine abdomen} : 0.08 \times 50 = 4 \, mGy = 0.4 \, cGy$$

For the chest field, the half-value layer (HVL) is approximately 3 mm aluminum (Al), whereas for the abdominal fields, 2.5 and 2.0 mm Al, respectively, are used. Then *from* Table 11.1 the embryo/uterine dose conversion factors are 2 mcGy/(cGy of ESE$_d$), 265 mcGy/(cGy of ESE$_d$), and 199 mcGy/(cGy of ESE$_d$). Multiplying these values by the ESE$_d$ for each projection gives a fetal dose estimate (FDE) for each, namely:

$$PA \text{ chest FDE} = 0.02 \times 2 = 0.04 \, mcGy \, (0.04 \, millirads)$$
$$Erect \, AP \text{ abdomen FDE} = 0.26 \times 265$$
$$= 69 \, mcGy \, (69 \, millirads)$$
$$Supine \text{ abdomen FDE} = 0.4 \times 199$$
$$= 79.6 \, mcGy \, (79.6 \, millirads)$$

(Note: 1 cGy = 1 rad and therefore 1 millicGy equals 1 millirad)

The total FDE is therefore 0.04 + 69 + 79.6 = 149 mcGy = 1.49 mGy. For diagnostic x-rays, 1 mGy is the same as an equivalent dose of 1 mSv, and consequently the calculated approximate EqD to the patient's embryo-fetus from her obstruction series is 1.49 mSv (149 millirem).

For reference purposes this value of EqD to the embryo-fetus is substantially less than the 5 mSv (500 mrem) recommended by the National Council on Radiation Protection and Measurements as a maximum EqD to the embryo-fetus during the 9 month gestation period.

Patient Motion and Motion Reduction Methods

Patient motion is frequently a problem in pediatric radiography. Due to the limited ability of very young children to understand the radiologic procedure and, in most cases, their imperfect ability to cooperate, these children are less likely to remain still during a radiographic or fluoroscopic exposure. To solve or at least minimize this problem, the radiographer must employ very short exposure times by selecting a high-mA (400 mA or greater) station and using effective immobilization techniques. For some examinations, such as chest radiography, individual pediatric motion restriction devices are available to hold the pediatric patient securely and safely in the required position (see Fig. 11.4). Such procedures and correct image postprocessing techniques dramatically reduce or eliminate the need for repeat examinations that will increase patient dose.

Gaining Cooperation During the Procedure

Combining technologists who have experience working with children with examination rooms specially designed for pediatric studies is very beneficial. These rooms contain not only appropriate restraint devices, if needed, but also suitable entertainment and distraction items such as cartoon posters and puppets. The examination efficiently progresses with the best chance of patient cooperation when the child feels less intimidated.

CASE 11.2   Modified Upper Gastrointestinal Examination

X-ray projection details:

Fluoroscopy: 115 kVp, 4.5 mA (mean values), 3.5 minutes

Spot images (4): 110 kVp, 200 mA, 20 msec (mean values)

Calculation:

Suppose that from measured data on the involved fluoroscopic unit, the entrance exposure rate dose to the patient is about 12.5 mGy per milliampere minute. Therefore the entrance skin exposure dose (ESE_d) for the delivered fluoroscopic radiation is obtained from the product:

$$12.5 \text{ mGy/mAmin} \times 4.5 \text{ mA} \times 3.5 \text{ min} = 197 \text{ mGy } (19.7 \text{ cGy}$$

From measured spot image radiation output, for the technique factors used in this study, let the x-ray output at the patient's entrance surface be 0.5 mGy/mAs.*

Therefore the total ESE_d for the four spot images is given by:

$$4 \times 0.5 \text{ mGy/mAs} \times 200 \text{ mA} \times 0.020 \text{ sec} = 8 \text{ mGy } (0.8 \text{ cGy})$$

Using half-value layer (HVL) values 4.0 and 3.5 mm aluminum (Al), respectively, the uterine dose rates *obtained from* Table 11.1 *are as follows:*

Averaged fluoroscopic irradiation: 56 mcGy/cGy = 56 mrem/cGy (entrance dose factor)

Spot image: 45 mcGy/cGy = 45 mrem/cGy (entrance dose factor)

The estimated approximate equivalent dose to the embryo-fetus from this modified upper gastrointestinal (UGI) study is then:

$$56 \times 19.7 + 45 \times 0.8 = 1139 \text{ mrem} = 1.14 \text{ rem} = 11.4 \text{ mSv}$$

For this modified UGI study on a heavy patient, a fetal EqD estimate has been obtained that is more than twice the National Council on Radiation Protection and Measurements recommended maximum fetal EqD of 5 mSv (0.5 rem). This result, however, is far below the range between 100 and 200 mSv (10 and 20 rem) at which therapeutic abortion has historically been considered. If the embryo-fetus were in its most sensitive stage (i.e., early first trimester), then possibly some genetic studies could be undertaken. Otherwise, in most situations, increased follow-up would be the course of action.

---

*For the spot images the entrance surface of the patient is only about 46 cm (18 inch) from the x-ray tube target, and that is why the value of mGy/mAs can be so high.

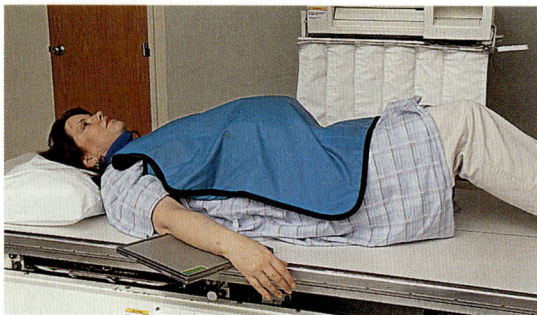

Fig. 11.9 To protect a developing embryo-fetus from unnecessary radiation exposure, place a lead apron over the female patient's lower abdomen and pelvic regions when these sites do not have to be included in the area to be irradiated.

Collimation

Precise collimation is especially significant in pediatric studies because of the increased possibility of late tissue effects occurring in these young patients as compared to in older patients. The automatic collimation system is designed to reduce the radiation field size to the dimensions of the image receptor, but because many pediatric patients are significantly smaller than the image receptor, further manual adjustment of collimation is often necessary. As in any other radiographic study, limiting the field size to the anatomic features of interest not only reduces patient exposure but also enhances the quality of the completed image by decreasing scatter. Wise selection of projection orientation is also essential. Female patients who may be imaged in either a PA or AP projection will receive significantly lower doses to the breast tissue if imaged in a PA projection.[21]

Patient Protection in Computed Tomography for Adults and Children: Similarities and Necessary Changes

Unfortunately, many facilities have, in the past, routinely used the same technical exposure factors for both adults and small children and continue to do so today. There has been an apparent unwillingness to develop new scanning protocols because of the conflicting demands of multiple pediatric protocols. Mindful of the overall enhanced vulnerability of children to ionizing radiation, all facilities and imaging personnel must make every conscious effort to develop and use low-dose pediatric protocols that are in the best interest of the children entrusted to their care.

IMAGE GENTLY CAMPAIGN

An initiative of the **Alliance for Radiation Safety in Pediatric Imaging** (as discussed in Chapter 1) is the **Image Gently Campaign**. The goal of this campaign is to change long-established practice by raising awareness about methods for lowering radiation dose during pediatric medical imaging examinations (Alliance for Radiation Safety in Pediatric Imaging, 2016.)[22] The Image Gently website, www.imagegently.org, provides information about pediatric imaging examinations for RTs, medical physicists, radiologist, pediatricians, and parents. Also, of value to RTs, the site includes protocols for reducing pediatric radiation dose during digital radiography, fluoroscopy, computed tomography examinations, interventional radiology procedures, and nuclear medicine studies. Radiographers and imaging facilities can "pledge" to Image Gently (see Appendix B for the pledge). As of 2020, over 64,000 RTs have taken the pledge.

IMAGE WISELY CAMPAIGN

A second initiative of the Alliance for Radiation Safety in Pediatric Imaging (as discussed in Chapter 1) is the **Image Wisely Campaign**. This campaign promotes lowering the amount of radiation used in medically necessary imaging procedures and eliminating unnecessary procedures in adult medical imaging. The Image Wisely Campaign includes on its website, www.imagewisely.org, information on radiography, fluoroscopy, computed tomography, and nuclear medicine examinations for radiologic technologists, medical physicists, radiologists, referring physicians, and all adults. Radiographers can pledge to Image Wisely (see Appendix B for the pledge). Over 40,000 RTs have taken the pledge.

DUAL ENERGY X-RAY ABSORPTIOMETRY (DEXA, OR DXA SCAN)

Of all naturally occurring materials in the human body, bone has the highest physical density. Bone is composed of numerous layers of tissues of various densities and contains a high calcium content that accounts for its overall mass and general strength. Cortical, or compact, bone that comprises the outer layer of bone is exceptionally dense, while trabecular, or cancellous, bone is composed of a spongy, less solid, or more porous inner layer. The size and shape of bones change as a person grows.[23] A marked loss of bone mass, however, commonly occurs in many individuals as aging progresses. This condition is termed *osteoporosis*, a systematic metabolic bone disorder.[24] Women older than 50 years are primarily affected by bone density loss, often resulting in pathologic fractures. Lately, it has also been noted that the condition unexpectedly has become more prevalent in younger adults and children. Methods have been developed to determine the degree of bone loss, by measuring bone mineral density (BMD). The most widely used test to accomplish this is called **Dual-Energy X-Ray Absorptiometry (DEXA, or DXA Scan)**.[25] The DEXA scan is a noninvasive x-ray procedure that can quantitatively predict the risk of bone fracture(s). For this scan two different low-energy level x-ray beams are utilized. Since denser bone absorbs more of the low-energy radiation than does less dense bone, the ratio of the transmission of the lower and higher energy beams in various osseous (bony) locations is used to calculate average scores for the densities of the patient's bone in those locations.[25] The results can then be evaluated by comparison with normal value ranges. An example of a DEXA scan is shown in Fig. 11.10.

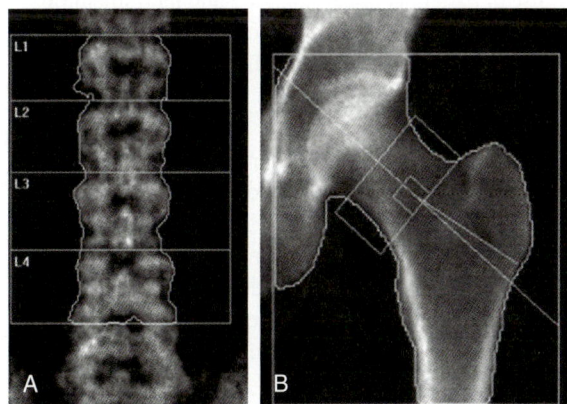

Fig. 11.10 DEXA images of the spine and hips. (From Lupsa BC, Insogna K: Bone health and osteoporosis, *Endocrinol Metab Clin North Am* 44(3):517–530, 2015.)

As mentioned previously, in terms of radiation safety, the benefit of exposing a patient to radiation in terms of diagnostic information obtained must outweigh any possible risk of biologic damage resulting from the exposure. When compared with other imaging procedures (e.g., conventional x-ray images, computed tomography), the DEXA scan results in substantially less radiation exposure for the patient. It is therefore considered a nonharmful radiation procedure.[26] As a result, DEXA scanning does not require protective shielding for the technologist or patients undergoing this procedure.[23]

SUMMARY

- Effective communication with the patient is the first step in holistic patient care.
- Imaging procedures should be explained in simple terms.
- Patients must have an opportunity to ask questions and receive truthful and clear answers within ethical limits.
- Adequate immobilization of the patient is necessary to eliminate or at least minimize any voluntary motion.
- Restraining devices are available to immobilize either the whole body or the individual body part to be imaged.
- Involuntary motion can be compensated for by shortening exposure time with an appropriate increase in mA and by using very-high-speed image receptors.
- Protective shielding may be used to reduce or eliminate radiation exposure of specific radiosensitive body organs and tissues.
- The guidelines for use of protective shielding with newer digital equipment in light of more recent analyses of radiation risks have been recently reexamined by professional societies and scientific advisory groups. Current recommendations now discourage routine use of patient gonadal shielding and fetal shielding.
- Appropriate technical exposure factors for each examination that ensure a diagnostic image of optimal quality with minimal patient dose must be selected.
- Standardized technique charts must be available for each x-ray unit to help provide a uniform selection of technical exposure factors. High kVp and lower mAs should be chosen whenever possible to reduce the amount of radiation received by the patient.
- When digital images are acquired, correct postprocessing is essential to produce a high-quality diagnostic image.
- Imaging departments should establish a quality control program that ensures standardization in the acquisition and postprocessing of digital images.
- An air gap technique can be used as an alternative to the use of a mid-ratio grid (8:1).
- Repeat radiographic exposures must be minimized to prevent the patient's skin and gonads from receiving a double dose of radiation.
- Radiographic examinations are to be performed only when patients will benefit from useful information gained from the procedure. Nonessential radiologic examinations should not be performed.
- The amount of radiation received by a patient from diagnostic imaging procedures may be specified as entrance skin exposure (ESE) (including skin and glandular), gonadal dose, or bone marrow dose.
- ESE is the most straightforward quantity to obtain and thereby the most widely used.
- The estimated genetically significant dose (GSD) for the population of the United States is approximately 0.20 mSv.
- Fluoroscopically guided positioning is an unethical and unacceptable practice that leads to increased patient radiation dose.
- "Abdominal radiologic examinations that have been requested after full consideration of the clinical status of a patient, including the possibility of pregnancy, need not be postponed or selectively scheduled."[16]
- The NCRP recommendations for elective abdominal examinations of women of childbearing years states that such examinations should be performed during the first few days after the onset of menses to minimize the possibility of irradiating an embryo.[17,18]
- A radiographer must carefully question female patients of childbearing age regarding any possibility of pregnancy before they undergo an x-ray examination.
- If irradiation of an unknown pregnancy occurs, a calculated estimate of the appropriate equivalent dose to the embryo-fetus as a result of the examination should be obtained. A radiological physicist performs this estimation.

- Children are much more vulnerable to late effects of radiation than are adults.
- Use a PA projection to protect the breasts of female patients.
- Adequate collimation of the radiographic beam to include only the area of clinical interest is essential, and effective immobilization techniques should be used when necessary. The use of a high mA station and a short exposure time also helps minimizes patient motion effects.
- A developing embryo-fetus is especially sensitive to exposure from ionizing radiation.
- Use the smallest technical exposure factors that will generate a diagnostically useful radiographic image, carefully collimate the beam to include only the anatomic area of interest, and cover the lower abdomen and pelvic regions with a suitable contact shield if they do not need to be included in the examination.
- The goal of the Image Gently Campaign is to change practice by increasing awareness about methods to lower radiation dose during pediatric medical imaging examinations.[21]
- Radiographers and imaging facilities can pledge to Image Gently.
- Radiographers can pledge to Image Wisely.
- The most widely used test to measure bone mineral density is Dual Energy X-Ray Absorptiometry (DEXA, or DXA scan).
- When compared with other imaging procedures such as conventional x-ray radiography or computed tomography, the DEXA scan results in much less radiation exposure for the patient and is therefore considered a non-harmful radiation procedure.[25]

GENERAL DISCUSSION QUESTIONS

1. What is meant by a holistic approach to patient care in radiology?
2. How can voluntary motion be minimized during a diagnostic radiographic procedure?
3. Why is gonadal shielding important in diagnostic radiology?
4. What role do appropriate radiographic technical exposure factors play in patient dose management?
5. How does immobilization contribute to reducing radiographic exposure for the patient?
6. What is the air gap technique, and how does it compare to using a mid-ratio grid?
7. What are the benefits of implementing repeat analysis programs in radiology?
8. Why is fluoroscopically guided positioning considered unacceptable practice?
9. What are the special precautions for protecting pregnant or potentially pregnant patients during x-ray examinations?
10. How does the Image Gently and Image Wisely campaigns contribute to patient radiation safety?

REVIEW QUESTIONS

1. What does a holistic approach to patient care in radiology emphasize?
   A. Technical skills of radiographers
   B. Financial aspects of healthcare
   C. Effective communication and patient comfort
   D. Quick turnaround times for imaging
2. How can voluntary motion be minimized during a radiographic procedure?
   A. Using longer exposure times
   B. Providing clear instructions and comfort
   C. Increasing the radiation dose
   D. Avoiding patient interaction
3. Which of the following techniques is used to minimize voluntary motion during radiographic procedures?
   A. Increasing exposure time
   B. Providing clear instructions to hold still
   C. Using higher kilovoltage
   D. Employing a grid
4. What role do appropriate radiographic technical exposure factors play?
   A. They increase patient discomfort
   B. They minimize image quality
   C. They optimize image quality while reducing patient dose
   D. They have no effect on patient safety

5. How does immobilization help in reducing radiographic exposure?
   A. It increases patient movement
   B. It allows for longer exposure times
   C. It prevents motion artifacts and reduces repeat images
   D. It makes the procedure more complicated

6. What is the air gap technique used for?
   A. To improve patient comfort
   B. To reduce scatter radiation without a grid
   C. To increase radiation exposure
   D. To enhance fluoroscopic imaging

7. What is a benefit of implementing repeat analysis programs in radiology?
   A. They increase the number of repeat images
   B. They help identify causes of repeat exposures
   C. They reduce the need for patient shielding
   D. They have no effect on patient safety

8. What is a key benefit of implementing repeat analysis programs in radiology?
   A. Increasing patient wait times
   B. Reducing the number of radiologists needed
   C. Identifying causes of repeat exposures
   D. Enhancing the aesthetic quality of images

9. What precautions are taken to protect pregnant or potentially pregnant patients?
   A. Use of alternative imaging methods when possible
   B. Increasing radiation dosage for better images
   C. Avoiding all imaging procedures
   D. No special precautions are needed

10. What is the goal of the Image Gently and Image Wisely campaigns?
    A. To promote higher radiation doses in imaging
    B. To increase the use of fluoroscopy
    C. To enhance patient safety and reduce unnecessary radiation exposure
    D. To standardize imaging equipment across facilities

Management of Occupational Radiation Dose

OBJECTIVES

After completing this chapter, the reader will be able to perform the following:

- Define all key terms.
- State the annual occupational effective dose limit for whole-body exposure of diagnostic imaging personnel during routine operations.
- Explain why occupational exposure of diagnostic imaging personnel is limited and state the reason for allowing a much larger equivalent dose for radiation workers than for the population as a whole.
- Identify the type of x-radiation that poses the most significant occupational hazard in diagnostic radiology and explain the various ways this hazard can be reduced.
- Explain how the various methods and techniques that reduce patient exposure during a diagnostic examination can also minimize exposure for the radiographer and any other personnel.
- Discuss the responsibilities of the employer for protecting declared pregnant diagnostic imaging personnel from radiation exposure.
- Describe the three underlying principles of radiation protection that can be used for personnel exposure reduction.
- State and explain the inverse square law, and solve mathematical problems applying this concept.

- Differentiate between a primary and a secondary protective barrier, and list examples of such barriers.
- Describe the construction of protective structural shielding.
- Discuss the protective garments that may be worn to reduce whole-body or partial-body exposure.
- List and explain the methods and devices that may be used to reduce exposure for personnel during routine fluoroscopic and interventional examinations.
- Specify the techniques that are useful for reducing the radiographer's exposure when performing a mobile radiographic examination.
- Explain the variation in dose rate caused by scatter radiation near the entrance and exit surfaces of the patient during C-arm fluoroscopy and discuss dose reduction methods for C-arm operators.
- List the three categories of radiation sources that may be generated in an x-ray room, list the considerations on which the design of radiation-absorbent barriers should be based, and explain the importance of each.
- Differentiate between a controlled area and an uncontrolled area.
- Discuss current approaches to shielding design.
- Describe radiation caution signage.

CHAPTER OUTLINE

KEY TERMS

Broad-beam x-ray transmission factor (B)	**distance**	**secondary protective barrier**
Bucky slot shielding device	**inverse square law (ISL)**	**shielding**
control-booth barrier	**leakage radiation**	**time**
controlled area	**occupancy factor (T)**	**uncontrolled area**
cumulative effective dose (CumEfD) limit	**primary protective barrier**	**use factor (U)**
	primary radiation	**workload (W)**
	scatter radiation	

Some x-ray procedures increase the radiographer's risk of exposure (Box 12.1) due to scatter radiation. This chapter presents an overview of methods that can be used to reduce exposure for imaging professionals during diagnostic x-ray procedures. Also, a brief explanation of the design of a diagnostic x-ray suite is presented.

BOX 12.1   Imaging Procedures That Increase the Radiographer's Risk of Exposure

- General fluoroscopy
- Interventional procedures that employ high-level control fluoroscopy (HLCF)
- Mobile examinations
- C-arm fluoroscopy

ANNUAL LIMITS FOR OCCUPATIONALLY EXPOSED PERSONNEL

Effective Dose Limits

Federal government standards, following a recommendation of the National Council on Radiation Protection and Measurements (NCRP), permit diagnostic imaging personnel to receive an "annual occupational effective dose (EfD) of 50 millisievert (mSv)"[1] for whole-body exposure during routine operations. However, in keeping with the ALARA (*as low as reasonably achievable*) philosophy and careful supervision of personnel cumulative radiation exposure records, no radiographer should approach this EfD level. The dose level referred to here, includes only occupational dose and does not include personal medical exposure that an employee may receive or the background exposure that all people receive.

To ensure that the lifetime risk of occupationally exposed personnel is not exceeded, an additional recommendation is that the *lifetime EfD* in mSvs should not exceed 10 times the person's age in years. Hence a cumulative effective dose (CumEfD) limit has been established for the whole body.

Annual Occupational and Nonoccupational Dose Limits

The annual occupational EfD limit of 50 mSv (5 rem) is an upper boundary limit. It is much higher than the annual EfD limit allowed for individual members of the general population not occupationally exposed. That limit is:

- 1 mSv (100 mrem) for *continuous or frequent* exposures from artificial sources other than medical irradiation and natural background radiation[1]
- 5 mSv (500 mrem) for *infrequent* annual exposure[1]

The 1 mSv annual EfD limit set for members of the general public is intended to limit that exposure to reasonable levels of risk that are comparable with risks from other familiar sources—that is, about 10^{-4} to 10^{-6} annually[1] (10^{-4} to 10^{-6} means an excess cancer risk of 1 chance in 10,000 to 1 chance in 1 million per year). The 5 mSv maximum annual EfD limit recommendation is made because annual exposures above the 1 mSv recommendation need not be regarded as especially hazardous, provided the average exposure to individuals in these groups does not exceed an average annual EfD of about 1 mSv.[1] Both these limits will maintain the annual equivalent dose to organs and tissues below levels of concern for tissue reactions.[1]

Allowance for a Larger Equivalent Dose for Radiation Worker

Valid reasons exist for permitting radiation workers to accumulate a larger equivalent dose (EqD). Among the most important of these reasons is that the workforce in radiation-related jobs is small when compared with the population as a whole. Therefore the expectation of any measurable increase in disease in the population, in individuals, or impact upon the gene pool is negligible. Thus, the amount of radiation received by this workforce can be substantially greater than the amount received by the general public without alteration in the genetically significant dose, the average annual gonadal EqD to members of the population who are of childbearing age. Although the radiographer and other diagnostic imaging personnel are allowed to absorb more radiation, the EqD received must be minimized whenever possible, reducing the potential for:

- Somatic damage
- Genetic damage

ALARA CONCEPT

The best manner for radiographers and radiologists to conscientiously employ the ALARA principle is to use all appropriate radiation-control procedures to minimize their exposure levels. Personnel should faithfully employ procedures such as:

- The principles of time, distance, and shielding
- Adequately collimating the radiographic beam Fig. 12.1)

DOSE-REDUCTION METHODS AND TECHNIQUES

Methods and techniques that reduce patient exposure can also reduce exposure for the radiographer, thereby limiting occupational exposure. Whenever a repeat image is performed because of human or mechanical error, the patient receives a double dose of primary radiation, while also increasing the radiographer's potential for exposure to scattered radiation.

Repeats in Digital Imaging

Because image contrast and overall brightness in digital imaging can be manipulated after image acquisition, the need for all repeats as a result of improper technical exposure factors has been eliminated. However, repeats

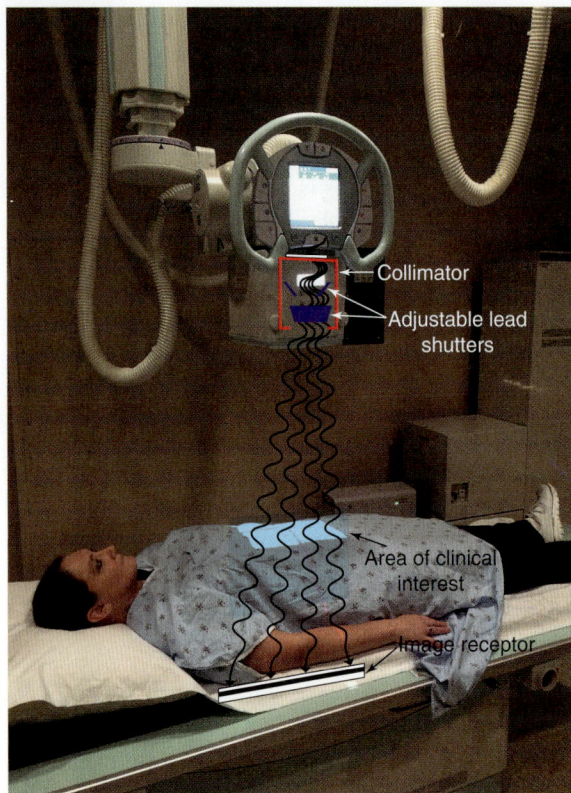

Fig. 12.1 Radiographic beam collimation (restricting the x-ray beam to the area of clinical interest) limits the production of scattered radiation. This radiation-control procedure helps keep the radiographer's occupational exposure as low as reasonably achievable (ALARA).

necessitated by mispositioning can still occur, causing additional radiation exposure to both the patient and possibly the radiographer. The radiographer must take the needed time to accurately position the patient prior to the exposure.

The Patient as a Source of Scattered Radiation

During any diagnostic x-ray examination, the patient becomes a source of scattered radiation as a consequence of the Compton interaction process. At a 90-degree angle to the primary x-ray beam, at a distance of 1 m, the scattered x-ray intensity is generally approximately 1/1000th of the intensity of the primary x-ray beam. This characteristic should always be kept in mind as an additional method of radiation protection.

Scattered Radiation—Occupational Hazard

Because scattered radiation poses the most significant occupational hazard in diagnostic radiology, the use of any device or imaging technique that lessens the amount of scattered radiation will significantly reduce occupational exposure of diagnostic imaging personnel. Beam constraint devices, such as automatic collimation, or positive beam limitation, restrict the dimensions of the radiographic beam so that its margins do not extend beyond the image receptor. This reduction in beam size decreases the number of x-ray photons available to undergo Compton scatter. Because scatter is reduced, the radiographer's potential for occupational exposure is decreased.

Filtration of the Diagnostic X-Ray Beam

When a radiographic beam is adequately filtered, non-useful low-energy photons are removed from the primary beam. Without proper filtration, a relatively high percentage of the customarily excluded low-energy photons will interact with the tissues of the patient's body. Some of these photons undergo Compton scatter. The radiographer's EqD could, therefore, increase as a result of exposure to this excess scattered radiation. Most of these low-energy photons, however, are absorbed in the patient, thereby increasing the patient's absorbed dose and contributing no useful diagnostic information to the image. Thus, filtration primarily benefits the patient.

Protective Apparel

Protective lead aprons (Fig. 12.2A) and, in their absence, shielded barriers (Fig. 12.2B) function as gonadal shields for diagnostic imaging personnel. These devices protect personnel from scatter and leakage radiation, which are types of secondary radiation.

Similar to protective gloves that are used to cover the hands of radiologists or radiographers when they must be in or near the primary x-ray beam, lead aprons are available in various thicknesses such as 0.25, 0.5, and 1 mm of lead equivalent.[2] Higher lead equivalents in protective apparel provide greater protection from radiation exposure. However, for practical use in the clinical setting, the weight of the garment and the approximate length of time that it will be worn must also be considered. An apron containing 1 mm lead equivalent may weigh as much as 12 kg.[2] Wearing this protective device for a lengthy procedure can, therefore, result in

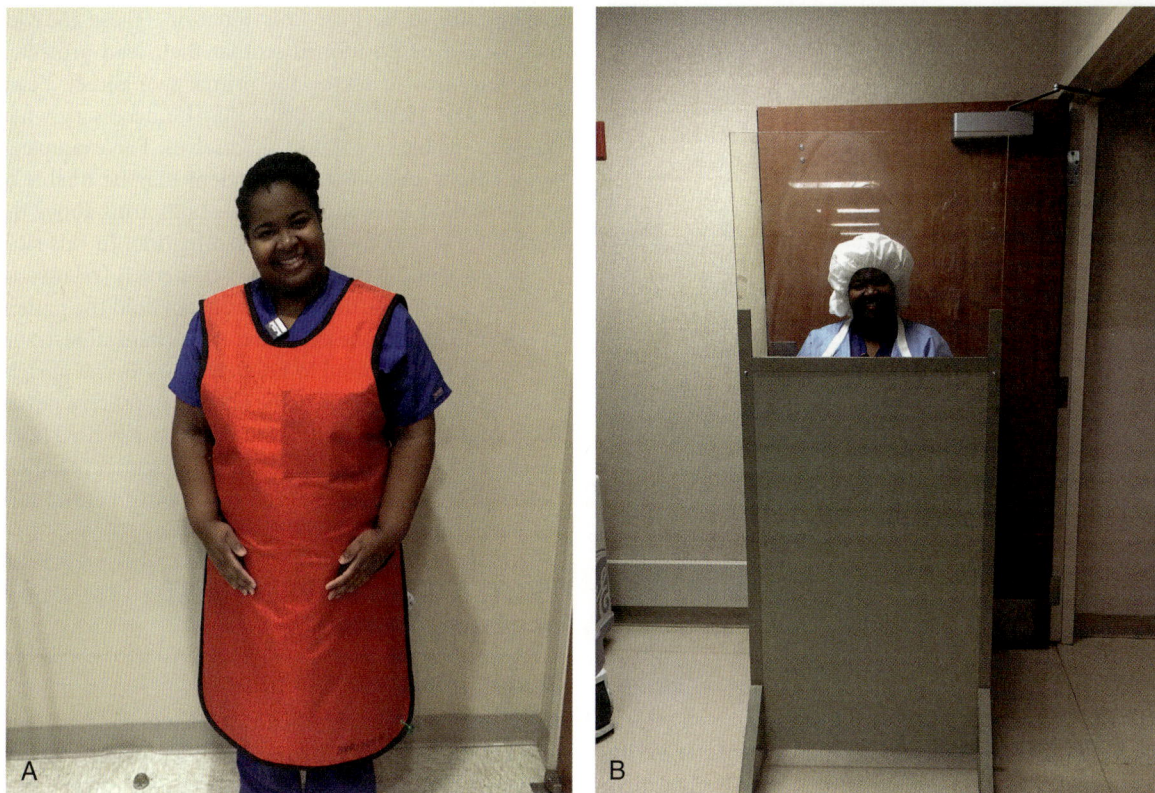

Fig. 12.2 (A) A lead apron protects occupationally exposed personnel from scattered radiation. (B) A lead mobile x-ray barrier of 0.5 or 1.0 mm lead equivalent provides protection from scattered radiation. It may be used during special procedures, in the operating room, and in cardiac units.

considerable back strain.* Depending on the energy range of the radiation for a specific procedure, an apron containing the lead equivalent of 0.5 mm or an apron containing the minimum required lead equivalent of 0.25 mm may be sufficient for use. The standard 0.5 mm lead equivalent apron, which has traditionally been worn during routine fluoroscopic procedures, weighs 3 to 7 kg. In contrast, the 0.25 mm minimum lead equivalent apron can weigh 1 to 5 kg.[2] Some physical attributes of protective lead aprons, including the percentage of x-ray

attenuation at selective peak kilovoltages (kVps), are listed in Table 12.1.

If any personnel could have the posterior surface of their body turned toward the x-ray source during a radiologic procedure, a *wraparound style apron* would be desirable to afford the best protection. When taking into consideration both the amount of protection provided by an apron and its weight, the 0.5 mm lead equivalent apron provides a good compromise for general use.

All protective apparel must be stored correctly when not in use to preserve the integrity of the garment. Lead aprons should be hung on racks or draped over a bar designed for storage to prevent unnecessary damage. They are never to be folded or crunched up in any fashion because this will lead to cracks or breaks in the lead-impregnated material, thereby compromising the device's effectiveness for protection from radiation. Regulatory requirements state that all aprons be

---

*To reduce the possibility of back or neck problems, other materials may be used in the protective apron to lessen its weight. Some garments, for example, are impregnated with tin[2] or similar metals because the electron shell structures of these substances offer advantages in terms of a more probable photoelectric interaction attenuation than does lead in the lower diagnostic x-ray energy range.

TABLE 12.1 Physical Attributes of Protective Lead Aprons

| | | PERCENTAGE X-RAY ATTENUATION | | |
| | | | KILOVOLTS AT PEAK | |
Lead Equivalent Thickness (mm)	Weight (kg)	50	75	100
0.25	1–5	97	66	51
0.50	3–7	99.9	88	75
1.00	5–12	99.9	99	94

At 100 kVp, x-ray attenuation for a 0.50-mm lead equivalent apron and a 1-mm lead equivalent apron is 75% and 94%, respectively.

Modified from Bushong SC: *Radiologic science for technologists: physics, biology and protection*, ed 12, St. Louis, 2021, Elsevier.

inspected annually for cracks or other defects either by fluoroscopy or by imaging the apparel with a high kVp technique.

Technical Exposure Factors

Technical exposure factors can influence the quantity of scattered radiation produced and thereby reaching imaging personnel. For lower kVps, more mA is needed to secure a high-quality image, and therefore more significant amounts of low-energy photons are present. These characteristics of the x-ray beam lend themselves to the production of increased large-angle scatter radiation. Conversely, higher kVp techniques:

- Increase the mean energy of the photons comprising the radiographic beam, leading to a decrease in large angle scatter
- Require lower incident photon beam intensity (i.e., lower milliampere-seconds [mAs])

Therefore with higher selected kVp values, less side-scattered radiation is available to strike imaging personnel, and the potential EqD is reduced.

Patient Restraint

Radiographers must *never* stand in the primary (useful) beam to restrain a patient during a radiographic exposure (Fig. 12.3A). When patient restraint is necessary, mechanical restraining devices should be used to immobilize the patient whenever possible. If mechanical means of restraint are not feasible, nonoccupationally exposed persons, wearing appropriate protective apparel, are to perform this function. These individuals should be positioned so that their lead-protected torsos are not struck by the primary, or direct, beam (Fig. 12.3B). Holding patients may be necessary when they are unable to support themselves. For example, a weak elderly male or female patient may be unable to stand without assistance and raise both arms above the head for a lateral chest x-ray examination. In this situation, a nonoccupationally exposed person (relative or friend) equipped with a lead apron can hold the patient in position during the exposure. A mechanical restraining device is often used to hold an infant in the upright position for chest images to be obtained. If such a device is not available, the child has to be physically held (usually by a parent) during the exposure. Pregnant women, however, are never to be permitted to assist in holding a patient at that time.

PROTECTION FOR PREGNANT PERSONNEL

Imaging Department Protocol

Pregnant staff members should be able to continue performing their duties without interruption of employment if they follow established radiation safety practices. Most health care facilities have policies for protecting pregnant personnel from radiation. Under these policies, an imaging professional who becomes pregnant first informs her supervisor. After this voluntary declaration has been made, the health care facility officially recognizes the pregnancy. The facility, through its radiation safety officer:

- Provides essential counseling
- Furnishes an appropriate additional radiation dosimeter for monitoring of any possible radiation exposure to the embryo-fetus

This additional dosimeter is to be worn at the waist level during all radiation procedures. When a protective lead apron is used, the dosimeter should be worn at waist level beneath the apron. The purpose of this additional monitor is to ensure that the monthly EqD to the embryo-fetus does not exceed 0.5 mSv. This EqD limit excludes:

- Medical radiation
- Natural background radiation

This practice is designed to significantly lower the total lifetime risk of leukemia and other malignancies in persons exposed in utero.

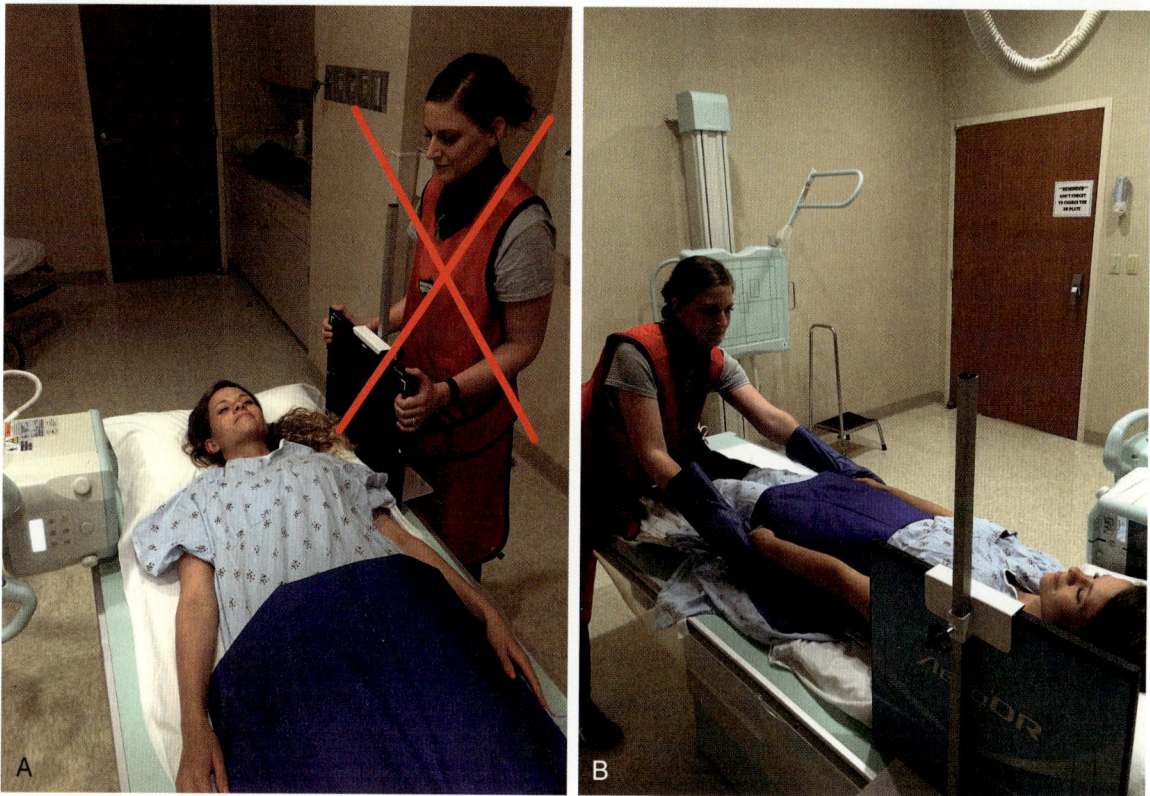

Fig. 12.3 (A) The radiographer should never stand in the primary (useful) beam to restrain the patient. (B) A nonoccupationally exposed person restraining a patient during a radiographic exposure should wear a lead apron, gloves, and thyroid shield and stand outside the primary beam.

Acknowledgment of Counseling and Understanding of Radiation Safety Measures

After receiving radiation safety counseling, the pregnant radiologic technologist must read and sign a form acknowledging that she has received counseling and understands the practices to be followed to ensure the safety of the embryo-fetus. For monitoring of pregnant personnel, a separate monthly report is provided to specifically document the exposure of the worker and the embryo-fetus. A copy of this report is sent to the facility's radiation safety officer.

Protective Maternity Apparel

Protective maternity apparel, when needed, should be available for pregnant radiologists and radiographers. Specially designed maternity protective aprons consist of 0.5 mm lead equivalent over their entire length and width. They have an extra 1 mm lead equivalent

protective panel that runs transversely across the width of the apron to provide added safety for the embryo-fetus.

Wraparound protective aprons of 0.5 mm lead equivalent can also be used during pregnancy. The overall physical size of the apron must be appropriate for the pregnant worker to ensure safety and provide reasonable comfort.

Work Schedule Alteration

In accordance with ALARA guidelines, work schedules are designed to distribute radiation exposure risk evenly to all employees. If a declared pregnant radiographer is reassigned to a lower radiation exposure risk area (e.g., removed from interventional fluoroscopy and assigned to general radiography), then the remaining radiographers in the higher-risk area who must fill in can be subject to increased risk. Therefore the declared pregnant radiographer does not necessarily need to be reassigned to a lower radiation exposure position as a direct consequence of a declared pregnancy. However, it is imperative that, while remaining in her current position, the EqD to the embryo-fetus does not exceed the NCRP recommended monthly EqD limit of 0.5 mSv or a total of 5.0 mSv during the entire pregnancy.

BASIC PRINCIPLES OF RADIATION PROTECTION FOR PERSONNEL EXPOSURE REDUCTION

As previously stated, the three basic principles of radiation protection are:

- Time
- Distance
- Shielding

Occupational radiation exposure of imaging personnel can be minimized by the use of these cardinal principles.

Time

The amount of radiation a worker receives at a particular location is directly proportional to the length of time the individual is in the path of ionizing radiation. During fluoroscopy, the reduced exposure time will decrease both:

- Patient exposure
- Personnel exposure

For this reason, fluoroscopic x-ray units are equipped with 5 minute timers to alert the radiologist or other authorized equipment operator that a specific amount of time has elapsed. To minimize radiation exposure, a radiographer should be present in a fluoroscopy room only when needed to perform appropriate patient care and to fulfill the duties associated with the procedure. Otherwise, the radiographer should remain behind a protective barrier.

Distance

Distance is the most effective means of protection from ionizing radiation. Because there is a significant decrease in the radiation level as a consequence of the dispersion or spread of the radiation beam with distance, imaging personnel will receive significantly less radiation exposure by standing farther away from a source of radiation.

Application of the inverse square law. When light is emitted from a source, such as a flashlight, the intensity

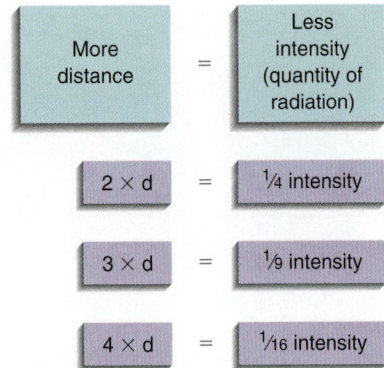

Fig. 12.4 As the distance between the source of radiation and any given measurement point increases, radiation intensity (quantity) measured at that point decreases by the square of the relative change in distance between the new location and the old.

decreases quickly with the distance from the source. X-rays act in the same manner, as the distance from the source increases, the intensity decreases. The **inverse square law (ISL)** expresses the relationship between distance and intensity (quantity) of radiation and is an important tool for limiting the dose received by personnel. The law is simply stated as: "The intensity of radiation is inversely proportional to the square of the distance from the source."

To be more explicit, as the distance between the radiation source and a measurement point increases, the intensity, or quantity of radiation measured at the more distant position decreases by the square of the ratio of the original distance from the source to the new distance from the source (Fig. 12.4). This lowering of radiation intensity physically occurs because the total x-rays emitted are spread over *a new area that has increased by the square of the relative distance change.* For example, when the distance from the x-ray target, a point source* of

---

*Point source: To correctly treat finite-sized radioactive sources as "point sources" so as to facilitate the calculation of exposure rates at points of interest, it is necessary that the distance of such points from the radioactive source be at least equal to 10 times the largest dimension of the source. As an example of this concept, consider a spherical radioactive source whose diameter is 2.5 cm. Then the smallest distance away from this source at which it may be accurate enough to regard it mathematically as a "point source" will be 25 cm.

radiation, is doubled, the radiation at the new location spans an area four times larger than the original area. However, because the same amount of radiation exists to cover this larger area, the intensity at the new distance consequently decreases by a factor of four (Fig. 12.5).

The formula for ISL is shown in the equation in Box 12.2. A mathematical example is also provided. The inverse square law should be used whenever possible to reduce the radiographer's exposure from sources of x-radiation. (This law also may be applied to sources of gamma and neutron radiation.)

Conversely, the ISL also implies that if a radiographer moves closer to a source of radiation, this individual's radiation exposure can dramatically increase. For example, if the radiographer stands 2 m away from an x-ray source instead of 6 m away, the radiographer's radiation exposure increases by a factor of $(6/2)^2 = 9$.

Shielding

When it is not possible to use the principles of time and/or distance to minimize occupational radiation exposure, **shielding** of appropriate thickness may be used to provide adequate protection from radiation. The most common materials used for structural protective barriers are:

- Lead
- Concrete

Accessory protective devices are made of lead-impregnated vinyl. These accessory devices include:

- Aprons
- Gloves
- Thyroid shields
- Protective eyeglasses

This apparel is to be used when it is not possible to remain wholly behind either a stationary or movable protective barrier. The ability of materials to attenuate radiation depends on their atomic number, density, and thickness.

Protective Structural Shielding. Structural barriers such as walls and doors in an x-ray room have been designed to provide radiation shielding for both:

- Imaging department personnel
- The general public

These barriers are necessary to ensure that occupational and nonoccupational annual EfD limits are not exceeded. Lead impregnated drywalls of appropriate thickness are used in the walls of the radiography

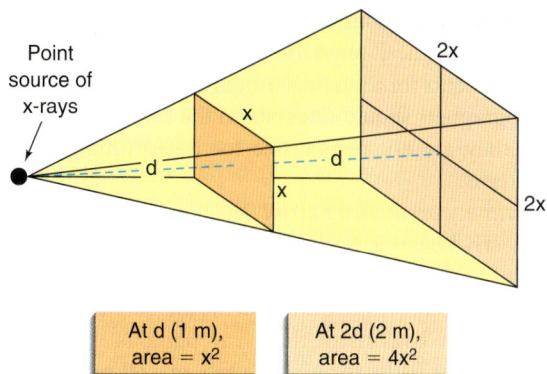

| At d (1 m), area = x^2 | At 2d (2 m), area = $4x^2$ |

Fig. 12.5 When the distance from a point source of radiation is doubled, the radiation at the new location spans an area four times larger than the original area. However, the intensity at the new distance is only one-fourth of the original intensity.

BOX 12.2 Inverse Square Law Formula and Example

$$\frac{I_1}{I_2} = \frac{(d_2)^2}{(d_1)^2}$$

where I_1 expresses the exposure (intensity) at the original distance, I_2 expresses the exposure (intensity) at the new distance, d_1 expresses the original distance from the source of radiation, and d_2 expresses the new distance from the source of radiation.

Example: If a radiographer stands 1 m away from an x-ray tube and is subject to an exposure rate dose* of 2 mGya per hour, what will it be if the same radiographer moves to a position located 2 m from the x-ray tube?

Answer:

$$\frac{I_1}{I_2} = \frac{(d_2)^2}{(d_1)^2}$$

$$\frac{2}{I_2} = \frac{(2)^2}{(1)^2}$$

$$\frac{2}{I_2} = \frac{4}{1} \text{ (Cross-multiply)}$$

$$4I_2 = 2$$

$$I_2 = 0.5 \text{ mGy}_a/\text{hr}$$

*Exposure rate dose, given in units of mGya per hour, is the same quantity as air kerma rate.

or fluoroscopy room to provide adequate shielding. A qualified medical physicist determines the exact lead requirements for a particular imaging facility. Although radiographers should understand the concept of shielding, they are not responsible for determining barrier thickness.

Primary protective barrier. The purpose of a **primary protective barrier** is to prevent direct, or unscattered, radiation from reaching personnel or members of the general public on the other side of the barrier. The primary beam consists of the x-ray photons that follow straight-line paths through all sets of collimator shutters. Primary protective barriers are located perpendicular to the undeflected line of travel of the x-ray beam (Fig. 12.6).

If the peak energy of the beam is 120 kVp, the primary protective barrier in a typical installation:

- Contains of 1.6 mm (1/16 inch) lead
- Extends 2.1 m upward from the floor of the x-ray room, when the x-ray tube is 1.5 to 2.1 m from the wall in question

Secondary protective barrier. Secondary radiation consists of radiation that has been deflected from the primary beam. Leakage from the tube housing (photons that pass through the housing) and scatter (primarily from the patient) make up the secondary radiation. A **secondary protective barrier** protects against leakage and scatter radiation. Any wall or barrier that is never struck by the primary x-ray beam is classified as a secondary barrier (see Fig. 12.6). This does not mean that secondary radiation cannot strike primary barriers as well. A secondary barrier should overlap the primary protective barrier by approximately 1.3 cm (1/2 inch). In a typical installation, the secondary barrier consists of 0.8 mm (1/32 inch) of lead.

Radiographic and fluoroscopic exposures should be made only when the doors to x-ray rooms are closed. This practice affords a substantial degree of protection for persons in areas adjacent to the room door because in most facilities room doors have attenuation for diagnostic energy x-rays equivalent to that provided by 0.8 mm (1/32 inch) of lead.

Control-booth barrier. X-ray rooms housing permanent radiographic equipment contain a **control-booth barrier** for the protection of the radiographer. This barrier must:

- Extend at least 2.1 m upward from the floor
- Be permanently secured to the floor

Diagnostic x-rays should scatter a minimum of two times before reaching any area behind this barrier. Because this booth is situated so that it intercepts leakage and scattered radiation only, it may be regarded as a secondary protective barrier. To ensure maximum protection during radiographic exposures, personnel must remain *entirely* behind the barrier. The radiographer may observe the patient through the lead glass window* in the booth (Fig. 12.7). This window typically consists of 1.5 mm (1/16-inch) lead equivalent. With the appropriate degree of shielding in the barrier, the radiographer's exposure will not exceed a maximum allowance of 1 mSv (100 mrem) per week; in actual practice in a well-designed

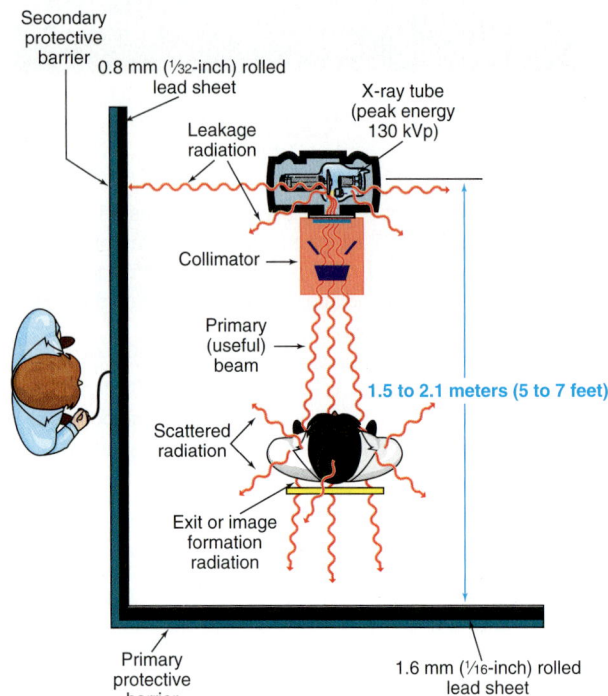

Fig. 12.6 Protective barriers are lined with lead to protect personnel and the general public from radiation. The primary protective barrier is located perpendicular to the undeflected line of travel of the x-ray beam. The walls that are not in the direct line of travel of the primary beam are called *secondary protective barriers* because they are designed to shield only against secondary (leakage and scattered) radiation.

---

*The wall barrier of the control booth should be at least 46 cm (18 inches) beyond the edge of the view window.

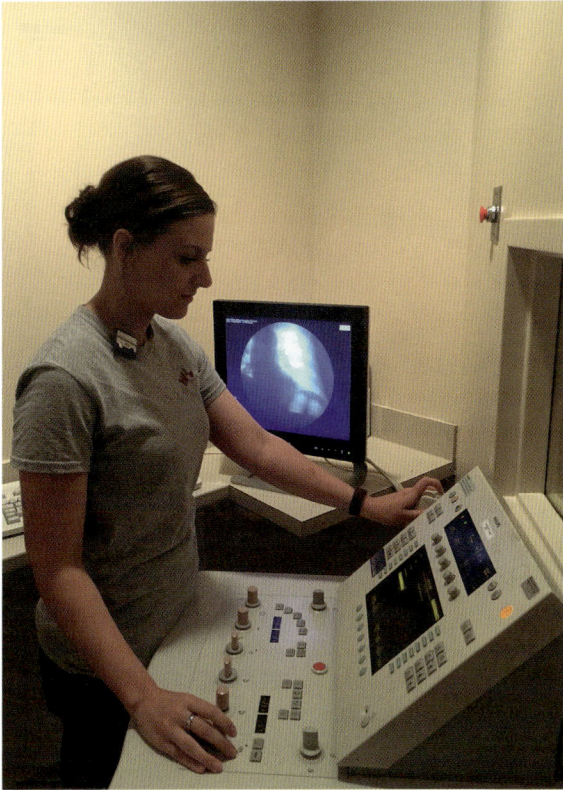

Fig. 12.7 While making a radiographic exposure with a stationary radiographic unit, the radiographer must remain completely within the control-booth barrier (behind the fixed protective barrier) for safety. The radiographer may observe the patient through the lead glass observation window in the control booth.

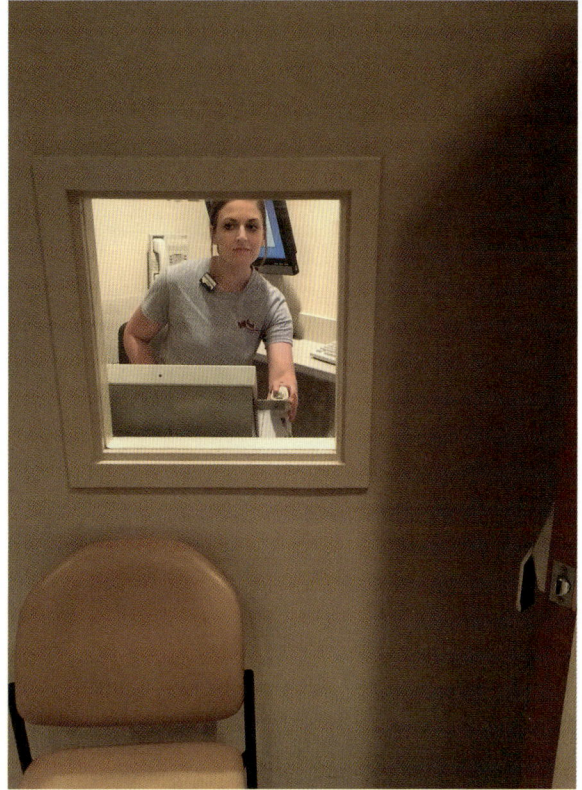

Fig. 12.8 A clear lead acrylic secondary protective barrier impregnated with approximately 30% lead lends a modern appearance to the facility.

facility, exposure should not exceed 0.02 mSv (2 mrem) per week. For further protection, the exposure cord, if one is present, must be short enough that the exposure switch can be operated only when the radiographer is completely behind the control-booth barrier.

Clear lead–acrylic secondary protective barrier. Clear lead–acrylic material impregnated with approximately 30% lead by weight may be fashioned into an effective secondary protective barrier, such as for the control booth (Fig. 12.8). This creates a modern appearance for the facility and permits a panoramic view, allowing diagnostic imaging personnel to observe the patient more completely. *Modular* or movable x-ray barriers:

- Are shatter-resistant
- Can extend 2.1 m upward from the floor
- Are available in lead equivalency from 0.3 to 2 mm

Clear lead–acrylic overhead protective barrier. Clear lead–acrylic protective barriers also can be used as overhead x-ray barriers providing an open view during special procedures and cardiac catheterization (Fig. 12.9). This shielding typically offers 0.5 mm lead equivalency protection.

Accessory protective devices. Accessory protective shielding includes aprons, gloves, and thyroid shields made of lead-impregnated vinyl. These protective garments are available in a variety of:

- Shapes
- Sizes
- Thicknesses

As lead equivalent thickness increases, attenuation of the x-ray beam also increases when kVp remains the same.

Requirements for lead aprons and gloves. If the radiographer's hands will be near the x-ray beam, leaded gloves should be used. A suitable lead apron is to be

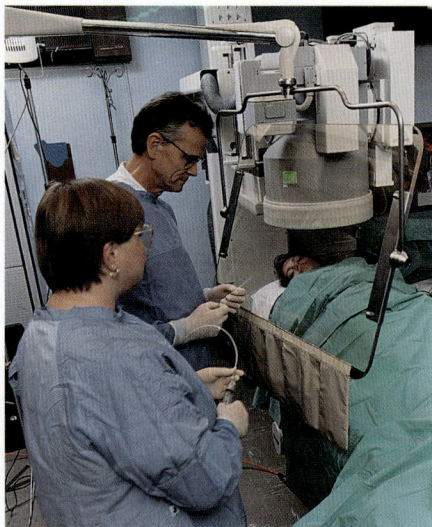

Fig. 12.9 A clear lead acrylic overhead protective barrier used during special procedures and cardiac catheterization. (From Fluke Biomedical.)

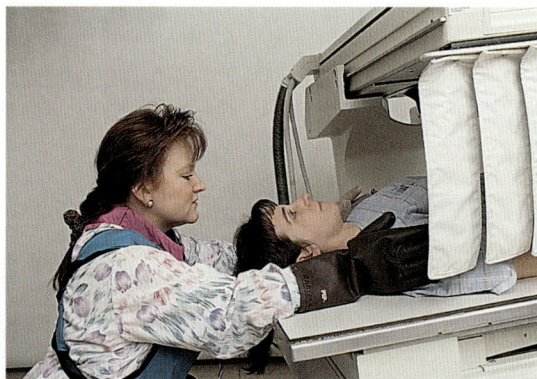

Fig. 12.10 A lead apron, gloves, and thyroid shield protect the radiographer from scattered radiation.

worn whenever the radiographer cannot remain behind a protective barrier during an exposure (Fig. 12.10). Historically, from regulatory doctrine, if the peak energy of the x-ray beam was 100 kVp, then a protective apron's attenuation must be equivalent to at least a 0.25 mm thickness of lead. An apron of 0.5 mm lead equivalent, however, affords much higher security and is the most widely used and recommended thickness in diagnostic imaging and is the minimum lead equivalent required for a protective garment worn by occupationally exposed individuals during fluoroscopic or interventional procedures. Regardless of the regulatory mention of 0.25 mm thicknesses of lead for some purposes, the need for 0.5 mm lead equivalent for fluoroscopy and interventional cases and the recommendations that 0.5 mm lead aprons are desirable for all purposes have prompted most facilities to stock 0.5 mm lead aprons only. This eliminates the possibility of personnel inadvertently selecting the wrong apron. Therefore 0.5 mm has become the all-purpose apron of choice and in many cases, should also be in a wraparound style. A lead apron with 0.25 mm of lead is, however, very appropriate for use in mammography.

Neck and thyroid shield. A neck and thyroid shield (Fig. 12.11) are employed to guard the thyroid area of occupationally exposed personnel during:

• General fluoroscopy
• X-ray special procedures

The neck and thyroid shield should be a minimum of 0.5 mm lead equivalent.

Protective eyeglasses. Scatter radiation to the lens of the eyes of diagnostic imaging personnel can be substantially reduced by the use of protective eyeglasses (Fig. 12.12), fitted with optically clear lenses that contain a minimal lead equivalent protection level of 0.35 mm. Side shields on the glasses are also available and useful for procedures that require turning of the head. A wraparound frame containing optically clear lenses with 0.5 mm lead equivalent may also be acquired.

X-RAY TUBE HOUSING CABLES

While the x-ray tube housing is massive enough to provide a significant degree of shielding from secondary radiation, it is also designed to protect the operator from the hazard of electric shock. Because of this, the radiographer must be both observant* and careful when handling this piece of equipment and its adjoining part, the collimator. While manipulating the tube housing assembly for a radiographic examination, the radiographer should avoid rough handling or severely bending the high-tension cables that connect to the positive and negative terminals of the x-ray tube. *No one should ever touch the tube housing or high-tension cables while a radiographic exposure is in progress.*

---

*Observant means looking at the physical condition of the cables and cable coverings to discern undue wear or stress effects that could lead to a serious hazard.

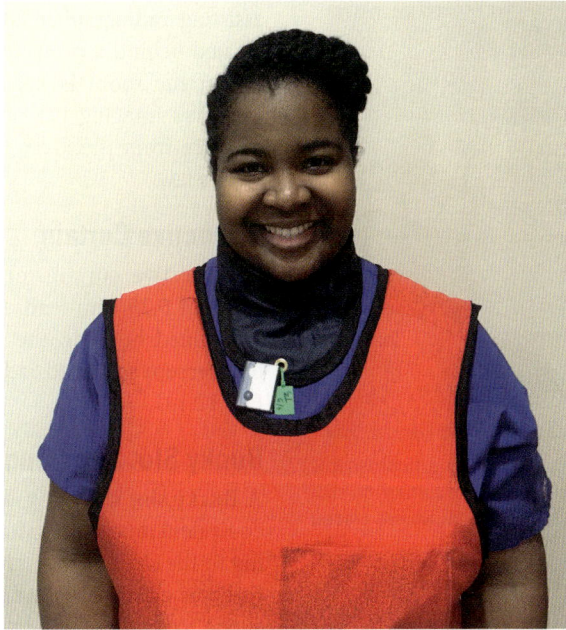

Fig. 12.11 The neck and thyroid gland can be protected from radiation exposure through the use of a 0.5-mm lead equivalent protective shield.

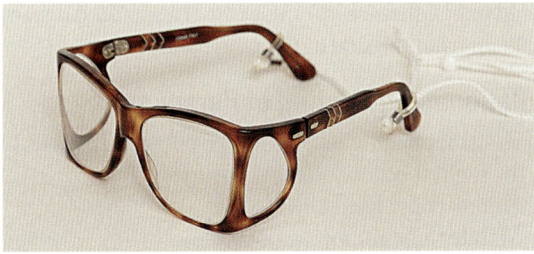

Fig. 12.12 Eyeglasses protect the lens of the eyes during general fluoroscopy and special procedures. (Shown are glasses with wraparound frames; other styles are also available.)

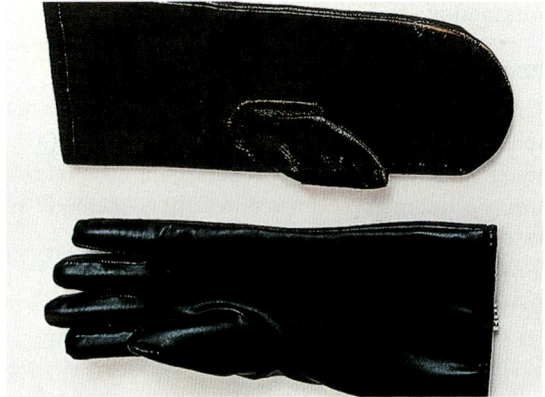

Fig. 12.13 Lead gloves.

PROTECTION DURING FLUOROSCOPIC PROCEDURES

Personnel Protection

To ensure protection from scattered radiation emanating from the patient during a fluoroscopic examination, the radiographer should:

- Stand as far away from the patient as is practical
- Move closer to the patient only when assistance is required

A protective apron of at least 0.5 mm lead equivalent must be worn during all fluoroscopic procedures.

Protective lead gloves of at least 0.25 mm lead equivalent should be worn whenever the hands must be placed near the fluoroscopic field (Fig. 12.13). Imaging personnel assisting during a fluoroscopic examination also should wear thyroid shields of 0.5 mm lead equivalent, especially if they are standing close to the patient being examined (Fig. 12.14). If immediate assistance during a fluoroscopic examination is not required, the radiographer should either stand behind the radiologist, who is also wearing protective

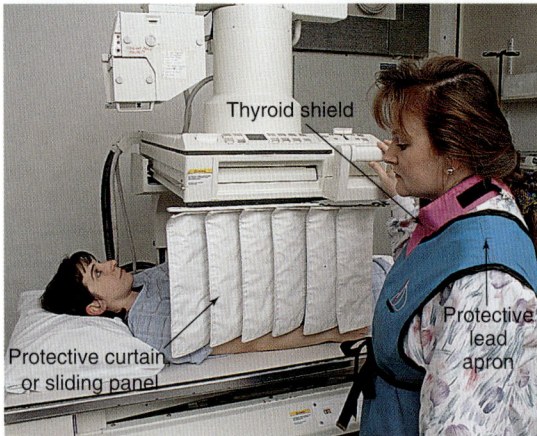

Fig. 12.14 Scattered radiation produced during a fluoroscopic examination can be absorbed by a protective curtain or sliding panel, with a minimum of 0.25 mm lead equivalent placed between the fluoroscopist and the patient.

apparel, or stand behind the control-booth barrier until services are required. A wrap-around protective apron is recommended to protect personnel who must move around the x-ray room during a fluoroscopic examination.

Dose-Reduction Techniques

Many of the methods and devices that reduce the radiographer's exposure when operating stationary (fixed) radiographic equipment also reduce the dose received during a fluoroscopic procedure. These methods and devices include:

- Adequate beam collimation
- Adequate filtration
- Control of technical exposure factors
- Appropriate source-to-skin distance
- Diagnostic-type protective x-ray tube housing

To ensure adequate protection for both the radiographer and the radiologist, some additional requirements are included in the federal government specifications for the use of fluoroscopic equipment. An example is use of a cumulative timing device that produces an audible signal after 5 minutes of total beam-on time has been exceeded.

Remote-Control Fluoroscopic Systems

The remote-control unit provides imaging personnel with the best radiation protection opportunity. Remote-control systems permit the radiologist, and assisting radiographer, to remain at a control console located behind a protective barrier until their presence within the room is needed. This system also further improves imaging personnel safety because the added distance from the x-ray tube makes use of the inverse square law.

Protective Curtain

A protective curtain, or sliding panel, with a minimum of 0.25 mm lead equivalent should typically be positioned between the fluoroscopist and the patient to intercept scattered radiation above the tabletop (see Fig. 12.14).

Bucky Slot Shielding Device

A Bucky slot shielding device of at least 0.25 mm lead equivalent must automatically cover the Bucky slot opening in the side of the x-ray table during a standard fluoroscopic examination when the Bucky tray is positioned at the foot end of the table (Fig. 12.15). This shielding device protects the radiologist and radiographer at the gonadal level. Without this device and the protective curtain in place, the exposure dose rate to the fluoroscopist could markedly exceed 1 mGya/hr at a standard distance of 0.6 m from the side of the x-ray table.

Rotational Scheduling of Personnel

Diagnostic imaging personnel are potentially subjected to the highest occupational exposure during:

- Fluoroscopy: fixed and mobile
- Mobile radiography
- Special procedures
- Interventional surgery

Scheduling radiographers to spend less time in these higher radiation tasks by arranging assignments to clinical areas in a rotational pattern can decrease this exposure. This practice, therefore, uses the cardinal safety principle of *time* as a means of additional radiation protection.

PROTECTION DURING MOBILE X-RAY EXAMINATIONS

Use of Protective Garments

Mobile radiographic systems create special radiation protection considerations for the radiographer. Some states require radiographers to wear lead aprons whenever they are performing mobile radiographic or

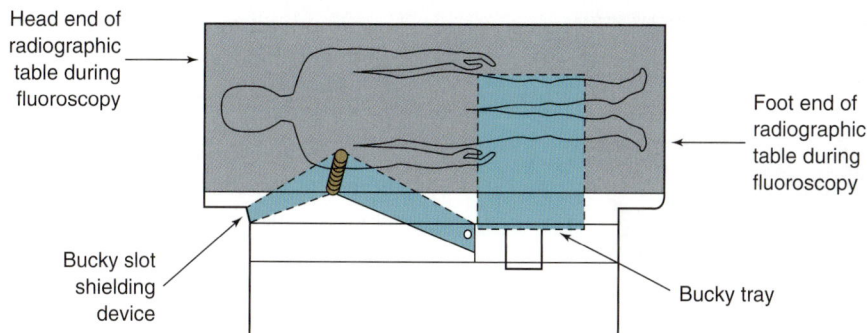

Fig. 12.15 To provide protection at the gonadal level for the fluoroscopist, the Bucky slot shielding device should be at least 0.25 mm lead equivalent.

fluoroscopic examinations. A protective apron should be assigned to each mobile unit so that it is immediately available for the radiographer.

Distance as a Means of Protection

The most recent mobile units are equipped with a remote-control exposure device. This permits the radiographer to leave the immediate vicinity and uses the cardinal principle of *distance* as an effective means of protection from radiation. Most mobile units are not remotely controlled. For those units the cord leading to the exposure switch must be long enough to permit the radiographer to stand at least 2 m from the:

- Patient
- X-ray tube
- Useful beam

If possible, the radiographer should also attempt to stand at a right angle (90 degrees) to the x-ray beam–scattering object (the patient) line. This is the location at which the least amount of scattered radiation is received (Fig. 12.16). However, because distance and shielding have much more influence on the reduction of exposure to the technologist, those factors should be addressed first.

PROTECTION DURING C-ARM FLUOROSCOPY

Personnel Exposure Resulting From Scattered Radiation

Safety procedures are particularly important when mobile fluoroscopy (C-arm) systems are used. Because patterns of exposure direction are less predictable and the equipment is frequently operated by physicians

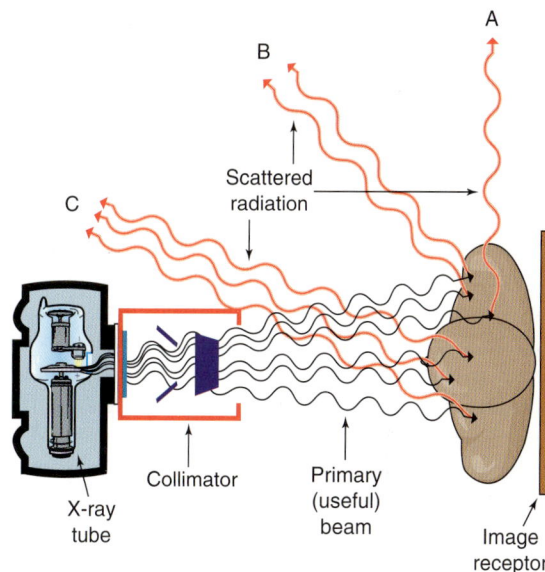

Fig. 12.16 When the protective factors of distance and shielding have been accounted for, the radiographer will receive the least amount of scattered radiation by standing at a right angle (90 degrees) to the scattering object (the patient) (in position *A*). The most scattered radiation would be received at point *C* because of backscatter coming from the patient. (Intensity, or quantity, of x-ray exposure at any given point is indicated in this picture by the number of scattered x-rays reaching that point.)

whose training and experience in radiation safety may not match those of an experienced radiologist, the radiographer should exercise special vigilance. For C-arm devices with similar fields of view, the dose rate for personnel located within a meter of the patient is comparable to that in routine fluoroscopy—approximately several milligray in air (mGya) per hour. The

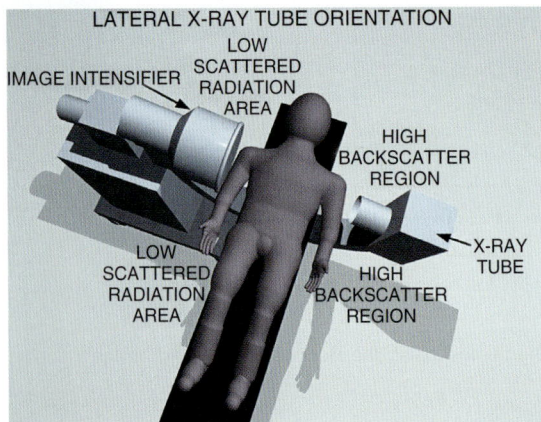

Fig. 12.17 Cross-table exposure during use of a C-arm fluoroscope. The exposure rate caused by scatter near the entrance surface of the patient (the x-ray tube side) exceeds the exposure rate caused by scatter near the exit surface of the patient (the image intensifier side). The location of lower potential scatter dose is on the side of the patient away from the x-ray tube (i.e., the image intensifier side). (From Mark Rzeszotarski.)

exposure of personnel is primarily caused by radiation scattered from the patient. During operating room procedures in which cross-table exposures are used (Fig. 12.17), an understanding of the patterns of x-ray scatter is particularly useful. The exposure rate caused by scatter near the entrance surface of the patient (the x-ray tube side) exceeds the exposure rate caused by scatter near the exit surface of the patient (the image intensifier side). The difference in the amount of scatter, typically a factor of 2 or 3, is caused by the higher radiation intensity at the entrance surface of the patient. Thus, the location of the lower potential scatter dose is on the side of the patient away from the x-ray tube (i.e., the image intensifier side). The radiographer should never encounter the actual useful beam.

Need for Protective Apparel for all Personnel and Monitoring of Imaging Personnel

The C-arm fluoroscope can be manipulated into almost any position and remain energized for lengthy periods to accommodate, for example, an orthopedic surgeon performing an open reduction of a fractured hip in the operating room or a vascular surgeon performing an interventional procedure. When radiographers and other medical personnel participate in procedures that require this unit to be energized for significant durations,

they are subject to increased radiation exposure. Also, the physical configuration of a C-arm fluoroscopic unit limits the methods that can be used to achieve protection from scattered radiation. For this reason, personnel who routinely operate a C-arm fluoroscope or those who are in the immediate area of the unit when it is energized must wear a lead apron instead of crowding behind a portable lead–acrylic shield. This garment should be 0.5 mm lead equivalent to ensure adequate protection. A neck and thyroid shield of 0.5 mm lead equivalent should also be worn. Appropriate monitoring of imaging personnel who are typically involved in C-arm fluoroscopic procedures is mandatory.

Positioning of the C-Arm Fluoroscope

The positioning of a C-arm fluoroscope influences the radiation exposure to the patient and the radiographer. From the perspective of increased radiation safety, it is best to reverse the C-arm to place the x-ray tube under the table and the image intensifier over the table (see Fig. 10.23).

Exposure Reduction for Personnel

At the start of each procedure, the unit's cumulative timer should be reset to zero so that it will be possible to be aware of the actual beam-on time.[3] When an image storage device (e.g., last image hold) is used, beam-on time decreases, and therefore exposure reduction increases. If the image intensifier (II) is positioned as close to the patient as possible, the required fluoroscopic x-ray beam intensity is minimized. This equipment–patient arrangement also permits the image intensifier to function more effectively as a scatter barrier between the patient and the person operating the C-arm fluoroscope. All these methods can lead to significant exposure reduction to both personnel and patient.

During a C-arm procedure, it is imperative that the patient's anatomic region of interest be oriented correctly, with minimal use of "positioning" the fluoroscope.[3] Furthermore, collimating the x-ray beam to the smallest anatomical area possible will decrease the amount of scattered radiation produced from the interaction of the x-ray beam with the patient, the actual scattering object.

Because distance from the source of radiation is the simplest method of protection for occupationally exposed personnel, C-arm operators should use it to their advantage whenever possible. Usually, this can be accomplished by using the foot pedal or the hand-held exposure switch, with the cables extended away from the machine as far as possible when making x-ray exposures.

For better visualization of small body parts, C-arm fluoroscopes can magnify the image. However, the use of magnification usually requires higher mA, which produces additional radiation exposure. *Mag mode* should be used only upon request by the physician performing the procedure.[3]

PROTECTION DURING HIGH-LEVEL CONTROL INTERVENTIONAL PROCEDURES

Increased Importance of Radiation Safety Technique

All of the previously mentioned standard precautions and procedures for the reduction of dose to personnel are applicable during *interventional* procedures. Here, these techniques take on increased importance because of the extended length of some of these procedures, the large number of digital images that may be taken, and, in particular studies, the frequent use of the high-level control (boost) mode of operation. In boost mode, the exposure rate may significantly exceed the rate used in routine fluoroscopy (e.g., maximum allowed entrance exposure rate dose to a patient in regular fluoroscopy is 8.8 cGY/minute [or 10 R/min exposure rate], whereas in high-level or boost mode this value can range upward to 20 to 40 cGy/minute).

Knowledge of Dose Reduction Techniques Required by the Radiographer

Although the duration of the procedure and the number of the exposures taken are under the control of the radiologist or other interventional physician, the radiographer should verify that all dose-reducing features are available and in good working order. These include the presence of:
- High-quality, low-dose fluoroscopy mode
- Pulsed beam operation (e.g., using 7.5, 15, or 30 radiation pulses/second in place of continuous fluoroscopy radiation)
- Manual collimation
- Correct beam filtration

- Removable grids
- Road-mapping*
- Time interval differences[†]
- Last image hold mode

As previously discussed, using the last image hold mode feature, the operator does not need to be exposed again to review the position of a catheter in relation to landmarks when no new information is required. Also, if possible, the patient beam entry side could be changed during the procedure to reduce the total dose to any one area of skin.

High-level control is to be used sparingly and only when increased visualization is necessary during a critical maneuver such as the deployment of stents[4] (tubular support device that can be inserted into a blood vessel, canal, or duct to relieve obstruction). Many standard and C-arm interventional fluoroscopic systems now possess the technical capability for standardized dose structure reporting.[5]

Road-mapping is a method of digital image subtraction in which the frame that contains the greatest amount of contrast material in vessels is identified and is then subtracted from all subsequent images. Live fluoroscopic images of the catheter moving through the vasculature can then be seen even after the vessels contain less contrast. By using this equipment feature, overlaying of two images can be accomplished (e.g., a stored image and a current image). Thus, there is a decrease of procedure time because fewer mask images (*masking* refers to a two-step imaging process that can be used to remove or obscure unwanted areas from the final or useful image by subtracting from a current image an initially or subsequently acquired reference image) are needed. This leads to some reduction in radiation dose. Choosing the road-mapping feature in place of *cineradiography* (a technique in which a camera is used to record continuous images, of nonstationary internal body structures, that are generated during selected intervals [e.g., 10 seconds] of nonstop radiation exposure) can also result in a lower radiation dose.

[†]*Time-interval difference (TID)* is a method of digital image subtraction in which each TID image results from subtracting a previously acquired regular image from one that is a few frames in advance (e.g., if a time-interval difference of five images is chosen, the first TID image to appear will be that obtained when frame one is subtracted from frame six. The second image will contain the subtraction of frame two from frame seven, etc.). This technique progressively reveals vessels containing material and suppresses soft tissue in the images. It is *less sensitive to patient motion* than when the first image is selected as the "mask" or reference image and is then subtracted from all successive images.

These systems automatically furnish reports that yield an equivalent dose record for every examination.

How the Radiologist or Other Interventional Physician Can Reduce Radiation Exposure

The radiologist or other interventional physician can reduce radiation exposure by the following means:

- Decreasing the duration of the procedure, thereby shortening fluoroscopic beam-on time
- Obtaining fewer digital images
- Reducing the use of continuous fluoroscopic mode relative to the pulsed mode of operation
- Retaining the protective curtain, if available, on the image intensifier or leaving the scatter shield in place during a procedure
- Regularly using the last image hold feature to view the most recent fluoroscopic image

These practices will substantially decrease exposure not only to all participating personnel but to the patient as well.

Extremity Monitoring

Because the hands and forearms of physicians performing interventional procedures can be subjected to significant radiation exposures if the safety protocol is not carefully followed—and sometimes this may not be possible—it is essential that extremities be monitored. Physicians need to be aware of the recommended dose limits that have been established for extremities. The NCRP currently recommends an annual EqD limit to localized areas of the skin and hands of 500 mSv (50 rem). To avoid remotely approaching this limit and consequently significantly increasing the possibility of future adverse effects, protective gloves should be worn whenever feasible by any physician whose hands will, of necessity, often be close to the fluoroscopic beam.

DIAGNOSTIC X-RAY SUITE PROTECTION DESIGN

Requirement for Radiation-Absorbent Barriers

To reduce the EfD to radiographers, nonoccupationally exposed personnel, and the general public to levels deemed statistically safe by both federal and

> **BOX 12.3   Radiation-Absorbent Barrier Design Considerations**
>
> - The mean energy of the x-rays that will strike the barrier
> - Whether the barrier is of a primary or a secondary nature
> - The distance from the x-ray source to a position of occupancy 0.3 m from the barrier
> - The workload of the unit
> - The use factor of the unit
> - The occupancy factor behind the barrier
> - The intrinsic shielding (e.g., tube housing attenuation) of the x-ray unit
> - Whether the area beyond the barrier is "controlled" or "uncontrolled"

international bodies, every radiography room must be equipped with radiation-absorbent barriers. The design of these barriers is based on considerations listed in Box 12.3.

Reason for Overshielding

The shielding design for radiographic rooms must include all of the factors identified in Box 12.3 to meet necessary radiation protection standards. In addition, the designer should plan conservatively to satisfy future regulatory limits that may be more stringent. These considerations and the ALARA principle are why many diagnostic x-ray facilities are overshielded. Spending extra money up front for additional shielding is far easier and much less expensive than adding shielding after the suite has been completed.

Radiation Shielding Categories

As mentioned in previous sections, three categories of radiation sources are generated in an x-ray room. They are classified as follows:

1. Primary radiation
2. Scatter radiation
3. Leakage radiation

The last two categories are collectively known as *secondary radiation*.

Primary radiation. Primary radiation emerges directly from the x-ray tube collimator (Fig. 12.18) and moves without deflection toward a wall, door, viewing window, and so on. Because of this property, primary radiation, also is known as *direct radiation*, is energy that has not

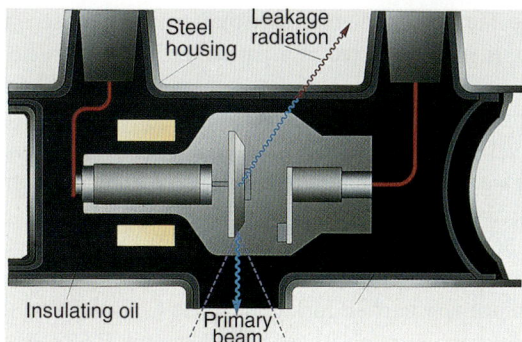

Fig. 12.18 Primary radiation emerges directly from the collimator and spreads throughout the room.

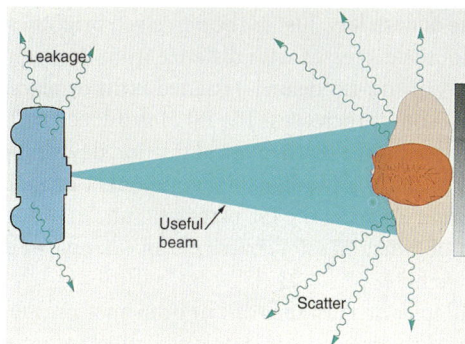

Fig. 12.19 Scatter radiation emerges from the patient and spreads in all directions.

been degraded by scattering, and substantial portions of the initial beam may not have been attenuated. Therefore, a wall in the path of direct radiation requires the most protective shielding to ensure the safety of personnel and the public. In a typical x-ray suite, the most crucial primary radiation barrier is that behind the wall Bucky unit.

Scatter radiation. Recall that scatter radiation results whenever a diagnostic x-ray beam passes through matter. Compton interactions between the x-ray photons and the electrons of the atoms within the attenuating object deflect x-ray photons from their initial trajectories. As a result, photons emerge from the object in all directions (Fig. 12.19). Scattered radiation is greatly reduced in intensity relative to the incident beam. It also is substantially weakened in energy and consequently in penetrating power. The amount of shielding required to protect against scatter radiation is, therefore, usually much less than that for primary radiation. In general, the patient is the major source of scatter radiation.

Leakage radiation. Leakage radiation is radiation generated in the x-ray tube that does not exit from the collimator opening but instead partially penetrates the protective tube housing and also, to some degree, the sides of the collimator (see Figs. 12.18 and 12.19). Leakage radiation is therefore always present in some amount. When shielding is planned for a secondary barrier, the potential contributions from leakage radiation must be added to those from the scatter radiation reaching that barrier.

Calculation Considerations

Workload. Because a diagnostic x-ray unit does not produce radiation 24 hours a day, 7 days a week, a parameter that reflects the unit's radiation-on time has been used in the determination of barrier shielding requirements. The quantity, workload (W), is essentially the radiation output-weighted time that the unit is delivering radiation during the week. It has also been called the unit's *duty cycle*. Workloads are specified either in units of milliampere-seconds (mAs) per week or milliampere-minutes (mA-min) per week. The following example illustrates this concept.

Example: A radiographic x-ray suite is in operation 5 days per week. The average number of patients per day is 20, and the average number of images per patient is 3. The mean technical exposure factors are 90 kVp, 300 mA, and 0.1 sec. Find the weekly workload.

Solution:

$$W = (300 \text{ mA} \times 0.1 \text{ sec}) \times (5 \text{ days/wk})$$
$$\times (20 \text{ patients/day}) \times (3 \text{ images/patient})$$
$$= 9000 \text{ mAs/wk}$$
$$= 150 \text{ mA} - \text{min/wk}$$

Note that the kVp is not used in the workload calculation. It is, however, an essential parameter in the calculation of barrier-shielding thickness. (This will be demonstrated later on in an example illustrating the calculation of shielding for a wall in an x-ray suite.)

Inverse square law. Just as the perceived brightness of a light source decreases with distance from its origin, the intensity of an x-ray beam is lessened as the displacement from its source increases. The ISL, introduced earlier in this chapter, is the mathematical relation describing this property and is a fundamental component of radiation protection. As such, the ISL plays a significant role in the design of radiation safety barriers. An example of its use is shown here.

Example: At a distance of 1 m from an x-ray tube target, the dose rate measured by a radiation survey meter was 4.5 mGy per hour. What would that instrument read if it were moved back an *extra* 2 m?

Solution: ISL is mathematically given by the following proportion:

$$\frac{I_1}{I_2} = \frac{(d_2)^2}{(d_1)^2}$$

If the given data are substituted into the relation and cross-multiplied, the following result is obtained:

$$3^2 \times I_2 = 4.5 \times 1^2$$
$$9I_2 = 4.5$$
$$I_2 = 0.5 \text{mGy/hr}$$

This result demonstrates a large reduction in radiation intensity. Its direct consequence is a greatly reduced barrier shielding thickness requirement.

The inverse square law is built into the combined mathematical and empiric (i.e., experimentally derived) formulas that determine primary barrier thickness values and secondary barrier thickness values. Because these relations are formulated to give answers for *broad-beam attenuation** rather than just for a very localized area, the ISL effect is slightly less than it would be for an idealized situation. A short discussion with an example illustrating the usage of this for a primary barrier is presented in the following pages. Before this discussion proceeds, however, several other concepts of fundamental importance in the design of appropriate shielding have to be introduced.

---

*As defined in NCRP Report 147 (see below), *broad-beam* attenuation refers to that effect occurring when the field area is large at the barrier and the point of measurement is near the barrier's exit surface.

Use factor. If radiation, whether primary or secondary, is never directed at a particular wall or structure, then conventional or existing construction is sufficient. Most structures in a diagnostic x-ray suite, however, are struck by radiation to some degree for some fraction of the weekly beam-on time. The **use factor (U)** was introduced to delineate this fractional contact time.

For primary radiation, the use factor represents the portion of beam-on time that the x-ray beam is directed at a primary barrier during the week. Consider a typical radiographic suite with a wall Bucky unit. If 50% of the x-ray examinations involve this device, the wall behind the Bucky unit has a U (*primary*) = 1/2.

Because scatter and leakage radiation emerge in all directions in the x-ray room, every wall, door, viewing window, and other surface will *always* be struck by some quantity of radiation. Therefore U (*secondary*) = 1 for all radiation-accessible structures. Furthermore, if a particular wall is considered a primary barrier and its required shielding is designed on that basis, then in virtually all situations no supplementary shielding need be added for the secondary radiation that may also be striking this barrier.

Table 12.2 presents the most current recommended use factor values. **U** also can be referred to as the *beam direction factor.*

Occupancy factor. Radiation barriers are installed to protect personnel and the general public from radiation exposure. If no one will ever be present beyond an existing wall in a particular area while the x-ray unit is being operated, the addition of extra shielding to that wall is unnecessary. For that location the shielding design statement would be that *existing construction is sufficient.* An example of this is an outside wall facing a courtyard that "always" has no occupancies. The opposite extreme is an area in which someone is always present. When planning radiation protection shielding for a diagnostic x-ray suite, the designer must consider not only zero and full occupancy cases but also the more common partial occupancy situations. The **occupancy factor (T)** is used to modify the shielding requirement for a particular barrier by taking into account the fraction of the work-week during which the space beyond the barrier is occupied. Table 12.3 lists the latest recommended values for T.

Controlled and uncontrolled areas. If a region adjacent to a wall of an x-ray room is to be used only by occupationally

TABLE 12.2 Use Factors Recommended by the International Commission on Radiological Protection

Use Factor	Primary Barrier
Full use (U = 1)	Floors of radiation rooms except dental installations, doors, walls, and ceilings of radiation rooms exposed routinely to the primary beam
Partial use (U = ¼)	Doors and walls of radiation rooms not exposed routinely to the primary beam; also floors of dental installations
Occasional use (U = 1/16)	Ceilings of radiation rooms not exposed routinely to the primary beam; because of the low use factor, shielding requirements for a ceiling usually determined by secondary rather than primary beam considerations

From International Commission on Radiological Protection (ICRP): *Report of committee III on protection against x-rays up to energies of 3 MeV and beta and gamma rays from sealed sources*, ICRP Publication No. 3, New York, 1960, Pergamon Press.

TABLE 12.3 Suggested Occupancy Factors*†

Location	Occupancy Factor (T)
Administrative or clerical offices; laboratories, pharmacies, and other work areas fully occupied by an individual; receptionist areas, attended waiting rooms, children's indoor play areas, adjacent x-ray rooms, image reading areas, nurses' stations, x-ray control rooms	1
Rooms used for patient examinations and treatments	½
Corridors, patient rooms, employee lounges, and staff rest rooms	$1/5$
Corridor doors‡	$1/8$
Public toilets, unattended vending areas, storage rooms, outdoor areas with seating, unattended waiting rooms, patient holding areas	$1/20$
Outdoor areas with only transient pedestrians or vehicular traffic, unattended parking lots, vehicular drop-off areas (unattended), attics, stairways, unattended elevators, janitors' closets	$1/40$

*For use as a guide in planning shielding where other occupancy data are not available.
†When using a low occupancy factor for a room immediately adjacent to an x-ray room, care should be taken to also consider the areas farther removed from the x-ray room. These areas may have significantly higher occupancy factors than the adjacent room and may therefore be more important in shielding design despite the larger distances involved.
‡The occupancy factor for the area just outside a corridor door can often be reasonably assumed to be lower than the occupancy factor for the corridor.
Adapted from National Council on Radiation Protection and Measurements (NCRP): *Structural shielding design for medical x-ray imaging facilities*, Report No. 147, Bethesda, MD, 2004, NCRP.

exposed personnel (e.g., radiographers), that location is designated a **controlled area**. Conversely, a nearby hall or corridor that is open to and frequented by the general public, is classified as an **uncontrolled area**. For the latter, the weekly maximum permitted equivalent dose (MPED) is equal to 20 microsieverts (20 μSv or 2 mrem); for controlled areas, it is a much more significant amount: 1000 μSv or 1 mSv (100 mrem). The main reason for allowing this huge disparity lies in the fact that the occupationally exposed population makes up only a tiny fraction of the overall population. Therefore the potential for detrimental radiobiologic effects in the general public as a whole (i.e., its genetically significant dose [GSD] value) as a result of the higher MPED to occupationally exposed personnel is

statistically negligible. Whether the area beyond a structure is designated as controlled or uncontrolled is clearly very significant in determining the amount of radiation shielding to be added to that structure. The following sections discuss the use of these concepts in the determination of radiation shielding requirements.

Calculating Barrier Shielding Requirements

For each wall, door, and other barrier in an x-ray room that is to provide protection from radiation, the product of W × U × T must be determined. The number of mA-minutes per week or *workload* is generally determined by overall utilization of the x-ray unit. In contrast, the *use* and *occupancy* factors are typically different

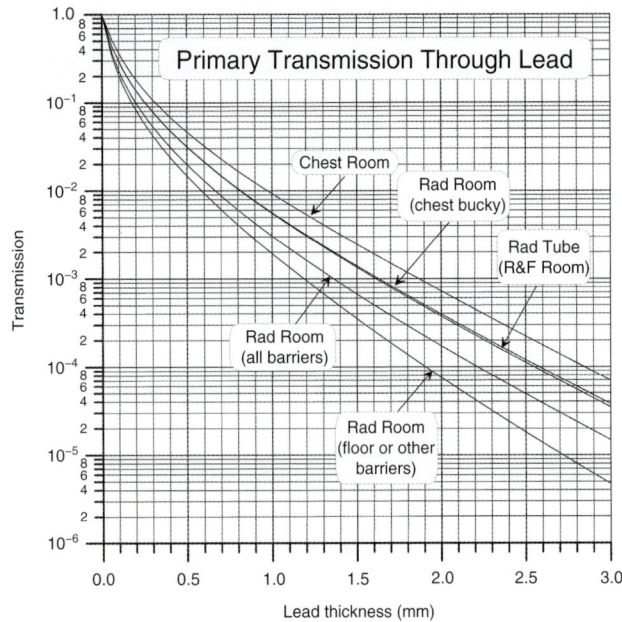

Fig. 12.20 Assorted plots of primary broad-beam transmission through lead. (From National Council on Radiation Protection and Measurements [NCRP]: *Structural shielding design for medical x-ray imaging facilities,* Report No. 147, Bethesda, MD, 2004, NCRP.)

among the various barriers. The shielding designer also must conclude whether the barrier is primary or secondary and whether the area beyond the barrier is controlled or uncontrolled.

With the publication of NCRP Report No. 147,[6] entitled *Structural Shielding Design for Medical Imaging Facilities*, the objective of a shielding calculation is now described as determining the thickness of a barrier sufficient to reduce the air *kerma** in a full or partially occupied area to a value that is less than or at most equal to the ratio **P/T** where the quantity **P** refers to the permissible weekly radiation dose (note: for diagnostic x-rays, dose, and equivalent dose are numerically equal) to that location, and **T** is the area's occupancy factor.

Primary barrier calculation. Using material from NCRP Report No. 147, the combined mathematical and empiric relation that was briefly mentioned in the section on the ISL is introduced. For primary, or direct, radiation only, the mathematical expression is given by:

$$B = P(d_p)^2 / (K_r \, NUT)$$

where **B** is by definition the **broad-beam x-ray transmission factor (B)** and is the ratio of air kerma (Ka) behind a barrier of material thickness "x" to the value of Ka at the same location with no intervening barrier; dp is the distance from the x-ray source to a representative location and distance behind the direct radiation barrier (e.g., one-third of a meter beyond the barrier is typical); Kr is the average unshielded air kerma per patient at *a reference distance of 1 m from the source*; N is the expected number of patients examined in the room per week; U and T are, as noted, previously, respectively, the use and occupancy factors; and P depends on whether the barrier is for a controlled or uncontrolled area. Once the value of B has been calculated for a particular situation, then plots (Fig. 12.20) of transmission factors (values of B) versus attenuating material thickness supplied in Appendix B of NCRP Report No. 147 may be used to obtain the required shielding thickness for the barrier.[6]

---

*Recall that air kerma (Ka) is essentially absorbed dose in air resulting from the passage of an x-ray beam through it. Its numeric value is specified in units of gray.

The primary radiation intensity for a selected kVp at a barrier location for an x-ray suite may be determined by making air kerma measurements on the suite's x-ray unit at a reference distance (e.g., 100 cm) from the x-ray tube target with the aid of a calibrated ionization chamber. This information can then be used to determine the amount of shielding necessary to attenuate the radiation to permissible levels for that x-ray energy. The following example demonstrates determination of the primary barrier shielding requirement associated with a wall Bucky from an average-usage radiographic room with an uncontrolled area existing behind the barrier (e.g., a public corridor).

Example:

Given the following specifications, determine the required shielding:

- The average kVp for the x-rays striking the barrier = 100.
- P = 0.02 mGy/wk because of the uncontrolled area.
- dp = 3 m
- 100 patients per week in this x-ray room.
- U = 1/2
- T = 1/4
- The measured value of Kr is 6 mGy per mA-min at 1 m at 100 kVp.

Solution:

Substituting the foregoing information into the expression for the transmission factor "B" gives:

$$B = (0.02)(3)^2 / [(6)(100)(0.5)(0.25)]$$
$$= 0.0024$$

From the graph in Fig. 12.20, using *the curve for radiographic room chest Bucky*, a shielding requirement of approximately 1.3 mm lead is obtained. Currently, in the United States shielding is specified in fractions of an inch of lead, most commonly, 1/32 and 1/16. The standard 1/32 inch is approximately 0.8 mm, and the standard 1/16 inch is equal to 1.58 mm. Because the calculation of shielding for the primary barrier required 1.3 mm lead, then in the United States the conservative choice would be to install 1/16-inch lead shielding for this barrier.

Secondary barrier calculation. Secondary barriers intercept both scatter and leakage radiation. As has been mentioned previously, *no additional shielding against secondary radiation is needed for areas already protected against primary radiation.* Because scatter and leakage radiation emerge in all directions, the use factor U for these is always = 1.

Scatter radiation. The intensity and energy of the scatter radiation at the location of a barrier are generally unknown because of all the potential variables involved. Therefore the following properties, typically, are assumed for the determination of scatter radiation barrier shielding:

1. The energy of the scatter radiation is conservatively considered to be equal to that of the primary radiation.
2. The intensity of radiation scattered at 90 degrees at a distance of 1 m from its source is reduced by a factor of 1000 relative to the primary radiation for a field size of 400 cm2 (20 cm × 20 cm).

The larger the x-ray field dimension at the source of the scatter radiation (usually the patient), the more significant will be the amount of generated scatter radiation. Also, notably of importance are the primary beam photon energy and the incident location of the x-ray beam on the patient. The ISL again plays a vital role in shielding requirements, but regarding scatter radiation, however, the distance is measured from the center of the irradiated portion of the patient (the prime source of scatter) rather than from the x-ray tube target.

Leakage radiation. Leakage radiation does not emerge directly from the collimator opening but instead seeps out or *leaks through* the x-ray tube housing walls and also partially penetrates the sides of the collimator when the x-ray beam is on. Leakage radiation is therefore an additional radiation output component that shielding designers must consider. Regulatory standards mandate that the maximum permissible leakage exposure rate at 1 m from the target of a diagnostic x-ray tube in all directions *cannot exceed 100 millitoentgens (mR) per hour or 0.88 milligray (mGy) air kerma per hour* when the tube is being operated continuously at its maximal permitted kVp and mA combination.

Because of the attenuation that occurs when leakage radiation penetrates the tube housing walls, any emerging radiation is essentially monoenergetic; thus, the basic concept of half-value layer (HVL) may be applied at barriers to reduce leakage radiation levels to permissible values. Data tables incorporating this concept have been developed to specify the amount of shielding needed to attenuate leakage radiation sufficiently at various distances from the x-ray tube. This value should be compared with that necessary to attenuate scatter radiation satisfactorily. Traditionally, if both shielding requirements do not differ substantially (i.e., are less than three HVLs of shielding material apart), then the conservative decision would be to install a composite that is the *sum of the required shielding for each radiation source.* However, if the needed barrier shielding for each of the two differs substantially (i.e., more than three HVLs), then, again conservatively, the larger value alone can be used for the shielding. The following example illustrates the method used in most existing diagnostic x-ray rooms for determining leakage radiation shielding requirements.

Example: If shielding must be added to a wall that is subject only to secondary radiation to protect a controlled area, then find the total thickness of lead needed, given the following information:

HVL for scatter and leakage radiation: 0.2 mm lead (Pb) for each. Shielding requirement for scatter radiation alone for a particular barrier: 0.75 mm Pb

Shielding requirement for leakage radiation alone for that barrier: 0.3 mm Pb

Solution: The difference in barrier shielding requirements for scatter and leakage = 0.45 mm lead, which is less than 3 HVL, which equals 3 × 0.2 mm lead, or 0.6 mm lead. Therefore the conservative total shielding thickness amount for the barrier would be 0.75 + 0.3 = 1.05 mm Pb.

Current Approaches to Shielding

Among the most current approaches to shielding design detailed in NCRP Report No. 147, a more rigorous workload analysis incorporates the range of kVps actually used. Also, the true role of leakage radiation in state-of-the-art equipment is now modeled explicitly, along with scatter. The traditional rule of adding an HVL if leakage and scatter barrier requirements are similar has now been abandoned in favor of exact calculations. Use factors at present reflect an actual percentage of the time that the beam is directed at various barriers. Some existing shielding that was generally ignored in older design calculations, such as the patient table, Bucky, and image receptor, is included in the new designs. Finally, the suggested occupancy factors have been reevaluated to approximate more closely the percentage of the time that

TABLE 12.4 Brief Summary of National Council on Radiation Protection and Measurements Report No. 147 New Shielding Guidelines

Item	New Approach
Workload	More realistic use of contemporary survey data
Leakage and scatter	Explicit barrier calculations
Use factor	Adjusted for beam direction data reflecting actual usage patterns
Occupancy factor	Realistic assumptions of occupancy of low-occupancy areas (e.g., stairwells)

Adapted from National Council on Radiation Protection and Measurements (NCRP): *Structural shielding design for medical imaging facilities*, Report No. 147, Bethesda, MD, 2004, NCRP.

workers are expected to be present (see Table 12.3). In NCRP Report No. 49,[7] a minimal occupancy factor of at least 1/16 was assumed. Under the revised guidelines, occupancy factors for areas such as closets and stairways may be placed as low as 1/40. Some of the changes in the revision of NCRP Report No. 49 are listed in Table 12.4.

RADIATION CAUTION SIGNS

The appropriate deployment of radiation signs or electronic notices is an essential component of safety in a radiology department. Specific rules and regulations vary somewhat according to the jurisdiction of the facility (i.e., state, federal, military, etc.). However, the main points concerning the type of signs and the circumstances under which posting is required are essentially the same. Each radiographer should check with the radiation safety officer in the institution where employed, concerning specific regulations that govern the facility where they work.

Beam-On Indicator Sign

Some states require specific imaging equipment installations, primarily computed tomography (CT) scanners, to include warning lights that are conspicuous near the door to the examination room from any corridor. The sign should read "x-ray beam on" or the equivalent and be self-illuminating whenever the x-ray equipment is energized. Some states require an

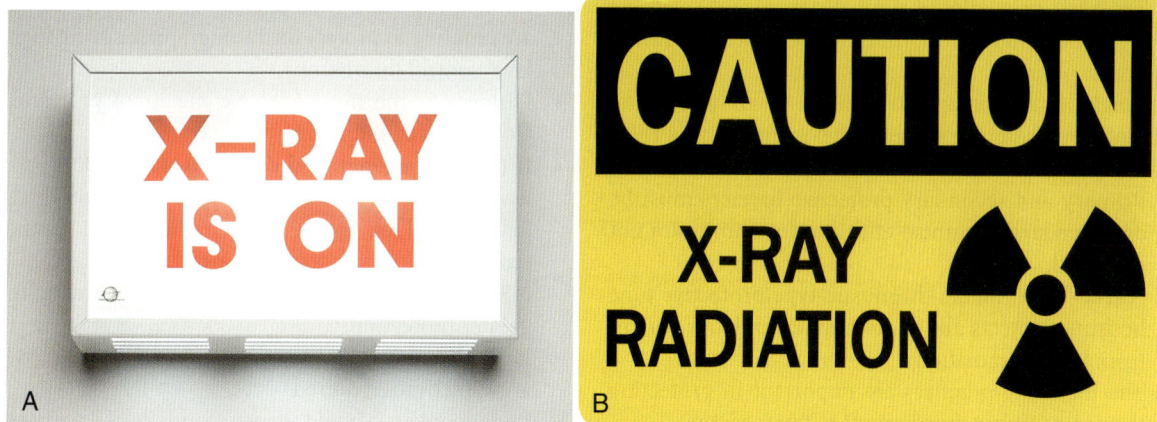

Fig. 12.21 Radiation warning signs typically found in a diagnostic radiologic facility. (A) A self-illuminated sign used outside the door to a computed tomography (CT) scanner. (B) A general radiation warning sign used to indicate the potential for exposure that may exceed 0.05 mSv at 30 cm from a source of radiation. (A, From Brian Struble/DigitalMomentStudios.com, © 2017.)

interlock such that exposure is terminated if the door is opened.

General Posting

Radiation warning signs are posted within controlled areas of the hospital or facility. They are typically found on the door to CT and interventional x-ray rooms, linear accelerator treatment rooms, and storage areas for radioactive materials. An example of the latter is shown on the right in Fig. 12.21. Such signs are required to be magenta or purple or black on a yellow background. Further specifications may be found in Recommended State Regulations of the Conference of Radiation Control Program Directors.[8] A sign reading "Caution Radiation Area" is usually adequate for rooms containing fixed diagnostic equipment. A radiation area is generally an area in which radiation exposures may exceed 0.05 mSv (5 mrem) in 1 hour at 30 cm from a source. Other categories of caution signage exist for areas in which radiation exposures may exceed those encountered in diagnostic radiology. These signs are required in radiation oncology or nuclear medicine departments and include the labels: High Radiation, Very High Radiation, Airborne Radioactivity, and Radioactive Materials.

SUMMARY

- An annual occupational effective dose of 50 mSv for whole-body exposure during routine operations and an annual effective dose of 1 mSv for individuals in the general population have been established.
- A CumEfd limits a radiation worker's whole-body cumulative occupational effective dose to his or her age in years times 10 mSv.
- Radiation workers can receive a higher equivalent dose than the general public without altering the genetically significant dose (GSD).
- Occupational exposure must be kept ALARA.
- The following methods of reducing scatter radiation also reduce the occupational hazard for the radiographer:
  - Use of beam-limitation devices, higher kVp and lower mA techniques, appropriate beam filtration, and adequate protective shielding.
  - Proper utilization of protective apparel (lead aprons, gloves, thyroid shields).
  - Reduction of repeat images.

- The basic principles of time, distance, and shielding are to be employed to minimize occupational radiation exposure.
- Pregnant radiographers can wear an additional monitoring device at waist level to ensure that their monthly equivalent dose does not exceed 0.5 mSv.
- Primary and secondary protective barriers must be designed so that annual effective dose limits are not exceeded.
- A lead-lined, metal, diagnostic-type protective tube housing protects the radiographer and the patient from leakage radiation.
- The following practices are important in protecting the radiographer during routine fluoroscopy:
  - The radiographer, in addition to wearing protective apparel, should stand as far away from the patient as is practical and move closer to the patient only when assistance is required.
  - A protective curtain and Bucky slot shielding device must be used.
  - The x-ray beam must be adequately collimated, and a cumulative timing device should be used.
- The following are required to protect the radiographer during mobile radiographic examinations:
  - The radiographer must wear protective garments.
  - The radiographer should stand at least 2 m from the patient, x-ray tube, and useful beam.
  - If possible, the radiographer should also stand at a right angle to the x-ray beam–scattering object (the patient) line.

- Limited exposure time and dose reduction features are required to protect the radiographer during high-level control fluoroscopy.
- Distance is the most effective means of protection from ionizing radiation.
- If the peak energy of the x-ray beam is 100 kVp, a lead apron of at least 0.25 mm lead equivalent thickness should be worn if the radiographer cannot remain behind a protective barrier. A lead apron of 0.5 or 1 mm lead equivalent thickness affords much greater protection.
- Lead gloves, a thyroid shield, and protective glasses are sometimes required.
- Radiographers should never stand in the primary beam to hold a patient during a radiographic exposure.
- When designing diagnostic x-ray suites, equivalent dose to radiation workers, nonoccupationally exposed personnel, and the general public must be taken into consideration.
  - Facilities must be equipped with radiation-absorbent barriers.
  - Occupancy factor, workload, and use factor must be considered when thickness requirements for a protective barrier are being determined. Whether an area beyond a structure is designated as a controlled or uncontrolled area is significant in determining the amount of radiation shielding to be added to that structure.
- Radiation caution signs are an important component of safety in an imaging department.

GENERAL DISCUSSION QUESTIONS

1. What is the annual occupational effective dose limit for whole-body exposure of diagnostic imaging personnel during routine operations?
2. Why is occupational exposure for diagnostic imaging personnel limited, and why are radiation workers allowed a higher equivalent dose compared to the general population?
3. What type of x-radiation poses the most significant occupational hazard in diagnostic radiology, and what methods can reduce this hazard?
4. How do methods that reduce patient exposure during diagnostic examinations also minimize exposure for radiographers and other personnel?
5. What responsibilities do employers have in protecting declared pregnant diagnostic imaging personnel from radiation exposure?
6. What are the three underlying principles of radiation protection for personnel exposure reduction?
7. Explain the inverse square law and provide an example of its application.
8. Differentiate between a primary and a secondary protective barrier, and provide examples.
9. What types of protective garments can be worn to reduce whole-body or partial-body exposure?
10. What are the three categories of radiation sources generated in an x-ray room, and what considerations should be taken into account for designing radiation-absorbent barriers?

REVIEW QUESTIONS

1. What is the annual occupational effective dose limit for whole-body exposure of diagnostic imaging personnel?
   A. 20 mSv
   B. 50 mSv
   C. 100 mSv
   D. 30 mSv

2. Why is the occupational exposure of diagnostic imaging personnel limited?
   A. To reduce costs
   B. To protect their health
   C. To improve image quality
   D. To comply with insurance regulations

3. What type of radiation poses the most significant occupational hazard in diagnostic radiology?
   A. Primary radiation
   B. Scatter radiation
   C. Leakage radiation
   D. Background radiation

4. How can scatter radiation hazards in diagnostic radiology be reduced?
   A. By increasing patient exposure
   B. By using protective barriers and distance
   C. By reducing image quality
   D. By using longer exposure times

5. What is one responsibility of employers regarding pregnant diagnostic imaging personnel?
   A. To require them to work longer hours
   B. To provide additional training
   C. To implement radiation exposure limits
   D. To assign them to higher radiation jobs

6. What is one consideration for designing radiation-absorbent barriers?
   A. The color of the barrier
   B. The energy level of the radiation
   C. The aesthetics of the room
   D. The type of imaging equipment used

7. What does the inverse square law state?
   A. Radiation intensity increases with distance
   B. Radiation intensity decreases with the square of the distance
   C. Radiation exposure is unrelated to distance
   D. Radiation exposure is constant regardless of distance

8. What is a primary protective barrier designed to do?
   A. Protect against scatter radiation
   B. Absorb leakage radiation
   C. Intercept the primary beam of radiation
   D. Enhance image quality

9. Which of the following is an example of a secondary protective barrier?
   A. X-ray tube housing
   B. Lead apron
   C. Wall of the x-ray room
   D. Lead-lined door

10. What type of protective garments can be used to reduce radiation exposure?
    A. Surgical scrubs
    B. Lead aprons
    C. Cotton uniforms
    D. Plastic gowns

Radiation Monitoring

OBJECTIVES

After completing this chapter, the reader will be able to perform the following:

- Define all key terms.
- Discuss the requirement for a personnel dosimeter and explain the function and characteristics of such devices.
- Identify the appropriate location on the body where the personnel dosimeter(s) should be worn during the following procedures or conditions: (1) routine radiographic procedures, (2) fluoroscopic procedures, (3) special radiographic procedures, and (4) pregnancy.
- Identify the sensing material in the thermoluminescent dosimeter ring badge.
- Describe the various components of the optically stimulated luminescence (OSL) dosimeter, and the

personnel direct ion storage dosimeter (DSI) and explain the use of each of these devices as personnel monitors.

- Explain the function of radiation survey instruments.
- List three gas-filled radiation survey instruments.
- Explain the requirements for radiation survey instruments.
- Recognize the operating regions of the following instruments: (1) ionization chamber–type survey meter (cutie pie), (2) proportional counter, and (3) Geiger–Müller (GM) survey meter.
- Identify the radiation survey instrument that can be used to calibrate radiographic and fluoroscopic x-ray equipment.

CHAPTER OUTLINE

KEY TERMS

control monitor

extremity dosimeter

Geiger–Müller (GM) survey meter

glow curve

ionization chamber-type survey meter (cutie pie)

optically stimulated luminescence (OSL) dosimeter

personnel direct ion storage dosimeter (DSI)

personnel dosimeter

personnel dosimetry

personnel monitoring reports

proportional counter

radiation survey instruments

thermoluminescent ring dosimeter (TLD)

To ensure that occupational radiation exposure levels are kept well below the annual effective dose (EfD) limit, some means of monitoring personnel exposure must be employed. The radiographer and other occupationally exposed persons should be aware of the various radiation exposure monitoring devices and their functions. This chapter provides an overview of both personnel and area monitoring. In addition, because radiation dosimetry reports still specify radiation exposure for workers in traditional units and subunits, traditional units' numerical values are identified in parentheses after International System (SI) units' numerical values. However, facilities may request that dosimetry reports employ SI units.

PERSONNEL MONITORING

Requirement for Personnel Monitoring

Personnel dosimetry refers to the monitoring of equivalent dose to any person occupationally exposed on a regular basis to ionizing radiation, which is recommended. It is *required*, however, whenever radiation workers are likely to risk receiving 10% or more of the annual occupational EfD limit of 50 millisievert (mSv) (5 rem*) in any single year as a consequence of their work-related activities. In keeping with the as low as reasonably achievable (ALARA) concept, most health care facilities issue dosimetry devices when personnel could receive approximately 1% of the annual occupational EfD limit in any month, or approximately 0.5 mSv (50 mrem). Radiation exposure monitoring is accomplished by wearing personnel dosimeters.*

Purpose of Personnel Dosimeters

The **personnel dosimeter:**
- Provides an indication of the radiation exposure working habits and working conditions of diagnostic imaging personnel
- Determines occupational exposure by detecting and measuring the quantity of ionizing radiation to which the dosimeter has been exposed over a period of time
- Does not protect the wearer from exposure because the instrument is only capable of detecting and measuring the amount of ionizing radiation to which it has been exposed

*Rem (radiation equivalent man) is the traditional unit for the quantity, equivalent dose (EqD).

Placement of Personnel Dosimeters

During Routine Radiographic Procedures. A personnel monitoring device records only the exposure received in the area where the device is worn. During routine radiographic procedures, when a protective apron is not being used, the primary personnel dosimeter should be attached to the clothing on the front of the body at collar level to approximate the location of maximal radiation dose to the following (Fig. 13.1):
- Thyroid
- Head
- Neck

Consistency of location in wearing the dosimeter is necessary and is the responsibility of the individual wearing the device. A list of the types of personnel monitors available to diagnostic imaging personnel is found in Box 13.1. A discussion of each

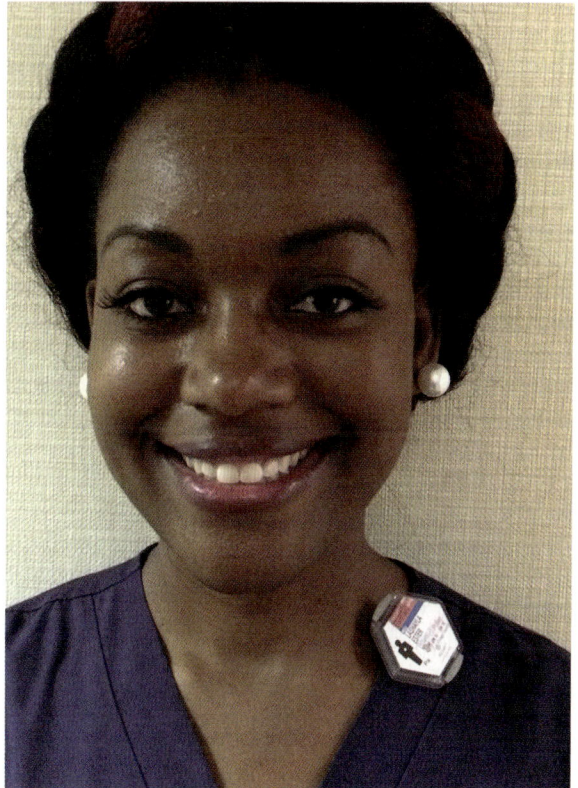

Fig. 13.1 To approximate the maximum radiation dose to the thyroid and the head and neck during routine radiographic procedures, the primary personnel monitor should be attached to the clothing on the front of the body at collar level.

of the personnel monitoring devices will be provided later in this chapter.

When a Protective Apron is Worn. Fluoroscopy, surgery, and special radiographic procedures produce the highest occupational radiation exposure for diagnostic imaging personnel. When a protective lead apron is worn during such procedures, the dosimeter should be placed outside the apron at collar level on the anterior surface of the body since the unprotected head, neck, and lenses of the eye receive 10 to 20 times more exposure than the protected body trunk. Located at collar level, the dosimeter provides a reading of the approximate equivalent dose to the exposed thyroid gland and eyes of the occupationally exposed person. If the lead apron's shielding integrity is not compromised, a dosimeter reading that is within acceptable limits outside of the apron ensures a minimal reading under the apron.

As a Second Monitor When a Protective Apron is Worn. During *lengthy interventional fluoroscopy procedures* (e.g., cardiac artery patency investigations), some health care facilities may prefer to have diagnostic imaging personnel wear two separate monitoring devices. As mentioned previously, the first, or primary, dosimeter is to be worn outside the protective apparel at collar level, whereas the second dosimeter should be placed beneath a wraparound-style lead apron at waist level to monitor the approximate equivalent dose to the lower body trunk. Commercially available lead aprons typically have either 0.5-mm or 0.25-mm lead equivalent shielding. Another version is also available with a 0.35-mm lead equivalent in the front and 0.25-mm shielding in the back. For those occupationally exposed personnel who utilize two radiation dosimeters, it is useful to have some knowledge of the difference in equivalent dose readings between the two dosimeters.

As a Monitor for the Embryo-Fetus. In addition to a primary dosimeter worn at collar level, pregnant diagnostic imaging personnel are typically issued a second

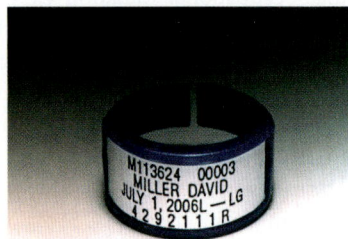

Fig. 13.2 An extremity dosimeter (thermoluminescent ring dosimeter [TLD]) can be used to monitor the equivalent dose to the hands. (From Landauer, Inc., Glenwood, IL.)

monitoring device (also worn beneath the protective apron, at waist level) to record the approximate radiation dose to the abdomen during gestation. This monitor, therefore, can provide an estimate of the equivalent dose to the embryo-fetus.

Extremity Dosimeter

An **extremity dosimeter**, typically a **thermoluminescent ring dosimeter (TLD)** (Fig. 13.2), should be worn by an imaging professional as a second monitor when performing fluoroscopic procedures that require the hands to be near the primary x-ray beam. Ring dosimeters are most commonly utilized by nuclear medicine technologists, due to the need for occupational handling of unsealed radioactive sources. Even though ring dosimeters are worn under gloves to avoid contamination, such extremity monitors have a laser-etched cover to ensure the retention of permanent identification of the wearer. The TLD element of the dosimeter is encapsulated within its engraved cover.

The TLD ring is a light-free device that contains a crystalline form (powder or, more frequently, small chips) of lithium fluoride (LiF), which functions as the sensing material of the dosimeter. When irradiated, some of the electrons in the crystalline lattice structure* of the LiF molecules absorb energy and are "excited" to higher energy levels or bands. The presence of impurities in the crystal causes electrons to become trapped within the bands. When the LiF crystals are passed through a special heating process for dosimeter reading

---

*A geometric arrangement of the points in space at which the atoms, molecules, or ions of a crystal occur. Also called *space lattice.*

TABLE 13.1 Occupational Exposure Values for a Typical Year

Category	NUMBER OF WORKERS (THOUSANDS)		AVERAGE ANNUAL EFFECTIVE DOSE (MSV)		Collective Effective Dose (Person-Sv)*
	All	**Exposed**	**All**	**Exposed**	
Medicine	584	277	0.7	1.5	416
Industry	350	156	1.2	2.4	380
Nuclear power	151	91	3.6	5.6	550
Flight crews, flight attendants	97	97	1.7	1.7	165
Other†					789
				Total	**2300**

*See NCRP Report No. 101, p 60.

†Includes workers in the US government (Department of Energy, US Public Health Service), uranium mining, well logging, miscellaneous workers, visitors to facilities, and so forth.

Data from National Council on Radiation Protection and Measurements (NCRP): *Exposure of the U.S. population from occupational radiation, Report No. 101*, Bethesda, MD, 1989, NCRP, pp 65–70.

purposes, the trapped electrons receive enough energy to rise above their present locations into a region called the *conduction band*. From there, the electrons can return to their normal state, with the emission of energy in the form of visible light. The energy emitted is equal to the difference between the electron-binding energies of the two orbital levels.[2]

Radiation dose determination is accomplished through the use of an electronic instrument known as a TLD analyzer. After the LiF crystals are heated to free the trapped, highly energized electrons, this instrument records the amount of light emitted by the crystals as the electrons return to their ground state. This amount is proportional to the dosimeter exposure. A graphic plot is constructed to demonstrate the relationship of light output, or emitted thermoluminesence intensity, to temperature variation of the LiF crystals. The plot, known as a **glow curve**, represents a unique signature of the exposure received by the TLD ring dosimeter.

Advantages of the TLD Ring Dosimeter. For the purpose of monitoring radiation in the hands, the TLD ring dosimeter is relatively accurate and reliable. The TLD ring dosimeter is small, and light-weight, and the LiF crystals interact with ionizing radiation in the same manner as human tissue.* Exposures as low as 1.3×10^{-6} C/kg (5 mR)** can be measured precisely. Because the

dosimeter is not affected by humidity, pressure, and normal temperature changes, it can be worn for up to 3 months and is reusable after a reading has been obtained. Therefore, ongoing use is reasonably cost-effective.

Disadvantages of the TLD Ring Dosimeter. Thermoluminescence readings will be lost if not carefully recorded. The readout process destroys information stored in the TLD, thus preventing the "read" TLD from serving as a permanent legal record of exposure. Calibrated dosimeters must be prepared before-hand and read with each group of TLDs as they are processed.

Record of Radiation Exposure

A record of radiation exposure should be included in the employment record of all radiation workers. Table 13.1 provides occupational exposures (gathered from personnel dosimeter readings) for a typical year. The listed values represent the corresponding average annual EfD to the whole body and the related collective effective dose.

PERSONNEL DOSIMETERS FOR OCCUPATIONAL MONITORING

Characteristics

A personnel dosimeter should be lightweight, easy to carry, and constructed of materials durable enough to tolerate normal daily use. The dosimeter must be able to detect and record both small and large exposures in a consistent and reliable manner. Outside influences such as very warm weather, humidity, and ordinary mechanical shock should not affect the performance of the instrument. The monitors should be reasonably inexpensive to purchase and maintain.

*The effective atomic number of LiF is 8.2, which is similar to that of human soft tissue (Z = 7.4).

**1 R = $2.58 \times (10)^{-4}$ C/kg by definition

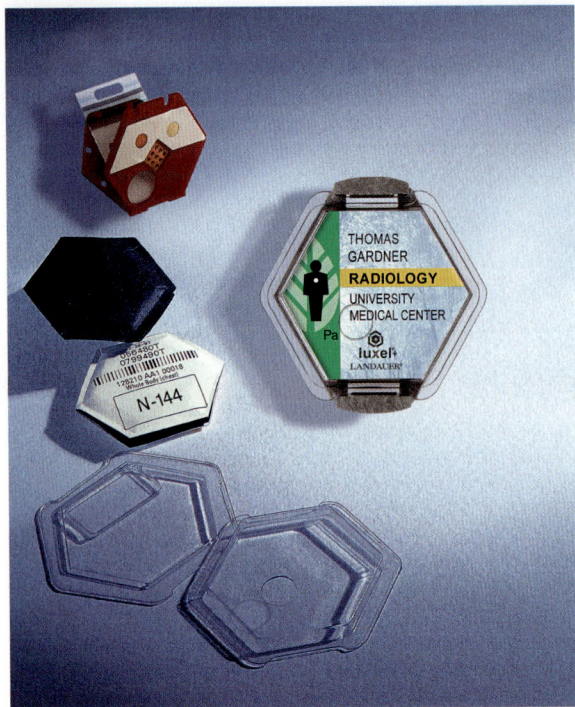

Fig. 13.3 Optically stimulated luminescence (OSL) dosimeter. Disassembled OSL dosimeter demonstrating components of the monitor: sensing material holder, preloaded packet incorporating an Al_2O_3 strip sandwiched within a three-element filter pack, which is heat sealed within a light-tight black paper wrapper that has been laminated to the white paper label. The front of the white paper packet may also be color-coded to facilitate correct usage and placement of the dosimeter on the body of occupationally exposed personnel. (All components are sealed inside a tamperproof plastic blister pack.) (From Landauer, Inc., Glenwood, IL.)

Types

Two types of personnel dosimeters are predominantly used to measure individual exposure of the whole body to ionizing radiation:

- Optically stimulated luminescence (OSL) dosimeters
- Direct ion storage dosimeter (DIS)

Optically Stimulated Luminescence Dosimeter. The optically stimulated luminescence (OSL) dosimeter for personnel monitoring offers excellent features (Fig. 13.3) while eliminating many of the disadvantages of its predecessors. The OSL is the most common type of device used for monitoring occupational exposure in diagnostic imaging and radiation therapy. The OSL

dosimeter has replaced earlier devices for personnel monitoring in essentially all health care facilities.

The OSL dosimeter shown in Fig. 13.3 contains an aluminum oxide (Al_2O_3) thin layer detector. An exposed dosimeter is "read out" by using laser light at selected frequencies. When such laser light is incident on the sensing material, the material becomes luminescent in proportion to the amount of radiation exposure received by the detector.

Although the OSL dosimeter can be worn continuously for up to one year, it is common practice for it to be worn without a reading for a period of one to three months. OSL dosimeters are typically shipped to a monitoring company for analysis and dose determination, a task that requires some time for the report of a reading to be communicated. An in-house reader may be purchased from a vendor. With the in-house reader, occupational exposure doses can be determined on the day of occurrence.

Energy discrimination. As seen in Fig. 13.3, three different filters are incorporated into the detector packet of the OSL dosimeter. The filters are, respectively, made of:

- Aluminum (Al)
- Tin (Sn)
- Copper (Cu)

Each filter blocks a portion of the radiation-sensitive aluminum oxide and causes a different degree of attenuation for any radiation striking the dosimeter, depending on its energy. The aluminum filter offers the least absorption, whereas the copper filter attenuates the most. When the exposed aluminum oxide layer of the OSL dosimeter is read out by a laser, the degree of luminescence detected in the areas from beneath the filters is a measure of radiation dose occurring within different energy ranges. Thus, a situation in which high-energy radiation strikes the dosimeter would demonstrate a similar reading through all three filters. Conversely, if the dosimeter had been subjected to only very low-energy radiation, the laser readout would have been much more pronounced in the region covered by the aluminum filter than in the other filter-blocked portions. Somewhat more energetic radiation would enhance the intensity of the region beneath the tin filter. This is the manner in which radiation energy discrimination is achieved by the OSL dosimeters. The varied energy ranges are typically classified as "deep," "eye," and "shallow" and physically correlate with different penetration depths and therefore different effective radiation energies, with "deep" being the most penetrating at a centimeter or more, "eye" at 0.3 cm, and "shallow" at the surface, or below 0.01 cm.

In the OSL dosimeter from one manufacturer* a "bare" or unfiltered portion of the aluminum oxide is used to detect dynamic exposures, that is, those received during rapid motion between the source of radiation and the dosimeter. Examination of the laser-produced glow curves from this bare region demonstrates a shift or spread in their light frequency that can be correlated with motion (technically classifiable as a Doppler shift*).

Optically stimulated luminescence dosimeter sensitivity. The OSL dosimeter provides an accurate reading as low as 10 μSv (1 mrem) for x-ray and gamma ray photons, with energies ranging from 5 kiloelectron volts (keV) to greater than 40 megaelectron volts (MeV). Because of this, the OSL dosimeter is actually very sensitive. The OSL's maximum equivalent dose measurement for x-ray and gamma ray photons is 10 Sv (1000 rem). For beta particles with energies from 150 keV to in excess of 10 MeV, dose measurement ranges from 100 μSv to 10 Sv (10 mrem to 1000 rem). For neutron radiation with energies of 40 keV to greater than 35 MeV, the OSL has a more limited dose measurement range: up to 200 μSv (20 mrem) for fast neutrons and up to 250 μSv (25 mrem) for thermal energy neutrons (eV energy range).

Control monitor. The vendor that supplies health care facilities with OSLs provides **control monitors** with each batch of dosimeters. These control monitors serve as a basis for comparison with the remaining OSL dosimeters after they have been returned to the company for processing. The control monitors must be kept in a radiation-free area within an imaging facility; therefore, their response should be minimal or zero. After processing, if the average control monitor reading is greater than zero, then the associated batch of OSLs may have been exposed to radiation while in transit. To ensure that false readings are not recorded, the control monitor reading is reported to the health care facility. This reading, if

different from zero, must be subtracted from each of the remaining OSLs in the batch to ensure accuracy in exposure reporting.

Advantages of the OSL dosimeter. The OSL is lightweight, durable, and easily worn. The OSL contains an integrated, self-contained, preloaded packet. Color-coding, graphic formats, and body location icons provide simple identification. This monitoring device has a tamperproof blister packet that is not affected by heat, moisture, and pressure. The OSL offers complete reanalysis in the event a health care facility believes that an error in reading the dosimeter has occurred. Because of the OSL dosimeter's sensitivity to as low as 10 μSv (1 mrem) for x-ray and gamma ray photons in the energy range 5 keV to 40 MeV, it is an excellent and practical monitoring device for employees working in low-radiation environments and for pregnant workers. This device can be worn for long periods of time (up to one year) to record occupational exposure.

Disadvantages of the OSL dosimeter. A disadvantage of the OSL is that occupational radiation exposure is recorded only in the body area where the device is attached. In addition, if the facility does not have an in-house reader, exposure cannot be determined on the day of occurrence. The OSL dosimeter is not an efficient monitoring device if it is not regularly used.

Personnel monitoring report. Results from **personnel monitoring reports** must be recorded accurately and maintained for review to meet state and federal regulations. To comply with such requirements, health care facilities use established dosimetry services. These monitoring services process various types of personnel dosimeters, such as the OSL dosimeter, and then supply written personnel monitoring reports to the health care facility (Fig. 13.4A). These statements, typically one for each hospital department that is being monitored, list the deep, eye, and shallow occupational exposure of each covered person on a monthly, quarterly, year-to-date, and lifetime equivalent basis. In addition, if requested, the total effective dose equivalent (TEDE) for persons of interest can be supplied at year's end. Information on the report is arranged in a series of columns. These columns include the items listed in Box 13.2.

The cumulative columns shown in Fig. 13.4A provide a continuous audit of the actual absorbed radiation equivalent dose. These totals can be compared with

---

Doppler shift refers to the apparent change in frequency of a light wave as observer and light source move toward or away from each other. This is similar to the increase in pitch of a train whistle experienced by a pedestrian as the locomotive moves toward the individual and its decrease in pitch noted by the pedestrian as the train moves away from the person.

LANDAUER®

Landauer, Inc. 2 Science Road Glenwood, Illinois 60425-1586
Telephone: (708) 755-7000   Facsimile: (708) 755-7016
www.landauerinc.com

luxel®

SAMPLE ORGANIZATION
RADIATION SAFETY OFFICER
1000 HIGH TECH AVENUE
GLENWOOD, IL 60425

RADIATION DOSIMETRY REPORT

ACCOUNT NO.	SERIES CODE	ANALYTICAL WORK ORDER	REPORT DATE	DOSIMETER RECEIVED	REPORT TIME IN WORK DAYS	PAGE NO.
103702	RAD	9920800151	06/11/04	06/07/04	4	1

PARTICIPANT NUMBER	ID NUMBER / NAME / BIRTH DATE / SEX	DOSIMETER	USE	RADIATION QUALITY	DEEP DDE	EYE LDE	SHALLOW SDE	DEEP DDE	EYE LDE	SHALLOW SDE	DEEP DDE	EYE LDE	SHALLOW SDE	DEEP DDE	EYE LDE	SHALLOW SDE	DEEP DDE	EYE LDE	SHALLOW SDE	RECORDS FOR YEAR	INCEPTION DATE (MM/YY)
					05/01/04 – 05/31/04			QTR 2			2004										
0000H	CONTROL / CONTROL / CONTROL	Ja / Pa / U	CNTRL / CNTRL / CNTRL	PN / P / NF	M / M / M	M / M / M	M / M / M											5	07/97 / 07/97 / 07/97
00191	ADDISON, JOHN (M)	Ja	WHBODY		90 / 60 / 30	90 / 60 / 30	90 / 60 / 30	90 / 60 / 30	90 / 60 / 30	90 / 60 / 30	100 / 70 / 30	100 / 70 / 30	100 / 70 / 30	200 / 170 / 30	200 / 170 / 30	200 / 170 / 30	5	07/97
00192	JORGENSON, MIKE (M)	Pa / U	WHBODY / RFINGR		M / M	M / M	M / M	M / M	M / M	M / M	M / M	M	M / 70	M / 100	M	M / 100	5	07/97 / 07/97
00193	THOMAS, LEE (M)	Pa / U	WHBODY / RFINGR		ABSENT / ABSENT			M	M	M	M	M	M / M	M / M	M	M / M	5	07/97 / 07/97
00196	WALKER, JANE (F)	Pa	WHBODY		3	3	3	12	11	11	12	11	11	22	21	21	5	11/97
00197	EDWARD, CHRIS (M)	Pa	WHBODY		M	M	M	M	M	M	M	M	M	M	M	M	5	01/98
00198	ZERR, ROBERT (M)	Pa	WHBODY / NOTE		40 CALCULATED	40	40	160	160	160	200	200	200	240	240	240	5	07/98
00199	ADAMS, JANE (F)	Pa	WHBODY		M	M	M	M	M	M	9	10	12	9	10	12	5	07/98
00200	MEYER, STEVE (M)	Pa / Pa / U	COLLAR / WAIST / ASSIGN / NOTE / RFINGR	PL	105 / M / 4	105 / M / 105	105 / M / 105	6	162	165	11	327	334	51	1247	1284	5	08/98 / 08/98 / 08/98
	ASSIGNED DOSE BASED ON EDE 1 CALCULATION						140			400			690			2180			
00202	HARRIS, KATHY (F)	Pa / U	WHBODY / RFINGR		M / M	M	M	M / M	M	M	M / M	M	M / 30	M / M	M	M / 30	4	02/99 / 02/99

QUALITY CONTROL RELEASE: VS

M: MINIMAL REPORTING SERVICE OF 1 MREM
ELECTRONIC MEDIA TO FOLLOW THIS REPORT

20 · PR 674 · RPT130 · N1

NVLAP®

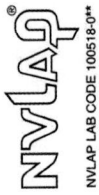

NVLAP LAB CODE 100518-0** · 02013

Fig. 13.4 (A) The personnel monitoring report must include the items of information shown here.

A

Fig. 13.4 cont'd (B) Modified report showing a summary of occupational exposure. (From Landauer, Inc., Glenwood, IL.)

BOX 13.2 Information Found on a Personnel Monitoring Report

1. Personal data: participant's identification number, name, (and may also include) birth date, and sex.
2. Type of dosimeter: *P* represents Luxel optically stimulated luminescence (OSL) dosimeter* for x-ray, beta, and gamma radiation; *J* represents Luxel OSL dosimeter for x-ray, beta, gamma, and fast neutron radiation; *U* represents a finger dosimeter used to monitor x-radiation and gamma and beta radiation.
3. Radiation quality (e.g., x-rays, beta particles, neutrons, combined radiation exposure).
4. Equivalent dose data, including current deep, eye, and shallow recorded dose equivalents (millirem) for the time indicated on the report (e.g., from the first day of a given month to the last day of that month).
5. Cumulative equivalent doses for deep, eye, and shallow radiation exposures for specific periods, the year to date, and lifetime radiation.
6. Inception date (month and year) that the monitoring company began keeping dosimeter records for a given dosimeter for an individual listed on the account who is wearing a monitoring device.

---

*Luxel OSL dosimeter is manufactured by Landauer, Inc., Glenwood, IL.

allowable values established by regulatory agencies. Whenever the letter *M* appears under the current monitoring period or in the cumulative columns, it signifies that an equivalent dose *below the minimum* measurable *radiation quantity* was recorded during that time. The minimal reporting levels vary according to the dosimeter type and radiation quality as follows:

X-ray, gamma	10 µSv (1 mrem)
Beta	100 µSv (10 mrem)
Neutron	200 µSv (20 mrem) *fast,* 100 µSv (10 mrem) *thermal*
Fetal	10 µSv (1 mrem)
Rings	300 µSv (30 mrem)

Change in employment by radiation worker. When changing employment, the radiation worker must convey the data pertinent to accumulated permanent equivalent dose to the new employer so that this information can be placed on file. Fig. 13.4B is an example of an appropriate summary of an occupational exposure report. A copy of such a report should be given to the radiation worker on termination of employment.

In health care facilities that have a well-structured radiation safety program, personnel monitoring reports are received and reviewed and, if necessary, because some readings have exceeded a certain threshold value set by the facility, investigated by the radiation safety officer (RSO). Such a process should be an integral component of the facility's radiation safety program. This practice is compatible with the ALARA policy.

Direction Storage Dosimeter. The **personnel direct ion storage (DIS) dosimeter** is a recent development, using electronic components developed in the 1990s and first applied to miniaturized personnel dosimetry systems in the early 2000s.[2] The DIS is basically a small (several mm³) ionization gas-filled dosimeter connected to a "solid state" device, with electrically erasable programmable read-only memory (EEPROM, or E²PROMs). EEPROMs are used in microcomputers and various consumer products to store small amounts of data while allowing some memory to be erased and reprogrammed to store more data. EEPROMs are used in voice-activated greeting cards, keyless entry systems, and various other "smart card" applications.

In the personnel dosimeter, (Fig. 13.5) when radiation ionizes the gas in the ionization chamber, the cumulative electric charge is stored in the EEPROM and will remain in the device indefinitely, until either added to by additional ionization or until "read out" by the introduction of a small control signal.[3] The amount of charge stored in the device is directly proportional to the amount of radiation exposure produced by ionization that has occurred in the chamber. Other memory chips within the DIS store information pertaining to the facility and the badge wearer.

The DIS dosimeter is read out through a physical connecting device such as a universal serial bus (USB) or via a wireless connection, and the data can then be stored electronically at the facility. However, it may also be read out by the device wearer via a cellphone application. Thus, the individual wearer may obtain an instantaneous readout while the facility is able to obtain their own reports, such as:

- Radiation exposure summary
- Exposure history
- Individuals who have not had their devices read

Advantages of the direct ion storage dosimeter. Advantages of the personnel DIS dosimeter include instant access to data and no need for the institution to collect individual dosimeters, mail them to the

A

Detector

Detector
battery

Communication
battery

B

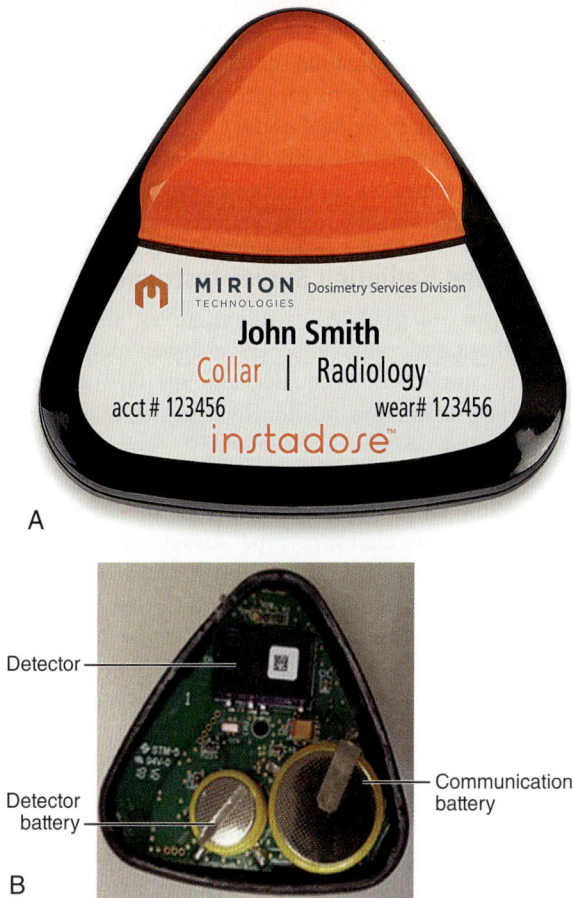

Fig. 13.5 Personnel direct ion storage dosimeter. (A) External (unopened) view. (B) Internal (opened) view. (From Mirion Technologies, Dosimetry Services Division, Irvine, CA.)

manufacturer for readout, and issue new dosimeters to the individuals. DIS dosimeters are also lightweight, durable, and can be dropped or scratched with little chance of harm to the device.

Disadvantages of the direct ion storage dosimeter. Radiation exposure cannot be determined if the dosimeter is not regularly used.

RADIATION SURVEY INSTRUMENTS FOR AREA MONITORING

Radiation Detection and Measurement

Radiation monitoring instruments are used for both individual monitoring and area monitoring.

Radiation survey instruments fall into three categories: those without a readout scale, those with a readout scale, and those that have a readout scale and are ionization-chamber-based.

The most common of these have a Geiger–Müller (GM) tube as their detector, the operation of which is described later in this chapter. Such instruments can be used in multiple conditions, depending on their level of calibration ("the adjustment of an instrument to accurately read the radiation level from a reference source"[4]) and associated components. The simplest version, lacking any readout scale but possibly allowing adjustable sensitivity levels, is only a "detector" used to indicate the presence of any radiation above the background. The detector will emit a repetitive sound, whose volume or repetitive frequency is directly associated with the intensity of radiation. Other versions, more fully equipped, contain calibrated readout scales, as well as audible indicators, and are typically used either as area or room monitors or as portable survey instruments for measuring exposure rates at any location or object of interest. These instruments, however, do not directly supply a cumulative radiation exposure reading. Finally, there are ionization chamber–based instruments, which are described in more detail later in this chapter. The most common type of survey meter that incorporates an ionization chamber as its radiation detector is the *cutie pie* (Fig. 13.6). The meter acquired this nickname

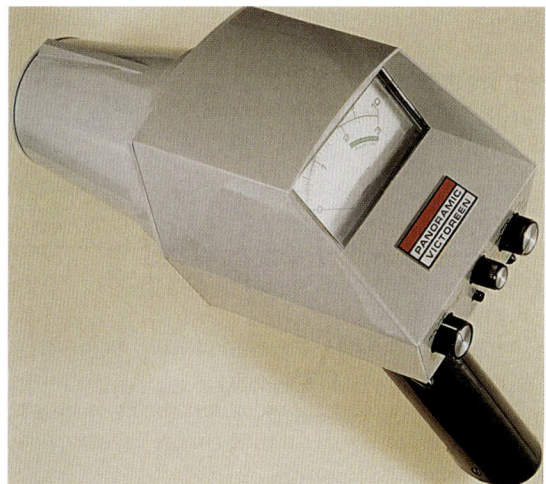

Fig. 13.6 Ionization chamber–type survey meter, or "cutie pie." (From Victoreen, Inc., Cleveland, OH.)

sometime during 1943 or 1944 "due to its diminutive size."[5] This instrument, when properly calibrated, is capable of measuring radiation exposure rates over a very wide range and also determining cumulative radiation exposure for the period of time the instrument is irradiated. In this regard, the cutie pie can be considered a dosimeter, as are all properly calibrated ionization chamber–based devices.

Types of Instruments

When in contact with ionizing radiation, survey instruments respond to the charged particles that are produced by the radiation interacting with and subsequently ionizing the gas (usually air) in the detector. These instruments measure either the total quantity of electrical charge resulting from the ionization of the gas or the rate at which the electrical charge is produced.

Gas-filled radiation detectors serving as field instruments include:

- Ionization chamber–type survey meter ("cutie pie")
- Proportional counter
- GM survey meter

All three detect the presence of radiation and, when properly calibrated, provide a reasonably accurate measurement. The cutie pie and the **proportional counter** measure both exposure and exposure rate, whereas the GM meter typically provides only exposure rate. Each of these instruments has its own special use, and they are not all equally sensitive in the detection of ionizing radiation.

Requirements

Radiation survey instruments for area monitoring should meet the following requirements:

1. Portable, so one person can carry and operate the device in an efficient manner for a period of time.
2. Durable enough to withstand normal use, including routine handling that occurs during standard operating procedures.
3. Reliable; accurately assess radiation exposure, or exposure rate, in a given area.
4. Interacts with ionizing radiation similar to how tissue reacts, thereby permitting a more accurate determination of tissue dose.
5. Detects all common types of ionizing radiation.

6. The energy of the radiation should not significantly affect the response of the detector, and the direction of the incident radiation should not affect the performance of the unit, ensuring consistency in unit operation among individual users.
7. Cost effective; the initial cost and subsequent maintenance expenses should be reasonably affordable.
8. Calibrated annually to ensure accurate operation.

Gas-Filled Radiation Survey Instruments

Three types of gas-filled radiation survey instruments exist: the ionization chamber–type survey meter (cutie pie), the proportional counter, and the GM detector. These instruments are individually discussed in the paragraphs below.

Ionization Chamber–Type Survey Meter (Cutie Pie).

The **ionization chamber–type survey meter (cutie pie)** is both a rate meter device (for exposure rate) used for area surveys and an accurate integrating or cumulative exposure instrument (see Fig. 13.6). The cutie pie measures x-radiation and gamma radiation, and, if equipped with a suitable window, can also record beta radiation.

Sensitivity ranges and uses. In the rate mode, the cutie pie can measure radiation intensities ranging from 10 to several thousand microgray per hour (1 mR/h to several thousand milliroentgens per hour); in the integrated mode, it can sum exposures from as low as 10 μGy_{-a} to a Gy_{-a} (1 mR to tens of R). This device is useful for monitoring radiographic x-ray installations and for measuring fluoroscopic and computed tomography scatter radiation exposure rates, when exposure timers exceed 1 second in duration. The cutie pie is typically the instrument of choice when determining exposure rates from patients containing therapeutic doses of radioactive materials and when assessing the exposure rates in radioisotope storage facilities. Finally, the cutie pie is especially valuable when quantifying the cumulative exposures received outside of protective barriers associated with radiation oncology treatment rooms.

Advantages and disadvantages. The advantages of the cutie pie include the ability to measure a wide range of radiation exposures within a few seconds over a broad expanse of radiation energies, exhibiting essentially the same response or sensitivity. The

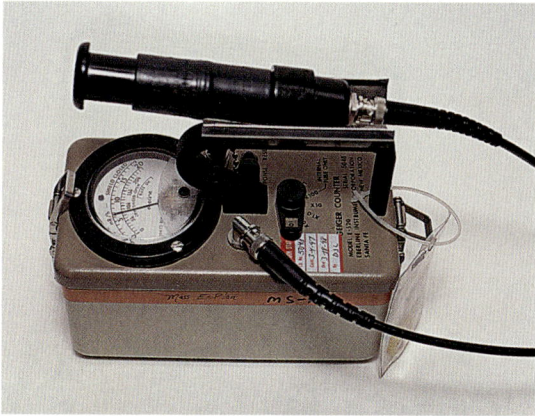

Fig. 13.7 Geiger–Müller (GM) survey meter.

delicate detector of the unit, however, may be considered a disadvantage. Another caveat is that without adequate warm-up time, its meter will drift on its most sensitive scales and thereby potentially produce an inaccurate reading. This device cannot be used to accurately measure exposures or exposure rates produced by typical diagnostic procedures because the exposure times are too short to permit the meter to respond appropriately.

Proportional Counter. The proportional counter serves no useful purpose in diagnostic imaging because it is generally used in a laboratory setting to detect alpha and beta radiation and small amounts of other types of low-level radioactive contamination. The proportional counter can discriminate between alpha and beta particles. Because alpha radiation travels only a short distance in the air, the operator of the proportional counter must hold the unit's probe close to the surface of the object being surveyed to obtain an accurate reading of the alpha radiation emitted by the object.

Geiger–Müller Survey Meter

Sensitivity and use. The **Geiger–Müller (GM) survey meter** serves as the primary portable radiation survey instrument for area monitoring in nuclear medicine facilities (Fig. 13.7). With the exception of alpha particle emission, the unit is sensitive enough to detect individual particles (e.g., electrons emitted from certain radioactive nuclei) or photons. Hence it can easily detect any area contaminated by radioactive material. Because

the GM survey meter allows rapid monitoring, it can be used to locate a lost radioactive source or low-level radioactive contamination. By utilizing its audio mode, the GM survey meter may also be employed to scan radiation barriers for shielding defects.

Components. The GM survey meter has an audible sound system (an audio amplifier and speaker) that alerts the operator to the presence of ionizing radiation. Metal encloses the counter's gas-filled tube or probe, which is the unit's sensitive ionization chamber. When the shield covering the probe's sensitive chamber is open, very low-energy x-radiation gamma radiation, and beta radiation can be detected. Meter readings are usually displayed in milliroentgens per hour. Because GM tubes tend to lose their calibration over time, the instrument generally has a "check source" of a weak, long-lived radioisotope located on one side of its external surface to verify its constancy daily.

Disadvantages. The scale reading of a GM survey meter is not independent of the energy of the incident photons. This means that photons of widely different energies cause the instrument to respond quite differently and thus, unless corrected for, provide erroneous readings. The cutie pie (ionization chamber–type survey meter), as mentioned previously, exhibits a much flatter, or more constant, response, with varying photon energies. In addition, the GM survey meter is likely to saturate or jam when it is placed in a pulsed (i.e., noncontinuous) high-intensity radiation area (e.g., that associated with a linear accelerator used in radiation therapy), thereby yielding a false reading.

INSTRUMENTS USED TO MEASURE X-RAY EXPOSURE

Ionization chambers can be used to measure radiation output from both radiographic and fluoroscopic x-ray equipment. As previously described, the cutie pie ionization chamber may be used for radiation protection surveys. If a cutie pie ionization chamber operating in "rate" mode were placed in the primary beam during a radiographic exposure, the electrical signal produced during the very brief (usually a fraction of a second) exposure duration would be too small to be recorded, and measured reliably. An *ionization chamber device specifically designed for such measurement conditions* consists of an ion chamber connected to an electrometer, a very fast-responding electrical instrument that can measure tiny electrical currents with high precision and accuracy, see Fig. 13.8. Both the ionization chamber and the electrometer system must be precisely calibrated periodically to meet state and federal requirements. A current listing of accredited calibration laboratories is available from the American Association of Physicists in Medicine.*

Medical physicists utilize ionization chambers, connected to electrometers to perform annual standard measurements required by state, federal, and health care accreditation organizations for radiographic and fluoroscopic devices. These annual measurements (usually referred to as a physics survey) include x-ray output in Gy or mGy, fluoroscopic radiation entrance rates in mSv/min or R/min, kVp setting accuracy, exposure timer exactness, and half-value layers or beam quality. From these measurements, important x-ray machine performance values such as µSv/mAs or mR/mAs as a function of selected kVp and linearity of machine radiation output are obtained. Data that can be utilized for determining radiation dose to patients are another by-product of this annual survey. The ion chamber and electrometer combination, but equipped with a specially calibrated *parallel plate shaped thin window ion chamber,* sensitive to the very low x-ray energies, is normally used for similar measurements for mammography x-ray units.

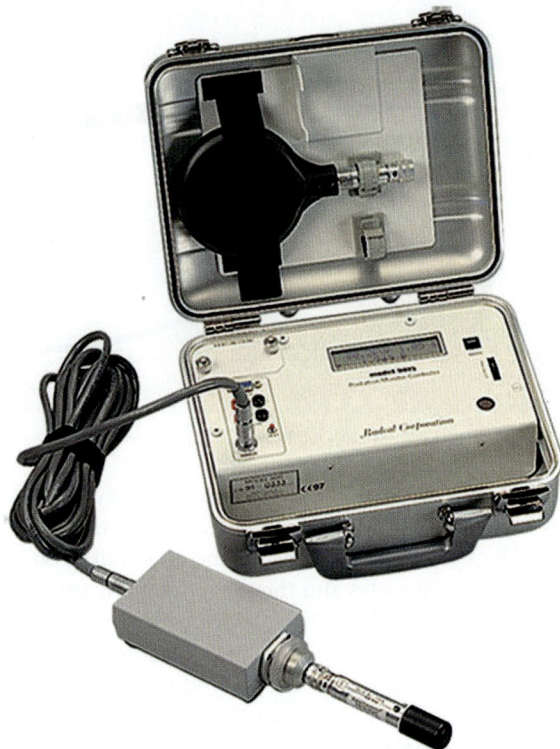

Fig. 13.8 Ion chamber connected to an electrometer. Ionization chamber (probe with a black sensitive element containing electrodes at its end) and electrometer (in carrying case) that may be used for measurement of x-ray machine output. Also shown (stored in the lid of the carrying case) is a larger, more sensitive disk-shaped ionization chamber that may be used for the measurement of scattered radiation. (Photo from RadCal Corp.)

*1631 Prince Street, Alexandria, VA 22314 or www.aapm.org.

SUMMARY

- Personnel monitoring ensures that occupational radiation exposure levels are kept well below the annual effective dose (EfD) limit.
- Personnel monitoring is required whenever radiation workers are likely to risk receiving 10% or more of the annual occupational EfD limit of 50 mSv (5 rem) in any 1 year as a consequence of their work-related activities.
- To keep radiation exposure ALARA, most health care facilities issue dosimeter devices when personnel could receive approximately 1% of the annual occupational EfD limit in any month, or approximately 0.5 mSv (50 mrem).
- The working habits and conditions of diagnostic imaging personnel with respect to radiation exposure can be assessed over a designated period through the use of the personnel dosimeter.
- Even when a protective apron is not normally required, a radiation worker should wear a personnel monitoring device attached to the clothing on the front of the body at collar level during routine radiographic procedures to detect any potential radiation dose to the thyroid and the head and neck.
- During high-level radiation procedures, imaging professionals are required to wear both a thyroid shield and a lead apron, with the dosimeter worn outside the front of the protective garment at collar level, to provide a reading of the approximate equivalent dose to the eyes and the head as a whole.

- Commercially available lead aprons typically have either 0.5 mm or 0.25 mm lead equivalent shielding.
- Pregnant radiation workers may wear a second dosimeter beneath a lead apron to monitor the abdomen during gestation to provide an estimate of the equivalent dose to the embryo-fetus. Many facilities provide pregnant radiographers with a second dosimeter for this purpose.
- An extremity dosimeter, which is commonly a thermoluminescent ring dosimeter (TLD) ring dosimeter, should be used as a second monitor when performing fluoroscopic procedures that require the hands to be near the primary x-ray beam.
- In general, personnel dosimeters must be lightweight, portable, durable, and cost efficient.
- Two types of whole-body personnel monitoring devices are now used. the optically stimulated luminescence (OSL) dosimeter, and direct ion storage dosimeter (DIS).
- Reports from personnel monitoring programs must be recorded accurately and maintained for review to meet state and federal regulations. A record of radiation exposure is required by regulatory agencies to be contained in the employment record of all radiation workers.
- Personnel monitoring reports list the deep, eye, and shallow occupational exposure of each covered person on a monthly, quarterly, year-to-date, and lifetime equivalent basis.
- Whenever the letter M appears under the current monitoring period or in the cumulative columns on a radiation monitoring report, it signifies that an equivalent dose below the minimum measurable radiation quantity was recorded during that time.
- In health care facilities that have a well-structured radiation safety program, personnel monitoring reports are received and reviewed by the Radiation Safety Officer (RSO).
- Area monitoring can be accomplished through the use of radiation survey instruments.
- When in contact with ionizing radiation, survey instruments respond because of the charged particles that are produced by the incident radiation interacting with and subsequently ionizing the gas (usually air) in the detector. These instruments measure either the total quantity of electrical charge resulting from the ionization of the gas or the rate at which the electrical charge is produced.
- Three different types of gas-filled radiation detectors serve as field instruments, including the ionization chamber–type survey meter ("cutie pie"), the proportional counter, and the Geiger–Müller (GM) survey meter.
- Radiation survey instruments for area monitoring must be durable, easy to carry, able to detect all common types of ionizing radiation, and not be substantially affected by the energy of the radiation or the direction of the incident radiation.
- Ionization chambers can be used to measure the radiation output from both radiographic and fluoroscopic x-ray equipment.
- Medical physicists use ionization chambers connected to electrometers to perform the annual standard measurements or qualified physicist survey required by state, federal, and health care accreditation organizations for radiographic and fluoroscopic devices.

GENERAL DISCUSSION QUESTIONS

1. What is the primary purpose of a personnel dosimeter, and why is it essential for radiation workers?
2. Where should personnel dosimeters be worn during routine radiographic procedures, and why is this placement important?
3. What are the recommended locations for wearing dosimeters during fluoroscopic procedures and special radiographic procedures?
4. What is the sensing material used in thermoluminescent dosimeter (TLD) ring badges, and how does it function?
5. What are the main components of an optically stimulated luminescence (OSL) dosimeter, and how does it work?
6. What is the function of radiation survey instruments, and why are they important in radiation safety?
7. Can you name three types of gas-filled radiation survey instruments and their applications?
8. What are the key requirements for radiation survey instruments to ensure accurate measurements?
9. What are the operating regions of the ionization chamber-type survey meter (Cutie Pie), proportional counter, and Geiger–Müller (GM) survey meter?
10. Which radiation survey instrument is typically used to calibrate radiographic and fluoroscopic x-ray equipment?

REVIEW QUESTIONS

1. What is the primary function of a personnel dosimeter?
   A. To enhance image quality
   B. To measure and record radiation exposure
   C. To calibrate x-ray equipment
   D. To protect patients from radiation

2. Where should a personnel dosimeter be worn during routine radiographic procedures?
   A. On the wrist
   B. At the waist level
   C. On the collar, at the level of the thyroid
   D. On the ankle

3. What is the sensing material used in a thermoluminescent dosimeter (TLD) ring badge?
   A. Aluminum
   B. Silicon
   C. Lithium fluoride
   D. Lead

4. Which component is part of an optically stimulated luminescence (OSL) dosimeter?
   A. Film badge
   B. Aluminum oxide detector
   C. Ionization chamber
   D. Geiger–Müller tube

5. What is the primary function of radiation survey instruments?
   A. To increase radiation output
   B. To measure radiation levels in the environment
   C. To improve patient comfort
   D. To assist in patient diagnosis

6. Which of the following is a type of gas-filled radiation survey instrument?

A. Photomultiplier tube
B. Ionization chamber
C. Radiographic film
D. Thermoluminescent dosimeter

7. What is one requirement for radiation survey instruments?
   A. They must be waterproof.
   B. They must be able to measure only alpha radiation.
   C. They must be calibrated regularly for accurate measurements.
   D. They must be lightweight for portability.

8. Which survey meter is commonly used for measuring high radiation levels and calibrating x-ray equipment?
   A. Proportional counter
   B. Geiger–Müller counter
   C. Ionization chamber (Cutie Pie)
   D. Film badge

9. What operating region is typical for a Geiger–Müller (GM) survey meter?
   A. High radiation range
   B. Moderate radiation range
   C. Low radiation range
   D. No radiation range

10. What is the purpose of using a dosimeter during pregnancy for radiation workers?
    A. To monitor the dose received by the fetus
    B. To increase the radiation dose during procedures
    C. To ensure the worker does not exceed their personal dose limit
    D. To calibrate equipment for better imaging

Radiation Safety in Computed Tomography

OBJECTIVES

After completing this chapter, the reader will be able to perform the following:

- Define all key terms.
- Explain why computed tomography examinations are of greater concern in terms of radiation safety in comparison with routine radiographic examinations.
- List two concerns that relate to patient dose in CT scanning and explain each.
- Compare the entrance exposure from a CT examination with the entrance exposure from a routine fluoroscopic procedure.
- Describe how interslice scatter affects the radiation dose to a patient.
- State the reason why direct patient shielding is not necessary during a CT examination.
- For spiral, or helical, CT, state how patient dose is affected when pitch ratio is adjusted.
- Identify various methods for reducing patient dose during a CT examination.
- Discuss the concept of computed tomography dose parameters.
- Explain how to calculate the effective CT dose.
- State the goal of CT imaging from a radiation protection point of view.
- Identify a simple equation that can be used for the calculation of a CT scan effective dose (EfD).
- Explain how x-ray beam collimation for a single slice CT scanner (SSCT) is accomplished.
- Identify the difference between detectors used for a single detector CT scanner versus a multidetector scanner.
- State the most direct advantages of MDCT scanners over SSCT scanners.
- With MDCT, identify the composition of slices.
- With MDCT, state the correlation to slice number.
- Describe what occurs as reconstructed slice thickness decreases.
- Identify the four major sections, or compartments, of the heart.
- Explain the difference between the diastole phase and the systole phase of the cardiac cycle.
- Identify the four major sections, or compartments, of the heart.
- Explain the difference between the diastole phase and the systole phase of the cardiac cycle.
- Identify what properties modalities must have to obtain useful images of a rapidly beating heart.
- In electrocardiogram (ECG) gated imaging, explain the details of the electronic link with the CT scanner and the final result that occurs.
- In the cardiac cycle, determine what must be transmitted for heart beats to occur at a regular pace.
- Identify the two components in spatial resolution in CT scanning.
- Identify the primary method used to increase vascular contrast resolution in CT scanning.
- List the factors affecting temporal resolution, spatial resolution, and contrast resolution for CT scanning.
- Understand how cone beam computed tomography (CBCT) differs from standard computed tomography (CT).
- Describe what types of medical procedures CBCT is most suited for.
- List some advantages and disadvantages of CBCT.
- Compare the patient radiation doses received from CBCT procedures with those from standard CT scans.

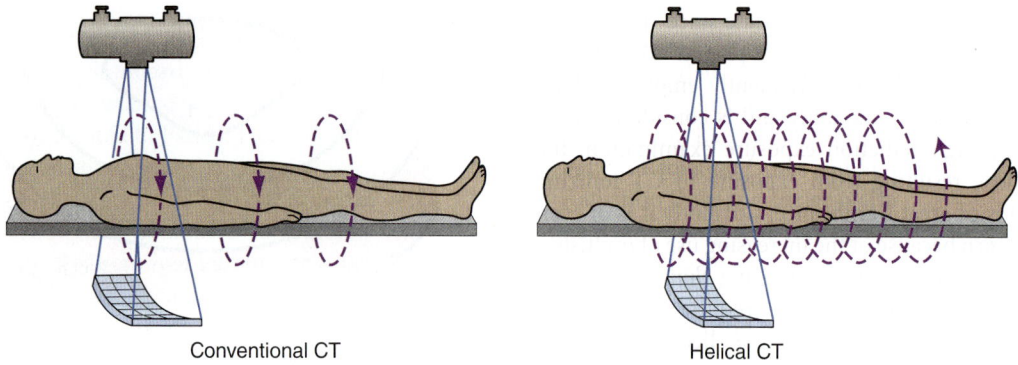

Fig. 14.2 Axial versus spiral (helical) CT scanning.

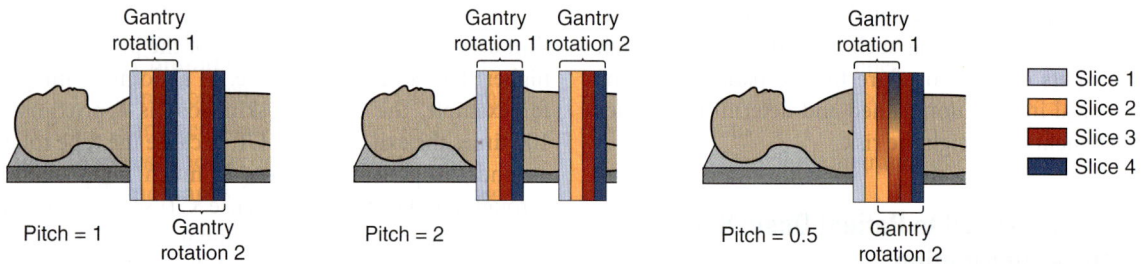

Fig. 14.3 Illustration of different pitch value scan sequences.

the anatomy outside the field of view is usually caused only by internal scatter. Therefore generally, in CT, anatomy does not appear in the primary x-ray beam unless it is part of the intended field of view.

Helical, or Spiral, Computed Tomography

Helical, or spiral, CT presents a more substantial challenge for assessing patient dose than conventional CT. Helical CT may be defined as a data acquisition method that combines a continuous gantry rotation with a selectable speed of continuous table advance forming a spiral path of data acquisition (Fig. 14.2).[1]

Such types of scans are often characterized by the quantity **pitch ratio** or just *pitch*. Pitch is the ratio of the movement or advance of the patient couch during a CT scan, also known as *table increment (I)*, to the x-ray beam collimator dimension (Z). Mathematically, it is expressed as the proportion: I/Z. When the spiral scan pitch ratio is approximately 1, the patient dose is comparable to that produced by nonhelical or *axial* CT. However, when the pitch ratio is higher (e.g., 2:1), the patient dose is reduced in comparison with ordinary axial CT because the same number of x-rays produced during each rotation of the tube is spread out over a

BOX 14.1 Optimization of Patient Dose in CT

- Tube current modulation
  - Longitudinal
  - Angular
- Iterative reconstruction
- Optimization of tube voltage and other scan parameters
- Correct patient centering

larger area of the patient. The reverse also is true: patient dose increases at a pitch less than one (Fig. 14.3).

METHODS FOR REDUCTION OF PATIENT DOSE IN CT

Box 14.1 provides a list of several dose reduction methods that lead to optimization of patient dose in CT. These methods are discussed in the sections that follow.

Tube Current Modulation

Recognizing that the x-ray tube current (mA) determines the rate of x-ray output from the tube, CT manufacturers utilize patient anatomical information

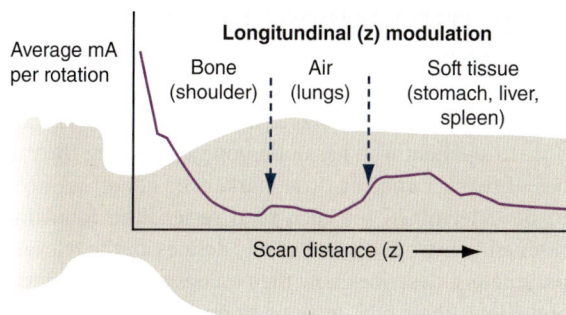

Fig. 14.4 X-ray tube current as a function of position superimposed on a CT projection radiograph illustrating the principle of longitudinal dose modulation. (From McCollough CH, Bruesewitz MR, Kofler JM: CT dose reduction and dose management tools: overview of available options, *RadioGraphics* 26(2):503–512, 2006.)

obtained from an initial "scout view" to vary or modulate the current as the tube moves along the longitudinal axis of the patient, usually referred to as the *z-axis*. Lower tube current is used in regions where there is decreased attenuation because the anatomy is thinner or less dense (e.g., the thorax), and higher tube current is used in regions where there is more attenuation due to the anatomy being thicker (e.g., the abdomen) (Fig. 14.4). This practice will reduce patient dose in regions where fewer photons are needed to acquire an image of acceptable quality. **Tube current modulation** is sometimes referred to as *automatic exposure control (AEC) for CT* in comparison with the AEC systems that are used in radiographic and fluoroscopic imaging systems.

Tube current may also be varied as the x-ray tube rotates about the patient to reduce dose to radiation-sensitive organs such as the breast that reside on the anterior surface of the patient rather than the midline. *Angular-based tube current modulation* reduces tube current while the x-ray tube is on the anterior side of the patient and maintains or increases dose as it rotates on the posterior side. This method has been shown to underdose the superficial anterior organs without adversely affecting image quality.[2]

In the past, external shields impregnated with radiopaque material such as bismuth have been used to reduce the dose to organs near the patient's surface. However, tube current modulation techniques have been found to be more effective and have less effect upon image quality.[3,4]

Iterative Reconstruction

Originally, CT scan data were reconstructed from data acquired during the scanning process through a technique known as **filtered back projection*** that was applied *only a single time*.

Recent advances in computer technology allow data to be acquired with lower patient dose. CT scan data can be reconstructed, modified, reconstructed again, modified, etc., until an image with the lowest noise possible

---

Filtered back projection: The standard method of reconstructing CT slices is called *back projection*. This involves reflecting back the projection across the image at the angle it was acquired. By reflecting back all of the projections associated with a complete revolution of the x-ray tube and detector system, a composite image (i.e., a summary of more and less intense detector signals (represented by *different gray levels*) can be built up, producing a reconstructed image. This image looks similar to the real picture but is blurry. To correct the blurring problem created by standard back projection, a filter is superimposed on all of the back projections, thereby producing what is known as a *filtered back projection image*. Filtering refers to changing the projection data before doing the back projections to remove blurriness. The simplest filter employed is a high-pass filter, or a sharpening filter. This type of filter preferentially picks up sharp edges within the projection (and thus, in the underlying slice) and tends to ignore flat areas. Because the high-pass filter creates negative pixels at the edges, it subtracts out the extra smearing caused by plain back projection. Thus the end result is a more accurate reconstruction. The high-pass filter, however, accentuates the noise already present in a CT image. To obtain a "cleaner" image, other "softer" filters have been developed to replace the high-pass filter for images that do not have very high contrast (with appreciation from xrayphysics.com/ctsim.html) created by standard back projection, a filter is superimposed on all of the back projections, thereby producing what is known as a *filtered back projection image*. Filtering refers to changing the projection data before doing the back projections to remove blurriness. The simplest filter employed is a high-pass filter, or a sharpening filter. This type of filter preferentially picks up sharp edges within the projection (and thus, in the underlying slice) and tends to ignore flat areas. Because the high-pass filter creates negative pixels at the edges, it subtracts out the extra smearing caused by plain back projection. Thus the end result is a more accurate reconstruction. The high-pass filter, however, accentuates the noise already present in a CT image. To obtain a "cleaner" image, other "softer" filters have been developed to replace the high-pass filter for images that do not have very high contrast (with appreciation from xrayphysics. com/ctsim.html).

is obtained. Such a repetitive process is referred to as **iterative reconstruction**. With filtered back projection alone, decreasing tube current may decrease dose, but at a price of increased quantum noise in the final image. Iterative reconstruction techniques, however, can be used to reduce dose to levels below those of filtered back projection while maintaining acceptable noise levels.[5,6]

Optimization of Tube Voltage

Changing x-ray tube voltage changes patient dose in CT as it does in radiography. However, the effect is the opposite. In radiography, increasing kVp tends to decrease patient dose because exposure time can be decreased. In CT, all other factors being equal, increasing kVp tends to increase patient dose.[7]

In general radiography, increasing kVp lowers the number of photoelectric interactions in the patient because the occurrence probability of photoelectric interactions decreases as photon energy is increased ($\sim 1/E^3$). So more photons pass through the patient to reach the image receptor, and the exposure time may be decreased. However, in CT, because of the higher effective energy of the x-ray beam (due to its greater filtration), both photoelectric *and Compton interactions* contribute substantially to the image. Thus if kVp is increased, the output of the x-ray tube increases during a set scan time, and the patient exposure due to the higher prevalence of Compton interactions actually increases. Controlling the variables of kVp, scan time, and tube current is a major part of most CT protocols for optimum use of patient dose.[8]

Patient Centering

Verifying that the center of the patient coincides with the center of the CT gantry is a significant part of dose reduction strategies that are under the control of the CT technologist. Miscentering of the patient by only a few centimeters can result in unnecessarily large differences in patient dose when the tube current modulation system or AEC is in use. If the patient is placed closer to the x-ray tube when the scout view (radiographic) image is obtained, then the image of the patient is magnified, causing the tube current modulation system to increase the tube current, thereby overdosing the patient. A miscentering of 2 centimeters can produce as much as a 25% unnecessary increase in patient dose.[9] Automatic patient miscentering correction software is becoming available to alleviate this problem.[10] Still, there is no substitute for proper positioning.

COMPUTED TOMOGRAPHY DOSE PARAMETERS

To approximate and characterize the effective radiation dose to a patient who has undergone a CT study, the values of two CT-specific dose markers or quantities need to be determined for each scan series. The following discussion introduces and briefly defines all the relevant parameters, describes how their values can be obtained, and shows their relationships to one another. The relevant **dose parameters** are as follows:

- Computed tomography dose index (CTDI)
- $CTDI_W$ (weighted CTDI)
- $CTDI_{vol}$ (CTDI volume)
- Effective milliampere-second (mAS)
- Dose length product (DLP)

DLP and $CTDI_{VOL}$ are the two most significant CT dose markers and have quantitative values that directly depend on the technical details of the performed CT scan. Both quantities are displayed by the scanner's software for each completed patient scan. There is a progressive relationship among all of the listed parameters, as demonstrated in the following paragraphs.

CTDI is determined by an ionization measurement using a 1cm diameter and 10 cm (100 mm) long, pencil-like, ionization chamber inserted into a cylindrical acrylic phantom (Figs. 14.5 and 14.6).

The phantom is similar in diameter to either an average human head (16 cm diameter) or human abdomen (32 cm diameter) and is scanned utilizing a *single axial* scan with technical factors (kVp, mAs, and slice thickness) that are *equivalent* to those used for an actual

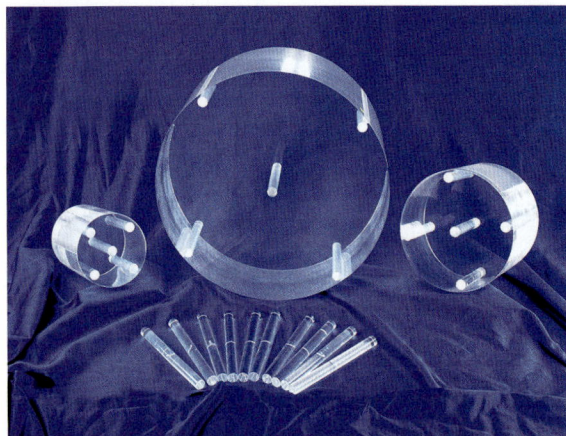

Fig. 14.5 Acrylic body and head CTDI dosimetry phantoms.

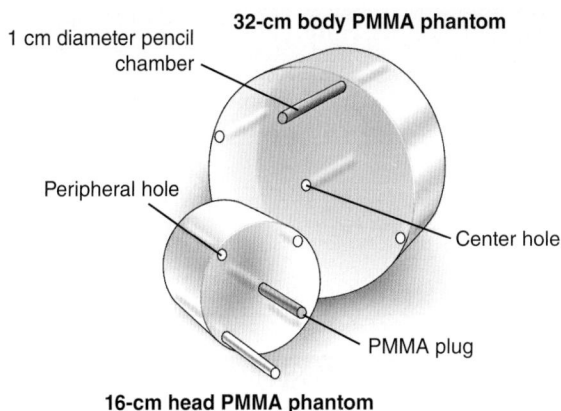

Fig. 14.6 Demonstrates the measurement process for obtaining CTDI$_w$ for both the body and head phantoms. The pencil chamber will be successively inserted into each of the 4 peripheral cavities and then into the central cavity and ionization measurements obtained. PMMA (poly methyl methacrylate) is an organic compound made up of carbon, hydrogen, and oxygen. It is the chemical name for what is commonly referred to as *acrylic* or *Lucite* or *Plexiglas*.

patient study that could be either helical or axial. The irradiated pencil chamber is attached to an electrometer whose ionization charge reading, when multiplied by several correction factors, will then be given in milligray (mGy) units. Dividing this number by the scan direction collimation* will make this ionization measurement *representative* of the localized dose from a multiple slice examination.

CTDIW is simply a weighted average of two measured CTDI values: one that is obtained with the pencil chamber placed in the central cavity of the acrylic phantom and the other derived from the average of four peripheral (1 cm depth from the cylindrical surface) cavity measurements that are located at the 3, 6, 9, and 12 o'clock positions (see Fig. 14.6). The mathematical expression for CTDI$_w$ is given by:

$$CTDI_W = \frac{1}{3}\left(CTDI_{center}\right) + \frac{2}{3}\left(CTDI_{periph}\right)$$

CTDIVOL is the average absorbed dose within the scanned volume. It takes into account whether the scan is axial or helical and its value is directly related to CTDI$_W$ by the following expression:

$$CTDI_{VOL} = CTDI_W / Pitch$$

For purely axial scans, such as those typically used in adult head scan sequences, the pitch (P) equals 1, and therefore $CTDI_{VOL} = CTDI_W$. For helical scans, however, the pitch is usually greater than 1 (e.g., 1.375 is quite common) but sometimes can be less than 1 when overlapping is desired, so the magnitude of CTDI$_{VOL}$ could be either less than the CTDI$_W$ or greater than the CTDI$_W$.

Effective mAS is simply the ratio of applied mAS to selected pitch:

$$Eff\ mAS \equiv mAS/pitch$$

Box 14.2 provides an example of the determination of effective mAs.

At the conclusion of each patient CT scan sequence, built-in computer software accesses a detailed measurement database that supplies a numeric value of the patient's CTDI$_{VOL}$ for that particular scan sequence. Also provided is the value of the quantity *dose length product* (DLP).

DLP represents the product of the CTDI$_{VOL}$ and the irradiated scan length. DLP is expressed in mGy-cm and characterizes the volumetric extent along the patient's body that has been irradiated with an average absorbed dose and therefore is representative of the total patient absorbed radiation energy. As such it has a greater significance than just the CTDI$_{VOL}$ alone for estimating future cancer risk as a result of radiation doses unavoidably delivered to sensitive organs from CT examinations. Mathematically*:

$$DLP* = CTDI_{VOL} \times irradiated\ scan\ length.$$

Scan length, which may be considered as *approximately* the superior-inferior extent of the patient's

---

*Scan direction collimation is equal to the product of the number of slices (N) used during one axial acquisition and the nominal slice width (T). For example, in a single detector row or single slice scanner for a 10-mm slice thickness, N = 1 and T = 10, so NT = 10. In a multislice CT scanner with selected scan thickness parameters 4 x 5 mm, then N = 4, T = 5, and NT = 20.

---

*Although CTDI$_{vol}$ is an accurate representation of the dose in the central slices within a long scan length, it is not an accurate measure of dose on the edges of the scan. DLP particularly implies that the CTDI$_{vol}$ values are exactly the same for the whole scan length. However, to be exact, because of the sharp dose gradients between the "on" and "off" values at the edges of the volume of interest, DLP just serves as an acceptable and useful first-approximation and guide to the entire actual physical situation.

BOX 14.2 Example of the Determination of Effective mAs

Which of the following five CT scan protocols would be expected to result in the highest $CTDI_{vol}$? (Note: KVP and beam collimations are all the same.)

1. mA = 400, rotation time = 0.5 sec, pitch = 1
2. mA = 100, rotation time = 1 sec, pitch = 0.5
3. Effective mAs = 200, pitch = 0.5
4. Effective mAs = 200, pitch = 1
5. There is no difference in CTDIvol for any of these

Solution: The value of $CTDI_{VOL}$ ultimately depends on the scan technique applied and this includes both mA, time, and pitch. The combination of the three is the Eff mAs. It is seen that this value is the same (200) for all four cases. Therefore the $CTDI_{VOL}$ will be the same also and choice #5 is the correct answer.

From Cagnon C, DeMarco J, Angel E: *Estimating patient radiation dose from computed tomography*, UCLA David Geffen School of Medicine, 2008. https://www.aapm.org/meetings/amos2/pdf/34-9723-93678-499.pdf.

irradiation, can be derived from the product of slice width times the number of slices times the pitch. Thus a helical scan that is composed of sixty 5-mm slices with a pitch of 1.5 has an approximate scan length of $60 \times 0.5 \times 1.5 = 45$ cm. If instead, this was a contiguous axial scan, the scan length would be just $60 \times 0.5 = 30$ cm. The length of the scan shown or calculated from the console is the distance between the centers of the starting and ending images. The irradiated length for such a set of images can vary from this distance, how much depending on the acquisition mode.

EFFECTIVE COMPUTED TOMOGRAPHY DOSE

Table 14.1 lists body scan region–specific conversion factors generated by the European Union[11] that when combined with the dose information supplied by the CT software for each delivered scan sequence will yield an effective dose (EfD) value for that CT scan. The simple expression to be used for the calculation of a computed tomography scan EfD is given by the following equation:

$$EfD = DLP \times EfDLP$$

where *EfDLP* is the normalized EfD associated with a specific scan region of the body. It is expressed in

TABLE 14.1 Scan Region Specific Conversion Factors

Body Region Scanned	Normalized Effective Dose (EfDLP) Factor
Head	0.0023
Neck	0.0054
Chest	0.017
Abdomen	0.015
Pelvis	0.019

CASE 14.1 Head Scan (Axial)

Scan data: $CTDI_{VOL}$ = 60.8 mGy, DLP = 373 mGy-cm (portion of scan series at 140 kVp)
$CTDI_{VOL}$ = 49.1 mGy, DLP = 351 mGy-cm (portion of scan series at 120 kVp)
From Table 14.1, EfDLP (head) = 0.0023.
Therefore the total EfD to this patient is given by the following equation:
$(373 + 351) \times 0.0023 = 1.67$ mSv (0.167 rem)

CASE 14.2 Chest Scan (Helical)

Scan data: $CTDI_{VOL}$ = 8.5 mGy, DLP = 323 mGy-cm
From Table 14.1, EfDLP (chest) = 0.017.
Therefore the EfD to this patient is given by the following equation:
$323 \times 0.017 = 5.49$ mSv (0.549 rem)

CASE 14.3 Abdominal Scan (Helical)

Scan data: $CTDI_{VOL}$ = 10 mGy, DLP = 460 mGy-cm
From Table 14.1, EfDLP (abdomen) = 0.015.
Therefore the EfD to this patient is given by the following equation:
$460 \times 0.015 = 6.9$ mSv (0.69 rem)

millisieverts per milligray-centimeter (mSv/mGy-cm) and represents a conversion factor from a patient's scan DLP to the effective dose received by the patient as a result of that scan. EfDLP values are given in Table 14.1.

Using those values and the information displayed on the dose page printout for a patient's CT scan, the EfD from that scan can be calculated. Several examples of using such data from actual patient CT scans are demonstrated in Cases 14.1 to 14.3. Typical effective dose value ranges for several frequent computed tomography examinations can be found in Table 14.2.

TABLE 14.2   Typical Effective Dose Values for CT Examinations

Examination	Effective Dose (mSv)
Head	1–2
Chest	2–6
Abdomen	5–8
Pelvis	3–6
Coronary artery calcification	0.1–3
Coronary angiography	1–18

In the early 2000s, various publications calculated individual and population risks of cancer from computed tomography procedures based upon risk estimates derived from the atomic bomb survivors' studies. These studies were used to predict the number of cancers in large populations due to medical procedures such as CT by multiplying the small risk estimates for individual procedures by the large population of patients undergoing such studies every year.

More recent analysis, however, has shown no increase in the risk of cancer or any other measures of early death from effective doses below 100 mSv (10 rem).[12,13] Routine head and body scans fall in the 1 to 10 mSv effective dose range, and CT angiography rarely exceeds 15 mSv (1.5 rem). Because there is considerable uncertainty in the estimation of risk below 100 mSv, many of the major scientific and advisory bodies concerned with radiation bioeffects (UNSCEAR, ICRP, NCRP) have discredited this practice.[14-16] In 2011 the American Association of Physicists in Medicine issued the following position statement[17]:

"Discussion of risks related to radiation dose from medical imaging procedures should be accompanied by acknowledgement of the benefits of the procedures. Risks of medical imaging at effective doses below 50 mSv for single procedures or 100 mSv for multiple procedures over short time periods are too low to be detectable and may be nonexistent. Predictions of hypothetical cancer incidence and deaths in patient populations exposed to such low doses are highly speculative and should be discouraged."

In summary, the goal of CT imaging should be to obtain the best image possible while delivering an acceptable level of ionizing radiation to the patient. In the *absence* of specifically designed scan protocols, the fulfillment of this responsibility lies with the technologist performing the examination.

MULTIDETECTOR COMPUTED TOMOGRAPHY (MDCT)

X-ray beam collimation for a single slice CT scanner (SSCT) is accomplished by employing physical pre- and post size restriction of the CT x-ray beam. Collimation is used to reduce scatter radiation to the patient and thereby decrease patient dose and improve image sharpness. Pre-patient collimation controls the aperture at the x-ray tube, directly limiting the x-ray beam to the desired width. Post-collimation can be used to limit penumbra effects. Therefore in SSCT, *slice width* is very much determined by x-ray beam collimators. The *slice number* refers to the amount of slice images the CT scanning machine can obtain per gantry rotation. It is equal to one for SSCT scanners.

Multidetector scanners employ numerous rows of CT detectors, unlike SSCT scanners, which only use one. MDCT's most direct advantages over SSCT scanners are faster scanning procedures with improved spatial resolution. For both SSCT and MDCT scanners there is a "fan-beam" geometry for the utilized x-ray beam (Fig. 14.7). The z-axis dimension is along the length of the patient and illustrates the longitudinal or axial extent of the scanner detectors, whereas the x–y plane corresponds to the cross-patient scan coverage.

To reconstruct an accurate image from a patient's scan, at least 180 rotational degrees of data must be acquired. The remaining 180 degrees of projections for a full 3600 rotation are simply a mirror image of the first 1800 because in whichever opposed direction a photon travels through a particular path length through the body, it will be overall attenuated by the same amount. Due to the fan beam geometry of the x-ray beam, however, it is necessary to measure an extra amount equal to the fan angle or transverse spread of the x-ray beam to wholly acquire all of the data needed. Any element of tissue must be included in all of the 180 degrees of projections to be reconstructed correctly.[18]

MDCT Collimation, Slice Width, and Slice Number

In MDCT systems the total number of *data channels* is simply equal to the total number of detector rows.

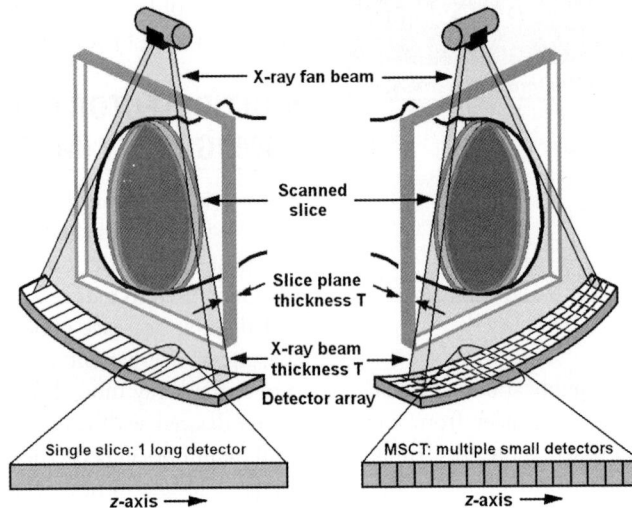

Fig. 14.7 Fan beam Geometry for 2 detector configurations. Single slice computed tomography (left) vs multislice computed tomography (right). The arc expanse of the x-ray beam is what constitutes the "fan-like" geometry. The fan angle of the emitted beam determines the extent of detector coverage in the transverse (cross-plane or x–y) dimension. (From Goldman LW: Principles of CT: multislice CT, *J Nucl Med Technol* 36(2):57–68, 2008. This research was originally published in the *Journal of Nuclear Medicine Technology*.)

The product of the selected detector configuration or the number of involved detector rows multiplied by the effective detector row thickness is equivalent to the *beam collimation*. For example, with a detector configuration of 60 detector rows, each row having a z-axis dimension of 0.5 mm, the beam collimation would be equal to 30 mm (i.e., 60 × 0.5 mm). Concerning the patient, the physical manifestation of the beam collimation is considered to be the x-ray beam size as defined at the gantry isocenter.

With MDCT, slices can be composed of a single detector row thickness or multiple adjacent detectors, and the effective slice thickness or *slice width* is therefore determined by the chosen detector configuration and not by physical x-ray beam collimation. Thus, for a 60 row, 0.5 mm MDCT, combining every two adjacent detectors would allow a set of thirty 1mm slices (30 × 1 mm) per rotation of the gantry. In contrast, a combination of 4 detector rows instead could yield fifteen 2 mm slices (15 × 2 mm). The *slice number* thus correlates to how many images the CT scanning machine can obtain per gantry rotation.

The selection of the detector imaging configuration should always be related to the type of study to be performed, the required slice thickness for diagnostically

useful multiplanar reconstructions, and whether there is also a need for three dimensional (3-D images). For routine acquisitions, without the need for 3-D imaging, very thin effective detector thicknesses (0.5 mm or 1 mm) are unnecessary. In such cases, if 3 mm thick images in the axial, coronal, and sagittal planes are sufficient for radiologist review, the effective detector thickness can be enlarged to a combination of six 0.5 mm units without a marked impact on image quality.[19]

MDCT Advantages

A significant difficulty that arose with early single-slice spiral (helical) CT scanning was the inverse relationship between scan length (z-axis extent) and spatial resolution along the head to toe axis (i.e., axial resolution) of the patient. Thus, because of the requirement for small scan lengths for adequate spatial resolution, using SSCT scanners for a volumetric acquisition with acceptable spatial resolution in all directions (i.e., isotropic) would be very difficult since only limited regions could be imaged during each breath-hold. A solution to this issue was to design a CT scanner with a detection system that would permit the acquisition of multiple thin (1.5 mm and less) simultaneous slices and also have an increased x-ray tube rotational speed. For example, even

BOX 14.3   Advantages of MDCT

Shorter Scan Duration
Reduced movement artifacts for:
- Children
- Trauma patients
- Acutely ill or dyspneic patients

Improved Contrast-Enhanced Scans
- Well-defined phase of contrast enhancement
- Reduced contrast volume for CT Angiography (CTA)
- More-homogeneous enhancement

Longer Scan Ranges Permitting CT
- Thoraco-abdominal aorta
- Carotids from arch to intracerebral circulation

Trauma
- Full spine examinations

Thinner Sections
Near Isotropic Imaging (any application):
- Arbitrary imaging planes
- Multiplanar reformations
- Three-dimensional rendering

From Prokop M: Multislice CT: technical principles and future trends. *Eur Radiol* 13:3–13, 2003; Prokop M: General principles of MDCT. *Eur J Radiol* 45(suppl 1): S4–S10, 2003.

a very early four-detector row scanner with a 0.5 second gantry rotation yielded a performance that was up to eight times greater than a 1 second single-slice scanner. These scanners allowed higher spatial resolution to be achieved over a longer scan range. Currently, most institutions employ scanners with 16, 64, or even greater numbers of detector rows instead of just 4, faster gantry rotational times, and sub-millimeter length detector rows. Therefore faster and more varied slice acquisitions can be achieved along with much improved z-axis resolution. Box 14.3 lists the multiple benefits of MDCT scanners over previous generation SSCT scanners.[20]

Slice Thickness and Reconstruction Interval

Detector configuration is the number of data channels being used in the z-axis direction and the effective detector thickness of each data channel. For example, a detector configuration of 128×0.5 mm would signify the use of 128 data channels in the z-axis, each of which has an effective thickness of 0.5 mm. As mentioned previously, MDCT slices can be composed of single detector row

thicknesses (for highest resolution) or from combinations of multiple adjacent detector rows. Images can also be acquired at selected intervals or separations.

The reconstructed slice width or thickness can be varied independently of the data set acquisition as long as the recreated width is not less than the slice collimation (SC). In other words, if slices of a certain thickness are used for scanning, it is not possible to later reconstruct thinner slices to obtain smaller detail. However, it is simple to reconstruct broader slices for more convenient clinical viewing, if thin slices were used for scanning.[21]

The reconstruction interval is the selected spacing between adjacent processed image slices of the patient. It is configured by the software from all of the raw data that was obtained during the patient scan. Reconstructed images can be obtained at any desired and reasonable separation. The slices remain the same thickness (z-axis dimension) for whatever partition is chosen, but their individual relative positioning changes. This simply means that the produced slice images can overlap or be contiguous (no spacing) or be noncontiguous (gapped) (Fig. 14.8).

The majority of multiplanar reconstructions will generally be *contiguous*, ensuring that there are no missing areas of anatomy which could occur with noncontiguous, or gapped, intervals. With overlapping scanning, more images than necessary are created and more radiation dose to the patient is delivered. Overlapped images, however, can be useful in certain situations. They are acquired when it is needed to track in fine detail small and/or tortuous objects (arteries, veins) such as are present in cardiovascular studies.

As the reconstructed slice thickness decreases, the number of photons within each voxel also decreases, resulting in increased relative **image noise**. Unfortunately, to maintain acceptable noise levels within an image with a smaller slice thickness, the radiation dose to the patient must then be increased, typically by increasing the mAS. Ultimately, slice thickness determines the trade-off in image quality between **spatial resolution** (how accurately small physical changes in the image can be differentiated) and *image noise* (the standard deviation of the image data). *Decreased slice thickness = increased spatial resolution and increased image noise.* It is also important to note that reducing the reconstruction interval (i.e., smaller gaps) can increase the visibility of small lesions that may otherwise be obscured by volume averaging. If the lesion is centered in the slice, there will then be less healthy tissue to average or smooth it out. Table 14.3

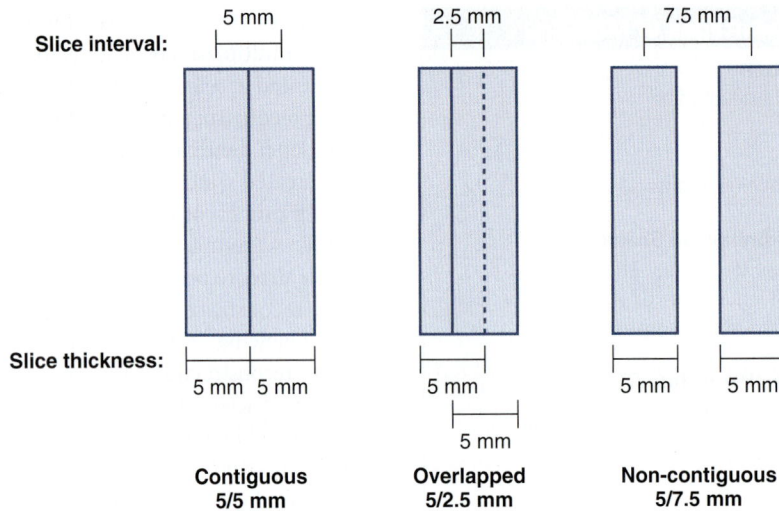

Fig. 14.8 Several slice reconstruction intervals for 5 mm slices. In the figure, the "mm" values represent the center to center spacing of the slices. (From Tristan Charles, RadTrain. Available from: www.radtrain.com.au.)

TABLE 14.3   Summary of CT Hardware and Parameters for State-of-the-Art CT Scanners from the Major CT Manufacturers

Scanner	X-ray sources, number	Detector rows, number	Detector-row z-axis dimension, mm*	Total nominal beam width, mm	Fastest gantry rotation time, sec	Temporal resolution for each cross-sectional image, sec[†]
GE Discovery CT750 HD	1	64	0.625	40	0.35	0.175
Hitachi SCENARIA	1	64	0.625	40	0.35	0.175
Phillips Brilliance iCT	1	128	0.625	80	0.27	0.135
Siemens SOMATOM Definition FLASH	2 (95° apart)	64	0.6	40	0.28	0.075
Toshiba Aquilion ONE	1	320	0.5	160	0.35	

*Values measured at scanner isocenter
[†]Values do not reflect the use of multi-segment reconstruction
From Halliburton S, Arbab-Zadeh A, Dey D, et al.: State of the art in CT hardware and scan modes for cardiovascular CT, J Cardiovasc Comput Tomogr 6(3):154–163, 2012.

below presents a summary of some (but *not the latest*) existing CT hardware and their characteristics.[22]

COMPUTED TOMOGRAPHY CARDIOVASCULAR IMAGING (CT CVI)

Complications in the usual functioning of the heart brought on by various anatomical changes or defects,

collectively known as coronary heart disease (CHD), is a major cause of morbidity and mortality. In the field of diagnostic radiology, cardiac imaging has become a commonplace procedure. In conjunction with a cardiologist, a trained cardiac radiologist supervises and then interprets various types of medical imaging to diagnose disorders of the heart such as: leaky heart valves, defects in the size and shape of the heart, and potential ruptures or tears or blockages in various structures. A cardiac radiologist can employ a variety of imaging techniques such as interventional fluoroscopy, ultrasound (e.g., echocardiograms), high-speed x-ray computed tomography scans, and magnetic resonance imaging (MRI) scans. All of these tests are used to screen for heart disease, determine the cause of various symptoms, monitor the heart's performance status, and, especially, to ascertain if a particular treatment is yielding positive results. The following sections focus only on CT imaging methods and systems to discover and examine cardiovascular maladies.

Basic Heart Anatomy and Processes

The heart is a multi-chambered muscle about the size of an average human fist. Essentially, it is a sophisticated pumping mechanism that consists of 4 major sections or compartments, named the *right atrium*, *left atrium*, *right ventricle*, and *left ventricle*. As shown in Fig. 14.9, the atria are the two upper or more cranially positioned chambers. The right atrium receives and holds oxygen-depleted blood emerging from venous channels. This blood is then sent down to the right ventricle (through the tricuspid valve), which in turn,

via a muscular contraction, pumps it through the pulmonary artery for recirculation through the lungs and consequent reoxygenation. The left atrium receives the newly oxygenated blood by transport from the lungs through the left and right pulmonary veins and immediately by contraction pushes the blood into the left ventricle (through the mitral valve). Subsequently, passage across a one-way valve (aortic valve) into the aorta artery followed by another contraction or "beat" of the heart muscle moves the oxygenated blood into whole-body circulation. This is known as the *cardiac cycle*. The cardiac cycle comprises a complete relaxation and contraction of both the atria and ventricles and lasts approximately 0.8 seconds.[23] Box 14.4 below contains explanations of the anatomic and medical terms that are used for CT CVI.

Phases of the Cardiac Cycle

At the beginning of the cardiac cycle, both the atria and ventricles are relaxed and the chambers fill with blood. This is the **diastole phase**. Blood is flowing into the right atrium from the superior vena cava and inferior vena cava and the coronary sinus. Blood flows into the left

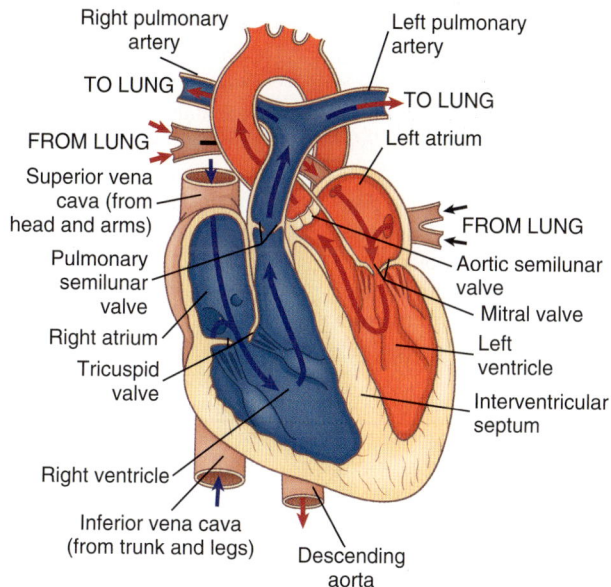

Fig. 14.9 Anatomy and blood flow through the heart. In this figure the *blue lines* and *blue arrows* show the direction in which oxygen-poor blood flows through the heart to the lungs while the *red lines* and *red arrows* show the direction in which oxygen-rich blood flows from the lungs into the heart and then out to the rest of the body through both the ascending (superior circular red segment) and the descending aorta. (From Stein L, Hollen CJ: *Concept–based clinical nursing skills*, ed 2, St. Louis, 2024, Elsevier.)

BOX 14.4   Explanation of Various Anatomic and Procedure Terms

Aneurysm: A rupture or tear in the outer wall of an organ.

Angina: Chest pain (such as squeezing or unusual pressure) or general discomfort caused when the heart muscle doesn't get enough oxygen-rich blood.

Aorta: The largest and most important artery in the body. The *aorta* begins at the top of the left ventricle, the heart's muscular pumping chamber. The heart pumps blood into the *aorta* through the *aortic* valve. The *aorta* ascends a little ways, bends over like a cane (i.e., arches) and then goes downward.

Cardiovascular disease: This most often refers to conditions that involve narrowed or blocked blood vessels that can lead to a heart attack, chest pain (angina), or stroke. Other heart conditions, such as those that affect its muscle, valves, or rhythm, also are considered forms of heart disease.

Cardiovasculature: The circulatory system which supplies the heart with nutrients and oxygen.

Coronary arteries: the network of lesser blood vessels that branch off the aorta to nourish the heart muscle itself with oxygen-rich blood. They are mainly composed of the left and right *coronary arteries*, both of which give off smaller branches. They are called the *coronary arteries* because they encircle the surface of the heart in the manner of a crown encircling royalty. The main arteries and all of their branches are often described as the "*Coronary Tree.*"

Coronary sinus: A collection of veins joined together to form a large vessel that collects blood from the heart muscle (myocardium). It delivers less-oxygenated blood to the right atrium, as do the superior and inferior vena cava.

CT angiography (CTA): ACT procedure that is used to diagnose and evaluate blood vessel disease or related conditions, such as aneurysms or narrowing or blockages.

Diastisis: The *middle stage of diastole* during the cycle of a heartbeat, where the initial passive filling of the ventricles has slowed down, but before the atria contract to complete the active filling.

Left ventricle: It is located in the bottom *left* portion of the heart below the *left* atrium, separated by the mitral valve. The *left ventricle* is the thickest of the heart's chambers and is responsible for pumping reoxygenated blood to the aorta, which delivers the blood to tissues all over the body.

Mycardial infarction (heart attack): A failure of the heart muscle which occurs when a portion of the heart is deprived of oxygen due to decreased blood flow as a result of blockage of a coronary artery. An artery supplying your *heart* with blood and oxygen becomes blocked by fatty deposits building up over time, forming plaques in the *heart's* arteries. If a plaque ruptures, a blood clot can form and significantly obstruct the arteries, leading to a *heart attack*.

Myocardium: The muscle tissue which forms the wall (or most of the wall) of the heart; also known as the *heart muscle*. The myocardium establishes a thick middle layer between the outer layer of the heart wall (the epicardium) and the inner layer (the endocardium), with blood supplied via the coronary circulation.

Perfusion: The passage of fluid through the circulatory system or lymphatic system to an organ or a tissue. As related to cardiac processes, perfusion is measured as the rate at which blood is delivered to tissue, or volume of blood per unit time per unit tissue mass.

Pulmonary arteries: The vessels carrying oxygen depleted blood from the right ventricle of the heart to the left and right lungs for reoxygenation.

Pulmonary embolism (PE): A blockage of an artery in the lungs by a substance that has moved from elsewhere in the body through the bloodstream (an embolism).

Pulmonary veins: The vessels carrying reoxygenated blood from the lungs to the left atrium of the heart.

Right atrium and left atrium: Akin to household foyers these are entrances to the heart. Blood enters the heart from different portions of the body through the two *atria*. Deoxygenated blood enters the *right atrium* through the inferior and superior vena cava and reoxygenated blood from the lungs enters the *left atrium* through the pulmonary vein.

Right ventricle: The lower right chamber within the heart that initiates the pumping of oxygen-depleted blood to the lungs.

Systole and diastole: Two phases of the cardiac compression/relaxation cycle. *Systole* occurs when the heart contracts to pump blood out, and *diastole* occurs when the heart relaxes or returns to its normal volume after contraction.

Vena cava (superior and inferior): Situated on the right side of the heart, these are the largest veins in the body. After the body's organs and tissues have exhausted the oxygen in the blood, the superior and inferior vena cava carry the oxygen depleted blood back to the right atrium. The superior vena cava moves oxygen-poor blood from the upper parts of the body, including the head, chest, arms, and neck while the inferior vena cava retrieves oxygen-poor blood from the lower parts of the body.

atrium from the four pulmonary veins. The two valves situated respectively between each atrium and each ventricle, the tricuspid and mitral valves, are both open, so blood flows unimpeded from the atria and into the ventricles. Approximately 70%–80% of ventricular filling occurs by this method, and the remainder is due to atrial contraction. Following this are secondary contractions involving the ventricles that the heart experiences while it pumps blood into circulation via the pulmonary and aortic valves. These are both one-way valves, thereby preventing the backflow of blood into the right and left ventricles from the pulmonary trunk on the right and the aorta on the left. This is the **systole phase** (see Fig. 14.9).

In summary, both the atria and ventricles undergo contraction and relaxation processes, and it is essential that these components be *precisely regulated and coordinated* to ensure that blood is pumped efficiently to all critical areas of the body.[23,24] It is to be noted that as with any muscle in the body, the cardiac cycle of the heart is essentially an electrical process involving *depolarization* (i.e., a reduction in voltage difference) of a muscle,* in this case the heart muscle.

CT CVI[5] and ECG Gated Imaging

To effectively image a rapidly beating heart, most imaging modalities must have very short image acquisition times. It is necessary to eliminate or at least significantly minimize the heart motion to be able to clearly visualize coronary arteries located close to the heart muscles. Since the most quiescent part of the heart cycle is the diastolic phase, cardiac imaging will be optimal if done during this period. Therefore the heart cycle, which is essentially an electrical process involving a periodic repetitive sequence of different magnitude millivolt electrical pulses associated with the different phases of

the cycle, must be precisely monitored throughout the scanning procedure. To do this, an **electrocardiogram (ECG)**, which is a graphical tracing or readout of these pulses or electrical activity with time, is acquired. Box 14.5 presents a brief discussion of ECG that will enhance understanding of the following material and Fig. 14.10 shows this graphically.[26,28]

In ECG gated imaging, the CT scanner is electronically linked to the patient's real-time electrocardiogram. CT image acquisition and reconstruction can then be coordinated with the quiescent heart phases associated with particular magnitude electrical pulses, thereby removing or minimizing motion artifacts. Thus, the scanner is programmed to initiate scanning and to scan only through a selected portion of the diastole phase in the cardiac cycle in which the heart is entirely at rest. As a result, there will be nonscanning delay periods during and after contractions of the ventricles (Fig. 14.11). But whenever the ECG voltage signal level regains a value associated with a specific part of the diastole phase, the scanner will be triggered to image the next section of the heart and scan until another voltage pulse is received that will stop the radiation and advance the table position.*

This technique is called prospective (i.e., delayed or future) gating and is essentially a step and shoot process since for most facility scanners the detector's limited longitudinal extent mandates that the scanner advances the table in between several quiescent phases of the heart.[25,27,28] This process is depicted in some detail in Fig. 14.11.

Fig. 14.11 exhibits a segment of a prospective ECG gated imaging cycle. The imaging acquisition is composed of four processes in sync with one another. The top of the figure indicates the desired transverse heart slices to be acquired in the patient during the step and shoot scan. The next portion shows a schematic time sequence of the scanner's (activation of x-ray tube and table movement) behavior during the acquisition process. The third row is the superimposed ECG voltage signal level pattern and demonstrates sychronization

---

*Normally, there is a difference in the amount of electrical charge in the form of alkali ions between the inside and outside of the plasma membrane of a muscle. This implies the presence of an electrical potential difference or voltage between inside and outside. Depolarization is a loss of that potential difference due to a change in permeability of the muscle wall that allows a *migration of sodium ions* to the interior leading to an electrical neutrality. Depolarization occurs in the four chambers of the heart: right atria first and then left atria, followed by both ventricles. A wave of electrical depolarization originates within the right atrium (RA) and then spreads through the RA and across the inter-atrial wall into the left atrium (LA).

---

*Instructions are built into the protocol to start the scanner's x-rays at a desired distance from the R wave peak of the ECG scan, for example, at 60% or 70% of the R-R interval duration (see Box 14.5). Thus the scanner, in congruence with the patient's ECG pulse, starts the scan at a preset point in the cardiac cycle, just after diastole commences, and the x-ray projection data are acquired for only part of the complete gantry rotation (i.e., a partial scan).

BOX 14.5 Electrocardiogram and the Cardiac Cycle

An *electrocardiogram* (ECG) is a test that measures the electrical activity of the heart. With each beat, an electrical impulse (or "wave") travels through the heart. This impulse causes various portions of heart muscle to squeeze and pump blood through and from the heart. The ECG is essentially a graph of voltage versus time of the electrical activity of the heart received from electrodes placed on the skin. The amplitude, or voltage, of the recorded electrical signal is expressed on an ECG in the vertical dimension and is measured in millivolts (mV). Abnormal heart beat patterns can be easily discerned by this procedure.

The normal cardiac cycle begins with spontaneous depolarization of the *sinoatrial (SA) node**, a small region of muscle situated in the top of the right atrium. A wave of electrical depolarization** spreads from the SA node through the right atrium and across the interatrial septum*** into the left atrium. This activates the AV (atrioventricular) node. In a normal heart the only route of transmission of electrical depolarization from atria to ventricles is through this node. The AV node thus acts as an electrical relay station between the upper and lower chambers of the heart. The AV node lies near the bottom of the right atrium, on the right side of the septum that divides the atria. When the impulses generated by the SA node reach the AV node, they are delayed for about a tenth of a second. This delay in the cardiac pulse is extremely important: It ensures that the atria have ejected their blood into the ventricles first before the ventricles contract. Then the wave of depolarization spreads down and into the right and left ventricles. With normal conduction of this electrical signal, the two ventricles will contract simultaneously. This is significant for maximizing cardiac efficiency.

In summary, the spread and evolution of this series of electrical impulses causes the four chambers of the heart to both contract and relax (i.e., to depolarize and repolarize) *in a coordinated fashion*. Studying these electrical impulses permits an understanding of how well the heart is functioning. The electrical impulses are characterized by distinct waveforms named: *P, QRS complex*, and *T*. P

and T occur by themselves while Q, R, and S sequentially occur in very rapid succession thus behaving essentially as a unit named the QRS complex (Fig. 14.10).

ECG WAVEFORM DETAILS

The P waveform or pulse results from the depolarization of the left and right atrium and thus signifies the contraction of the atria. The P wave is small in amplitude and typically lasts no more than 0.11 seconds.

The second waveform is the QRS complex. The QRS complex represents the electrical impulse as it spreads through the ventricles and indicates the ventricular depolarization leading to the contraction of the large ventricular muscles. The latter causes the pressured outflow of blood from the heart into the large arteries exiting the heart. Under normal circumstances, the duration of the QRS complex in an adult patient will be between 0.06 and 0.10 seconds. The Q and S portions are always negative while the R pulse is the positive waveform of the complex. It is the most prominent signal spike seen on an ECG graph, representing the required electrical stimulus that passes through the main portion of the muscularly dense ventricular walls.

The ***T*** wave follows the QRS complex and indicates *ventricular repolarization* or relaxation. A T wave will normally have the same voltage direction or polarity as the QRS complex that preceded it. Should a T waveform demonstrate an opposite polarity or direction to that of the QRS complex, this generally indicates some sort of cardiac pathology.

In brief summary, the *R* waveform or large signal spike of the *ECG* is conveniently used as a reference point. data acquisition by the scanner is normally initiated following a brief delay after the *R* wave and continues only during the heart quiescence. To encompass the entire heart, the images are usually created from data collected over a series of R to R intervals (the time between QRS complexes). The instantaneous heart rate or time between heart beats can be calculated from the time between any two QRS complexes. Normal values for RR interval range from 0.6 to 1.2 seconds.

---

*SA node is a small body of specialized muscle tissue situated in the top tissue wall of the right atrium of the heart that acts as a pacemaker by producing a contraction signal at regular intervals.

**Depolarization, in more detail, is an electrical process involving the movement or migration of potassium ions within the heart muscle membrane that causes it as a whole to become less negatively charged approaching a neutral electrical potential. This type of electrical activity physically leads to contraction of the heart muscles and happens automatically in a functioning heart.

***The septum is the wall of tissue that separates the left and right atria of the heart. From Cardiology Teaching Packages and Cardiac Conduction System Learning Resources, School of Health Sciences, University of Nottingham, UK.

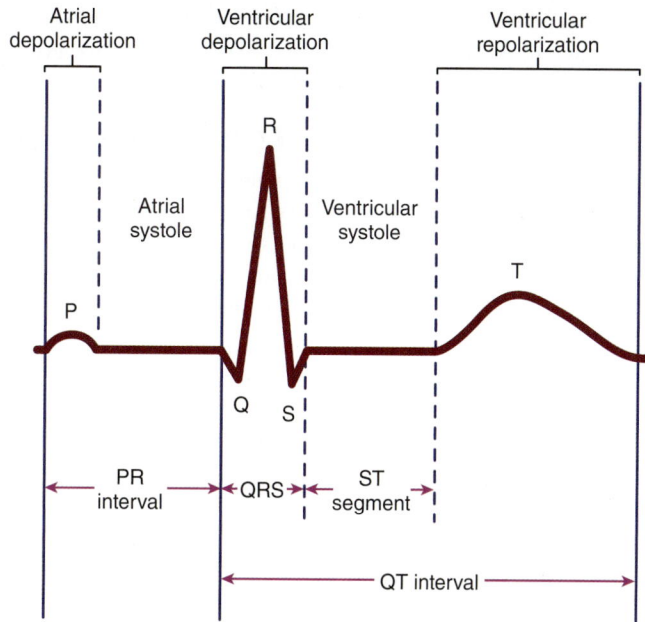

Fig. 14.10 The major segments or phases of the cardiac cycle. (From Urden LD, Stacy KM, Lough ME: *Critical care nursing*, ed 9, St. Louis, 2022, Elsevier.)

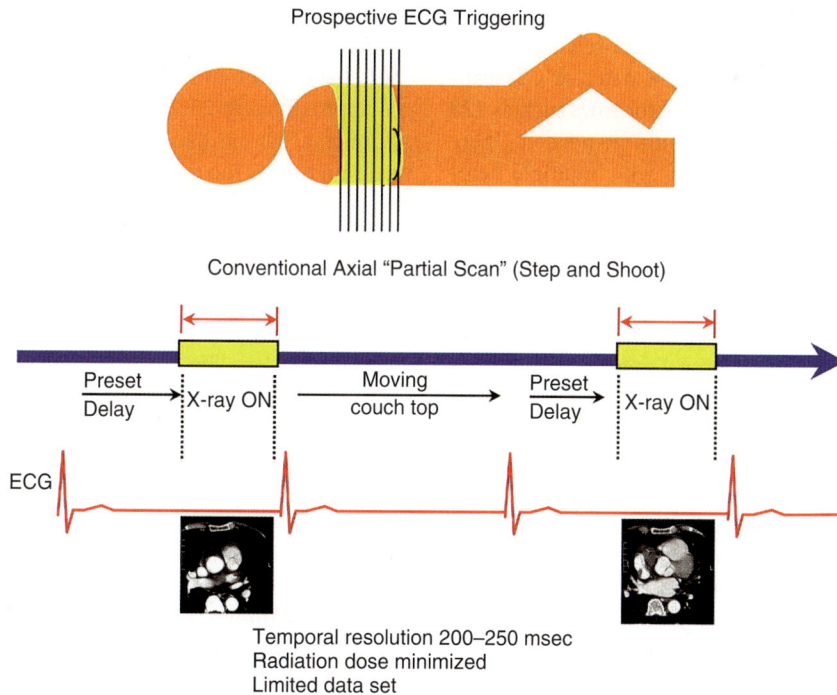

Fig. 14.11 Prospective ECG gating imaging. (From Mahesh M, Cody DD: Physics of cardiac imaging with multiple-row detector CT, *Radiographics* 27(5):1495–1509, 2007.)

with the scanner's movements and x-ray beam-on times. The bottom part of the diagram presents images of the successive anatomic portions of the heart anatomy and immediate surrounding structures that are being acquired as the prospective gating procedure progresses.[25]

As shown in Fig. 14.11, data are acquired for a brief period, the table is translated to the next rest position, and, after a short delay while inactive heart status is reached, the scanner then acquires more projections. This cycle repeats itself until the desired scan length for complete coverage of the heart is reached.

Heart Beat Rate

As long as the depolarization and repolarization electrical impulses in the cardiac cycle are transmitted normally, the heart beats (pumps) at a regular pace.

To complete a cardiac CT image acquisition, the entire heart needs to be covered. Adding more rows of detectors permits the whole heart to be fully imaged in fewer beats. For example, with a 64 detector row CT scanner, having 64 data acquisition channels each being 0.625 mm wide, a scan length of 64×0.625 mm = 40 mm can be achieved per gantry rotation. Typically, since the cardiac region ranges from 120 to 150 mm in the z-axis dimension, it can be covered entirely in three to four gantry rotations with a 64-row detector CT scanner. With a higher number of detector rows such as 128 and 256, even fewer rotations would be needed. There are potential problems, however, with multiple heart beats occurring during an imaging study: for example, the patient could move between the beats and if the full scan is slow, the patient may need to take another breath. Both of these situations can alter the position of the heart in the chest and may cause the acquired images to be unusable. Therefore the most optimum solution is to capture the heart's entire superior-inferior expanse with high resolution in one disastolic phase.

Heart rate, the average number of beats per minute (bpm), is a critically important parameter for obtaining useful cardiac CT imaging since it determines the required temporal resolution of the scanner. It is observed that a patient's diastolic, or heart rest interval, adjusts to coordinate with the patient's beat rate. Thus with faster heart rates, there are shorter diastole durations. A normal heart rate for an average adult is about 60 to 80 beats per minute. For rates from 60 bpm up to 80 bpm, the diastolic interval as a whole lasts from

250 msec to about 175 msec. For heart rates closer to 100 bpm, there is, however, only around 100 msec for diastole.

CT CVI Imaging Metrics[29]

Temporal Resolution (TR). The ability to distinctly resolve (i.e., remove blur from) fast-moving objects, comparable to the shutter speed capability of a camera, is called temporal resolution. For most applications of CT, very high-speed image acquisition is not of great importance because the structures of interest have minimal or no motion. However, excellent TR is vital during cardiac CT, particularly for evaluating the coronary arteries that are most clearly imaged when there is the least cardiac motion. This occurs during the heart's rest periods, of which the optimum component is typically in the mid-diastole phase (diastasis). As heart rate increases, diastole as a whole shortens relative to systole, and diastasis (i.e., optimum quiescence) abbreviates substantially. The cardiac optimum rest period, if defined as the time with a coronary artery displacement of <1 mm, has a mean duration of 120–160 msec, but can range from 66 to about 330 msec depending on the heartbeat rate.[29]

High temporal resolution in cardiac CT is primarily achieved through short gantry rotation times and *partial scan image reconstruction*. Current generation CT scanners have minimum gantry 360 degree rotation times of approximately 250 msec (somewhat less in newer scanners). For cardiac CT, however, a 250 msec gantry rotation time is too long. Attempting to reduce this time by increasing tube rotational speed has an engineering limitation due to overall gantry weight, which during tube rotations exerts very powerful centrifugal forces on the gantry ring.[27] To overcome this, a partial scan reconstruction from a 180-degree gantry rotation plus the fan beam angle (see Fig. 14.7) is used. Employing partial scan reconstruction will bring the temporal resolution into the range of 125–135 msec.[29] This improved TR significantly reduces cardiac pulsation artifacts on the CT images. With half of the full rotation scans, heartbeat rates in the 80s are about the largest for which standard gating can obtain motionless images.

Spatial Resolution (SR). Spatial resolution in CT scanning has two components: *axial, or longitudinal, SR* and *cross-plane, or transaxial, SR* (Fig. 14.12).

Axial resolution is associated with the z-axis extent of the individual detector element or element combinations

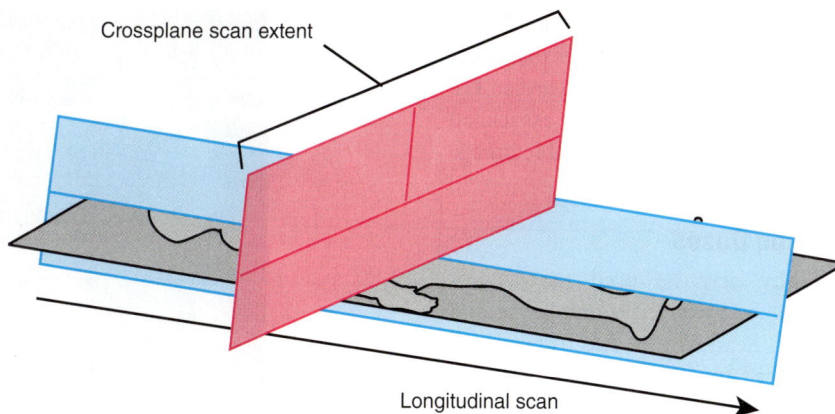

Fig. 14.12 Spatial resolution geometry.

employed to produce a slice (e.g., a 64 slice CT scanner has 64 detector element rows, each 0.625 mm in z dimension, which can be configured to generate slices as thin as 0.625 mm or in multiple combinations: 1.25 mm, 2.5 mm, 5 mm, etc. yielding different degrees of spatial resolution). As a whole, the z-axis spatial resolution is influenced by the detector size, the reconstruction thickness, and other factors such as pitch. It ranges from 7 to15 line pairs per centimeter.

Transaxial, or crossplane, SR is determined by the number of x-ray projections available for reconstruction, the field of view (FOV), and the image matrix size* selected (e.g., usually 512 × 512 pixels or 1024 × 1024 pixels). Spatial resolution in the x-y plane has always been quite high, about 20 line pairs per centimeter (or 2 line pairs per mm) or even greater in the newest designs.

Current CT scanners typically have a limiting spatial resolution of 0.5–0.625 mm along the z-axis, and approximately 0.5 mm in the x and y-axes. For 3-D reconstructions, it is essential to achieve isotropic spatial resolution, which means that the resolution in the

transaxial plane (*X–Y* plane) and in the longitudinal direction (*Z* direction) are all the same.

Contrast Resolution (CR). CT **contrast resolution** is the ability to distinguish between small x-ray attenuation differences in a CT image. The primary method used to increase vascular CR is to intravenously administer iodinated contrast material,* providing that it is tolerated by the patient. After doing this, image intensity differences in vascular areas with a larger concentration of contrast media relative to surrounding structures are often enhanced enough so that subtle differences in specific details may be perceived. The contrast resolution of CT can also be improved by decreasing image noise. Using higher mAS per slice is one way of doing this, but any of the methods employed to improve the signal to noise ratio must keep the radiation dose to the patient within acceptable ALARA boundaries.

Metrics Summary. Factors affecting **TR** include gantry rotation time, acquisition mode, and reconstruction mode. Factors affecting **SR** include detector size, selected detector configurations, FOV, and reconstruction interval. Factors affecting **CR** include detector noise and relative degrees of radio-opacity amongst areas to be examined. Knowledge and understanding

---

*In a digital image, the resolution is limited by the pixel size associated with the image matrix, that is, *the smallest resolvable object cannot be smaller than the pixel size.* The pixel size is determined by the sampling distance, which is just the size of the field of view (FOV). When the FOV is 320 mm, the theoretical size of 1 pixel in an image matrix is 0.625 mm for a 512 × 512 matrix of pixels because for 512 pixels in a 320 mm length there will be 320/512 = 0.625 mm of length per pixel. Similarly, for a 1024 × 1024 matrix each pixel will now be 0.313 mm in length.

---

*Iodinated contrast is a form of intravenous molecular agent that is mostly made up of stable iodine ($^{127}_{53}$I). This material is often used in CT procedures because, with its much higher atomic number, its degree of photoeletric interaction with incident CT x-rays is much greater (i.e., it is more radio-opaque) than that of surrounding noniodinated tissues.

of the trade-offs between the various scan parameters (technique factors, pitch, etc.) and the metrics that affect image quality are the keys to establishing cardiac CT protocols that minimize the radiation risks associated with CVI studies while delivering acceptable image quality.[21,31]

CT CVI and Radiation Doses

Computed tomography may be used for screening and follow-up evaluation of the entire aorta and vascular anatomy from head to toe. The usual drawbacks of CT as compared to other potential imaging modalities such as MRI and ultrasound include its use of ionizing radiation and intravenous injections of iodine-containing contrast which can be damaging to the kidneys. Current high-speed computed tomography is independent of patient characteristics or stringent patient cooperation concerning very extended breath-holding and has become the most applied technique for visualization of the arterial tree. The spatial resolution, and contrast between blood and soft tissue, provided by computed tomography are superior to that of magnetic resonance imaging. Therefore the evaluation of small and convoluted vessels is improved with CT. Due to recent technical developments, the radiation and contrast media doses given to the patient have decreased substantially. They are still a point of significant concern, however, in patients who require frequent follow-up scans throughout their entire life. To follow the ALARA principle, for both initial and follow-up exams, the image acquisition should always be made in the same cardiac phase, as there can be a difference of up to 5 mm in aortic diameter between systole and diastole. For extended aorta investigations, the measurements are usually performed in an oblique sagittal orientation which will also encompass the candy-cane shaped geometry of the thoracic aorta (Fig. 14.13). The imaging technologist must always be mindful of motion, streak, or metallic artifacts that could adversely influence the measurements. When the prophylactic surgical repair of an aortic aneurysm is considered, preprocedural precise and accurate information regarding the length and width of the diseased segment and its relationship with any side branches are needed. CT is the most frequently used technique for preprocedural imaging, since it noninvasively provides accurate and detailed anatomical information and can also detect regions with calcifications.

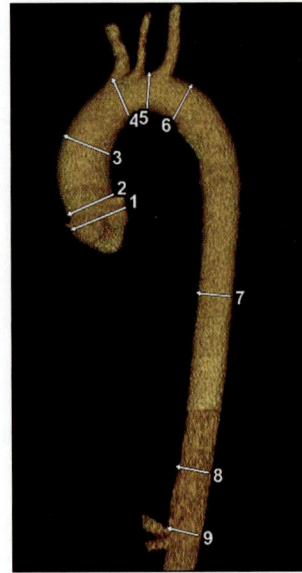

Fig. 14.13 Candy-cane shape of the thoracic aorta. Normal anatomy of the thoracic-abdominal aorta with standard anatomic landmarks for reporting aortic diameter as illustrated on a volume-rendered CT image. Some of the numbered anatomic locations are *1*, Aortic sinuses (widenings); *3*, Mid ascending aorta; *5*, Mid aortic arch (between left common carotid and subclavian arteries); *6*, Proximal descending thoracic aorta (begins approximately 2 cm distal to the left subclavian artery); *7*, Mid descending aorta; *8*, Aorta at the diaphragm (The muscle at the base of the chest that separates the abdomen from the chest. It contracts and flattens during inhalation); *9*, Abdominal aorta at the origin of the celiac artery. (The celiac artery, also known as the celiac axis, is a major artery in the abdominal cavity supplying blood to the stomach.) (From Hiratzka LF, Bakris GL, Beckman JA, et al: ACCF/AHA/AATS/ACR/ASA/SCA/SCAI/SIR/STS/SVM guidelines for the diagnosis and management of patients with thoracic aortic disease: executive summary, *J Am Coll Cardioly* 55(14):1509–1544, 2010.)

Prospective ECG-gating enables acquisition of data by selectively activating the x-ray tube only in a specific cardiac phase triggered by the associated ECG signal, and then deactivating the x-ray tube during the remainder of the R-R cycle.* A significant advantage of this scanning protocol is lower patient radiation dose because x-ray exposure only takes place during a selected cardiac phase rather than throughout the entire cardiac cycle. A

---

*R-R cycle is essentially the time between successive specific ECG voltage signals of the cardiac cycle associated with heart beats. For normal R-R cycles the time interval is between 0.6 and 1.2 seconds. In prospective gating, the x-ray beam-on time will typically be about 25% of the R-R interval period.

typical range of effective dose for prospective gating "64 channel cardiac CT was found to be 6.2 .is ± 2.0 mSv (620 ± 200 mrem)."[21]

Patient Radiation Doses and Volume Scanning

Typical multidetector CT scanners (64 detector rows and less) acquire cardiac data over an interval of time during which the patient table translates enough so that the scanner's detectors obtain data from the most superior to the most inferior portion of the heart. If it were possible to image the entire extent of the heart within just one heartbeat period, this *volume scanning* process would eliminate artifacts due to seams or gaps between image sections caused by inter-heartbeat variations in the locations of coronary arteries. Equally important, because of the brief duration during which the x-ray tube must remain activated (as little as 0.35 seconds for a full gantry rotation), extended volume scanning can result in a markedly decreased patient radiation dose when compared with traditional helical scanning. This is because in former standard or traditional cardiac CT imaging methods, the need for both high spatial and high temporal resolution required the pitch values in helical scanning to be as low as 0.4–0.2, resulting in a radiation beam overlap of nearly 60%–80%, respectively. Such an overlap can increase the patient's radiation dose *up to a factor of five times* compared to scanning using a pitch of 1.

The demand for higher temporal resolution has led to the development of a 320 × 0.5 mm row detector CT scanner. In a CT scanner with this capacity, with 0.5 mm minimum detector row sizes, the 320 detector rows in the longitudinal direction can cover a body region of up to 16 cm axial length per gantry rotation and therefore encompass the full extent of the heart in one gantry rotation, eliminating the need for overlapping pitch and thereby reducing both radiation dose and motion artifacts.

Table 14.4 lists EfD range values for some standard non-CT imaging procedures in comparison with Cardiac CT effective doses.

Radiation Dose and Image Noise

Image noise* increases as the slice section collimation is reduced. To keep the noise low, either the mA should be increased, thereby raising the radiation dose level, or thicker sections should be reconstructed yielding a greater signal. Because of the complexity of the latest MDCT configurations, it is advisable to design scanning protocols that are not based on previous milliampere settings used for 16 or fewer slice scanners but rather on dose indicators such as the calculated $CTDI_{vol}$. The latter are now displayed on the user interface of all current MDCT scanners.** As a consequence of the careful selection of parameters, the average increase in radiation dose with

---

*Image Noise: A deterioration in image quality due to a decrease in the ratio of "true" data relative to random nondata effects in the individual pixels (two-dimensional) and voxels (three-dimensional) comprising the overall image.

**Some limitations to the $CTDI_{100}$ formalism, which serves as the basis for $CTDI_{VOL}$ determinations, as regards measurement and specification of dose in MDCT for the current axially longer detector configurations by using only a 100 mm long ion chamber, have been discussed in a number of scientific publications and may lead to some new and more appropriate terminology concerning CT dose. The statements in this section comparing dose among different scanning configurations, however, are not expected to be significantly changed by these new approaches.[30,31]

TABLE 14.4	**Some Imaging Modalities' Effective Dose Range Values**	
Imaging Procedure	**Modality**	**Effective Dose Range (mSv)**
Cardiac Procedures		
CTA	Multiple row detector CT	6.0–25
Nuclear medicine with 99mTc	Single photon emission tomography (SPECT)	6.0–15
Coronary angiography (diagnostic)	Fluoroscopy	2.1–6.0
Routine CT Procedures		
Head CT	Multiple row detector CT	1.0–2.0
Chest CT	Multiple row detector CT	5.0–7.0
Abdominal and Pelvic CT	Multiple row detector CT	8.0–11.0

CT, Computed tomography; *CTA*, Computed tomography angiography.
From Mahesh M, Cody DD: AAPM/RSNA physics tutorial for residents: physics tutorial for residents, physics of cardiac imaging with multiple-row detector CT, *Radiographics* 27(5):1495–1509, 2007.

extended MDCT can be minimized and only becomes more pronounced if very thin-section images of high quality are required. A lower kVp setting may be used to increase the CT attenuation of iodinated contrast material and thus improve the contrast of these perfused structures. Any resulting gain in signal-to-noise ratio permits a lowering of radiation dose while maintaining a diagnostically acceptable image quality. The technique works best in the chest (e.g., in CTA of pulmonary embolism).

CONE BEAM COMPUTED TOMOGRAPHY (CBCT)

There also exists another form of computed tomography, much less familiar to the general public, but which is commonly used for varied image-guiding purposes in multiple areas of radiography and radiation oncology. This alternate form of tomographic imaging is called cone beam computed tomography or, in short, CBCT.

Specifically, CBCT has become indispensable in treatment planning and diagnosis in implant dentistry, oral surgery, orthopedics, and interventional radiology (IR), among other applications.

Integrated CBCT is also essential for precise patient positioning and verification in radiation image-guided radiation therapy (IGRT).

Radiation Beam Characteristics for CT and CBCT

There are numerous distinctions between CT and CBCT but possibly the most fundamental is the shape of the x-ray beam utilized for image production. In CT a fan beam that is very thin in the Z-axis dimension, usually ≳1 mm, is employed. As shown on the right side in Fig. 14.14, CBCT uses a broad beam that covers the entire Z-axis range of the patient that is to be scanned. This beam is directed through the volume of interest (VOI) at a large rectangular detector (also known as a flat panel detector), and *all volumetric data about the patient is gathered in a single rotational pass* of the x-ray tube and detector. This property makes the CBCT device much quicker and much more compact than standard CT systems and enables an ability to additionally focus the radiographic exam.

CBCT vs. CT Imaging Details and Image Quality

In Fig. 14.15 the schematic on the left explicitly shows that CBCT radiation geometry involves *simultaneous* multitudinous x-ray projections through the VOI producing the imaging data at the flat plane detector from which orthogonal planar images are subsequently reconstructed. Alternatively, in fan beam or conventional CT geometry, as displayed on the right side of Fig. 14.15, the initial reconstruction of data produces *individual* millimeter or sub-millimeter thick fan-shaped x-ray beams in a helical progression to acquire very fine individual image slices of the field of view (FOV) which are then combined by a secondary reconstruction process to create orthogonal planar images. Thus it can be seen that each of the standard CT acquisitions typically requires multiple rotational scans and a separate 2D

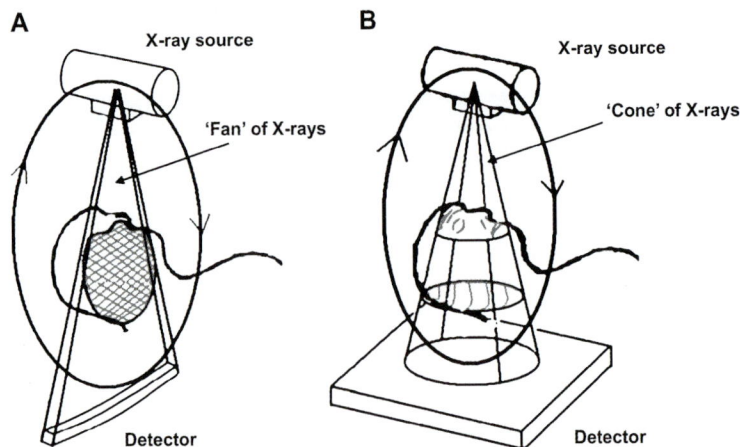

Fig. 14.14 Imaging methods for CT and CBCT scanning. (From Scarfe WC, Farman AG, Sukovic P: Clinical applications of cone-beam computed tomography in dental practice, *J Can Dent Assoc* 72(1):75–80, 2006.)

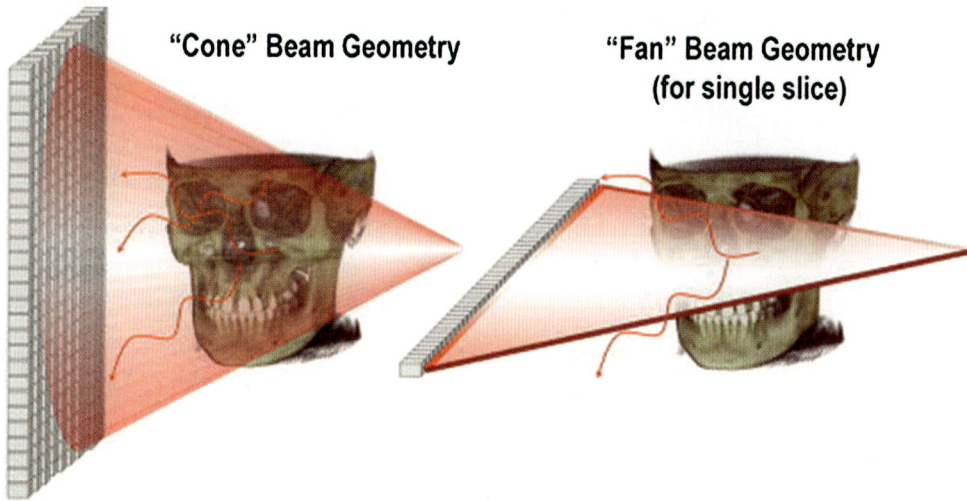

Fig. 14.15 CBCT vs. CT scan geometry and FOV. (From Scarfe WC, Farman AG: What is cone-beam CT and how does it work, *Dent Clin N Am* 52(4):707–730, 2008.)

reconstruction. Because a CBCT exposure, instead, initially incorporates the entire FOV, only one rotational sequence of the gantry is necessary to acquire enough data for the desired *acceptable* image reconstruction.

Disadvantages and Advantages of CBCT

With CBCT, as with any x-ray procedure, there is unavoidably some degree of scatter radiation. The amount of scatter radiation (illustrated in Fig. 2 by the wavy lines) generated and recorded by cone beam image acquisition, however, is substantially higher, because of the larger volume of the patient irradiated simultaneously, than that resulting from the tightly confined (thin section or slice) of conventional CT x-rays. Inserted attenuation filters of various shapes and sizes can be utilized with cone beam radiation, predominately applied in radiation therapy procedures, to reduce this radiation scatter while preserving and improving image quality.

Disadvantages

- Cone Beam Computed Tomography exhibits inferior contrast resolution compared to standard CT, due to the increased scatter, resulting in soft tissues not being as optimally viewed as with traditional CT.
- In CBCT imaging, streaking and motion artifacts are possible and, because they are not completely removable by the CBCT algorithms, can appear to some extent in the final image.

A certain amount of noise due to the previously mentioned radiation scatter will appear in the generated image, causing a further decrease in image quality.

It is therefore of interest to ask why should CBCT be employed? Below are presented situations for when using CBCT is quite advantageous.

Advantages

- Cone beam CT procedures offer a lower total radiation dosage to the patient than conventional CT.
- Cone beam CT, unlike standard CT, can be used with movable 3D C-arms expanding immobile patient usage. There is however the following caveat: because of a high amount of scatter radiation during the typical thirty second scan time, extra radiation safety precautions must be employed to protect occupational personnel.
- CBCT is very proficient in the evaluation of hard or bony tissues.
- In general, radiation exposure to the patient per exam with CBCT is just a fraction of that delivered by traditional CT.
- CBCT imaging exhibits fewer metallic object artifacts than standard CT imaging.

CBCT Radiation Detection

For cone beam computed tomography the conical x-ray beam that passes through the patient is detected by a

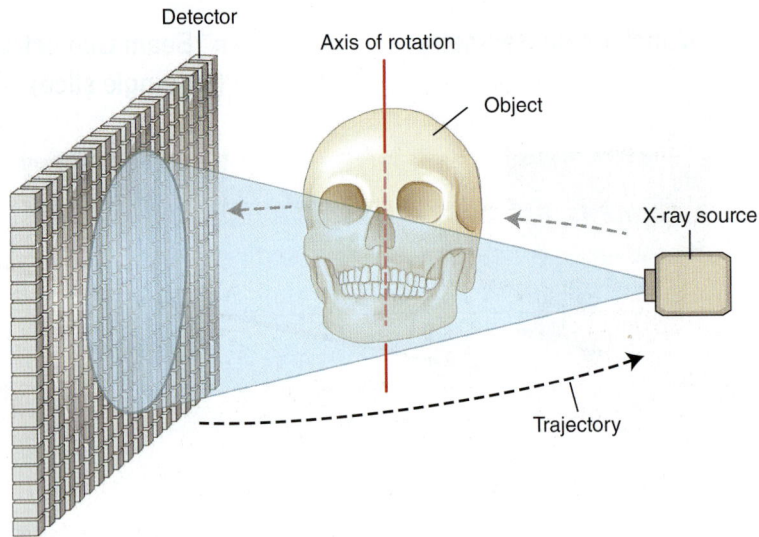

Fig. 14.16 Rotational CBCT imaging process. (From White SC, Pharoah MJ: *Oral radiology: principles and interpretation*, ed 7, St. Louis, 2014, Elsevier.)

large rectangular or square-shaped flat panel detector (typically with 12" to 15" dimensions). Physically, a CBCT device is far more compact than standard CT systems and because all data is gathered in a single pass around the patient, a CBCT procedure is much quicker (<1 minute). There is also the ability to determine the orientation of the exam during acquisition because the patient is not confined within a fixed gantry as in CT. Fig. 14.16 schematically indicates a CBCT imaging physical setup.

In a cone beam tomographic imaging revolution, the **flat panel detector** upon capturing x-ray photons must quickly send signals to the processing computer and perform these actions hundreds of times within a single rotation. A full rotation of the cone beam normally occurs within a duration not larger than 30 seconds. This brief period necessitates frame rate image acquisition times in milliseconds.

Flat Panel Detectors (FPD)

High-resolution **flat-panel detectors** (also used in digital mammography) have become the standard for cone beam computed tomography. FPDs are typically composed of a large area or wide field pixel array of amorphous silicon thin-film transistors (TFTs) coupled to a scintillation (light flashing) detector such as a layer of thallium-doped cesium iodide (Fig. 14.17). The incident

x-rays are first detected utilizing the scintillator, which absorbs and then converts the x-rays into visible light. These light photons are subsequently taken up and *registered* in the photo diode array located immediately beyond.

Although this particular detector design arrangement yields a wide dynamic range and reduces peripheral distortion, it does so at the cost of requiring a slightly greater radiation exposure than that of an image intensifier (II) device used in general fluoroscopy.

Trade-Offs: Image Quality vs. Scan Time and Patient Dose

The number of images generating the projection data throughout the cone beam scan is determined by the number of images acquired per second, the extent of the trajectory arc, and the duration of the rotation. In state-of-the-art scanners, the number of projections comprising a single scan may be varied. More projections yield additional information to reconstruct the image, allow for greater spatial and contrast resolution, increase the signal-to-noise ratio producing *cleaner* images, and reduce metallic artifacts. The downside is that more projection data usually necessitates a longer scan time, a higher patient dose, and a longer primary reconstruction time. To remain in accordance with the ALARA

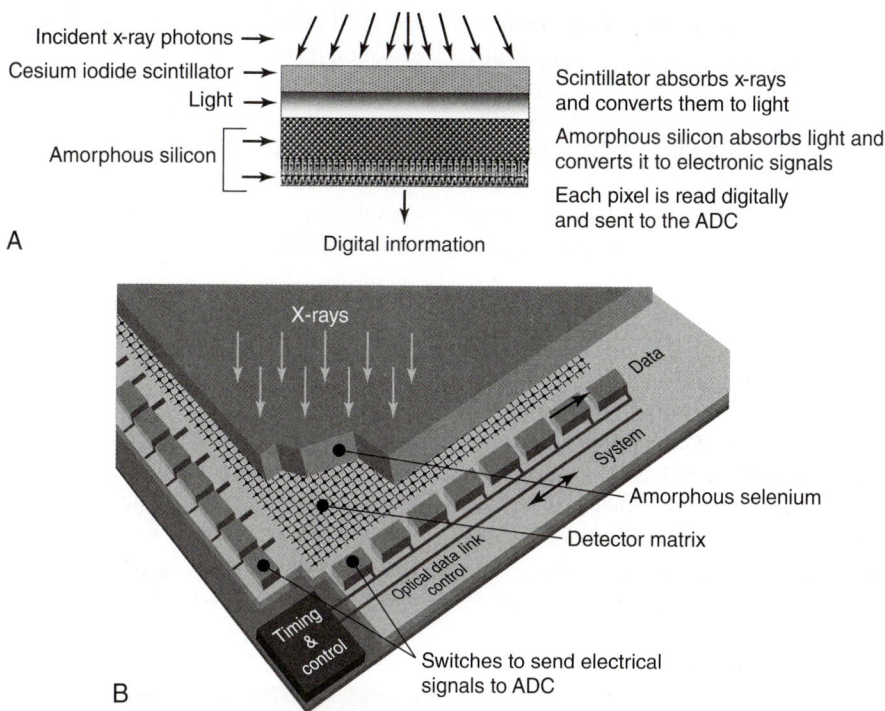

Fig. 14.17 (A) Cross-sectional drawing of an indirect conversion detector showing the scintillator, the light given off, and the amorphous silicon layer that converts the light into the electric signal. (B) Flat-panel detector in a direct conversion system in which the x-ray energy is converted directly to an electric signal. Amorphous selenium layer is shown. (*From Frank ED, Ehrlich RA: Radiography essentials for limited scope, ed 7, St. Louis, 2026, Elsevier.*)

principle while obtaining satisfactory diagnostic quality imaging, there must always be a balancing compromise between patient-received dosage and acquiring a sufficient number of basis images.

CT and CBCT X-ray Tubes

Regular computed tomography (CT) scanners employ conventional-anode x-ray tubes such as found in non-fluoro general-purpose x-ray rooms to produce the radiation needed for standard diagnostic imaging. The only difference between the typical x-ray room, x-ray tube, and a CT scanner x-ray tube is that a traditional CT scanner utilizes a *high-radiation output* X-ray tube whose anode or target has been especially designed to have a much larger heat capacity tolerance.

Cone beam CT devices utilize instead a partially modified low power medical fluoroscopy x-ray tube capable of continuous imaging throughout the scan. The fluoroscopic tube generates less radiation than standard CT but still in sufficient amounts to produce high-quality imaging. A lower power level also produces lower scatter radiation around the patient.

Focal spot sizes in fluoroscopic tubes can be as small as 0.3 mm in diameter (when high spatial resolution is required and only low radiation output is needed) and as large as 1.0 or 1.2 mm when higher heat capacity is needed and decreased resolution is acceptable. Many fluoroscopy systems have movable "wedge" filters that are partially transparent to the X-ray beam. These differentially attenuate the beam in selectable regions to reduce entrance dose and excessive image brightness. Several such filters are routinely used in CBCT daily imaging setup verification in radiation therapy.

Reconstructing 3D Objects from Cone-Beam Projections

Traditional radiology computed tomography typically utilizes millimeter or less thick axially fan-shaped x-ray beams in a helical progression to acquire individual image slices of the FOV and then stacks these slices to obtain a 3D representation. Each standard CT slice thus requires a separate scan and a separate 2D reconstruction employing the filtered back projection (FBP) technique discussed earlier in this chapter. Because a CBCT exposure, instead, always initially *incorporates the entire FOV*, only one or at most two slightly differentiated rotational sequences of the gantry are necessary to acquire enough data for image reconstruction.

For CBCT, with its 2D x-ray area detectors and its specific cone-beam geometry, a 3D volume must be assembled just from the acquired multi-angular 2D projection data. To facilitate this, various modified and complex filtered back projection methods have been devised to reliably reconstruct data to minimize artifacts incurred in various selected imaging geometries. An explanation of these mathematical reconstruction algorithms is beyond the scope of this textbook.

CBCT in Dental Radiography and Radiation Exposure

In dental radiography, a **cone-beam CT** exam permits the evaluation of the anatomy of a patient's jaws in all three planes (axial, sagittal, and coronal). Typically, a dental cone beam rotation includes many (several hundred) sequential planar projection images of the FOV (see Fig. 14.15) all of which are acquired in a complete (360⁰), or sometimes lesser arc. For implants, this is the examination of choice to determine patient-specific anatomical relationships. The radiation equivalent dose received from a cone-beam CT of the jaws can vary from approximately 20 to up to 200 µSv, depending on various factors such as the extent of the field of view, the desired resolution of the images, the patient's size, the location of the region of interest, and also the manufacturer's instrument settings. Considering all of this, it is still evident that dental CBCT scans are very low dose procedures.

As a specific example, let us assume that for a **cone-beam CT** of the jaws taken for purposes of an implant, the patient's received radiation equivalent dose is 200 µSv. Compare this to the average radiation dosage amount that a person naturally receives on the Earth every day. According to NCRP 2003, the daily background radiation equivalent dose received from the environment is approximately 8.2 µSv per day or 3 mSv (300 millirem) per year in the United States. Therefore

the maximum dental implant **cone-beam CT** received radiation is similar to that accumulated on average from natural sources for approximately 24 days. By comparison, a medical CT adult brain scan has a typical effective equivalent dose of about 2 mSv or 2,000 µSv.

Fig. 14.18 shows a state-of-the-art CBCT dental radiography unit (Carestream model 9300) employed by a periodontist facility.

Cone Beam CT in Interventional Radiology

Although it was not before the late 1990s that CBCT with x-ray image intensifiers as detectors was first tried out, it was not until the advent and general deployment of flat-panel x-ray detectors, which offered improved contrast and spatial resolution, that cone beam computed tomography became feasible for regular clinical use in interventional radiology procedures. At present many fixed and even mobile C-arm fluoroscopy systems are now capable of CBCT acquisitions and are invaluable,

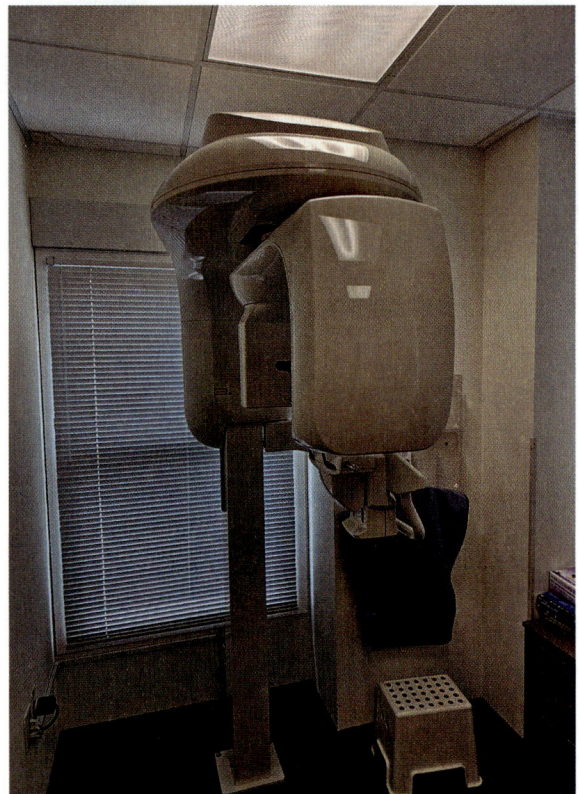

Fig. 14.18 CBCT dental radiography unit. (Courtesy Sky Perio Peridontists, Cherry Hill, New Jersey.)

for example, with respect to image guidance during the treatment of various orthopedic procedures.

Since a CBCT scanner can be physically mounted on a C-arm fluoroscopy unit in the interventional radiology (IR) suite, there is no need to transfer a patient from the IR suite to a conventional computed tomography scanner location for supplementary image reconstruction data. The possible clinical applications of CBCT in IR, to name a few, include device or implant positioning and assessment, intra-procedural localization, abscess drainage, prostatic artery embolization for benign prostatic hypertrophy, and a host of other procedures. An added benefit is that using CBCT before fluoroscopy potentially reduces patient radiation exposure because of the CBCT image guidance.

Cone Beam CT in Radiation Oncology

In radiation therapy departments, before commencing a treatment, patient position accuracy verification was traditionally achieved by megavoltage (typically 6MV) portal images with, commonly, AP/PA and lateral views. Unfortunately because of the very high energy used, these obtained images provide very poor contrast for soft tissues. This deficiency is compounded for obese patients. To remedy this situation it was necessary to design and install new types of imagers that were much more suitable for precise correction of motion and setup errors of patients undergoing radiotherapy. This became especially crucial as it was found that achieving a high therapeutic ratio* for previously considered untreatable areas of malignancy, requiring high doses of radiation but surrounded by critical radiosensitive structures, could be accomplished and be effective in treating the malignancy. In place of using megavoltage x-rays for positioning verification, these new positioning devices employ kilovoltage radiation which with its photoelectric interaction predominance offers vastly better soft tissue or tissue equivalent materials' contrast than does the Compton interaction (inversely proportional to the

photon energy and nearly independent of the atomic number, Z) dominated traditional megavoltage portal imaging systems.

Such a kilovoltage imaging system has been physically integrated into all current state-of-the- art therapeutic linear accelerators. Fig. 14.19 displays the on-board imager (OBI) of a Varian Medical Systems (Palo Alto, CA) linear accelerator. An OBI usually consists of a kilovoltage (kV) x-ray source and a kV amorphous silicon detector mounted in a synchronously connected fashion on the gantry of the linear accelerator using robotic arms. This enables 3D cone beam computed tomography acquisitions when the kilovoltage source and detector panel rotate once around the patient on the treatment couch. The acquired CBCT images provide soft tissue and bony structure information in three dimensions. In addition, these systems usually enable registration of the CBCT images with the corresponding patient CT and structure sets transferred from the treatment planning workstation. Any positional errors can then be estimated so that couch position adjustments can be downloaded to the linear accelerator for remote couch movement.[32] Thus, CBCT imaging has become an essential tool for high-dose precision radiotherapy and its usage is designated as **image-guided radiation therapy (IGRT)**.

IGRT Summary

CBCT was developed in the late 1990s and first commercially available in dentistry for dentomaxillofacial imaging in 2001. In the early 2000s, it was subsequently found to be clinically very advantageous for radiotherapy as it could significantly reduce patient set-up errors before each treatment session.

Over the past 20 years, successful treatment outcomes for various critically located tumor sites by utilizing very high dose complex treatment methods such as multi-angular anatomically conformal arc radiotherapy (known as VMAT*) and other varieties of intensity-modulated radiotherapy delivery (IMRT) has imposed a very great need for increased accuracy to ensure the protection of closely adjacent but noncancerous organs and structures during a therapeutic treatment regimen. An additional complication associated with these gains in tumor control is that the sizeable dose distributions delivered to the site of interest can be and usually are highly irregular architecturally with steep dose gradients. Consequently,

---

*Therapeutic ratio denotes the relationship between the probability of tumor control and the likelihood of normal tissue damage. An improved therapeutic ratio represents a more favorable tradeoff between tumor control and toxicity to nondiseased structures and/or tissues. Thus if it is possible to deliver a deadly radiation dosage to a tumor while maintaining dose levels to surrounding tissues at their nontoxic levels, a good therapeutic ratio has been achieved and a potential successful treatment outcome can result.

---

*VMAT is shorthand for volume modulated arc therapy.

any slight change in target organ volume or position during each treatment fraction can significantly alter the actual dose delivered to both the target and, unfortunately, any nearby surrounding normal tissues. In general, in orthodox radiation therapy, it is the *therapeutic ratio* that is of prime significance. Therefore an increase in the target dose to effect a potential cure is only feasible by *strictly minimizing radiation field margins*, thereby sheltering as much as possible noncancerous and potentially critical adjacent areas from destructive radiation levels. The x-ray *field* margin, commonly called the PTV (planned treatment volume) and its precise maintenance is thus the limiting factor in a successful and safe radiation treatment coverage of the entire tumor *and its almost inevitable slight displacements.*

Achieving these stringent accuracy goals necessitates deploying advanced **image-guided radiation therapy** (IGRT) throughout the treatment course. Employment of the latest CBCT devices and their modifications has substantially enabled regular precision three-dimensional positioning reproducibility for patients. IGRT also opens up the possibility of *real-time reoptimization of treatment plans for Adaptive Radiotherapy* (ART). Specifically, *ART is the process of radiation treatment during which the treatment plan can be modified, if necessary, just before each treatment fraction based on current anatomy.* This can be facilitated employing Artificial Intelligence boosted treatment planning and radiation delivery control. It seems clear that AI will be featured prominently moving forward in successful radiation therapy treatment programs.

In a radiation therapy treatment facility, every current linear accelerator treatment machine (LINAC) is now equipped to do modern image-guided radiation therapy (IGRT) with an attached CBCT scanner (see Fig. 14.19). During the rotation of the therapy accelerator's gantry, the laterally mounted imaging x-ray source produces divergent cone-shaped radiation, while the aligned linked flat panel x-ray receptor records the residual x-rays reaching the detector after the x-ray beam is attenuated by patient tissues. The robotic arms permit the optimum positioning of a 360^0 or lesser scanning arc relative to the patient's treatment region.

IGRT Radiation Doses

For noncomplex treatments, CBCT positioning verification may be done only once or twice per week but for complex treatment deliveries, patient position accuracy

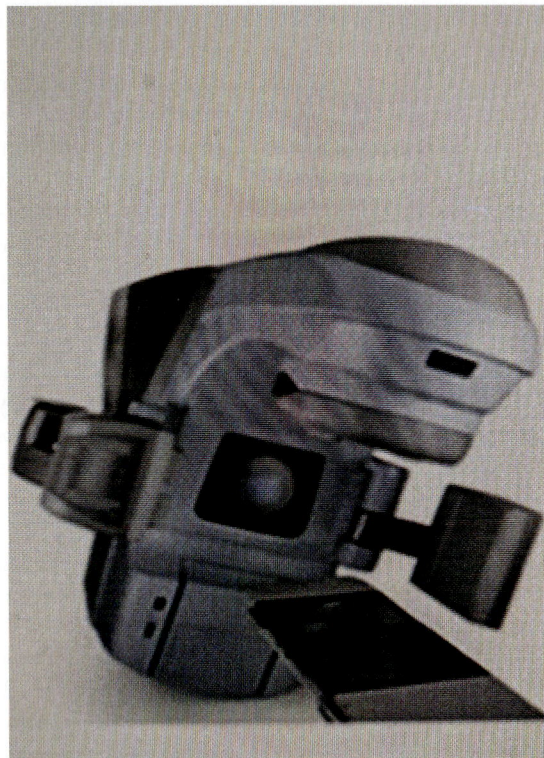

Fig. 14.19 Medical LINAC and CBCT device. The fluoroscopic x-ray tube is on the left side in the figure and the flat panel detector is on the right side. (Image courtesy of Varian Medical Systems, Inc. All rights reserved.)

using IGRT is performed prior to every treatment. A lengthy complex treatment course involving critical sites, requiring 2 to 3 mm accuracy for safety, therefore could add a nonnegligible amount of radiation dose to all of the exposed portions of the patient. As an example, for radical IMRT treatments involving the prostate, the total number of fractions, that is, treatment deliveries, using a LINAC, can range from 35 to 40 fractions. In that case, the CBCT effective dose to patients outside of the treatment area can clearly be nonnegligible.

Typical effective doses from *standard mode** CBCT for head and neck imaging is about 10 mSv (1 rem) per scan and about 23 mSv (2.3 rem) per scan for chest, and pelvis. If we just considered the treatment region, these

---

*Standard Mode CBCT in Radiation Therapy localizations typically uses the following technic factors: 125 KVP, 80 mA, 25 ms, and the scan itself could be as much as 25 seconds in duration.

scan doses, although vastly higher than dental radiography procedures, are completely insignificant when compared to the magnitude of the total treatment dose (in the range of multiple tens of thousands of millisieverts) that will be received by the patient in that location. There is, however, a significant caveat to this. According to existing studies by the National Institutes of Health and other investigative bodies, a potential *secondary cancer risk* of from 2% to 4%, in adjacent noncancerous CBCT direct and scatter radiation exposed areas, can result from frequent and/or daily patient position

verifications by *standard mode* CBCT. As a result of this determination, strong efforts were undertaken during the past decade to substantially lower the size of daily imaging doses in radiation therapy procedures. Revised *low-dose mode* CBCT techniques were developed and have been routinely employed, when applicable, resulting in almost an *80% unwanted radiation dose* reduction from that caused by the previous standard mode CBCT method. Lower mAs settings, if feasible, should therefore always be considered for daily CBCT, especially when bony anatomy is the main interest.[33]

SUMMARY

- Computed tomography is a frequently employed diagnostic x-ray imaging modality that is considered to be a relatively high radiation exposure examination.
- With higher radiation exposure to the patient, there is potentially an increased associated cancer risk.
- Skin dose and dose distribution are two concerns related to patient dose in CT scanning.
- CT examinations generally expose a smaller mass of tissue than that exposed during an ordinary x-ray series.
- The entrance exposure from a CT examination may be compared with the entrance exposure received during a routine fluoroscopic examination.
- When a series of adjacent slices is obtained, some radiation scatters from the individual slices being made into the adjacent slices. This is called *interslice scatter.*
- Direct patient shielding is not typically used in CT.
- When the spiral scan pitch ratio is approximately 1, the spiral CT patient dose is comparable to that produced by conventional or axial CT.
- Tube current modulation in CT scanning can help to reduce patient dose.
- Recent advances in computer technology allow scan data to be reconstructed, modified, reconstructed again, modified, etc., until an image having the lowest noise possible is obtained. Such a repeat process is referred to as *iteration* and used in iterative reconstruction in CT.
- In CT, all other factors being equal, increasing kVp tends to increase patient dose.
- A miscentering of 2 centimeters can produce as much as a 25% increase in patient dose.[9]

- $CTDI_{VOL}$ and DLP are required dose markers.
- EfDLP is expressed in millisieverts per milligray-centimeter (mSv/mGy-cm).
- For routine head and body CT exams, effective doses fall in the 1 to 10 mSv effective dose range.
- From a radiation protection point of view, the goal of CT imaging should be to obtain the best possible image while delivering an acceptable level of ionizing radiation to the patient.
- For the calculation of a computed tomography scan EfD, the equation, $EfD = DLP \times EfDLP$, can be used.
- X-ray beam collimation for a single slice CT scanner (SSCT) is accomplished by employing physical pre- and post- size restriction of the CT x-ray beam.
- Multidetector CT (MDCT) scanners employ multiple rows of CT detectors instead of only just one as in SSCT scanners.
- MDCT's most direct advantages over SSCT scanners are faster scanning procedures with much improved spatial resolution.
- With MDCT, slices can be composed of a single detector row thickness or multiple adjacent detectors and the effective slice thickness or slice width are therefore determined by the chosen detector configuration and not by physical x-ray beam collimation.
- With MDCT, the slice number correlates to how many images the CT scanning machine can obtain per gantry rotation.
- As reconstruction slice thickness decreases, the number of photons within each voxel also decreases, resulting in increased relative image noise.
- The four major sections, or compartments, of the heart are the: right atrium, left atrium, right ventricle, and left ventricle.

- During the diastole phase of the cardiac cycle the heart relaxes. It contracts during the systole phase.
- To obtain useful images of a rapidly beating heart, most imaging modalities must have very short image acquisition times.
- In ECG gated imaging, the CT scanner is electronically linked to the patient's real-time electrocardiogram and CT image acquisition, and reconstruction can then be coordinated with the quiescent heart phases associated with particular magnitude electrical pulses, thereby removing or minimizing motion artifacts.
- As long as depolarization and repolarization electrical impulses in the cardiac cycle are transmitted normally, the heart beats (pumps) at a regular pace.
- Spatial resolution (SR) in CT scanning has two components: axial or longitudinal SR, and cross-plane or transaxial SR.
- The primary method used to increase vascular contrast resolution (CR) in CT scanning is to intravenously administer iodinated contrast material providing that it is tolerated by the patient.
- Factors affecting temporal resolution (TR) include gantry rotation time, acquisition mode, and reconstruction method. Factors affecting spatial resolution (SR) include: detector size, selected detector configuration, the field of view (FOV), and reconstruction interval. Factors affecting contrast resolution (CR) include detector noise and relative degrees of radio-opacity amongst areas to be examined.
- To keep the patient's radiation dose ALARA, for both initial and follow up examinations, the image acquisition should always be made in the same cardiac phase, as there can be a difference of up to 5 mm in aortic diameter between systole and diastole.
- CBCT differs primarily from standard CT in the method of producing and resulting shape of the useful x-ray beam.
- Some disadvantages of CBCT are nonoptimum soft tissue contrast resolution and some unavoidable imaging artifacts.
- Cone beam CT, unlike standard CT, can be used with movable 3D C-arms expanding immobile patient usage.
- CBCT is very proficient in the evaluation of hard or bony tissues and therefore is of great value in dental radiography for evaluation of tooth implants.
- Image guided radiation therapy or IGRT is crucial for the successful treatment of malignancies that are nearby or adjacent to nonafflicted critical structures.
- Typical effective doses from *standard mode* CBCT for head and neck imaging were about 10 mSv per scan and about 23 mSv per scan for chest and pelvis, but these values have been substantially lowered in recent times.

GENERAL DISCUSSION QUESTIONS

1. Why do CT examinations generally expose a smaller mass of tissue than what occurs during an ordinary x-ray series?
2. What is interslice scatter?
3. Recent advances in computed tomography allow scan data to be reconstructed, modified, reconstructed again, modified again, etc., until an image having the lowest noise possible is obtained. What is this repeat process referred to as?
4. What are two concerns related to patient dose in CT scanning?
5. Why should ordering physicians weigh the benefits and risks of a CT scan procedure for a patient?
6. What is tube current modulation?
7. What are two required dose markers used in CT?
8. In what unit is EfDLP expressed, and how is EfDLP determined?
9. In the early 2000s, various publications calculated individual and population risk of cancer due to CT based upon risk estimates from studies of what group of people?
10. What is the goal of CT imaging from a radiation protection point of view?
11. With MDCT, of what can slices be composed?
12. What are the advantages of an MDCT scanner over a SSCT scanner?
13. What are the four major sections, or compartments, of the human heart?
14. Considering the cardiac cycle, what is the difference between the systole phase and the diastole phase?
15. To usefully image a rapidly beating heart, what must most imaging modalities have?
16. In ECG gated imaging, to what is the CT scanner electronically linked?

17. What are the two components of spatial resolution in CT scanning?
18. What is the primary method used to increase vascular contrast resolution?
19. For patient's who require frequent follow up CT scans, what should be done to keep their radiation dose ALARA for both the initial and follow up examinations?
20. During a CT CVI procedure, what needs to be done to keep image noise low?

21. What is the fundamental difference between CBCT and CT?
22. How does CBCT compare with standard CT in terms of patient radiation exposure?
23. What type of radiation detector is used in CBCT devices?
24. Image quality in CBCT is best for what type of anatomical structures?
25. List some advantages of CBCT over CT.
26. What is IGRT and discuss where is it most beneficial and why?

REVIEW QUESTIONS

1. Direct patient shielding is not typically used in:
   A. Computed tomography
   B. Digital fluoroscopy
   C. Computed radiography
   D. Digital radiography
2. As much as what percent of unnecessary increase in patient dose can a miscentering of 2 centimeters cause during a CT examination?
   A. 15%
   B. 25%
   C. 50%
   D. 75%
3. In CT examinations, which of the following interactions of x-radiation with matter primarily affect the image?
   A. Coherent scattering and photodisintegration
   B. Compton scattering and pair production
   C. Photoelectric and Compton interactions
   D. Photoelectric and coherent interactions
4. In what mSv *effective dose* range do routine head and body CT examinations fall?
   A. 1 to 10
   B. 15 to 25
   C. 30 to 40
   D. 45 to 60
5. The entrance exposure from a CT examination may be compared with which of the following procedures?
   A. An interventional x-ray procedure
   B. A mammography examination
   C. A single chest x-ray performed with a mobile x-ray unit
   D. A routine fluoroscopic examination

6. When the spiral CT scan pitch ratio is approximately 1, to what is the spiral CT patient dose comparable?
   A. To that produced by conventional or axial CT unit
   B. To that produced by a magnetic resonance imaging machine
   C. To that produced by a dedicated mammographic unit
   D. To that produced by a routine diagnostic x-ray unit
7. Regarding Multiple Detector CT scanners, which of the following is correct?
   A. A scanner with a 16-detector array typically employs a total of sixteen 10 mm long detectors
   B. The scan-time is determined only by the gantry speed
   C. The slice width selected can be larger than the physical size of an individual detector row
   D. The spatial resolution is less than that of previous single-detector row CT scanners
8. To acquire a useful set of CT cardiovascular images, it is necessary that:
   A. The radiation dose be allowed to increase as is needed to neglect any quantum noise
   B. The patient can hold their breath for long times
   C. The spatial resolution must be in the centimeter range
   D. The three metrics of CT image quality be satisfactorily met
9. Radiation dose to the patient in current CT CVI does *not* depend upon:
   A. The patient's ability to hold their breath for long times
   B. Whether ECG gating is employed or not

    C. The pitch of a helical scan is less than or greater than one

    D. The size of the detector rows employed in obtaining slices

10. Which of the following would generally result in the lowest *effective dose* to the patient?

    A. CTA

    B. Routine Head CT

    C. Routine Chest CT

    D. Routine Abdomen and Pelvis CT

11. For potential tooth implants which of the following is the best modality?

    A. Magnetic resonance imaging

    B. Dual energy computed tomography

    C. Cone beam computed tomography

    D. Interventional radiography

12. The main difference between CT and CBCT is:

    A. the shape of the radiation beam employed for imaging.

    B. the number of technical personnel required to perform such procedures.

    C. the radiation dose received by technical personnel.

    D. the portions of the body scanned by each modality.

13. Terminology that can be associated with CBCT does not include:

    A. IGRT

    B. FPDs

    C. Fan Beams

    D. Nonportability

14. In a CBCT examination performed by a dental specialist, the radiation dose to a patient

    A. is the same as that of a standard CT head scan.

    B. is equivalent to a 3D mammogram absorbed dose.

    C. is much lesss than what would be received annually from background radiation.

    D. is about one half of that from an MRI head scan.

Radiation Safety in Mammography

OBJECTIVES

After completing this chapter, the reader will be able to perform the following:

- Define all key terms.
- Explain the value of mammography for the detection of breast cancer.
- State the maximum dose to the glandular tissue of a 4.5-cm compressed breast using a digital system.
- Explain the reason why the age recommendation for a screening mammography is controversial.
- Cite examples of how radiation dose in mammography can be reduced.
- Recognize the value of digital mammography for imaging of patients with dense breasts.
- Identify the benefit of using the two most common metallic elements employed as filters in mammographic units.
- Describe the process of digital breast tomosynthesis (DBT), and explain the advantages of this procedure.
- Discuss the concept of radiation dose associated with DBT.

CHAPTER OUTLINE

Mammography and Breast Compression
  Patient Dose in Mammography
  Mammography Screening
  Dose Reduction in Mammography
  Filtration for Mammographic Equipment
Digital Breast Tomosynthesis/3D Mammography
  Tomography
  Digital Breast Tomosynthesis (DBT)
  Effects of Tomographic Angular Scan Range

Image Reconstruction (IR)
Advantages of DBT
Artifacts in Digital Breast Tomography
Properties of DBT Summarized
DBT Imaging Unit Characteristics
DBT Procedure: Steps and Details
Radiation Dosage
DBT Summary
Summary

KEY TERMS

baseline mammogram
compression
digital tomosynthesis
false-positive readings
full field digital detector

full-field digital mammography (FFDM)
mammography
mean glandular dose (MGD)
molybdenum filter

rhodium filter
shift and add algorithm (SAA)
signal-to-noise ratio (SNR)
spatial resolution

Some types of radiographic examinations require special consideration for radiation safety. This chapter addresses these concerns for standard mammography and digital breast tomosynthesis (3D mammography).

MAMMOGRAPHY AND BREAST COMPRESSION

During every current mammography procedure, there is an important component that produces an uncomfortable physical sensation for the patient which is present throughout all of the required x-ray exposures. This is firm compression* or flattening of the breast against the image receptor assembly platform by an acrylic paddle. It will be unpleasant for most patients and quite painful for more than a few. Usage of some radiolucent cushioning between the breast and the support plate of the machine, however, can noticeably reduce the degree of pain experienced by a sensitive patient. Alternatively, there has been found to be very helpful, and is available at some facilities, the option of patient self-compression wherein under the guidance of the mammographic technologist the patient physically controls the amount of compression pressure. Two x-ray views of each breast (craniocaudal direction [CC] and mediolateral oblique direction [MLO]) are taken in a standard screening mammogram evaluation. Therefore, there will always be some amount of radiation dose to the patient's breasts during mammographic examinations.

Mammography radiographers typically adjust the applied compression force based on breast size, skin tightness, any existing defects, and the patient's tolerance. This indicates that both the *compression force* and the *examination pressure* used during a mammogram can vary from patient to patient and also that protocols founded upon compression pressure which takes into account breast surface area will be a more realistic guide to better and less uncomfortable mammograms.

---

*Mammography systems normally display the compression force in traditional units generally from 20 to as high as 40 pounds (lbs) or in SI units 9 to 18 decanewtons (daN) applied by compression paddle to the breast (1 daN = 2.25 lbs). The force per unit area or *pressure*, however, is a better indicator for the degree of tissue compression. The pressure is defined to be the applied compression force divided by the contact area between the breast and the compression paddle and is specified in pounds per square inch (psi) in traditional units and in kilopascals (kPA) in SI units (1 kPA = 0.145 psi).

Research statistics acquired in one study[1] involving over 430 patients with varying breast sizes and varying existing physical conditions have shown that there was a range in compression pressure from 4.4 psi to 0.44 psi or about 30 kPA to 3 kPA. The mean applied compression force with a full-size paddle was about 20 lbs or 9 daN. It was also repeatedly noted that women with larger breasts tolerated a greater force of compression. Flattening and reducing breast thickness prior to a mammographic radiation exposure is necessary because of the following advantages:

- It ensures that the x-ray beam producing an image passes through much less breast tissue. This will generate less scatter radiation and thereby produce *a sharper image.*
- Less tissue to penetrate reduces the amount of incident radiation exposure that must be used and, therefore facilitates *a lower patient absorbed dose per exposure.*
- With less tissue packed together, overlapping of healthy tissues will be reduced and so will reduce their chance of *concealing a cancer* (i.e., it goes undetected) or alternatively, *simulating a false cancer.*

Patient Dose in Mammography

Mammography is a low-kilovoltage radiographic examination of the breast used to detect a breast cancer that is not palpable by physical examination (Fig. 15.1). Experts agree that yearly mammographic screening of women 50 years of age and older leads to earlier detection of breast cancer. Earlier treatment of the disease saves lives and reduces suffering. The value of mammography in younger women is somewhat controversial. The controversy has little to do with radiation risk (induction of breast cancer by radiation). Although it is still mentioned occasionally in the popular press, cancer researchers generally agree that radiation risk resulting from the small doses associated with mammography is negligible in all women.[2–4] Federal regulations for US Food and Drug Administration (FDA) certification of screening mammography facilities state that the mean dose to the glandular tissue of a breast that is compressed to a thickness of 4.5 cm using a digital dedicated mammography system should not be >3 mGy_t per view.[5] Studies have shown that well-calibrated mammographic systems are capable of providing excellent imaging performance with an average glandular dose of not more than 2 mGy_t.[6] The age recommendation for screening is controversial because mammography is less accurate in the detection of breast cancer in younger

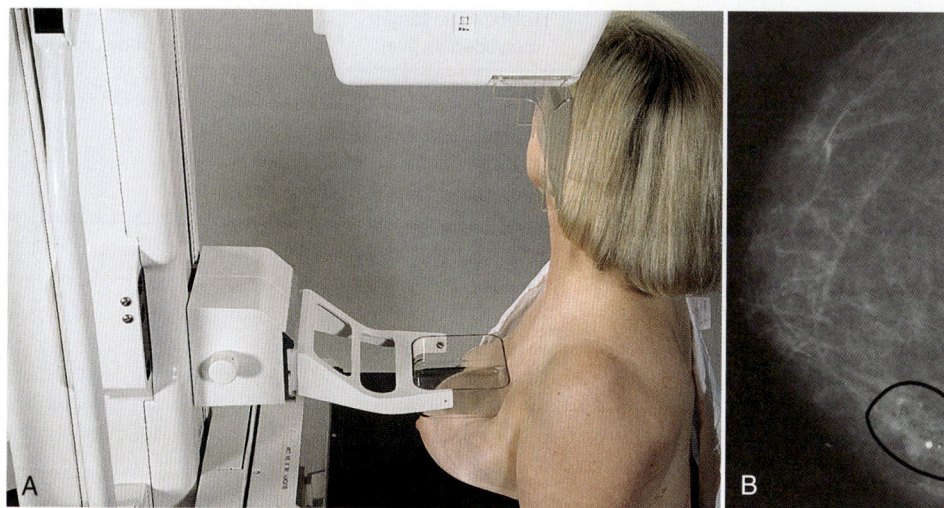

Fig. 15.1 (A) Mammography of the breast using the craniocaudal projection. (B) Mammography can be used to detect breast cancer.

women and is likely to result in many **false-positive readings**, leading to unnecessary biopsies in that population. The increased density of the breast of younger women tends to reduce radiographic contrast in the completed image. Digital mammography units which can enhance contrast with image gray-level manipulation, offer substantial improvement for patients with dense breasts. Such units combined with a newer irradiation technique known as **digital tomosynthesis** (discussed later in this chapter) will lower the percentage of false-positive readings caused by very dense breasts and consequently, permit a more effective screening of younger women. Earlier detection will save lives in general.

Mammography Screening

The authors of this textbook support the recommendations of the American College of Radiology, the American Cancer Society, and the American Medical Association. These groups advocate annual mammography screening or mammography screening at least every other year for women age 40 to 49 years. Before the onset of menopause, a **baseline mammogram** is also highly recommended for comparison with mammograms taken at a later age. The interested reader should contact these organizations for their latest policy statements on this subject.

Dose Reduction in Mammography

Dose reduction in mammography can be achieved by limiting the number of projections taken or by lowering the dose associated with each projection. In standard mammography, axillary projections should be done only on request of the radiologist. If standard mammography is performed as a routine screening procedure, it is prudent to perform only craniocaudal and mediolateral oblique projections of each breast with adequate compression to demonstrate breast tissue uniformly from the nipple to the most posterior portion.

Filtration for Mammographic Equipment

Appropriate attenuation is necessary for mammographic equipment, which by design produces photons with an energy range of 17 to 23 keV. Metallic elements such as molybdenum ($_{42}Mo^{96}$) and rhodium ($_{45}Rh^{103}$) have most commonly been employed as filters for these low-energy x-ray beams. When the x-ray tube target is made of molybdenum, either a 0.03-mm **molybdenum filter** or a 0.025-mm **rhodium filter** may be selected.[7] For rhodium x-ray tube targets, only rhodium filters are used. These filtration and target materials facilitate a satisfactory level of contrast in the obtained radiographic image over the clinical extent of compressed breast thickness. This is accomplished by employing specific filters that preferentially select or permit passage of a particular range or window of energies from the emerging x-ray spectrum that is very favorable for the photoelectric interaction. Molybdenum filters allow a lower energy window (17 to 20 keV) than rhodium filters (20 to 23 keV) (Fig. 15.2). Molybdenum filters are, therefore,

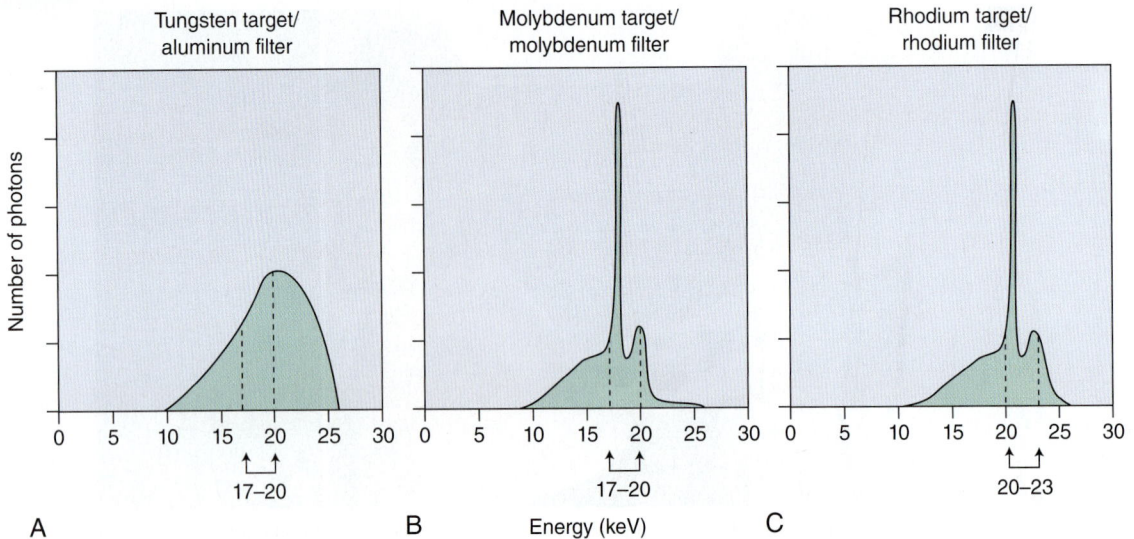

Fig. 15.2 (A and B) X-ray emission spectra for tungsten and molybdenum anodes. Note that tungsten produces a high volume of x-ray photons above the 17 to 20 keV range considered ideal for mammography. These photons merely degrade the quality of the recorded image. The molybdenum anode, however, produces few x-ray photons above the ideal energy range, thereby initiating a higher contrast on the finished image. (C) A rhodium anode produces a higher average energy x-ray beam than does the molybdenum anode. The energy range for rhodium-produced photons is 20 to 23 keV. Photons from this energy range can provide better penetration of larger, denser breasts. (From Ballinger PW, Frank ED: *Merrill's atlas of radiographic positions and radiologic procedures*, ed 9, St. Louis, 1999, Mosby.)

suitable for small and average breast thickness, whereas rhodium filters used with a molybdenum or rhodium anode are better for larger (i.e., compression thickness of 6 cm and greater) or dense breasts because they will produce an x-ray beam with more penetrating energy. Systemic use of such materials has the effect of reducing the **mean glandular dose (MGD)*** in firm breast tissue.

Maintaining and enhancing subject contrast are of paramount importance in mammography. Beryllium ($_4Be^9$) takes the place of the glass in the window of the low-kVp x-ray producing mammographic x-ray tube to accommodate this need.[7] This light, strong alkaline earth metal permits the relatively soft characteristic radiation important for enhancing contrast to exit the tube without undergoing any significant attenuation.

Recently, it has been shown that newer, **full-field digital mammography** systems and **digital tomosynthesis** systems provide better images with tungsten targets

($_{74}W^{184}$) with rhodium filtration (W/Rh) for most breast thicknesses and tungsten targets with silver ($_{47}Ag^{108}$) filtration (W/Ag) for thicker breasts. Digital detectors are better able to separate out image features in mammography when presented with the broader spectra provided by the tungsten targets.

Molybdenum x-ray tube targets with molybdenum or rhodium filtration are being replaced in newer digital systems by tungsten targets with rhodium or silver filtration.[8,9]

DIGITAL BREAST TOMOSYNTHESIS/3D MAMMOGRAPHY

Tomography

The method used for generating an in-focus two-dimensional (2D) image of a slice or cross-section through a three-dimensional (3D) object is called *Tomography*. Traditional x-ray tomography achieves this result by simply moving an x-ray source in a preselected arc in one direction (i.e., clockwise or counterclockwise) as a mechanically linked x-ray detector traverses in a constant plane in the opposite direction (right to left or left to right) during

---

*MGD is a convenient parameter that can be used to characterize the average absorbed dose to the breast as a result of a mammographic x-ray exposure. It will be discussed in detail later in this chapter.

the exposure. This facilitates a sharpening of structures in the focal plane while causing structures in other planes above or below to appear blurred. Typically, selected arc angles have ranged from 15 degrees up to 45 degrees. In the past, this technique was used to acquire more detail of specific structures within the patient, such as solid tumors. This practice has been almost totally superseded by the development of computed tomography.

Digital Breast Tomosynthesis (DBT)[10]

In standard digital mammography, the 3D breast structure is projected onto a detector plane perpendicular to the x-ray source, and the multiple tissues and structures of the compressed breast appear overlapped in the acquired projection image. This has two detrimental effects on a radiologist's ability to detect subtle lesions from these usual mammography images: first, malignant lesions or tumors may be obscured by the presence of overlapping normal glandular tissue, producing *false negatives*; second, the superimposition of normal tissues might combine into a structure that appears to be an abnormality, thereby signaling a *false positive*. This lowering of sensitivity and specificity in conventional mammography caused by tissue superimposition is often called "anatomical" or "structure" noise. DBT has the ability to overcome anatomical noise *by adding depth resolution to a mammogram*. This technique was first approved by the US FDA in 2011.

Digital breast tomosynthesis is an imaging technique which generates multiple planar images or views of the breast from a series of low-dose x-ray projection images acquired by a **full field digital detector*** while the x-ray tube rotates within a limited arc about the patient's breast.

***Full field digital detector** historically refers to: When digital imaging was introduced as an alternative to analog film-screen radiography, technology enabled only small field of views in breast imaging. This new technology was used primarily to obtain small "spot views" during stereotactic biopsies and wire locations, thus bypassing the time-consuming process of developing film-screen images and greatly expediting these procedures. Larger digital detectors were subsequently developed that permitted imaging an entire small breast, but multiple images were required for larger breasts, requiring added radiation and time. The latter limitation was partially overcome by mammographic equipment using fan-beam technology. Eventually, larger digital detectors became available, thus enabling full-field imaging.[13]

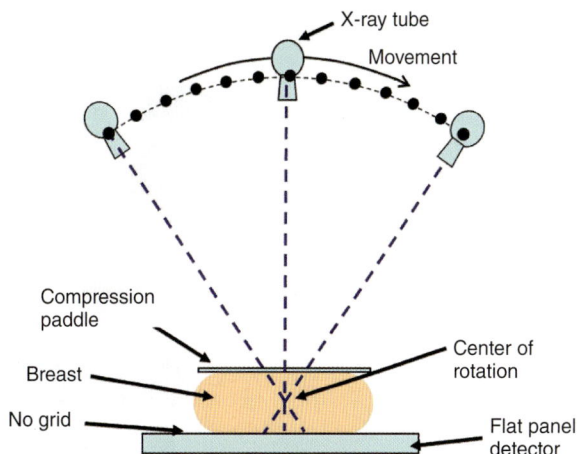

Fig. 15.3 DBT imaging configuration. The vertical direction is along the z-axis and the plane of the detector (also known as in-plane) corresponds to the x and y axis direction. (From Vaughan CL: Novel imaging approaches to screen for breast cancer: recent advances and future prospects, *Med Eng Phys* 72:27–37, 2019.)

This is physically achieved by modifying a standard digital mammography platform so that the gantry containing the x-ray tube assembly is able to rotate about an axis located above the breast support within the breast, while the compressed patient's breast and the mammography detector remain stationary. Breast positioning in DBT is the same as is used for conventional digital mammography, with the breast compressed, but often *to a lesser degree*, on a stationary support situated directly above the detector assembly to permit different oblique views.[11,12] Fig. 15.3 is a schematic of a standard mammographic imaging setup as used for DBT with the x-ray tube at several angular orientations.

Digital breast tomography is often referred to as "3D" mammography because mammographic images can be reconstructed at arbitrary angles from the many different x-ray projections. The DBT image creation technique uses the same algorithms* as those for computed tomography (CT). The images are not of the same quality, however, as CT images, since those are acquired from a full 360-degree x-ray projection, but the technology and algorithms are improving. In typical Digital Breast Tomography, the third axis (z-direction) is stereoscopically

---

*Algorithm refers to a finite sequence of computer-implementable instructions used by a computer to solve a class of problems or to perform a computation.

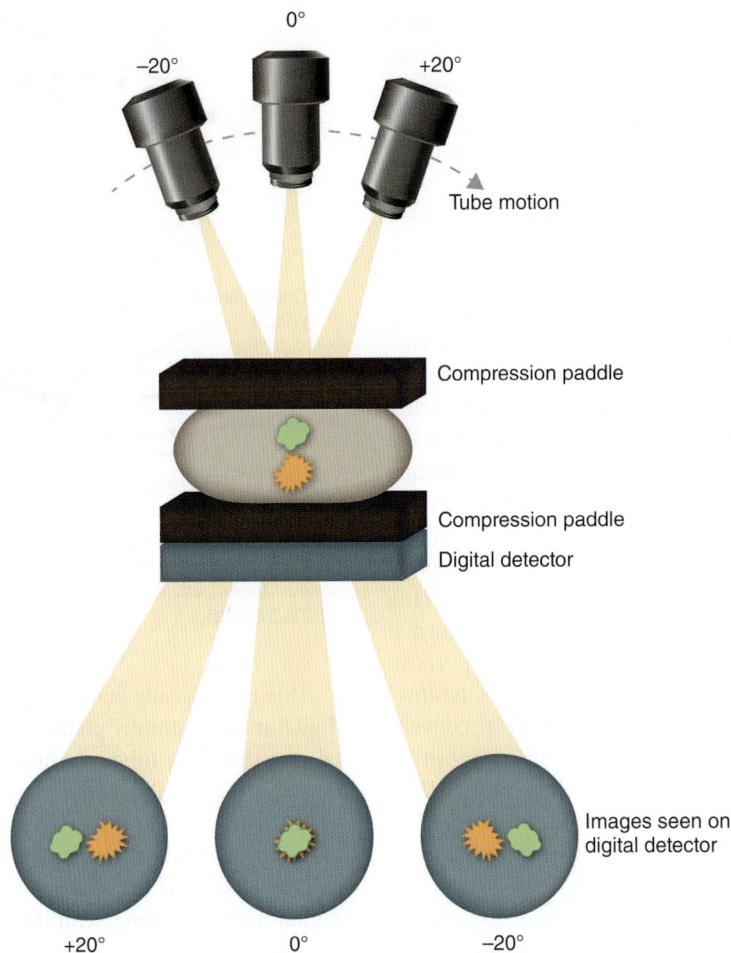

Fig. 15.4 Multiple gantry angle effects and depth resolution. (From Ikeda DM, Miyake KK: *Breast imaging: the requisites*, ed 3, St. Louis, 2017, Elsevier.)

extracted from the overall two-dimensional data. At different x-ray tube angles, objects at different heights in the breast are projected at different locations onto the detector with their detector separation increasing as the x-ray tube gantry angle increases (Fig. 15.4). The subsequent image reconstruction process leads to a stack of synthesized nonblurred slice images (similar in general appearance to 2D mammography planar images) of different depth layers in the breast parallel to the detector surface. The degree of overall resolution is predominantly determined by the detector's characteristics, the reconstruction algorithm used, and the total angle of rotation of the x-ray tube. The in-plane (x-y) sharpness, or resolution, of the image is much higher than the resolution in the z-axis or the direction between adjacent slices (called

depth resolution) due to the incomplete sampling of the object from a relatively small angular scan range. As of 2016, the best z-axis **spatial resolution*** obtained has been 2.3 mm using a 50-degree arc.[11]

Effects of Tomographic Angular Scan Range

On the Depth Resolution of Structures. A standard 2D **full field digital mammogram (FFDM)** gives no specific information of the depth in the breast (z-axis location) of a particular mass or abnormal structure, implying that it could

---

*Spatial resolution refers to the ability to distinguish spatially close objects as distinct separate objects and is given by a limiting number (e.g., in millimeters or in line pairs resolved per millimeter) that quantifies that limit.

be at any depth. But as can be observed from Fig. 15.4 with a sufficient gantry angular displacement, the lesion can be clearly distinguished on a detector from adjacent structures. A small tomosynthesis arc yields only a poor separation of vertically close objects (i.e., slight z-axis separation) while a large angle tomosynthesis arc provides a good visual separation of these objects and, therefore, a more precise vertical localization of the lesion or mass.[12]

On In-Plane Image Quality. If an x-ray source moves through a larger angular range, the obtained in-plane (x-y) image quality increases, at least initially. A larger angular range allows for extra view directions, which can improve the quality of the reconstructed image since the inside of the breast can be inspected more thoroughly. This is of importance since for many types of breast masses there is not much variation or differentiation from one laterally adjacent position to the next. Thus, image contrast is improved. However, if the total allowable breast dose is fixed while the number of views is increased, there is a deterioration in the overall image quality in each view because of increased image noise due to a lessening of the x-ray exposure per view (i.e., too low a **signal-to-noise ratio [SNR]**). The best performance for all tomosynthesis angles occurred when from one x-ray projection to the next, the angular increment was about 2.75 degrees.[14,15]

Effects Summary. The following quantities depend on acquisition geometry, scan parameters, and system hardware components[12]:
- Resolution
- Detector Noise
- Artifact level
- Patient Dose
- Accessible image volume
- Examination time

Optimal image acquisition geometry, therefore, should be a compromise that accounts for the effects of total tomosynthesis angle, angular increment, and the number and distribution of projections on[14]:
- correctly identifying architectural distortions and soft tissue lesions
- the perception of calcifications
- increased motion blur with increased scan time.

Image Reconstruction (IR)

Each DBT arc acquisition sequence may typically consist of from 15 to 25 separate x-ray projections. From the data generated by these, many well-defined planar views (their number depends on the compressed breast thickness) can be obtained after computer processing. These synthesized *slices* can subsequently be viewed either individually or in a continuous sequence, thereby generating a "movie." This latter option, called *cine mode,* offers a clinician an approximate three-dimensional scan of the breast which can yield an improved examination of suspicious architecture. Because only a limited arc angle inspection is available (e.g., from 15 up to 50 degrees depending on the mammographic unit), depth resolution through the breast of various objects or structures will also be dependent upon the depth range (z-axis extent) spanned by them. Thus, for structures such as microcalcifications that typically only persist across a few tomosynthesis planes, the image fidelity will be high.

Due to the breast's highly inhomogeneous volume, typical required viewing voxel* dimensions in tomosynthesis are 100 μm × 100 μm pixels in-plane (x-y plane) by 1 mm in depth (z-direction) to adequately resolve variations of interest in the breast. As a result of this resolution, the 3D distribution of attenuation that is entirely projected into just one image in conventional mammography can in DBT be separated into many 1 mm thick layers, thereby increasing the visualization of features that are often obscured by overlapping structures in a 2D single projection view.

As the x-ray projections are obtained, the raw image digital data is exported into the data processing computer's reconstruction algorithm. The conventional method of image reconstruction used in digital tomosynthesis is the **Shift and Add Algorithm (SAA).**[14] As shown in Fig. 15.4, objects within the image sample that are at different heights above the detector will be projected to different positions on the detector as the x-ray tube moves. It then becomes possible for the computer by properly *registering** these images to both shift and add them so

---

Voxel is a term used for a discrete image *volume element* (a 3D measure), and *pixel* is a term used for a discrete image *area element.*

**Registration of imaged structures is the procedure of precisely aligning two or more images of the same object. One image of the object always is classified as the *reference image.* Then, geometric transformations or local displacements (i.e., a shifting) are applied to all of the other images similar to the reference image so that they align with the reference image.[14]

that similarly catalogued structures in a particular plane are all lined up and are thus reinforced and those non-similarly registered structures are distributed over the image (misaligned) and are thereby blurred. As a result, for each reconstructed or synthesized plane, there is *in sharp relief* only the structures belonging to that plane, while other structures located in adjacent planes are out of focus in the plane of interest. Fig. 15.5 gives a pictorial summation of the acquisition and reconstruction processes. This combined method of acquisition and reconstruction significantly *reduces anatomical noise*, promoting easier and more reliable lesion detection.

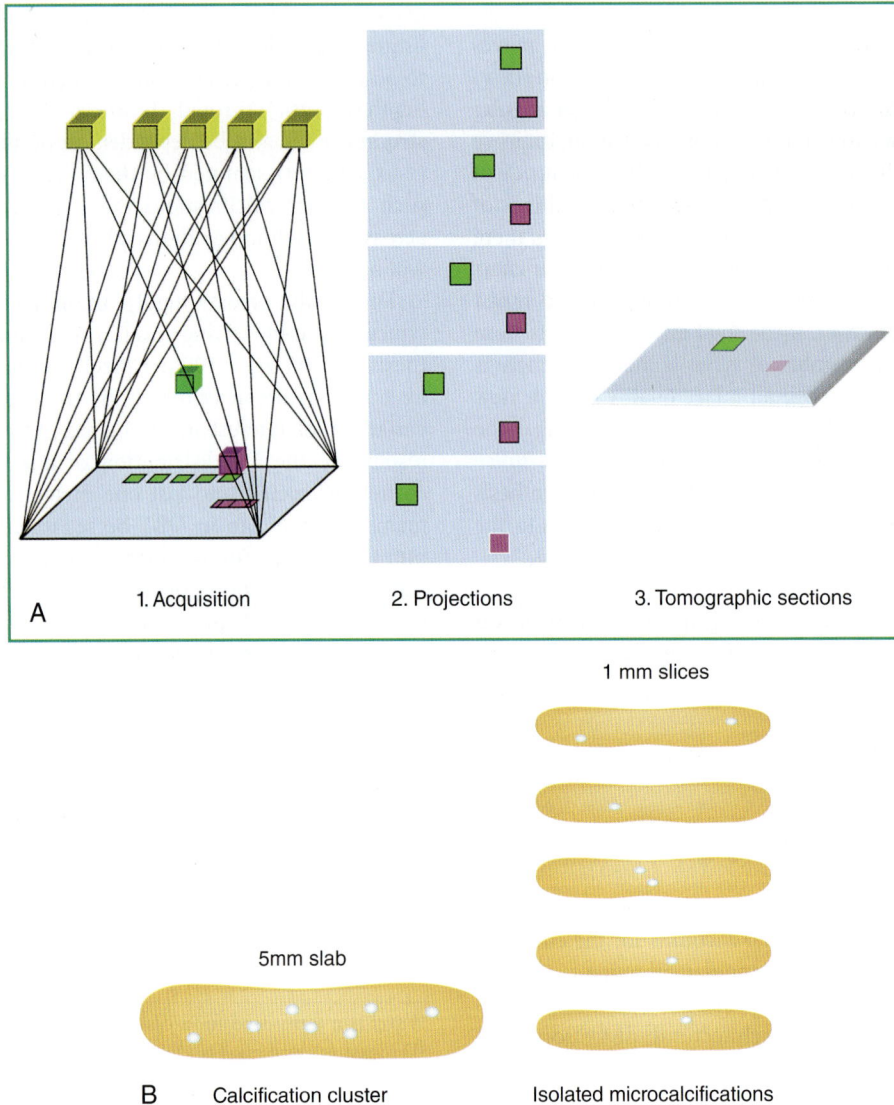

Fig. 15.5 (A) Shift and add method for tomographic image reconstruction. (B) By combining several thin slices together like a pancake, the existence of a *calcification cluster* whose components were spread out over several adjacent 1 mm reconstructed slices is now apparent. Consequently, the production of a slab composed from adjacent thin slices has led to a diagnostic result indicative of the potential presence of a nearby cancer. (A, From Blum A, Noel A, Regent D: Tomosynthesis in musculoskeletal pathology. *Diagn Interven Imaging* 99(7–8):423–441, 2018.)

All of the projection images are included in every synthesized planar image and all of these "planes," each parallel to the detector surface, are generated through the entire breast from just a small number of x-ray projection images. Typically, the generated view planes are spaced 1.0 mm center to center apart. A 4.5-cm thick compressed breast reconstructed at 1 mm spacing will, therefore, yield a group of 45 images.

In the acquisition process shown in Fig. 15.5A, an x-ray tube moves to five discrete positions.

Objects situated at two different levels are projected onto the detector at different locations due to parallax. The five projection images are shifted and added together to cause either of the objects in one of the two levels to be in sharp focus, depending on the magnitude of the shift for that object. Other types of images which can be reconstructed from tomosynthesis are *slabs, that is,* broader slices obtained by merging together a multiple number of adjacent tomographic reconstructed planes (see Fig. 15.5B). Slabs, therefore, have a substantial thickness, typically 1 cm or more, and are particularly useful for detecting microcalcification bunches. In fact, microcalcifications usually seen grouped in clusters in standard 2D mammography may not be as well visualized along the z-axis direction (depth) in the thin tomographic reconstructions and so not be obvious as making up a cluster. Furthermore, if some type of potentially pathological feature is detected in cine mode, then image slabs, because of their much fewer number, allow a quick spot review of the entire breast volume, prior to getting into the fine details of reviewing the numerous 1-mm synthesized tomographic planes.[11]

Advantages of DBT

DBT mammographic examinations may be used to diagnose breast cancer in people *who have no overt signs or symptoms.* Also, it can more sensitively investigate the cause of some breast problems, such as localized or distributed pain and nipple discharge. When a DBT series is combined with 2D standard mammogram projections, the combination may be able to yield the following benefits.[15]

Reduce the Need For Follow-up Imaging. Should abnormalities be detected on standard mammogram images, additional imaging will usually be recommended. This can be very stressful besides taking extra time and leading to additional costs. Performing a 3D mammogram along with a standard 2D mammogram at the same appointment, however, will reduce the need for follow-up imaging.

Detect More Cancers Than a Standard Mammogram Alone. Multiple studies indicate that performing a 3D mammogram along with a standard mammogram can result in about one more breast cancer found for every 1000 women screened when compared with a standard mammogram alone. At the expense of some increased patient radiation dosage, this amounts to finding a substantial number of otherwise undiscovered cancers when one considers the number of women annually screened.

Improve Breast Cancer Detection in Dense Breast Tissue. A DBT mammogram offers advantages in detecting breast cancer in patients with *dense breast tissue.* It has been noted that about 45% of all women receiving screening mammography are found to have either *heterogeneously dense* or *very dense* breasts. Breasts are normally considered to be dense if there is present a much greater concentration of fibrous or glandular tissue than fatty tissue. With standard 2D mammograms, nonfatty breasts pose challenges to accurately identifying the presence of cancer since irregularities can often be efficiently concealed or masked within the dense tissue. With a DBT mammogram, however, breast tissue can be scrutinized slab by slab or even thin layer by thin layer, overcoming the obscurity effect and making it easier to detect cancer in an early stage. It should be noted that data collected on many patients has shown that *the degree of breast density is not a major indicator for risk of breast cancer.*[15]

In Fig. 15.6B are shown planar images that might be reconstructed from an obtained DBT data set as displayed in Fig. 15.6A. The image planes depicted in Fig. 15.6A,B are at different distances above the breast support plate. As contrasted with the compacted 2D image shown in Fig. 15.6C, each of these tomographic planes clearly demonstrates a separate structure, whereas the 2D projection in Fig. 15.6C only exhibits a composite compacted image.

This ability to select multiple specific individual tissue planes in which various structures of interest are visually enhanced can significantly increase both the detection rate and the level of diagnostic confidence with respect to apparent abnormalities.[12] To summarize, DBT images may be reconstructed as thin planes or as slabs depending on the desired fineness of z-axis resolution. Another significant advantage of DBT is shown in Fig. 15.7.

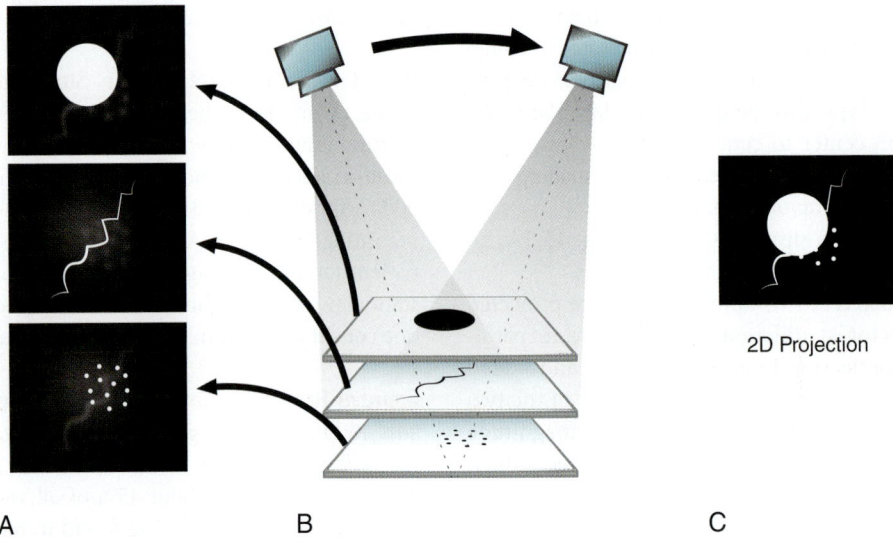

Fig. 15.6 DBT acquired breast slice views at three different depths. (From Abrahams RB, Huda W, Sensakovic WF: *Imaging physics: case review series*, St. Louis, 2020, Elsevier.)

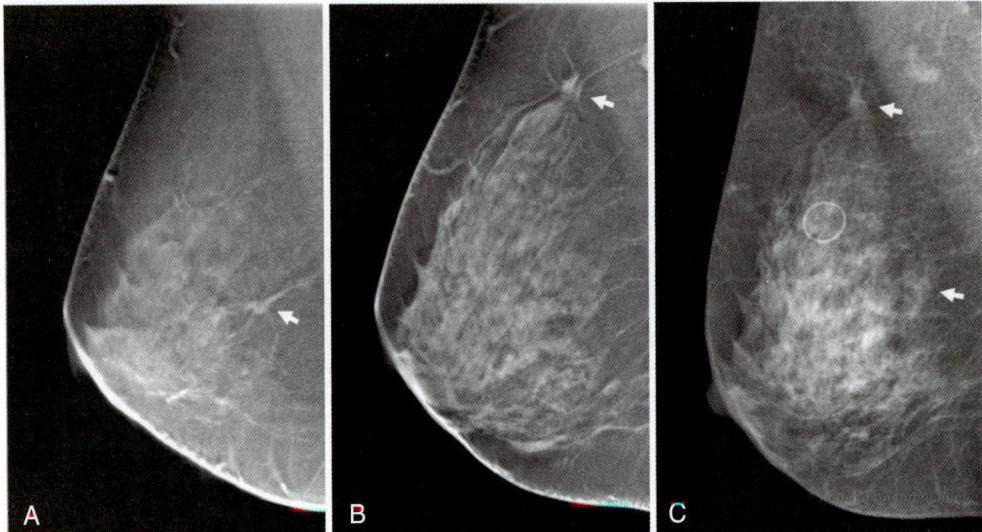

Fig. 15.7 Comparison of positive conventional mammogram and DBT images. The DBT slices in (A) and (B) readily demonstrate the presence of two distinct abnormalities, while the standard digital mammogram pictured in (C) offers a poorer or less clear indication. (From Chan HP, Helvie MA, Hadjiiski L, et al.: Characterization of breast masses in digital breast tomosynthesis and digital mammograms: an observer performance study. *AcadRadiol* 24(11):1372–1379, 2017.)

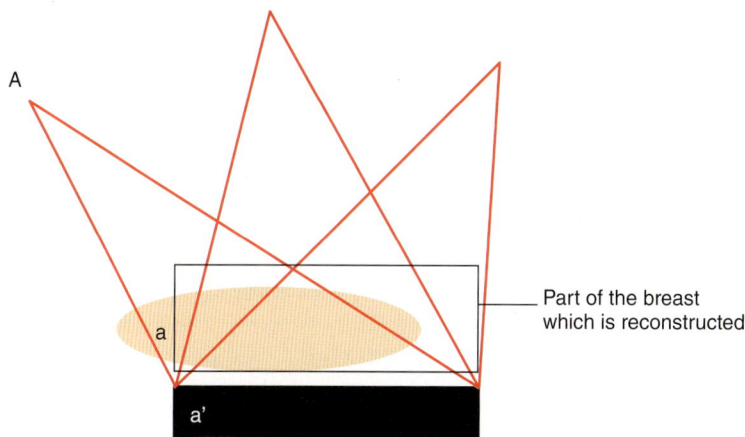

Fig. 15.8 Incompleteness in DBT imaging scan. The area marked *(a)* attenuates the beam when the tube is in position *(A)* and is projected to area *(a')* on the detector. The attenuation caused by this area is only added to the most peripheral part of the breast tissue included by the detector. As seen, not all of the breast is captured by the detector. (From Rangarajan K, Hari S: Artefacts in digital breast tomosynthesis, *ECR 2013 Poster C-1711,* 2013. © European Society of Radiology.)

Artifacts in Digital Breast Tomography[16,17]

Artifacts Due to Motion. The x-ray tube can move in either a continuous or a step-and-shoot motion.* With continuous motion, x-ray exposures must be short enough to avoid image blurring due to focal spot motion. If step-and-shoot motion is employed, the gantry must come to a complete stop at each angular location before delivering x-rays, otherwise vibrations will blur the image. It is also important that the total scan time be not too prolonged, so as to reduce the possibility of patient motion that can degrade the visibility of microcalcifications and small *spiculations* (lumps of tissue with spikes or points on the surface). A grid is generally not used during tomographic acquisitions since the varying irradiation angles essentially do the work of a grid.

Artifacts due to method of acquisition. Acquisition artifacts are primarily *truncation artifacts* that arise due to the limited physical size of the detector and the greater extent of oblique x-ray beams causing incomplete coverage of the breast in multiple views (Fig. 15.8).

Some major examples of these are:

a. *Bright area artifact*—Appearing at extreme ends of the image where the detector cannot see.
b. *Staircase artifact*—Presence of multiple lines at one of the ends of the image, creating a staircase-like

appearance or artifact *where the beam cannot see.* At each tube position there is a corresponding part of the breast tissue that would not be projected back by the detector. The breast seemingly ends at different places for different tube positions, leading to the production of lines at the edges of the image. This is schematically shown in Fig. 15.8.

Artifacts Due to Z-Axis Resolution Deficiency. For digital breast tomosynthesis, the attainable *in-plane (x-y) resolution* for a particular cross-section or breast slice is very good but the limited angle of rotation of the x-ray tube (up to about a maximum of 60 degrees) and the limited number of x-ray projections restricts the z-axis resolution. This produces an incomplete cancellation of objects outside of the plane of interest and is the source of most artifacts.[16] Consequently, the precise localization of an extended depth object will be less than perfect and some elongation of the suspicious object may also be present.

Fig. 15.9 depicts this situation.

Artifacts Due to Reconstruction Process.[16]

a. *Ripple*—This arises from a poorly but still visualized structure of high density (e.g., a calcification) being observed in different slices from those in which it is actually located.
b. *Halo artifact*—Manifestation of a very-low-intensity signal (dark) appearing to circle around high-intensity objects such as calcifications (white) leads to the creation of a halo or crown. Halos are particularly pronounced along the sweep direction of the x-ray tube.

---

*Microcalcifications are small calcium deposits in breast tissue that on a mammogram look like white specks.

*In step-and-shoot mode, the x-ray tube moves to a predetermined position (angle), makes an exposure, and then proceeds to the next position and so forth.

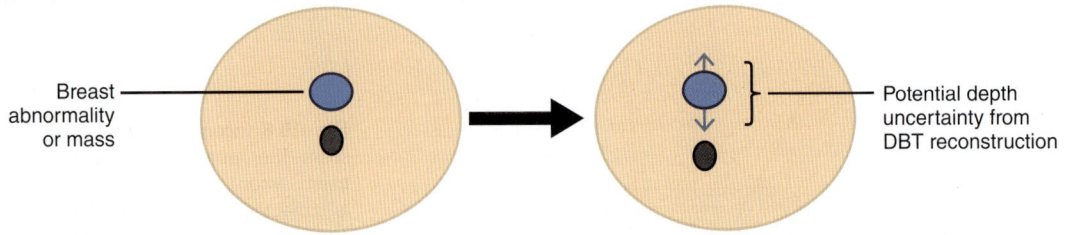

Fig. 15.9 Location uncertainty of a mass due to DBT limitations. (From Rangarajan K, Hari S: Artefacts in digital breast tomosynthesis, *ECR 2013 Poster C-1711*, 2013. © European Society of Radiology.)

Properties of DBT Summarized[18,19]

Expanding the Angular Sweep of the X-ray Tube

- Improves z-axis or depth resolution and the blurring of out of plane objects.
- Permits finer or thinner reconstruction slices.
- At larger angles can begin to degrade in-plane or x-y sharpness but allows better out-of-plane resolution for larger objects such as masses that occupy multiple planes.

Increasing the Number of Projections for a Given Angular Range

- Lowers the visibility of artifacts.
- Increases the patient's absorbed dose if the same exposure settings (i.e., technique factors) are used.
- Increases the relative importance of detector noise if, however, the total dose is held constant.

Number of Projections Required Depends On

- The angular extent of x-ray tube rotation.
- The number of image pixels or individual pixel size.
- The characteristics of the full field detector.
- The degree of differences in contrast of absorbing objects within the breast.

DBT Imaging Unit Characteristics[18]

Shown below in Fig. 15.10 are preparatory and operational pictures of a typical 3D mammography system. Table 15.1 is an inventory of the physical characteristics and operational parameters of several available commercial DBT units.

DBT Procedure: Steps and Details

For a DBT examination, the patient's breast is positioned the same way as it is in a conventional mammogram procedure. The radiologist may specify what the focal distance or location of the axis of rotation will be but typically the axis of rotation will be positioned in the center of the compressed breast. The scan itself takes less than two to three seconds per x-ray projection and there can be as many as 25 views taken. The entire procedure from the patient entering the examination room up to leaving it will usually take about 20 minutes. Box 15.1 lists the various steps during the radiation exposures process for a typical commercial DBT unit.[18]

With DBT alone, a compression force only great enough to securely retain the breast in a stable position during the procedure may suffice. For this situation, it is more feasible to use a *flexible compression paddle*, which will be less uncomfortable for the patient. In fact, it is possible that some DBT examinations could be performed using only half of the compression force employed currently in standard 2D digital mammography, leading to a substantial reduction in perceived and/or actual patient pain while incurring no clinically significant change in breast imaging fidelity and tissue coverage.[19,20] The effects of decreased compression were extensively examined in a study done with phantom images generated by using computer modeling methods that simulated three dissimilar breasts, each having two different compressed thicknesses (4 cm and 6 cm) as compared with a lesser compressed pair (4.5 and 6.75 cm compressions). Using *lesion conspicuity** as the metric of choice for masses and calcifications, the authors found no significant observational difference with the lesser

---

*The concept of **lesion conspicuity** is used to objectively quantify radiographic observational error. It is defined as a ratio between lesion contrast and the surroundings. Experiments have been done to determine whether this ratio or measure can be well correlated with the probability of detecting faint lesions.[22]

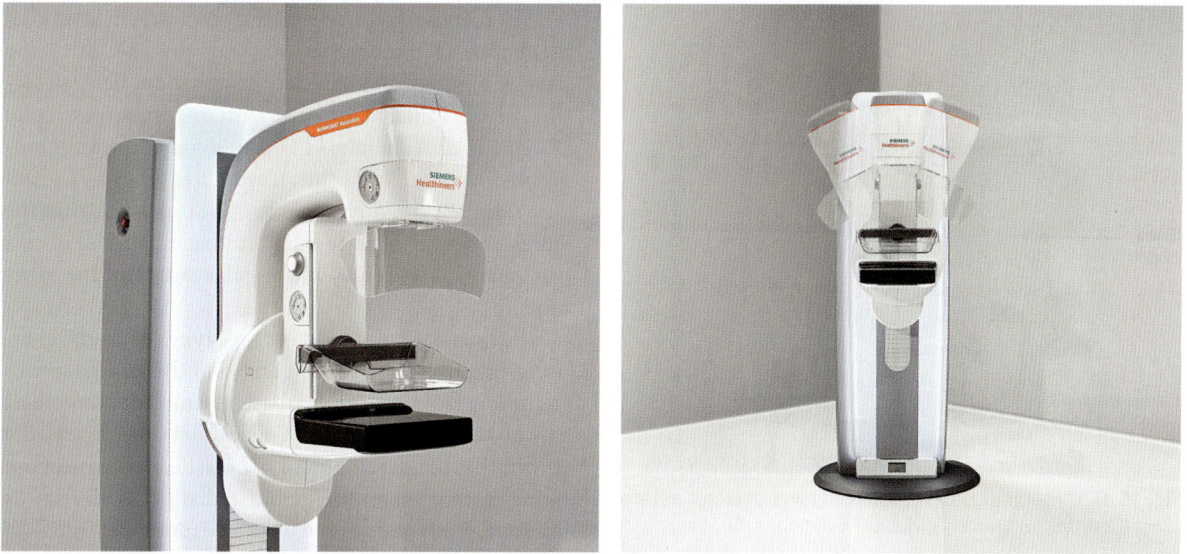

Fig. 15.10 Operational views of a DBT system. (Courtesy of Siemens Medical Solutions USA, Inc.)

TABLE 15.1 Physical Characteristics of Five Manufacturer's Digital Breast Tomosynthesis Units[10]

Manufacturers:	Fuji	GE	Hologic	IMS	Siemens
Anode Material:	W	Mo or Rh	W	W	W
Filter Material:	Al or Rh	Mo or Rh	Ag	Ag	Rh
Detector:	a-Se FPD*	CsI FPD**	a-Se FPD	a-Se FPD	a-Se FPD
Pixel size (μm):	150/100	100/50	100/140	85	85
Pixel shape:	Hexagonal	Square	Square	Square	Square
Tube motion:	Continuous	Step and shoot	Continuous	Step and shoot	Continuous
Sweep angle (°):	15/ 40	25	15	40	50
No. of projections:	15	9	15	13	25
Dose/projection:	Uniform	Uniform	Uniform	Variable	Uniform
Antiscatter grid:	No	Yes	No	No	No

*Amorphous selenium flat panel detector
**Cesium iodide flat panel detector

BOX 15.1 Siemens Mammomat DBT

Twenty-five views are acquired in an angular range from −25° to +25°. The exposure release button on the control box or on the foot or hand switch must be pressed and held during all exposures. Following proper positioning and compression of the patient's breast, the steps of the image acquisition process are:

1. Initially, the swivel arm is in the 0° position.
2. The first view is acquired for automatic exposure control settings.
3. Swivel arm then moves to -25° and a second exposure is taken.
4. The swivel arm subsequently covers the entire angular range from -25° to +25° while an exposure is taken at every 2° for a total of 50 projections.
5. Swivel arm returns to the start position.

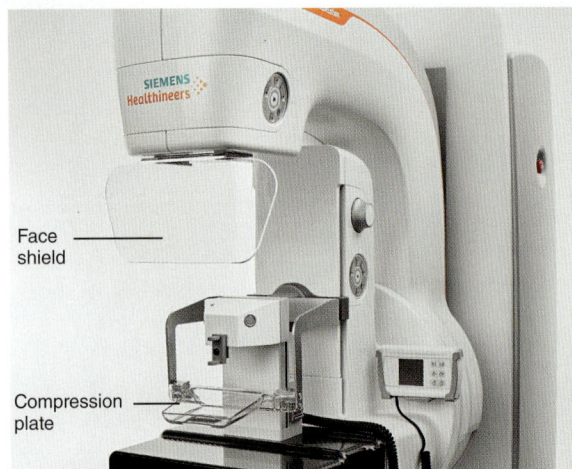

Fig. 15.11 Closeup of breast positioning and detector assemblies. (Courtesy of Siemens Medical Solutions USA, Inc.)

compressions when the exposure parameters were varied to maintain a constant dose to the breasts.[19–21]

To ensure radiation safety, a restricting *face shield must be used* during tomographic examinations (Fig. 15.11). The face shield is present because there is a risk that the patient's head can drift into the x-ray beam path if not prevented from doing so. Note that the face shield also moves when the swivel arm moves. The patient's head must, therefore, not lean against the face shield during the arc rotation.

RADIATION DOSAGE

The x-ray spectrum used for tomosynthesis is generally similar to that employed in standard digital mammography, and the selected peak kilovoltage (kVp) depends on the thickness and density of the compressed breast. If the x-ray energy is increased slightly, thereby sacrificing some degree of image quality, then it is possible to reduce the absorbed dose just by using less mA. Another option, especially for thicker breasts, for *reducing dose while maintaining image quality*, is to have additional filtering of the x-ray beam. This inherently increases the mean beam energy and consequent *net radiation penetration*. It can be achieved by selecting in place of the standard molybdenum/molybdenum (Mo/Mo) or molybdenum/rhodium (Mo/Rh) x-ray target/filter combinations, other pairings such as tungsten/rhodium (W/Rh), tungsten/aluminum (W/Al), or tungsten/silver (W/Ag).

For mammography, a useful and practical implementation of tomography was not possible until the development of digital flat panel wide field detectors which initiated **full field digital mammography (FFDM)**. Subsequently, FFDM was coupled with tomographic motion. With this, *any desired image slice and slice thickness could be computer reconstructed* from the stored multiple angle projection images, and all of this was obtained with just one angular sweep of the x-ray tube.[12,19]

The breast is composed of three types of tissue: glandular, adipose (fatty tissue), and skin. Because statistics stemming from a large database assembled from breast cancer screenings by many institutions has repeatedly shown that the development of breast cancer in adipose tissue is rare, mammographic radiation dosimetry is predominantly concerned with the dose deposited in the glandular tissue of the breast. Therefore, the parameter that has been chosen for both standard and 3D digital mammography to estimate and represent effective dose in x-ray breast imaging is the **mean glandular dose (MGD)**.

MGD is used to characterize the absorbed dosage to the radiosensitive fibroglandular breast tissue. Quantitively, it is determined from measurements which employ a special design (thin window circular parallel plate) ionization chamber to measure the air kerma or exposure *incident* on the breast or on a breast-equivalent phantom. To obtain the MGD from such measurements, the ion chamber readings must be multiplied by special conversion factors derived from data generated by complex randomized computer modeling of radiation interaction processes in the breast. These factors are referred to as the *normalized glandular dose coefficients*. For each ion chamber measurement, there is a particular coefficient value that is directly associated with the x-ray beam quality (HVL) employed as determined by the x-ray tube target/filter combination and the selected kVp. Tables for the latest determined coefficients are listed in the current American College of Radiology Mammography Quality Assurance Manual.

The angular range and number of exposures taken over the x-ray tube arc during the DBT scan are additional variables that need to be optimized with respect to balancing patient radiation dose and acceptable image quality. In general, it would seem that taking more exposures during a DBT procedure will generate reconstructions with fewer artifacts. However, doing this must be weighed against the consideration that for a patient receiving a full mammographic examination,* it is still desired to limit the total MGD to 3 mGy (0.3 cGy). More DBT angles will then mandate lesser irradiation per exposure and consequently smaller detector signals for each of the individual tomographic projections. For low enough exposures, image receptor inherent noise will start to become a nonnegligible component of the raw image and thereby may noticeably degrade reconstructed image quality. A greater number of exposures also increases raw data size which produces longer reconstruction times.

During a DBT acquisition process, the total delivered radiation dose is apportioned among the multiple single x-ray views with every projection contributing about only 5% to 10% of a normal single-view mammogram absorbed dose.[12,19] Because each image voxel is *ultimately overall* probed or irradiated by essentially the same number of x-ray quanta as in a standard 2D mammography acquisition, a quality tomosynthesis scan, in total, should deliver approximately the same MGD as a conventional mammogram. A major prerequisite for this to be achieved, however, is that the image receptor has a high detective quantum efficiency** (DQE). *Rapid imaging processing* is also another requirement for the DBT detector.

Usually it is assumed that within a normal breast there is a homogeneous mixture of adipose and glandular tissue surrounded by a layer of skin. In reality, it

---

*A total or full mammographic examination in a facility that has a DBT unit usually includes the standard stationary 2D x-ray projections as well as the DBT series of projections.

Detective quantum efficiency, or **DQE, refers to how efficiently a detection system translates incident x-ray photons into a *useful* signal relative to random noise within that image. In *medical radiography*, the listed DQE describes percentage-wise the degree to which an x-ray imaging system can produce an image with a high **signal-to-noise ratio (SNR)** relative to that delivered by an ideal detector whose efficiency is by definition taken to be 100%. This specification can also be considered an alternate measure of the *radiation dose efficiency* of a detector, since the needed amount of radiation exposure to a patient decreases as the system DQE is increased for the same image SNR and physical exposure conditions. Compared with film/screen imaging, a digital detector with high DQE has the potential to deliver significant object-detectability improvements at the same equivalent dose or an identical degree of detectability at a lower patient dose.

> ### BOX 15.2   Typical Mean Glandular Dose Values from Breast Phantom Measurements for Individual and Combined DBT and Standard 2D Exposures
>
> - Radiation dose for a single standard 2D mammogram is about 1.2 to 1.4 mGy or 1.3 mGy (130 mrads) on average.
> - Radiation dose for a 3D or DBT sequence of projections is about 1.3 to 1.5 mGy or 1.4 mGy (140 mrads) on average (no grid)
> - Total MGD for the combination is thus about 2.7 mGy or 270 mrads (ACR recommends that total MGD not exceed 3 mGy [300 mrads] per examination)

is found that the glandular dose deposited in various regions can differ considerably and that, especially, is why the *mean* glandular dose was adopted as a useful and practical parameter of mammographic absorbed dose. Some typical numerical values for mammographic procedures are shown in Box 15.2.

DBT SUMMARY

Breast tomosynthesis is a three-dimensional imaging technology that involves acquiring a dozen or more images of a stationary compressed breast at multiple angles of incidence during a partial rotational scan of the x-ray tube about an axis located within the breast. With these multiple diverse x-ray projections or views, objects at varying depths in the breast will be projected onto different locations on the detector. At any desired depth in the compressed breast, a reconstructed plane can be obtained by using the *Shift and Add method* or other techniques to properly combine all registered x-ray projection views for that location. Thus, in a particular reconstructed or synthesized tomosynthesis plane, a structure that is actually located at the corresponding depth will be in-focus, whereas structures lying above or below that plane are blurred.

Because there is a practical and technical limit to the angular extent of the projection acquisitions, DBT does not have isotropic spatial resolution, that is, there will be a very high spatial resolution within the planes parallel to the detector (x-y), and a considerably less fine plane by plane discrimination in the perpendicular direction (z-axis). The depth resolution, however, that has been achieved in present 3D systems is deemed to be good enough to substantially reduce the 2D mammography issue of tissue superposition, thereby noticeably lowering its negative impact on sensitivity and specificity.[23]

To keep the radiation dose to the breast from a single DBT procedure at levels comparable to a standard 2D mammography breast examination (e.g., a mediolateral view), the total x-ray tube radiation output is spread out over multiple projections, so that each individual projection delivers only a small fraction of the radiation dose of a standard 2D mammogram. This necessitates the usage of detectors with a high DQE at low air kerma or exposure levels and has led to the development of detectors specifically designed for DBT imaging.*

---

*Besides meeting the ordinary requirements for 2D digital mammography, detectors for DBT need to have additional capabilities. These include: (i) faster reading time, to keep the total acquisition time of all projections to a minimum; (ii) minimal *ghosting* (the reduction of sensitivity caused by previous exposure history of the detector) and minimal *lag* (the carryover of signal from a previous image); and (iii) minimal reduction in detective quantum efficiency at much lower exposures (a consequence of the need to divide the total exposure over multiple projections).[23,24]

Following irradiation, the individual images are reconstructed using sophisticated algorithms into a large number of thin (~1 mm) or much fewer slab-like (~1 cm) high-resolution slices that can be displayed individually or in a ciné mode. Note that additional acquisitions at a different focal distance are not required to enhance the visibility of objects *at any desired depth—* one set of acquired data can be reprocessed to generate the entire 3D volume set. It should always be kept in mind that "*there is no free meal in tomosynthesis—imaging parameters are a trade-off between z-axis accuracy, spatial resolution and importantly, radiation exposure to the breast.*"[16] In conclusion, digital breast tomosynthesis provides the following benefits relative to other modalities:

- Enhances conspicuity of abnormalities by minimizing the obscuring effects of overlying structures
- Permits cross-sectional imaging (i.e., planes of view) with high resolution
- A lower radiation dose as compared to CT mammography
- Lower cost as compared with CT and magnetic resonance imaging

SUMMARY

- Nonpalpable breast cancer may be detected through mammography.
- Flattening and reducing breast thickness prior to a standard mammographic radiation examination is necessary for producing a sharper image and reducing patient dose.
- Protocols founded upon compression pressure which takes into account breast surface area will be a more realistic guide to better and less uncomfortable mammograms.
- Two x-ray views of each breast (craniocaudal direction [CC] and mediolateral oblique direction [MLO]) are taken in a standard screening mammogram evaluation.
- The American College of Radiology, the American Cancer Society, and the American Medical Association advocate annual mammography screening or mammography screening at least every other year for women age 40 to 49.
- Federal regulations state that the mean dose to the glandular tissue (MGD) of a 4.5-cm compressed breast using a digital mammography system should not exceed 3 mGyt per view.
- Studies have shown that well-calibrated mammographic systems are capable of providing excellent imaging performance with an average glandular dose of not more than 2 mGyt.[22]
- Dose reduction in mammography can be achieved by limiting the number of anatomical projections taken.
- Axillary projections in mammography should only be done on request of the radiologist.
- Metallic elements such as molybdenum (Z = 42) and rhodium (Z = 45) are commonly employed as filters in mammography, enabling lower incident x-ray energy ranges that are more effective for breast imaging.
- Beryllium (Z = 4) takes the place of glass in the window of the low-kVp mammographic x-ray tube.
- Digital mammography units with image gray-level manipulation offer visualization improvement for patients with dense breasts.

- The method used for generating an in-focus two-dimensional image of a slice or cross-section through a three-dimensional object is called Tomography.
- Standard digital mammography can lead to both false positives and false negatives because the multiple tissues and structures of the compressed breast appear overlapped in the acquired projection image.
- Digital Breast Tomography (DBT) is an imaging technique, which generates multiple planar images acquired while the x-ray tube rotates within a limited arc above the patient's breast.
- The introduction of full field digital detector mammography (FFDM) was the primary technical breakthrough that enabled the wide-spread usage of DBT.
- Because in Digital Breast Tomography a third axis (z-direction) is stereoscopically extracted from the overall two-dimensional data, DBT is often referred to as "3D" mammography when mammographic images are reconstructed at arbitrary angles from the many different x-ray projections.
- Each DBT arc acquisition sequence may typically consist of from 15 to 25 separate x-ray projections. From the data generated by these, many nonblurred planar views can be obtained either individually or in a continuous sequence, thereby generating a "movie."
- The ability of DBT to decrease both false positives and false negatives as well as better image evaluation of dense breasts is due mainly to the enhanced z-axis resolution achievable by the tomographic method.
- The conventional method of image reconstruction used in digital tomosynthesis is the Shift and Add Algorithm (SAA).
- Artifacts present in DBT are primarily due to patient motion, the method of image acquisition, and imperfect z-axis or depth resolution.
- With DBT used alone, a compression force only great enough to securely retain the breast in a stable position during the procedure may suffice.
- For thicker breasts, a method of reducing patient dose while maintaining image quality is to employ additional filtering of the x-ray beam. This can be achieved by selecting in place of the standard molybdenum/molybdenum (Mo/Mo) or molybdenum/rhodium (MoRh) x-ray target/filter combinations, other pairings such as tungsten/rhodium (W/Rh), tungsten/aluminum (W/Al), or tungsten/silver (W/Ag).

GENERAL DISCUSSION QUESTIONS

1. What is the value of mammography for the detection of breast cancer?
2. What is the maximum dose to the glandular tissue of a 4.5-cm compressed breast using a digital system?
3. Why is the age recommendation for screening mammography controversial?
4. How can radiation dose in mammography be reduced?
5. What is the value of digital mammography for imaging patients with dense breasts?
6. What benefits do the two most common metallic elements used as filters in mammographic units provide?
7. Describe the process of digital breast tomosynthesis (DBT) and explain its advantages.
8. Discuss the concept of radiation dose associated with DBT.
9. What steps are involved in the DBT procedure?
10. What are the summarized properties of digital breast tomosynthesis (DBT)?

REVIEW QUESTIONS

1. What is the primary value of mammography in breast cancer detection?
   A. It reduces treatment costs.
   B. It provides early detection of tumors.
   C. It eliminates the need for biopsies.
   D. It is a noninvasive procedure.

2. What is the maximum dose to the glandular tissue of a 4.5-cm compressed breast using a digital system?
   A. 1 mGy
   B. 3 mGy
   C. 5 mGy
   D. 10 mGy

3. Why is the age recommendation for screening mammography considered controversial?
   A. There is no controversy.
   B. Different organizations have varying guidelines.
   C. It depends on breast size.
   D. It is based on patient preference.
4. Which of the following is a method to reduce radiation dose in mammography?
   A. Using thicker compression
   B. Increasing exposure time
   C. Employing digital mammography systems
   D. Decreasing breast compression
5. What advantage does digital mammography offer for patients with dense breasts?
   A. It requires less time.
   B. It provides clearer images.
   C. It eliminates the need for follow-up.
   D. It is less expensive.
6. What are the two common metallic elements used as filters in mammographic units?
   A. Aluminum and copper
   B. Molybdenum and rhodium
   C. Silver and gold
   D. Lead and iron

7. What does digital breast tomosynthesis (DBT) involve?
   A. Taking a single x-ray image
   B. Taking multiple x-ray images at different angles
   C. Using ultrasound to capture images
   D. Performing a biopsy
8. What is a key advantage of DBT compared to traditional 2D mammography?
   A. Higher radiation dose
   B. Improved detection of small cancers
   C. Longer examination time
   D. Lower image quality
9. How does DBT compare to conventional mammography in terms of radiation dose?
   A. DBT has a significantly lower dose.
   B. DBT has a similar dose.
   C. DBT has a higher dose on average.
   D. DBT has no radiation dose.
10. What is the first step in the DBT procedure?
   A. Analyzing the images
   B. Positioning the patient
   C. Taking a biopsy
   D. Compressing the breast

Radiation Safety in Nuclear Medicine

OBJECTIVES

After completing this chapter, the reader will be able to perform the following:

- Define all key terms.
- Explain how cancerous growths or tumors can either be eliminated or at least controlled by irradiation.
- Name some therapeutic isotopes, identify their properties, and describe how they are used.
- Explain the process of electron capture.
- Identify the two best radiation safety practices to follow for patients having therapeutic prostate seed implants.
- Explain the process of beta decay.
- Discuss the radiation hazards that may be encountered by personnel caring for a patient who is receiving iodine-131 therapy treatment for thyroid cancer.
- Explain how isotopes that are used as radioactive tracers in nuclear medicine work.
- Explain how the immune system may be used along with certain radioisotopes to treat cancer.
- Review dosimetry and radiation safety associated with radioimmunotherapy.
- Discuss how residual isotopes and radioactive materials may be properly disposed of.
- Identify the most common radioisotope used in nuclear medicine diagnostic studies.
- Explain the concept of diagnostic reference levels (DRLs) and their significance.
- Identify and describe the types of radiation events that are used in positron emission tomography (PET).
- Identify the most common isotope used for PET scanning.
- Explain the benefit of the combined imaging device called a PET-CT scanner.
- Describe radiation safety concerns associated with the design of a PET-CT imaging suite, and explain how radiation protection has been provided.
- Identify what factor the success of radioimmunotherapy depends upon.
- Explain how monoclonal antibodies are made.
- Identify organs of the human body that belong to the immune system.
- Discuss what theranostics is and how it works.
- Discuss the concept of radioimmunotherapy, its potential advantages over conventional radiation therapy, and identify groups of patients for whom this can be an important choice of treatment for certain types of cancer. Also identify professionals who are usually involved in radioimmunotherapy procedures.
- Discuss the reasons for concern over the use of radiation as a terrorist weapon, and identify what action most hospitals have taken for handling emergency situations involving radioactive contamination.
- Explain what a radioactive dispersal device, or "dirty bomb," is, and discuss the possible consequences of the detonation of such a device.
- Describe the procedure for external decontamination from radioactive materials.
- State the dose limit per event for individuals engaged in both nonlifesaving and lifesaving activities during a radiation emergency.
- State the reason why the Environmental Protection Agency (EPA) sets limits for radioactive contamination.
- Discuss the medical management of persons experiencing radiation bioeffects.
- Describe various strategies used to treat internal radiation contamination.

CHAPTER OUTLINE

KEY TERMS

annihilation radiation
beta decay
decontamination
diagnostic reference levels (DRLs)
electron capture
Environmental Protection
  Agency (EPA)
flourine-18 (^{18}F)
fluorodeoxyglucose (FDG)
Geiger-Müller (GM) detectors
half-value layer (HVL)

immune system
internal contamination
iodine-123 (^{123}I)
iodine-125 (^{125}I)
iodine-131 (^{131}I)
isotopes
monoclonal antibodies
neutrino
nuclear medicine
PET-CT scanner
positron

positron emission tomography
  (PET)
radiation therapy
radioactive contamination
radioactive dispersal device, or
  "dirty bomb"
radioimmunotherapy (RIT)
radioisotopes
surface contamination
technetium-99m (^{99m}Tc)
theranostics

Atoms that have the same number of protons within the nucleus but have different numbers of neutrons are called isotopes. Most elements in the periodic table (see Appendix C) have some associated isotopes, and quite a few of them have many. However, not all the nuclei of these isotopes represent stable groupings of protons and neutrons (i.e., the most secure bonding or the lowest energy configuration). A few have too many protons for stability, whereas others have too many neutrons, and some are just formed in higher energy states. Because of this, such isotopes spontaneously undergo processes or transformations either to rectify their unbalanced arrangement or to achieve a lower state of energy or both. All atoms whose nuclei behave in this manner are referred to as radioisotopes.

This chapter describes the application of some radioisotopes in both diagnostic and therapeutic medical procedures, including associated relevant radiation safety issues. The concept of diagnostic reference levels (DRLs) is introduced and some associated data presented. There is also an extended discussion of Radioimmunotherapy (RIT), which involves specialized radioisotope usage in conjunction with the action of the body's immune system. As an extra related and very current procedure, the concept of theranostics, which includes radioimmunotherapy, is introduced, explained, and its substantial importance for successful cancer therapy revealed and an example provided.

The chapter concludes with an examination of the role of radiation as a terrorist weapon, and some fundamental principles for dealing with radioactive contamination in a health care setting.

Common usage of English vs. metric units varies in different clinical settings. Therefore to assist the reader, both systems of units are used in this chapter.

MEDICAL USAGE

Radiation Therapy

As discussed in previous chapters, well-oxygenated, rapidly dividing cells are very sensitive to damage by radiation. This sensitivity is the foundation on which the branch of medicine commonly known as radiation therapy is based. Many cancerous growths or tumors can be either eliminated, or at least controlled, by sufficient irradiation of the area containing the growth. Radiation treatments are normally delivered externally using devices called accelerators that produce focused high-energy beams of x-rays or charged particles such as electrons and protons. However, for certain types of cancer, radiation can be delivered more effectively by infusion or by internal implantation of certain radioisotopes. These forms of therapeutic isotope procedures comprise a branch of radiation therapy known as brachytherapy. The isotopes used in brachytherapy are characterized by relatively long half-lives that are measured in terms of multiple days, months, or years and, except for a few of them, by relatively high-energy emissions. This radiation emanation may be in the form of gamma rays (photons emerging from the nucleus of an atom as contrasted to x-ray machine produced photons) and/or fast electrons (called beta radiation when coming from a nucleus). Several of the most important therapeutic radioisotopes are briefly described here.

Iodine-125. Iodine-125 ($^{125}I_{53}$) is an unstable and therefore radioactive isotope of the element iodine. It has been used quite extensively since 2000 in the form of titanium-encapsulated cylindrical seeds (4.5 mm long and in cross-section about the diameter of a paper clip [Fig. 16.1]) to give a tumoricidal radiation equivalent dose to cancers that are confined within the prostate gland. With the aid of computerized treatment planning and real-time ultrasound imaging, the seeds are permanently inserted into the gland in a calculated prescribed arrangement. The goal is to deliver 145 gray (Gy) to at least 90% of the prostate's volume while limiting radiation dose as much as possible to adjacent structures such as the urethra, bladder, and anterior rectal wall. The insertion process is done in the operating room and typically takes about 2 hours. This is a same-day procedure, and the patient is usually discharged within 4 to 5 hours afterward.

Iodine-125 has 53 protons and 72 neutrons in its nucleus and a half-life of 59.4 days. The nucleus decays physically by a process called **electron capture**, wherein an inner-shell electron interacts strongly with one of the nuclear protons, followed directly by the two combining to produce a neutron. There also occurs, as part of the process, the emission of energy in the form of a 27 keV characteristic x-ray generated because of the filling of the inner-electron shell vacancy by an outer low-energy electron. The nucleus now has one less proton, and thus the decay process has led to the formation of a different element called *tellurium-125* ($^{125}Te_{52}$). Tellurium-125 is produced in an unstable, excited energy state which immediately regains stability by its nucleus emitting the excess energy in the form of a 35 keV gamma ray. Both the 27 keV characteristic x-rays and the 35 keV gamma rays arising from the decay of the Iodine-125 nuclei deliver the radiation equivalent dose to the prostate gland. The decay process leading to the useful therapeutic radiation can be written as:

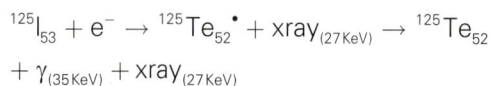

$$^{125}I_{53} + e^- \rightarrow {}^{125}Te_{52}^{\bullet} + xray_{(27 KeV)} \rightarrow {}^{125}Te_{52}$$
$$+ \gamma_{(35 KeV)} + xray_{(27 KeV)}$$

where the "•" indicates an excited state of the atom and the symbol "γ" signifies a gamma ray.

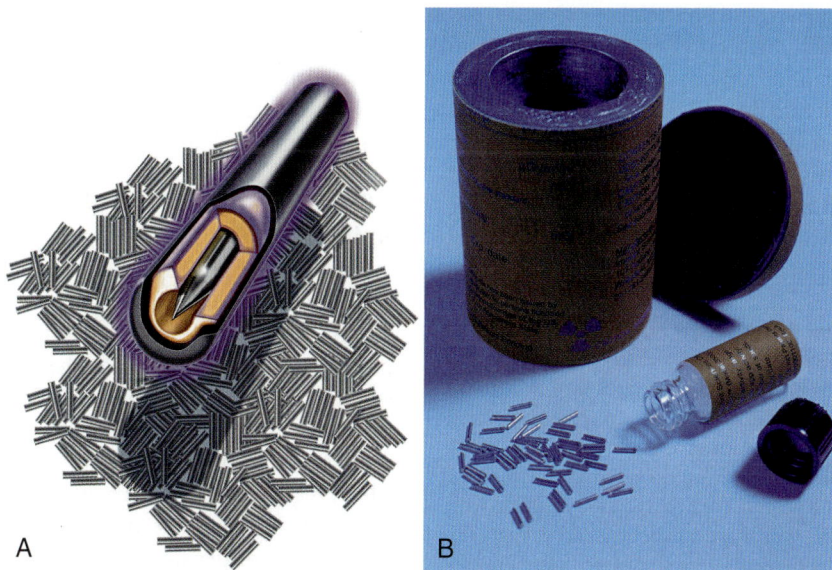

Fig. 16.1 (A) Iodine-125 (^{125}I) titanium–encapsulated cylindrical seed. (B) ^{125}I seeds before encapsulation. (From Implant Sciences Corporation.)

Because these radiation emissions have little penetrating power, a very high percentage of the radiation energy remains concentrated in the prostate gland. Essentially all of the remaining radiation is absorbed by the patient except for some small but detectable amount on the patient's physique, which emerges. At a distance of 1 meter, the *radiation exposure rate* for virtually all prostate seed implants is less than 0.5 milliroentgens per hour (mR/hr), increasing, however, to 15 to 20 mR/hr at the patient's lower abdominal surface. In terms of international or SI units, these values correspond to *equivalent dose rates* of approximately 5 microsieverts/hr (μSv/hr) at 1 meter and 150 to 200 μSv/hr at the abdominal surface.

The concepts of distance and time are the best radiation safety practices to be followed for these types of therapeutic implants. A typical safety recommendation is that patients with ^{125}I implants should significantly limit the durations of close contact (less than 30 cm or less than 1 foot) with small children and pregnant women for a period of 6 months (three half-lives) after the implant procedure. They may then resume completely normal behavior.

Iodine-131. **Iodine-131** ($^{131}_{53}$I) is another unstable isotope of the element iodine, but with 53 protons and 78 neutrons in its nucleus. It has a half-life of 8 days. As a consequence of its radioactive decay process (**beta decay***), it generates both electrons with an approximate mean energy of 192 keV and relatively high-energy assorted gamma rays (mean energy of 365 keV).

^{131}I can be joined chemically with sodium to form the chemical compound sodium iodide (NaI^{131}), which is radioactive and can be orally administered in the form of tablets. For a patient who has thyroid cancer, it is desirable to strongly irradiate any residual thyroid tissue not removed by surgery to destroy any remaining cancerous areas while significantly sparing surrounding tissue and other organs. Because the thyroid gland tends

---

*Beta decay is a process that normally occurs within a nucleus of certain unstable isotopes and is represented as: neutron -→ proton + electron + neutrino. A neutrino is a particle that has no electric charge and almost a negligibly small mass which in the beta decay process ensures conservation of energy by its kinetic energy carrying away any excess energy not accounted for by the electron and proton. For accuracy, the neutrino with the superscript symbol which appears in beta decay is actually an antineutrino, the anti-matter version of a neutrino. Further discussion of this distinction is not necessary in the scope of this text and so will not be mentioned again.

to highly absorb any iodine in the blood, administration of ^{131}I-labeled sodium iodide tablets is an efficient way of delivering a destructive radiation dose to the remainder of the thyroid. The relatively low energy electrons are the prime destructive agents.

Although the much more penetrating gamma rays deliver some radiation dose to more distant body sites, these rays primarily exit the body and present a radiation protection hazard to both nursing personnel and nuclear medicine technologists.

As discussed in earlier chapters, the concepts of time, distance, and shielding should be applied. If the patient is hospitalized (usually no more than 2 days), a large, up to 25 mm or 1 inch-thick, movable lead shield can be positioned between the patient and any attending personnel for protection. Such patients are also encouraged to drink lots of fluids so that as much ^{131}I, and therefore high-energy gamma radiation, can be removed from the body by urination in as short a time as possible.

The radioiodide tablets dissolve in the bloodstream, thus permitting an escape of some radioactivity through the pores of the skin, through urination, and in some special cases from vomiting. Thus, this poses another radiation safety hazard and a possible lengthy cleanup task. Consequently, hospital rooms for ^{131}I therapy patients are usually isolated, with restricted entry for general safety considerations and carefully prepared with well-placed absorbent cloths on top of nonporous flooring to facilitate a relatively easy cleanup of any radioactively contaminated surfaces. Only trained oncology nurses and nuclear medicine personnel should be allowed in the patient's room. Both groups should be wearing personnel dosimeters when they do so.

Proper Handling and Disposal of Radioactive Materials

The presence of partially used or unused radioisotopes and any items that they have contaminated necessitates that an institution follows appropriate procedures for their handling and disposal. Such procedures should be detailed within the fully documented radiation safety program of the institution and they must be in complete accord with the guidelines provided by state and federal regulations (e.g., Part 20 of Title 10 of the Code of Federal Regulations). All personnel involved in the handling and dispensing of radionuclides, as well as the removal of any remaining isotopes and any radioactively contaminated items, must wear gloves if the isotopes are in liquid form, be equipped with personnel dosimeters (whole body and extremity, the latter in the case of close handling), and follow the cardinal rules of radiation protection (time, distance, and shielding) where applicable. No solid encapsulated radioactive source is ever to be touched directly by hand. Instead, long tongs, which add distance as a safety measure, should be used.

Following a brachytherapy or a diagnostic radionuclide procedure, any residual isotope is to be returned to its shielded container. That container should then be labeled with how much activity remains and the current date. Also, any contaminated items as detected by a survey meter (e.g., gloves, clothing articles, absorbent pads, etc.) are to be placed in a sealed plastic bag that is labeled with the name of the radioisotope and the current date. After this is done, all involved personnel are to be checked with the survey meter to ensure that they have not been contaminated. Then the remaining isotope (if it is not to be returned to its supplier) and the packaged contaminated items are to be placed into a secure, shielded, and posted* storage area where they must be held for a period of 10 half-lives** before being suitable for disposal in ordinary trash. An exit survey, which should indicate background radiation levels, is to be conducted at that time. If any activity readings above background levels are found, the disposal must be delayed until the reading is at background levels. A record of the storage and disposal of the residual radionuclide and contaminated items must be kept for review by regulatory inspectors.

Nuclear Medicine

Nuclear Medicine is the branch of medicine that employs radioisotopes, also known as radionuclides, to study organ function in a patient, to detect the spread

---

*Posting should include a prominent display, at the entrance of the storage area, of the *Caution Radioactive Materials* sign, as well as emergency contact numbers for key personnel and regulatory agencies such as the state department of Environmental Protection and/or the Nuclear Regulatory Commission local office.

**For example, for an Iodine-125 brachytherapy case, any unused seeds would have to be held for a period of 10 half-lives = 10 × 59.4 days or 1.63 years before permissible disposal in ordinary trash, whereas for nuclear medicine procedures using radionuclides having very short half-lives such as, for example, 6 hours, the required storage time is only 60 hours or 2.5 days.

of cancer into bone, and to treat certain types of diseases. Diagnostic imaging techniques in nuclear medicine typically make use of short-lived radioisotopes as radioactive tracers. These radionuclides have been attached to biologically active substances or chemicals and form radioactive compounds that predominantly diffuse into certain regions or organs where it is medically desired to scrutinize particular physiologic processes.

Iodine-123. One of the most common examples of process monitoring makes use of **iodine-123** ($^{123}I_{53}$), yet another unstable isotope of the element iodine. ^{123}I undergoes radioactive decay by the process of *electron capture* (described in the section on iodine-125) and has an average half-life of 13.3 hours. When chemically coupled with sodium, it forms the radiotracer compound NaI^{123}. This compound, like the therapeutically used NaI^{131}, preferentially passes into the thyroid gland and achieves levels of concentration there that can be directly correlated with the thyroid gland's performance status. Thus, measurement of radioactivity in the region of the thyroid gland, which results from the relative *degree of uptake* by the thyroid of ^{123}I-labeled sodium iodide, makes it possible to determine the percentage of remaining functioning thyroid tissue.

Technetium-99m. By far the most common radioisotope used in nuclear medicine diagnostic studies (as much as 80% of all procedures) is **technetium-99m** (^{99m}Tc). This radionuclide is generated from the radioactive decay of another unstable isotope (molybdenum-99 [$^{99}Mo_{42}$]), which undergoes beta decay, during which (as discussed previously) an excess neutron transforms itself into a proton, with the emission of a fast electron from the nucleus. Having an additional proton within the nucleus means a change in atomic number and consequently a different element. The new element in this case is $^{99m}Tc_{43}$, with 43 protons and 56 neutrons. The beta decay of molybdenum produces technetium in a higher energy state than its ground state, and as a result it, too, is not stable. Most isotopes generated in this manner immediately shed their excess energy. However, some delay in doing so for a short period, and these relatively more enduring isotopes are given the designation *m*, which stands for *metastable* (meaning "more lasting"). ^{99m}Tc has a half-life of 6 hours and becomes stable by emission from its nucleus of a gamma ray photon (γ) with energy of 140 keV. The details of the overall decay process are:

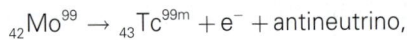

$$_{42}Mo^{99} \rightarrow {}_{43}Tc^{99m} + e^- + antineutrino,$$

followed by: $_{43}Tc^{99m} \rightarrow {}_{43}Tc^{99} + \gamma \, (140 \, keV)(T^{1/2} = 6 \, hr)$

^{99m}Tc is an extremely versatile radioisotope because it can be chemically incorporated into a wide variety of different compounds or biologically active substances, each with a specificity for different tissues or organs of the body. For example, in combination with a tin compound, technetium binds to red blood cells and the emitted radiation distribution is useful for mapping circulatory system disorders; in combination with a sulfur compound, it is absorbed by the spleen, thus making it possible to image the structure of the spleen; in another chemical combination, ^{99m}Tc concentrates in bone and permits evaluation of potential cancer spread to bony areas; it is also very commonly used along with treadmill stress testing to evaluate heart function. All these studies are possible because either a deficiency of radioisotope uptake (i.e., a cold spot in radioactivity) or an excessive uptake of radioisotope-labeled compound (i.e., hot spots of radioactivity) signals abnormal organ behavior. Because of such capabilities, nuclear medicine offers to a physician diagnostic input relating to *function* that goes substantially beyond the information provided by ordinary x-ray techniques.

Positron Emission Tomography

In Chapter 3, in which the pair production interaction is discussed, a diagnostic modality called **positron emission tomography (PET)** is also mentioned. Although this modality does not require the occurrence of *x-ray induced* pair production interactions, it does make use of **annihilation radiation** events. In the case of PET, the annihilation radiation is initiated by the radioactive decay of the nucleus of an unstable isotope. The instability in this case is associated with too many protons residing within the nucleus. Nuclei such as these usually spontaneously undergo a reaction in which the excess proton is transmuted into a neutron and a positively charged electron (**positron**). This conserves electric charge because the neutron has none. To conserve energy as well, the process, as in beta decay, includes the emission of a **neutrino**. As mentioned previously,

neutrinos have no electric charge and almost negligible mass, but their energy of motion (kinetic energy) balances the energy of the reaction. Neutrinos very rarely interact with anything and are therefore exceptionally difficult to detect.*

A positron, classified as antimatter, when passing close, and slowly, to an electron—normal matter—will interact destructively with the electron. In the process, both particles will disappear, having *annihilated* one another. Their respective masses are converted into energy that will be carried off by two photons emerging from the annihilation site in opposite directions (to conserve linear momentum) each with a kinetic energy of 511 keV. These energies correspond to the rest mass energies of the former positron and electron.

Imaging. If there is a volume (e.g., a human torso) in which many of these annihilation events are taking place, and if this volume is surrounded by a ring of densely packed detectors that are specifically tuned to 511 keV photon energies, then it is possible, in a manner analogous to that used in computed tomography (CT), to reconstruct useful (but not of CT quality) images of the regions within the encompassed volume from which the annihilation photons are coming. Such images, often called *hot spots*, can reveal the performance status of a physical process. This is the basic concept of, and rationale for, PET scanning.

Fluorine-18. By far the most important isotope in PET scanning is the radioisotope positron emitter **Fluorine-18**, which symbolically can be depicted as $^{18}F_9$. Thus, nine protons and nine neutrons are present in its nucleus. Nine neutrons, however, are not enough to maintain a stable arrangement along with 9 protons within this nucleus. The unstable nucleus will

---

*Elaborate facilities, located in multiple countries in deep underground caverns typically in abandoned salt mines, are used to detect neutrino fluxes. Within each such cavern are placed huge deep pools of water that are densely filled with rows of specialized scintillation detectors. These detector locations ensure that cosmic rays do not contribute to detection events. With these underground facilities, very large neutrino fluxes such as caused by and predicted for various significant astronomical events involving stars have led to unambiguous neutrino detection.

consequently undergo a change in which one less proton is present. This process, known as positron decay, can be simply detailed as:

$$p \rightarrow n + e^+ + \nu$$

where the Greek character "ν" (pronounced as nu) is the symbol for a neutrino. The positron will subsequently come into contact with an ordinary electron, resulting in an annihilation reaction leading to the production of two high-energy photons of 511 keV each.

The process as a whole can be summarized as:

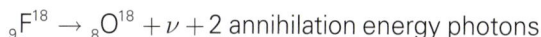

$$_9F^{18} \rightarrow \ _8O^{18} + \nu + 2 \text{ annihilation energy photons}$$

where $_8O^{18}$ is a stable isotope of oxygen with 8 protons and 10 neutrons.

Positron emission tomography is a very important imaging modality because it can be used to examine *metabolic processes within the body*. It can do so because the atoms that produce positrons can bind with molecules such as glucose, which is a primary component of metabolic reactions. The ability to detect changes in metabolism is particularly relevant to the detection of cancer cells. Such cells seek to reproduce without end and to do so requires a great deal of sugar, or glucose, to supply the energy for this unlimited growth. Therefore a radioactive molecule that is very similar to a glucose molecule, can be used to detect the presence of sites of excessive glucose metabolism that may be associated with cancer cell proliferation.

The great significance of the isotope ^{18}F is that it can be chemically attached to a glucose molecule, yielding a compound called **fluorodeoxyglucose (FDG)**. FDG has the chemical compound description: $C_6H_{11}F^{18}O_5$. FDG is a *radioactive tracer* that is very similar in chemical behavior to ordinary glucose, and so it is readily taken up or metabolized by cancerous cells and undergoes positron emission decay with subsequent generation of oppositely traveling annihilation photons. The presence of disproportional glucose metabolism regions can thereby be discerned by detecting areas of abnormally high radioactivity. These annihilation event sites are physically localizable through the PET scanner's patient-surrounding ring of coincidence detectors.

If a PET scanner is mechanically joined in a tandem configuration (e.g., like a two-person bicycle) with a

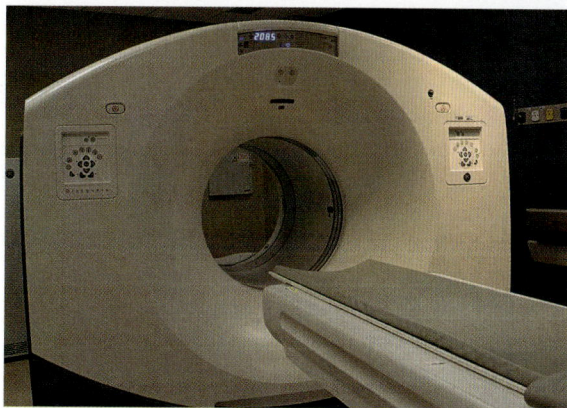

Fig. 16.2 Combined positron emission tomography/computed tomography (PET/CT) system. (From Rollins JH, Long BW, Curtis T: *Merrill's atlas of radiographic positioning and procedures*, ed 15, St. Louis, 2023, Elsevier.)

CT scanner to produce a single joint imaging device, then in essence a facility gains not only the ability to detect the presence of abnormally high regions of glucose metabolism, yielding evidence of cancer spread (metastasis) into other body areas, but also the means to obtain detailed information about the anatomic location and extent of these lesions or growths. Such a combined imaging device is called a **PET-CT scanner** (Fig. 16.2). The radiation safety aspects required of a PET-CT facility will be discussed later on in the chapter.

Diagnostic Reference Levels (DRL)

The concept of *diagnostic reference level* was initially introduced in the International Commission on Radiation Protection (ICRP) Publication #73 (Feb. 2014).[1] Numerically, a diagnostic reference level in Nuclear Medicine is the amount of activity in megabecquerels* (MBq) (or traditionally in millicuries [mCi]) of a

---

*The **becquerel** (symbol: **Bq**) is the SI unit of radioactivity and is defined as one nuclear disintegration per second. It officially replaced the curie (Ci), the unit in the superseded CGS system, in 1975. MBq is an abbreviation for megabecquerels (millions of Bq). 1MBq is a standard unit of radioactivity in Nuclear Medicine that numerically corresponds to 1 million nuclear disintegrations per second (dps). Since 1 curie (Ci) is equivalent to $3.7(10)^{10}$ dps, then 37 MBq is equivalent to an activity of 1 mCi.

particular radionuclide compound of the radioactive material that is administered (through injection or by swallowing) to the patient.

DRLs are essentially a tool which is related to the expected radiation dose received by an average-sized patient undergoing a given ionizing radiation imaging examination. As such, DRL values can aid in the enhancement of protection in the medical exposure of patients for radiation employed diagnostic and interventional processes. In ICRP Publication #135 (2017),[2] existing guidelines and clinical applications of DRLs and appropriate intervals for their updates are detailed.

Diagnostic Reference Levels are not used in all nuclear medicine departments, but have been recommended by advisory groups such as the National and International Councils on Radiation Protection and Measurements because of their implications for assurance of an appropriate balance of benefit and risk in nuclear medicine procedures.

By virtue of a large and possibly international database, the concept of the diagnostic reference level is used in medical imaging that employs ionizing radiation to indicate whether, in routine conditions, the patient administered radioactivity from a specified procedure is unusually high or low for that procedure. It follows naturally that the approach used most frequently in discussions among physicists, radiologists, and radiographers on how to accomplish optimization of radiation protection to both patient and technical personnel is to achieve compliance with the mean DRL value for the particular examination. However, it should be understood that DRL quantities are not pure descriptors of image quality. Median values of DRL quantities at a health center that are above or below a particular value do not necessarily indicate that images are adequate or inadequate for a particular clinical purpose. In general, it can be said that diagnostic reference levels are a required safety-inspired radiation dosage optimization tool for medical imaging procedures whose values *detail* a safety restriction on the amount of radioactivity received by an average-sized patient undergoing a given imaging procedure that will still yield diagnostically useful imaging.[3]

Nuclear Medicine Procedure DRLs

In ICRP Publication 135, existing guidelines and clinical applications of DRLs and appropriate intervals for their updates are specified. These are listed below.

- Quantities used for DRLs should assess the amount of ionizing radiation applied to perform a medical imaging task.
- DRL quantities should be easily measured or determined.
- DRL quantities, in general, gauge the amount of ionizing radiation useful for a medical imaging procedure and not the absorbed dose to a patient or organ (one exception is mammography, for which the mean glandular dose concept may be used).
- DRL quantities should be appropriate to the imaging modality being evaluated, to the specific study being performed, and to the specific size of the patient.
- The ICRP stresses that the radiation protection quantity "effective dose" *should not be used as a DRL quantity*. It introduces extraneous factors that are neither necessary nor pertinent for the purpose of a DRL.
- Setting a fixed maximum administered activity for very obese patients may also be considered. It is recognized that, in many countries, a standard activity is used in clinical practice for adult patients.

According to the ICRP, radiation metrics used for diagnostic reference levels should be directly related to the imaging modality being evaluated, should in general not exceed the quantity of ionizing radiation sufficient to satisfactorily perform a medical imaging task, and should be easily measured or determined. When two different imaging modalities are used for the same procedure (e.g., PET/CT), it is appropriate and required to set and present DRLs for both modalities independently. The numerical value of any DRL should be founded upon well-defined clinical and technical requirements for the selected medical imaging task. However, administered activities correlated with a patient's body weight is not recommended for examinations where the radiopharmaceutical is concentrated predominantly in a single organ (e.g., thyroid scans, lung perfusion scans). The ICRP further acknowledges that the administered activity for examinations of individual patients may be adjusted upwards only when there are sound clinical reasons for this increase.[2]

A Table of DRL Values

Table 16.1, established from a 2024 survey,[3] is a partial listing of DRL values for some very common Nuclear Medicine imaging procedures. Each column shows the mean DRL value in MBq for a particular regional

TABLE 16.1 Diagnostic Reference Levels for Common Nuclear Medicine Studies

Radiopharmaceuticals (procedures)	NCRP Recommended DRLs (MBq)
^{18}F-FDG (tumor)	461–710
[99m]Tc-diphosphonate (bone)	848–1185
^{99m}Tc-MIBI or TF (MPI, stress)	Tc: 945–1402 TF:1007–1459
^{99m}Tc-RBC (gated cardiac blood pool, planar)	916–1301
^{99m}Tc-MAG3 (renal dynamic)	283–379

NCRP, National Council on Radiation Protection and Measurements

Brink JA, Boone JM, Feinstein KA, et al.: NCRP Report No. 172—reference levels and achievable doses in medical and dental imaging: recommendations for the United States. https://ncrponline.org/shop/reports/report-no-172-reference-levels-and-achievable-doses-in-medical-and-dental-imaging-recommendations-for-the-united-states-2012. Accessed 15 April 2024.

sample of facilities. This table is not a final established table for all facilities but rather an averaged sampling of a number of facilities in multiple geographical regions.

DRL Summary

It is possible to assess the risk of carcinogenesis in groups of patients, considering absorbed doses in organs, general cancer incidence, and mortality rates. A calculational method that allows the establishment of DRL values and the associated risk of cancer induced by administered radioactive compounds through the estimation of associated absorbed doses in specific organs and based on the risk methodology of BEIR VII[4] is precisely what is needed. Such resulting absorbed doses were estimated based on the dose conversion factors of the radiopharmaceuticals used commonly in Nuclear Medicine procedures. This was published by the International Commission on Radiological Protection adjusted for multiple patient groups over multiple geographical regions. It was based on data from 2256 patients who underwent diagnostic procedures at the National Cancer Institute between 2017 and 2019. The program considered patient-specific data such as age, sex, and body mass index (BMI). The methodology developed in this work allows regional Nuclear Medicine services to keep their data available and updated regarding local DRLs, in addition to allowing the nuclear physician to know the risk of each procedure performed, extracted by

individual characteristics of the patient. A risk versus benefit analysis must always be present and this is fundamentally the basis upon which recommended diagnostic reference levels are founded.

Radiation Protection and the PET-CT Scanner

Positron emitters result in the production of high-energy radiation. Each ^{18}F nuclear transformation by positron decay yields two highly penetrating 511 keV photons. These cannot be shielded by an ordinary lead apron. Because the thickness of lead needed to attenuate such high-energy radiation by 50% (i.e., its **half-value layer [HVL]**) is approximately 0.5 cm (0.2 in.), adequate shielding at close distances could require up to 2.5 cm or an inch of lead. Therefore the design of a PET-CT imaging suite is complex, involving significant radiation safety concerns. A detailed discussion of the radiation safety design difficulties concerning the PET-CT technologist for an occupationally permissible facility follows. It is based on material presented at the 2004 American College of Medical Physics Annual Meeting in Scottsdale, Arizona by Melissa C. Martin, MS, FACR in a workshop entitled: *PET-CT Site Planning and Shielding Design*.

Unlike the usual diagnostic imaging suites in which the designer concentrates on protection from the radiation produced by ordinary radiographic and fluoroscopic units, the design of a PET-CT imaging suite presents unique additional radiation safety challenges. For a PET-CT facility, the scatter radiation generated by the CT scanner portion is only a secondary difficulty for the shielding designer. Of much more importance is the high-energy annihilation photons emanating in all directions from the patient while having the PET-CT scan. Furthermore, the presence of yet a third source of radiation, also of high energy, must be considered. Every patient who is to have a PET-CT scan requires what is called a "prep" time. During this time ^{18}F, in the form of FDG with an initial activity usually of approximately 15 mCi* (555 megabecquerels** [MBq]) is injected into the patient. The patient typically remains in the injection or prep

---

*1 curie $\equiv 3.7 (10)^{10}$ disintegrations (decays) per second (dps). Therefore 1 mCi = $3(10)^7$ dps.

**Since a becquerel (Bq) is defined as 1 disintegration per second, 1 mCi = 3.7 $(10)7$ Bq and 15 mCi = $15 \times 3.7 (10)7$ Bq = 55.5 $(10)7$ Bq = $555(10)6$ Bq = 555 Mbq.

room in a semi-reclining position for 45 to 60 minutes so that the FDG gets distributed throughout the body. This implies that to have a smooth-flowing, coordinated patient through-put, it will be necessary that while one "hot" patient is being scanned, a second "hot" patient is reclining in a nearby room waiting to be scanned. Therefore during this procedure the technologist and other personnel, as well as the general public, must be protected from at least two sources of high-energy photon radiation in addition to the scatter x-radiation from the CT scanner. Also, the change of activity during the prep and scan times due to the short half-life of most PET isotopes should be taken into account.

All of this makes the calculations for a practical space-limited shielding design anything but trivial. These problems are greatly simplified, however, when a facility can be designed from the beginning instead of being retrofitted into limited existing space. Unfortunately, most often the latter is the case. Earlier it was stated that it takes a considerable amount of lead to attenuate photons with 511 keV energy. Thus, unless other mitigating factors can be applied, the amount of lead shielding needed to ensure acceptable radiation safety could become unreasonable. However, mitigating factors for lessening the needed shielding do exist. They involve employing the concepts of weekly workload (W), occupancy factor (T), the decrease in activity of the ^{18}F during the prep and scan times, self-attenuation by the patient, and, significantly, the distance to each area of occupancy which strongly brings into play the inverse square law.

For simplification, just the requirements for the satisfactory radiation protection of the PET-CT radiographer in a new PET-CT suite will now be considered in detail. A workload for a busy facility with one scanner could be 7 PET-CT patients per daily shift, which amounts to 35 patients per work week, with each patient receiving at the start of prep time an activity of 15 mCi of ^{18}F doped FDG. The larger a weekly workload is, the greater the shielding that will be needed to stay within permissible equivalent dose levels to personnel and the public. ^{18}F has a short physical half-life of 110 minutes; therefore by natural decay alone, the patient's degree of radioactivity will diminish throughout the prep time, losing approximately 25% to 30% by the time of scanning. This process will continue during the 45 to 50-minute scan time, with the remaining amount of ^{18}F having decreased through physical decay alone to approximately 50% of its initial activity

by the conclusion of the scan. The patient's radioactivity is further lessened by any voiding that may take place just before the scanning procedure. The two processes taken together constitute what is known as the *effective half-life* (T_{eff}), which can be much less than the physical half-life of 110 minutes. As a result, the patient's remaining or residual radioactivity will typically be about one-fourth of its initial value after the scan is completed. This is important for the radiation safety of the general public and any family members at the patient's home. Such patients at discharge produce a measured midline *surface* radiation exposure rate of 40 to 50 mR/hr, which corresponds to about 0.4 to 0.5 millisieverts per hour (mSv/hr) equivalent dose rate. At a distance of 30 cm (approximately 1 foot), this decreases to approximately 15 mR/hr exposure rate or 0.15 mSv/hr equivalent dose rate. Usually, it is recommended that PET-CT patients maintain a one-meter separation from others as much as possible for the remainder of the day. After returning home, the patient is encouraged to drink plenty of fluids so that with frequent urination and little permanent tissue retention, the residual ^{18}F radioactivity will be almost negligible 1 day later. After this time, the patient may resume normal contact with all.

A well-designed facility should be arranged so that no areas of full occupancy are immediately adjacent to a high-energy radiation source; the prep room and scanning location of the patient are the most important areas from which to have ample separation. A secondary but less significant site is the patient's toilet, which could accidentally acquire some contamination.

To determine the equivalent dose rate (specified in µSv/hr at a particular distance from a person injected with a specific amount of ^{18}F), the shielding planner must make use of a "measured" quantity called the *dose rate constant*. Its measured value is 6.96 µSv/hr at a distance of 1 meter per millicurie (mCi) of ^{18}F. Thus, if the patient did not self-attenuate any of the ^{18}F radiation, then just after a 15 mCi injection, the equivalent dose rate 1 meter away would be approximately $7 \times 15 = 105$ µSv/hr. At greater distances, the inverse square law can be applied to obtain a value. For example, at a separation of 4 meters (approximately 13 feet), the initial high-energy photons' equivalent dose rate in the absence of any shielding or attenuation reduces to:

$$105/4^2 = 6.6 \, \mu Sv/hr \, (0.66 \, mrem/hr)$$

Distance is thus seen to be a very powerful tool of radiation protection. A well-designed facility takes especial advantage of this. Returning to the injected patient, there are other facilitators of radiation protection at hand. Both the patient and nature are responsible for this. It has been found from multiple measurements that the body can absorb a substantial amount of ^{18}F annihilation radiation.

Thus the mean maximum equivalent dose rate at 1 m from the patient per mCi (37 MBq) injected just after the injection is *not* 6.96 μSv/hr, as it would be for an unshielded point source of radiation; rather, it has been determined to be approximately 3 μSv/hr per mCi due to average *patient self-attenuation*.[5] At a distance of 4 m from the patient just after a 15 mCi injection, the equivalent dose rate is now given from the inverse square law by:

$$(15 \times 3)/4^2 = 2.8\,\mu\text{Sv/hr}$$

Nature's contribution to the radiation protection effort is that ^{18}F has a short half-life.

Therefore the 15 mCi dose injected at 2:00 p.m. will, because of natural radiation decay, be approximately 69%* as strong 60 minutes later for a 3:00 p.m. scan starting time. In actuality, the equivalent dose delivered by the "hot" patient while waiting during the prep time at a distance of 4 m is less than 2.8 μSv because of the continuing decrease of the Fluorine-18 activity. If not 2.8 μSv, then what dose equivalent would a person at this 4-meter distance *on average* receive in 60 minutes? It must be some percentage that lies between 100% and 69% of 2.8. Using the mathematics of radioactive decay** yields a mean value of approximately 83%, or a correction factor of 0.83. Consequently, the equivalent dose at a distance of 4 m that could be received by a technologist who is continuously present at this 4-meter location (i.e., occupancy level T = 1) from a 1-hour prep patient in the absence of any added shielding is:

$$0.83 \times 2.8 = 2.3\,\mu\text{Sv}$$

Over the course of a week, assuming a total of 35 patients, then, with all other conditions remaining the same, this technologist will accumulate from prep patients an equivalent dose of:

$$35 \times 2.3 = 81\,\mu\text{Sv}\,(8.1\,\text{millirem})$$

Over 50 weeks, this would add up to about 4000 μSv (400 mrem) from prep patients alone. However, prep patients are not the only sources of high-energy radiation dose to PET-CT personnel. There is also the scan patient and, to a much lesser extent, the patient's toilet and the hot lab. The contributions of all sources of radiation dose need to be factored into the facility's design and shielding plan.

Consider the scan patient in some detail. As always, it is desirable to have a good distance, if at all possible, between personnel and the radiation source. That is usually not feasible, especially if the PET-CT suite is being fit into a preexisting area. So, considering the scanned patient first, let it be assumed that there is a separation of only 3.3 m from the scan patient's midline to the location of the PET-CT technologist. In the absence of additional shielding, what could be the equivalent dose rate from this patient? The first factor to be aware of is the lesser activity remaining in the patient due to physical decay, namely, about 69% of the original 15 mCi. However, this is not the whole story. The prep patient is encouraged to void just before being scanned. What this means is that the residual ^{18}F in the patient's body at the start of the scan is less than 69% of the original activity. If it is assumed that approximately 20% more was removed by voiding, then at the start of the scan, the activity within the patient is roughly just 50% of the original activity, namely: $0.5 \times 15 = 7.5$ mCi. If there were no other considerations*, then *at the start of the scan* the equivalent dose rate at the location of the technologist with no shielding would be:

$$(7.5\,\text{mCi} \times 3\,\tfrac{\mu\text{Sv}}{\text{hr}}\text{ per mCi})/(3.3)^2 = 2\,\mu\text{Sv/hr}$$
$$(0.2\,\text{mrem/hr})$$

However, the radioactivity within the patient continues to decay all throughout the approximate 1 hour between voiding and his or her departure. Therefore

---

*Radioactive decay factor after a full 60 minutes is obtained from: correction factor = $e^{-[0.693 \times 60/110]} = 0.69$.

**Mean decay correction factor *over a period of 60 minutes* = $[1.443 \times (110/60) \times (1 - 0.69)] \approx 0.83$ where 1.443 is the average lifetime of the Fluorine-18 nucleus in a radioactive sample.

---

*In this situation, any degree of shielding provided by the scanner itself is being neglected.

the mean equivalent dose to the technologist from the scanned patient during this additional hour of isotope decay, as determined before, will actually be $0.83 \times 2 \ \mu Sv/hr = 1.7 \ \mu Sv$. Over the course of a week, this approximately amounts to: 35 patients $\times$ 1.7 = 60 μSv. At 50 weeks, this totals 3000 μSv (300 mrem). Then, the *unshielded technologist* could receive an annual equivalent dose of 4000 + 3000 = 7000 μSv (700 mrem) in this facility from the prep and scan FDG patients. Shielding can be installed to decrease this amount significantly. As an exercise, determining how much shielding would need to be installed to reduce this technologist equivalent dose of 7000 μSv to a total of 1300 μSv (130 mrem) per year or about 110 μsv/month (11 mrem/mo) will be discussed. The value used in this example is far below the occupational annual MPD of 0.05 Sv (5 rem). Fig. 16.3 depicts a facility layout schematic that will be referred to for shielding calculations. For simplicity, the calculations will not be for the entire suite but will be limited to what is required for protection of the PET-CT radiographer. In addition, the task will be further confined to just the contributions from the patient occupying the prep room and the patient being scanned. The hot lab and the patient's toilet will have to have their own substantial shielding installed to protect other regular facility occupants and the general public.

Beginning with the *scanned patient*, let it be required that both the technologist viewing window and the surrounding wall be shielded so that the 3000 μSv (300 mrem) high-energy annual equivalent dose contribution from scan patients decreases one-fourth of its unshielded value, namely to 750 μSv (75 mrem). As mentioned earlier, the amount of lead needed to decrease the intensity of this high-energy radiation by 50% (HVL) is equal to 0.5 cm (approximately 0.2 inch) of lead. One HVL will bring the equivalent dose down to 1500 μSv (150 mrem), and 2 HVLs will cut it to 750 μSv (75 mrem). The two HVLs amount to installing: $2 \times (0.5 \ cm)$ of lead = 1.0 cm ($\approx$ 0.4 inches) of lead. This must be placed in the wall surrounding the view window, and the view window itself must be composed of the equivalent amount of lead acrylic. This thickness of lead is far more than would be required to shield the

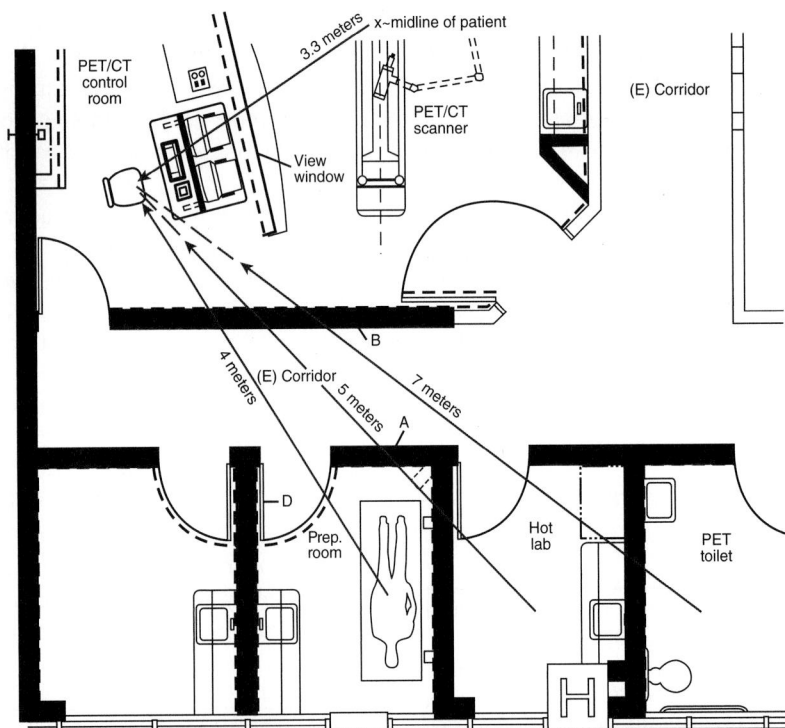

Fig. 16.3 Layout diagram of a positron emission tomography/computed tomography (PET/CT) imaging facility.

operator from the much less penetrating CT scatter radiation (typically about 1/16" Pb). Therefore the CT scatter radiation does not have to be additionally accounted for. For the patient in the prep room, the goal is to interpose enough shielding so that the 4000 µSv (400 mrem) annual equivalent dose contribution to the technologist location decreases to 500 µSv (50 mrem); this decrease by a factor of 8 requires 3 HVLs, or 1.5 cm (0.59 inches) of lead. Examining the diagram, it is seen that this amount of shielding can be distributed between the prep room corridor wall and door (labeled *A* and *D*, respectively) and the scan suite corridor wall (labeled *B*). Excluding personnel other than the operator and discounting any other circumstances, a practical solution is to place 1/2" of lead in A and D and add 1/8" of lead in the portion of B necessary to shield the technologist. This amounts to installing: 0.5" + 0.13" = 0.63"which is close enough to the calculated 0.59" Pb.

In conclusion, it is clear that there is much to be considered when radiation shielding is designed for a PET-CT facility. Other areas that are frequented by personnel and/or the general public must also be protected from the high-energy radiation. Their protection involves lower permissible equivalent dose limits than for the occupationally exposed radiographer. If there is the opportunity to construct the facility from the beginning, then with an intelligent design the required shielding can be greatly reduced; if not, then the calculations and the amount and variations of needed shielding can be sizable.

THERANOSTICS AND RADIOIMMUNOTHERAPY

Theranostics is a general term for the combined use of therapy by radiation and information localization by diagnostic imaging. An explanatory schematic is shown in Fig. 16.4.

The general principle of theranostics is that low-dose imaging is used to reveal information that indicates whether cancer cells will be or have been successfully treated when high-dose, targeted radiation therapy has been delivered. The imaging part of theranostics is carried out with PET or SPECT (single photon emission computed tomography) systems to reveal the distribution of specialized radionuclides in tissues at a molecular level or with MRI (magnetic resonance imaging) to reveal tissue properties, such as adequate blood

THERANOSTICS

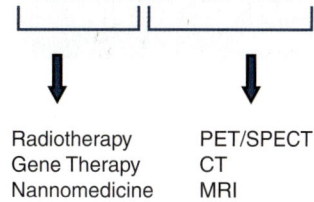

Radiotherapy	PET/SPECT
Gene Therapy	CT
Nannomedicine	MRI

Fig. 16.4 Composite meaning of theranostics.

perfusion,* that indicate a potential for successful radiation dose treatments. The therapy part of theranostics may involve cutting-edge directed treatments such as gene therapy to alter the function of cells or the use of nanoparticles to release therapeutic doses of cancer-killing materials.[6] In the material that follows we will examine the therapeutic technique that is used most frequently at present. It is called *Radioimmunotherapy*.

Radioimmunotherapy (RIT)

Radioimmunotherapy makes use of the capabilities of a patient's own immune system to attack cancer cells. This is a particularly powerful method of delivering radiation to cancer cells that are difficult to treat by external radiation therapy, such as those located in poorly oxygenated regions of tumors or in dispersed locations, as in leukemia and lymphoma. In formal terms, Radioimmunotherapy (RIT) is a specific treatment protocol for cancer by cytotoxic (cell-killing) radioisotopes conjugated (i.e., joined together or coupled) to specially designed immune system antibodies. This process will be explained in detail in the sections that follow.

The Immune System

Brief explanations of some of the major organic entities involved in the operations and reactions of the body's immune system are presented in Box 16.1.

This body complex is essentially an alliance between cells and proteins that work together to provide defenses against infection. The immune system is not a

---

*Blood perfusion is the local fluid flow through the capillary network and extracellular spaces of living tissues. It is characterized as the volumetric flow rate per volume of tissue. Blood perfusion is vital for normal tissue physiology and is responsible for the transport of oxygen, nutrients, and waste products.

> **BOX 16.1   Organic Entities Involved in the Operations and Reactions of the Body's Immune System**
>
> **Antigens** are protein molecules that are not recognized by the body and therefore seen as foreign by the immune system, thereby stimulating the system's production of antibodies or immune cells.
>
> **Antibodies (Ab)** are molecules produced by B-lymphocytes (white blood cells originating in bone marrow) that circulate in the blood and will chemically bind with and can interact destructively with antigens. These are among the key agents of the body's immune system.
>
> A **conjugate** refers to a compound formed by the joining of two or more *chemical* compounds.
>
> A **conjugated antibody** (also known as a tagged, loaded or labeled antibody) is one which has been attached to a substrate (the surface or material on or from which an organism lives, grows, or obtains its nourishment) such as an enzyme, toxin or inorganic compound.
>
> **Monoclonal antibodies (**mAb or moAb) are antibodies that are made by identical immune cells that are all clones of a unique parent cell. Thus, *monoclonal antibodies* are cells derived by cell division from a single ancestral cell.
>
> **Pathogens** are a bacterium, virus, or other microorganism that can cause disease. A pathogen may also be referred to as an infectious agent, or simply a germ.

broad categories of immune responses: those originating with *the innate immune* system and those associated with the *adaptive immune* system.

Innate immune responses rely on cells that require no additional modifications to do their jobs. These cells include *neutrophils*, natural killer (NK) cells, and a set of proteins termed the complement proteins. Innate responses to infection occur rapidly and reliably. Even infants have exceptional inherent immune responses.

Adaptive immune responses, however, involve T-cells and B-cells, cell types that do require an "educational" modification to prevent them from attacking harmless cells. The advantages of the adaptive responses are their long-lived memory and the ability to adjust to *new germs*. Central to both categories of immune responses is the ability to distinguish foreign invaders (things that need to be attacked) from the body's own tissues, which of course need to be protected. Because of their ability to respond rapidly, the innate responses are usually the first to react to an "invasion." This initial response serves to alert and trigger the adaptive response, which can take several days to fully activate.[7,8]

Monoclonal Antibodies

Monoclonal antibodies (MABs) are antibodies that have *monovalent affinity* which means, simply, that they preferentially bind always to a specific part of an antigen that is recognized by the antibody. To be more specific, MAB works by identifying and locating specific proteins on cells. Each MAB is attracted to one particular protein of the many that are on the cell and each MAB works in different ways depending on the foreign appearing protein (antigen) they are targeting (Fig. 16.5 and 16.6).

Specifics of Radioimmunotherapy

Radioimmunotherapy (RIT) is a combination of radiation therapy and immunotherapy. In basic (i.e., non RIT) immunotherapy, a *laboratory-produced* specialized antibody is "engineered" to recognize and bind to the surface of cancer cells. These specialized antibodies mimic the antibodies naturally produced by the body's immune system that attack invading foreign substances, such as bacteria and viruses.

Radioimmunotherapy goes a step further and uses such a *specialized antibody* that is also labeled or chemically combined with a radionuclide to deliver cytotoxic

single organ but rather is a collection of organs dispersed throughout the body whose purpose is to provide rapid responses to foreign agents. It includes organs such as the liver, thymus gland, bone marrow, lymph nodes, spleen, and even the tonsils. The bone marrow and thymus gland are important source locations for two key cells of the immune system called B-cells and T-cells, respectively. Box 16.2 contains a listing and description of the various cell types that comprise the immune system. The development of all cells of the immune system begins in the bone marrow with a blood-forming "stem" cell. The name stem cell is appropriate since all of the other specialized cells arise from it. Because of its ability to generate an entire immune system, this blood-forming cell is the cell that is most important in a bone marrow or hematopoietic (i.e., blood-forming tissues) cell transplant.

Although all components of the immune system interact with each other, it is typical to consider two

BOX 16.2 Cells of the Immune System

Bone marrow: The site in the body where most of the cells of the immune system are produced as immature or stem cells.

Stem cells: These cells have the potential to differentiate and mature into the different cells of the immune system.

Thymus: An organ located in the chest which instructs immature lymphocytes to become mature T-lymphocytes.

Cytotoxic (killer) T-cells: These lymphocytes mature in the thymus and are responsible for killing infected cells.

Helper T-cells: These specialized lymphocytes "help" other T-cells and B-cells to perform their functions.

B-Cells: These are lymphocytes that arise in the bone marrow and differentiate into plasma cells which in turn produce immunoglobulins (antibodies).

Plasma B-Cells: These cells develop from B-cells and are the cells that make immunoglobulin for the serum and the secretions.

Serum and plasma: Both come from the liquid portion of the blood that is left over once the blood cells are removed. *Serum* is the liquid that remains after the blood has clotted. *Plasma* is the liquid that remains when clotting is prevented with the addition of an anticoagulant.

Essentially, plasma is equal to serum minus clotting agent.

Immunoglobulins (Ig): These highly specialized protein molecules, also known as antibodies, fit foreign antigens, such as polio, like a lock and key. Their variety is so extensive that they can be produced to match all possible microorganisms in our environment.

Immunoglobulin G (IgG): Representing approximately 75% of serum antibodies in humans, IgG is the most common type of antibody found in blood circulation. IgG molecules are created and released by plasma B cells.

Neutrophils: A type of white blood cell (leukocytes) that is one of the first cell types to travel to the site of an infection. Neutrophils help fight infection by ingesting microorganisms and releasing enzymes that kill the microorganisms. Neutrophils are the most plentiful type, making up 55% to 70% of your white blood cells.

Complement proteins: The complement system is a secondary part of the immune system produced in the liver that enhances the ability of antibodies to clear microbes and damaged cells from an organism, promotes inflammation, and attacks the pathogen's cell membrane. It is essentially a "backup" complex system of more than 30 proteins that when triggered act in concert to help eliminate infectious microorganisms. Specifically, the complement system causes the bursting of foreign and infected cells and the ingestion of foreign particles.

Red blood cells: The cells in the blood stream which carry oxygen from the lungs to the tissues.

Platelets: Small cells in the blood stream which are important in blood clotting.

Dendritic cells: Important cells in presenting antigen to immune system cells.

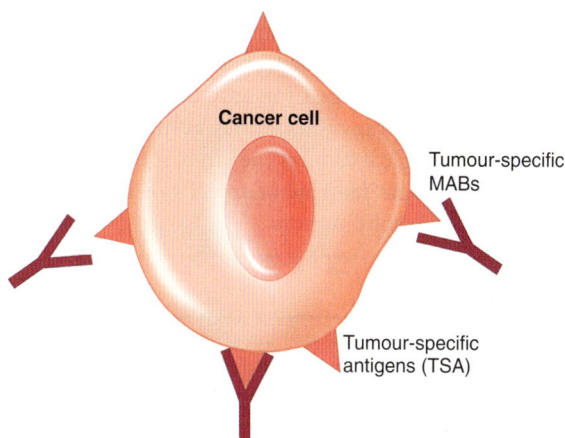

Fig. 16.5 Attack by the immune system on specific protrusions of a cancer cell. (From Lilly LL, Harrington S, Snyder JS: *Pharmacology for Canadian health care practice*, ed 2, Milton, Ontario, 2011, Elsevier Canada.)

(cell-killing) radiation to a target cell. Thus, for RIT cancer therapy, a radioactive antibody combination with specificity for a tumor-associated antigen is used to deliver a lethal dose of radiation to the tumor cells. The ability of the antibody to preferentially bind (i.e., attach itself) to a tumor-associated antigen increases the radiation dose delivered to the tumor cells while decreasing the dose to normal tissues. By its nature, effective RIT, ideally, requires a tumor cell to express or display an antigen that is unique to the *neoplasm* (an abnormal growth of tissue) or is not widely accessible in normal cells. Otherwise, RIT would not be practical. Therefore RIT is very dependent upon there being made available and then using precise focused entities such as monoclonal antibodies.

As an explicit example, an antibody known as an *immunoglobulin* (IgG), is a large, Y-shaped protein (shown in Figs. 16.5 and 16.6), produced mainly by

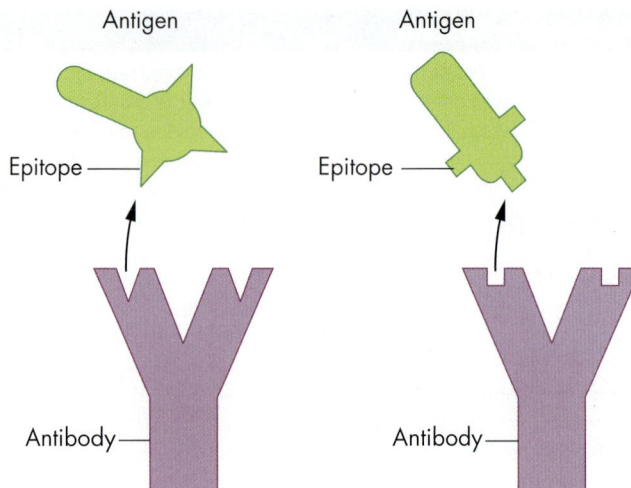

Fig. 16.6 Enlarged view of a "lock and key" interaction between an antibody and a protrusion of a cancer cell recognized as a foreign protein or antigen by the Immune system. (From Worsfold P, Poole C, Townshend A, et al.: *Encyclopedia of analytical science*, ed 3, Oxford, 2019, Elsevier Ltd.)

plasma cells, that is employed by the immune system to neutralize germs such as pathogenic bacteria and viruses. IgG is sensitive to a unique molecule or antigen of the pathogen. Each tip of the "Y" of an antibody contains a *paratope* (analogous to a lock, a paratope is a part of an antibody which recognizes and binds to an antigen) that is specific for one particular structure (similar to a key) on an antigen, allowing these two structures to join together with precision (see Fig. 16.6). Using this binding mechanism, an antibody can mark a microbe or an infected cell for attack by other parts of the immune system, or can neutralize its target directly (for example, by inhibiting a part of a microbe that is essential for its invasion and survival). Cancer cells naturally produce cancer-associated biological molecules, which are adaptive features of malignant change that possess multiple foreign-appearing (antigenic) binding sites in relatively high abundance as in comparison to normal tissues.

As mentioned before, in RIT a radioactive isotope (typically a short-range, high-energy beta-emitter) is chemically bound to a target-specific monoclonal antibody forming a radioactive *conjugate* or team which combines the excellent targeting specificity of the immune system with the known cancer killing power of high-energy radiotherapy. These *radioantibodies* are introduced into the blood or into a body cavity such as

the peritoneum, pleura,* and intrathecal space,** and are subsequently carried to the antigen-binding sites or targets on the tumor cells by blood flow, diffusion, or the wholesale flow of fluid. Thus, when injected into your bloodstream, appropriate radionuclide-linked monoclonal antibodies travel to and bind to cancer cells, cumulatively causing a high dose of destructive radiation to be delivered directly to the tumor cells while at the same time *limiting* radiation effects on neighboring healthy cells. Systemic radiotherapy with radiolabeled immuno-conjugates delivers a nonuniform, low dose rate irradiation over a prolonged period of time, in contrast to external beam radiotherapy which is usually engaged for only minutes at a time. Radioimmunotherapy thus far has been more successful in hematological cancers (i.e., in blood forming tissues such as bone marrow or in cells of the immune system) than in solid tumors.

*The pleura is a thin tissue that lines the chest cavity and surrounds the lungs, and the pleural space is the thin fluid-filled area between two layers of the pleura. The fluid in the pleural space helps the layers of the pleura glide smoothly against each other when you breathe.
**This is the fluid-filled space between the thin layers of tissue that cover the brain and spinal cord. Drugs can be injected into the fluid or a sample of the fluid.

TABLE 16.2 Some Radioisotopes Used and Considered for RIT

Radioisotope	Energy (MeV)	Range	Half-life
Beta-Particle Emitters			
[67]Copper	0.58	2.1 mm	2.6 d
[90]Yittrium	2.28	12.0 mm	2.7 d
[131]Iodine	0.61	2.0 mm	8.0 d
[186]Rhenium	1.07	4.5 mm	3.7 d
[188]Rhenium	2.12	10.4 mm	16.9 hr
Alpha-Particle Emitters			
[211]Astatine	6.8	80 µm	7.2 hr
[213]Bismuth	8.3	84 µm	46 min
[225]Actinium	6.0~8.0	60~90 µm	10.0 d
Auger-Electron Emitter			
[125]Iodine	varied	2~500 nm	59.5 d

Data from Kawashima H: Radioimmunotherapy: a specific treatment protocol for cancer by cytotoxic radioisotopes conjugated to antibodies, Sci World J 2014:492061, 2014.

RIT Agents

Radioimmunotherapy drugs that rely upon an alpha particle-emitting isotope (e.g., Bismuth-213 or Actinium-225), rather than a beta emitter, as the killing source of radiation tend to be more effective. The most developed drug in this category thus far is directed toward treating acute myeloid leukemia (AML).* Other types of cancer for which RIT has *therapeutic potential* include prostate cancer, metastatic melanoma, ovarian cancer, various types of leukemia, and high-grade brain tumors. Table 16.2 provides a list of some radioisotopes used or considered for RIT.

Irradiated cells absorb substantial amounts of energy in the form of photons or charged particles, which promote both direct macromolecular harmful alterations as well as indirect damage due to the generation of reactive oxygen and/or nitrogen species (free radicals, etc. [see Chapter 6 for a detailed discussion of irradiation induced molecular changes]). Both free radicals and molecular oxygen can alter DNA strands, and the damage induces not only the onset of apoptosis (programmed cell death) but also significant necrosis (the

death of most or all of the cells in an organ or tissue due to disease, injury, or failure of the blood supply).

For minimizing collateral injury of nearby normal cells from the radiation used for therapy, alpha particle or short-range beta particle emitters are preferable. There have also become available some monoclonal antibodies that are coupled with radioisotopes that emit very short-range *Auger* electrons (see Chapter 3).

Because an alpha particle gives its energy to the surrounding molecules within a very narrow range (<100 µm, equivalent to a few cell diameters), it leads to a much more concentrated energy transfer within the target and therefore less collateral effect to nontarget tissues as compared to antibodies labeled with beta-emitters. In addition to an alpha particle's very high LET, which results in a large relative biological effectiveness (RBE), *the cytotoxic (cell-killing) efficacy of an alpha particle is independent of the local oxygen concentration and cell cycle state.*

The success of radioimmunotherapy depends on the selective accumulation of cytotoxic radioisotopes at affected areas. Fundamental properties required for effective agents against a particular bio-target are: (1) high binding affinity to the intended mark, (2) high specificity, (3) high metabolic stability, and (4) low body self-rejection or immunogenicity*. From the viewpoint of those molecular characteristics, MABs have been regarded as very suitable vehicles for the delivery of therapeutic radioisotopes.

One of the most intriguing advantages of RIT over external x-ray beam radiotherapy is the ability to attack not only the primary tumor but also lesions systemically metastasizing or spreading. Thus, targeted radiotherapy treatments using specific vehicle agents can be effective in cases of (1) residual micrometastatic lesions,

---

*Acute myeloid leukemia (AML) is a cancer of the blood and bone marrow. It is a type of cancer in which the spongy tissue of the bone marrow makes *abnormal* myeloblasts (a type of white blood cell), red blood cells, or platelets.

---

*Currently, "biologic" drugs provide more treatment options for various diseases. But even these newer drugs have flaws, because in a small percentage of patients, there is *a self-immune response to the drug*, and so its effectiveness over time may be compromised. That undesirable response is called "immunogenicity." The challenge for researchers is to develop biologic drugs that don't provoke that kind of self-immune response, so that all patients can be treated with these medicines. At this time, it is difficult or impossible for physicians to predict which patients are going to end up with an immunogenic response, which makes it tricky to monitor them and prescribe the right treatment.[9]

(2) residual tumor margins after surgical resection, (3) tumors in the circulating blood including hematologic malignancy, and (4) malignancies that present as free-floating cells. Certain types of cancer, therefore, which are not well-handled by conventional means (i.e., external x-ray irradiation and/or chemotherapy) may well have much better potential probabilities for resolution with RIT.

How RIT Is Performed

A nuclear medicine physician and a radiation oncologist and other healthcare professionals, such as a medical physicist, a nuclear medicine technologist, and an oncology nurse, usually make up the team involved in radioimmunotherapy procedures. In general, a patient will receive a treatment either by an injection under the skin (subcutaneous injection) or through a drip (infusion) into a vein. RIT usually consists of several such procedures. For some drugs the first treatment will be into a vein, and then remaining treatments will be delivered subcutaneously. In either way, the "radioantibody" is introduced into the blood or a body cavity such as the peritoneum, pleura, or intrathecal space, and from there it is carried to its natural target or antigen-binding site on the tumor cell by blood flow, diffusion, or the bulk flow of fluid.

In general, for the patient, the most serious and most common side effect of RIT therapy is a decrease in blood counts due to various degrees of unavoidable collateral damage. This side effect may be present as late as several months after treatment but can be medically managed.

Radiation Safety Considerations in RIT Based Theranostics

The diagnostic stage of theranostics is carried out in the same environment that is used for nuclear medicine imaging. Since the types and amounts of diagnostic radionuclides used in theranostics falls within the range of what is used in typical nuclear medicine imaging procedures, there are no special shielding requirements. However, the therapeutic administration must be carried out in an environment that is designed to allow careful monitoring of the specialized radioactive sources because these therapeutic sources are capable of delivering relatively large doses of radiation to the skin of the patient or medical personnel who are present. The infusion of the

therapeutic radiopharmaceutical is in a liquid form and often involves more liquid than may be administered by a single injection. Radiation safety manipulation of containers of radioactive materials in liquid form is required. This necessitates that procedures be in place to keep track of administered activity, storage and ultimate safe disposal of any residual activity, and cleanup measures established for the possibility of radioactive spills. A dedicated room is usually set aside for the purpose of administering the therapeutic doses of radiolabeled pharmaceuticals.

Radiation Safety Example: Yittrium-90 (Y^{90}) Microspheres

Because there are multiple drug-radionuclide combinations that have been used or are in test trials (all of which have alpha or beta or gamma emissions or some combinations thereof), it is therefore practical for this textbook's educational purposes to just consider, as an example, the radiation safety and dosimetry characteristics of one of the most commonly used combinations, namely beta-emitter Yittrium-90 (Y^{90})* microspheres** which are chemically bonded to *Immunoglobulin-G (IgG)*. Representing approximately 75% of blood plasma antibodies in humans, IgG is the most common type of antibody found in the blood circulation.

IgG molecules are created and released by plasma B cells (see Box 16.2).

A practical and efficient agent for the above is Y^{90} combined with the immunoglobulin Ibritumomab Tiuxetan (trade-name *Zevalin*). For Zevalin, other than a lead and acrylic shielding combination about 4 cm in overall diameter around the syringe, only standard

---

*Y^{90} Characteristics: pure beta emitter, decay energy 0.94 MeV, maximum range in tissue 11 mm (2.5 mm average), $T^{1/2}$ = 64.2 hours. Two production methods: (1) Nuclear Reactor, (2) A $_{38}Sr^{90}/_{39}Y^{90}$ generator ($_{38}Sr^{90}$ [Strontium-90] decays by beta decay into $_{39}Y^{90}$ which then undergoes beta decay itself yielding an isotope of Zirconium $_{40}Zr^{90}$).

**A microsphere is a spherical shell that is usually made of a biodegradable or resorbable plastic polymer, that has a very small diameter, customarily in the micron or nanometer range, and that is often filled with a substance (such as a drug or antibody or radionuclide conjugated to an antibody) for release as the shell is degraded.

universal precautions for personnel are required to administer the drug, and strict patient isolation is unnecessary because of the significant self-absorption of the emitted radiation by the patient's body in general. After the radiolabeled antibodies bind to receptors/tumor antigens expressed on the surface of cancerous tissue, cells within an anatomic region reached by the radioactive emissions (beta particles in the case of Y^{90}) will be killed.

RIT with Zevalin is currently most often used to treat non-Hodgkin's B-cell lymphoma* (NHL) for newly diagnosed patients and for patients who have not responded to chemotherapy procedures.[10]

Patients who have had prior bone marrow transplantation or failed stem cell collection *should not receive* RIT. Y^{90}-microsphere treatment is a multiple interdisciplinary treatment modality.

Treatment planning and execution can jointly involve interventional radiology, radiation oncology, and nuclear medicine. *Microbrachytherapy*, a term used by radiation oncologists, originates from the approval of Y^{90} microspheres by the U.S. Food and Drug Administration (FDA) as medical devices. The actual use of Y^{90} microspheres, however, is as a radiopharmaceutical. The material is prepared in a solution and its activity is assayed in a nuclear medicine dose calibrator. The treatment prescription is specified in units of activity (typically gigabecquerels [GBq] or millicuries [mCi]). Absorbed dose to the tumor target is not used in the treatment prescription. As mentioned previously, the agent is administered by use of a syringe or injector via a catheter into an artery. For Zevalin, there is, however, some radiation that is detectable outside of the patient's body which can lead to radiation exposures of others at close distances. This is caused by an escaping

bremsstrahlung radiation component due to high-energy electrons interacting with larger atomic number materials in the patient such as bone.

Consequently, it is recommended that treated patients generally maintain at least a one-meter distance from others, especially young children and pregnant women for over a week (multiple half-lives of Y^{90}) after application of Zevalin. Furthermore, the beta radiation component, almost entirely absorbed by the body, can, however, in the case of a nursing mother via breast milk ingestion compromise a nursing infant and consequently nursing should cease for at least 5 half-lives of Y^{90} (about 2 weeks). Microspheres typically measure between 20 and 30 microns in diameter and are infused with Y^{90} at a specific activity of 2400–2700 Bq per sphere. Typical total treatment activities are in the range of 2 to 6 GBq (approximately 50–160 mCi).*

Y^{90} microsphere therapy is regulated by the NRC, pursuant to 10 CFR 35.1000, and patient release must follow the requirements in 10 CFR 35.75. A licensee may release patients, regardless of administered activity to that patient, if it can be demonstrated that the *total effective dose equivalent* (TEDE) to another individual from exposure to a released patient is not likely to exceed 5 mSv (0.5 rem). In addition, pursuant to 10 CFR part 35.75(b), licensees must provide a released patient with written instructions on actions recommended to maintain ALARA doses to other individuals if the dose to any other individual is likely to exceed one mSv.

For radiation safety regulatory purposes to others, only the bremsstrahlung radiation component need be considered here because the involved direct beta dose would be negligible. The following empirical equation can be used to estimate the total dose that an individual is likely to receive from exposure to a released patient at a distance r measured in centimeters:

$$DE(\infty) = (34.6\Gamma\ A\ T_p OF)/r^2$$

where in this equation: $DE(\infty)$ is the external exposure dose equivalent, attributable to bremsstrahlung radiation, up to total decay (i.e., out to infinite time) in

---

*Both Hodgkin's lymphoma and non-Hodgkin's lymphoma are a type of cancer that begins in a subset of white blood cells (lymphocytes). Lymphoma can develop when the number of lymphocytes (white blood cells that fight infection) increase out of control. This is caused by genetic changes in the cells that mean they no longer "listen" to signals that control their growth and death. The main difference between Hodgkin's lymphoma and non-Hodgkin's lymphoma is in the specific lymphocyte each involves. If upon examining the cells under a microscope there is detected the presence of a specific type of abnormal cell called a Reed-Sternberg cell, the lymphoma is classified as Hodgkin's.

---

*1 GBq = 10^9 disintegrations per second which is equivalent to 27 mCi of activity. Therefore 6 GBq would be equivalent to 162 mCi.

millisieverts; Γ^* is the specific bremsstrahlung equivalent dose rate constant* for Y^{90} in soft tissue equal to $1.52(10)^{-3}$ mSv/cm²/MBq/hr at 1 cm; A is the administered activity in megabecquerels (MBq); T_p is the physical half-life of the radionuclide in days (2.67 days for Y^{90}); OF is the assumed practical occupancy factor at 100cm (usually 1/4 or 0.25); and r is distance from the patient in centimeters.[10]

The above equation can be considered to be an approximation because it was derived under the idealized assumptions of instantaneous patient activity uptake, uniform activity deposition through the patient, and no biologic elimination. It can be solved for the maximum allowable administered activity for authorizing patient release on the basis of the 5 mSv (500 mrem) regulatory dose limit. In compliance with the public dose limit in 10 CFR 35.75(a), licensees may release patients from their control if the activity administered to *each* treated patient is no greater than 1420 GBq. Patient instructions are required only if the dose to other individuals is likely to exceed 1 mSv (0.1 rem). This dose equivalent would correspond to one fifth of the maximum allowable release value, corresponding to an administered activity of 284 GBq. Since all patients treated with ⁹⁰Y-microspheres receive a treatment activity that is *enormously lower* than this value, all such patients can be released and no records or instructions are required by the NRC.[11,12]

The same equation can also be used to calculate a projected potential TEDE to a family member who for a quarter of the time of the implant duration maintains a distance of one meter from a patient who has received a treatment dosage of 6 GBq (162 mCi). The family member is assumed to spend negligible time closer to the patient than 100 cm. Substituting into the equation the various parameter values, we then obtain:

$$\text{TEDE (family member)} = 34.6 \times 1.52 \, (10)^{-3}$$
$$\times 6000 \times 2.67 \times 0.25/(100)^2$$
$$= .022 \, \text{mSv} \, (.0022 \, \text{rem})$$

Although the 6 GBq or 162 mCi dosage is greater than the normal Y^{90} dosage used (see below), it is seen

to produce a TEDE to an informed family member that is substantially below the NRC regulatory limit.

Because of calculations such as the above and associated radiation protection survey results, it is well recognized that Y-90 Zevalin therapy can be safely done on an outpatient basis using only standard universal precautions. The *typically administered dose of Y-90 Zevalin* is between 777 and 1110 MBq (21–30 mCi), with a maximum of 1184 MBq (32 mCi).

Theranostics Imaging and RIT

The therapy aspect of RIT is usually coupled with a nuclear medicine imaging component to ascertain the actual targeting efficacy of the monoclonal antibody (MAB) employed. Nuclear medicine scanners cannot image the actual radioactive distribution of an agent from beta or alpha emissions because those radiations are absorbed locally to such a high degree that there is a negligible external signal for a nuclear medicine camera* to detect. Instead, a pre-treatment dose of pharmaceutical in which the MABs are tagged with technetium Tc⁹⁹ᵐ (emits easily detectable 140 keV gammas) is administered and thereby generates an image of the biological distribution of that pharmaceutical. Based upon the biodistribution seen in the technetium image, the amount of radionuclide (such as the beta emitter Y^{90}) to be injected into the patient is selected so as to deliver a tumoricidal dose that will not cause unacceptable harm to healthy tissues (Table 16.3). Injected 99mTc-serum albumin labeled antibody distribution activity in liver and lung in a patient with liver carcinoma. ROIs (in red) around lungs and liver demonstrate respective number of organ counts, which, for a calibrated imaging technique can be translated into a quantitative estimate of the likely distribution of an alpha particle emitting radiopharmaceutical to be administered later for therapeutic purposes (Fig. 16.7).

---

*An experimentally determined value based upon the mean bremsstrahlung energy.

---

*Nuclear Medicine camera, also called a *scintillation camera*, is an energy selective device used mainly to image *gamma* radiation emitting radioisotopes. It precisely records the distribution of radiation emitted from a chemical compound containing a radionuclide that is attracted to specific organs or tissues and thereby can be used to quantitatively ascertain the amount of radionuclide taken up by various scanned regions of interest.

TABLE 16.3 Some Imaging (Dx) and Therapeutic (Rx) Radionuclides That Are Used in Theranostics

Cancer	Radiouclide	Emission	Imaging
Prostate	Dx: ^{18}F	β plus	PET
	Rx: ^{177}Lu	β minus	
Liver	Dx: ^{99m}Tc	γ	SPECT or gamma camera
	Rx: ^{90}y	β minus	
Bone metastases	Dx: ^{99m}Tc	γ	SPECT or gamma camera
From Prostate Ca	Rx: ^{223}Ra	α	

"β plus" signifies a positron
"β plus" signifies an electron
"γ" signifies a gamma ray photon particle

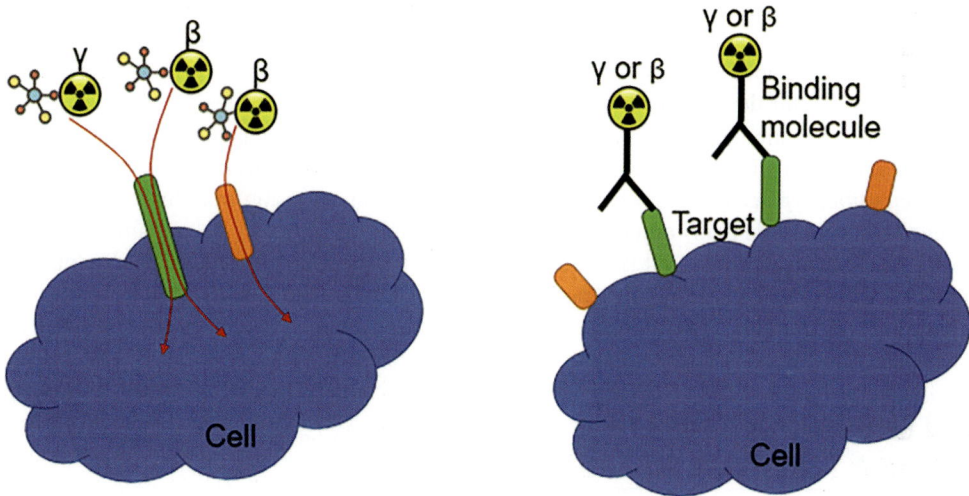

Targeted radionuclide therapy　　**Radioimmunotherapy**

Fig. 16.7 Schematic representation of the two approaches to therapy that define theranostics in nuclear medicine. Targeted radionuclide therapy uses more traditional radiochemicals and radiopharmaceuticals in which the pathway to localization of the diagnostic and therapeutic tracers might be the same (e.g., iodine-123 [^{123}I] NaI and iodine-131 [^{131}I] NaI) or the mechanism of localization may be similar but not the same (e.g., technetium-99m methylene diphosphonate and strontium-89 chloride). Radioimmunotherapy adopts monoclonal antibodies or fragments thereof. Consequently, the same binding molecule is used (via a linker or linking molecule) for diagnostic and therapy radionuclides. (Courtesy Geoff Currie, Charles Sturt University. From Gilmore D, Waterstram-Rich KM: *Nuclear medicine and molecular imaging*, ed 9, Philadelphia, 2023, Elsevier.)

Summary of Theranostics

The challenge for effective theranostics is that the radioisotopes that are normally used for imaging are different from the radioisotopes that could deliver sufficiently effective high doses to local regions of the body.

Theranostics has become clinically useful, however, in the last decade through the development of specialized radiopharmaceuticals that may be labeled with one radioisotope that emits long range radiation for imaging and another radioisotope that emits short range radiation to deliver therapeutic doses to neighboring cancerous molecules and cells.

Since the exact distribution of a radiopharmaceutical in a patient is not precisely predictable in advance, theranostics is necessarily *a two-step process*. First, a radiopharmaceutical that is tagged with a radioactive isotope *suitable for imaging* is injected into the patient and the distribution of the radiopharmaceutical reveals where the carrier molecules will appear in the patient. Then, the same carrier molecules are chemically combined with sufficient amounts of a therapeutic radioactive isotope and injected into the patient to deliver destructive radiation doses to desired targets.

Some cancer cells produce types of proteins called antigens that are rarely or never present in normal cells. Antibodies are molecules that bind to these antigens so as to inactivate or damage those cancer cells. Radiopharmaceuticals have been developed that use these antibodies as carrier molecules for the radionuclides. When the radionuclide emits radiation that can be detected by imaging devices, such as PET scanners or gamma cameras, then the radiopharmaceutical may be used for imaging. When the radionuclide emits radiation that is locally absorbed, the radiopharmaceutical is useful for therapy. *Carrier molecules that can be tagged by both an imaging radionuclide and therapeutic radionuclides, in a one or two step process are the essence of theranostics.*

RADIATION EMERGENCIES: USE OF RADIATION AS A TERRORIST WEAPON

After the attack on the World Trade Center by hijacked airplanes on September 11, 2001, the possibility of the use of other terrorist weapons, such as radiation, became a public health concern. Today, most hospitals have elaborate crisis plans for handling emergency situations involving **radioactive contamination**. Radiologic technologists should become aware of the radiation emergency plans that exist in the facilities in which they work. In this section, some fundamental principles of dealing with radioactive contamination in a health care environment are discussed.

Contamination

A **radioactive dispersal device, or "dirty bomb,"** is a radioactive source mixed with conventional explosives. It is intended to contaminate an area with radioactive material and thereby cause panic. The actual long-term

health effects of a dirty bomb are likely to be minimal. If the radioactive material remains in a small area, few people may be affected. However, if enough explosives are used to spread the same amount of radioactive material over a broader area, then the radioactivity will be diluted and may not be much higher than background levels.

For example, it would be difficult for terrorists to accumulate as much radioactive material as existed in the Chernobyl nuclear reactor. Even if they were able to do this and were to explode the device with the same force as the explosion at Chernobyl, the actual number of radiation injuries would probably be quite small. At Chernobyl, no cases of acute radiation syndrome (ARS) were caused by exposure outside the immediate vicinity of the reactor. The only cases occurred in emergency workers, primarily firemen, who worked for nonbrief periods *very near* to the reactor. They had little training and essentially no protective gear to prepare them for a radioactive emergency. In the United States at the present time, emergency responders are equipped to monitor and continuously assess the degree of personnel exposure on-site.

After an explosion of a dirty bomb, some individuals would unavoidably be contaminated with dust and debris, a portion of which could contain radioactive materials. The procedure for **decontamination** is surprisingly simple. Removal of contaminated clothing and immersion in a shower comprise the best method. If a wound contains radioactive material, a simple rinse of the area is usually sufficient to allow medical personnel to provide medical attention. Most hospitals are stocked with **Geiger–Müller (GM) detectors** (described in Chapter 5), and emergency personnel are trained to provide guidance concerning contamination levels. The facility's radiation safety officer would also be present to numerically assess contamination levels.

It is unlikely that a dirty bomb would cause contamination with so much radioactive material that a victim could not receive medical attention. The key here is that the same personnel need not be near patients for any length of time. Most emergency room treatments do not require the staff to be near patients for as long as an hour. Even if a GM detector shows readings of two to five times natural background radiation, this means an effective dose rate of only 0.06 to 0.15 mSv/hr would be experienced by a physician who is in direct contact with the patient. Therefore a physician could treat this patient under these circumstances without exceeding normal dose limits. Normal dose limits, though, do not apply in radiation crisis situations.

The **Environmental Protection Agency (EPA)** suggests that during such an emergency, individuals engaged in nonlifesaving activities work under a dose limit of 50 mSv (5 rem) per event. For individuals engaged in lifesaving activities, the dose limit is permitted to rise to 250 mSv per event.[13] Because it may be difficult to monitor all workers involved in a radiation emergency, a dose rate criterion is often used. In this case, if the dose rate in the area is less than 0.1 mSv/hr, emergency personnel may enter an area to perform critical tasks. If the dose rate exceeds 0.1 mSv/hr, emergency personnel should await specific instructions from radiation experts on how to proceed.[14,15]

Cleanup of a Contaminated Urban Area

The EPA sets limits for radioactive contamination that assume that a *1 in 10,000* risk of causing a fatal cancer is unacceptable. This type of regulation requires hospitals, educational facilities, and industries to control accidental exposures so that the health of the population cannot be measurably affected. It also assumes that many other carcinogens are present and that all are regulated to a similar low level.

However, if radioactive contamination were to result from a dirty bomb, it is hoped that a more realistic evaluation of actual risk would be used. Unnecessary use of resources to clean a large inhabitable area (e.g., at the heart of a major city) to unreasonably stringent standards would be an unfortunate outcome requiring the expenditure of vast resources that could be used to benefit the public elsewhere. For example, *a 1 in 10,000 probability of causing a fatal cancer corresponds approximately to a 2 mSv (200 mrem) effective dose*. Recall from Chapter 2 that the annual effective dose resulting from average natural background radiation is approximately 3 mSv. Therefore cleanup of a contaminated site to levels associated with normal radiation protection standards would require heroic measures, such as:

- Removal of topsoil
- Digging up of roadways

A practical compromise should be made to allow land use after a reasonable cleanup.

Medical Management of Persons Experiencing Radiation Bioeffects

If **surface contamination** is suspected, personnel should wear gowns, masks, and gloves when working with the patient. The same procedures that control the spread of infection are useful to prevent the spread of radioactive contamination. The clothing of individuals who have been contaminated should be placed in plastic containers and set aside for later evaluation. Removal of surface contamination involves removal of the patient's clothing and the use of a shower to cleanse the skin.

The various stages of ARS are discussed in Chapter 8. (A complete discussion of procedures for handling acute radiation syndrome is beyond the scope of this text. The interested reader is referred to recent publications on this subject.)[16] In dealing with patients with ARS, some estimate of the amount of exposure they have received helps predict the clinical course of the syndrome (Table 16.4). There are many methods other than ARS symptoms that may be used to determine the amount of radiation dose received during acute exposure. Biodosimetry is a general term used to refer to analysis of biological fluids such as blood and urine to look for actual internal contamination, changes in blood components, and for genetic analysis. Physical dosimetry methods include analysis of physical components of the body and surroundings. These include optically stimulated luminescence of teeth, implanted ceramics, plastic cards, and even fabric samples. These techniques may be used to provide information to aid in triage immediately after an accident or to modify treatment by refining dosimetry estimates at a later time. They have been compiled recently by the International Council on Radiation Protection and Units.[17] For exposures localized to specific regions of the body, medical management involves the prevention of infection and control of pain and potential skin grafts. If substantial amounts of beta-emitting radioactive material settle on a patient's skin, the dose is still superficial, and skin grafts may be successful in repairing very damaged areas. Gamma-emitting materials, however, can produce a deeper dose that could interfere with quick healing.

During the first 48 hours of ARS, symptoms such as nausea and vomiting occur. Medical management at this time is simply to treat the symptoms and try to prevent dehydration. The bone marrow becomes depleted (leukopenia and thrombocytopenia) after a few weeks. Bone marrow transplants (such as hematopoietic stem cell transplants) may be effective in replacing the function of damaged bone marrow. Such activities require special expertise and, in the event of a radiation emergency, would be coordinated by the Radiation Injury Treatment Network.[18]

TABLE 16.4   Dose Effect Relation After Acute Whole-Body Radiation from Gamma Rays or X-Rays

Whole-Body (Gy$_t$)	Absorbed Dose Effect
0.05	No symptoms
0.15	No symptoms but possible chromosomal aberrations in cultured peripheral blood lymphocytes
0.5	No symptoms (minor decreases in white blood cell and platelet counts in a few persons)
1	Nausea and vomiting in approximately 10% of patients within 48 hr after exposure
2	Nausea and vomiting in approximately 50% of persons within 24 hr, with marked decreases in white blood cell and platelet counts
4	Nausea and vomiting in 90% of persons within 12 hr and diarrhea in 10% within 8 hr; 50% mortality in the absence of treatment
6	100% mortality within 30 days because of bone marrow failure in the absence of treatment
10	Approximate dose that is survivable with the best medical therapy available
>10–30	Nausea and vomiting in all persons in less than 5 minutes; severe gastrointestinal damage; death likely in 2 to 3 weeks in the absence of treatment
>30	Cardiovascular collapse and central nervous system damage, with death in 24 to72 hours

Data from Gusev I, Guskova AK, Mettler Jr. FA, editors: *Medical management of radiation accidents*, ed 2, Boca Raton, FL, 2001, CRC Press.

In the event of **internal contamination**, various strategies are used, depending on the clinical and radiologic form of contamination. Some of these methods include:

- Dilution (forcing fluids)
- Blocking absorption in the gastrointestinal tract (administration of emetics, charcoal, laxatives)

If the radionuclide contamination is iodine, administration of potassium iodide to block further uptake in the thyroid is possible if no more than a few hours have elapsed since the contamination.

The National Library of Medicine and the National Institutes of Health (NIH) maintain a website that contains a wealth of information on dealing with radiation emergencies. It contains:

- Both basic and advanced methods for decontamination
- Methods to reduce exposure
- Specific medical emergency procedures for various situations

The website may be found at www.nlm.nih.gov/medlineplus/radiationemergencies.html.

SUMMARY

- Isotopes are atoms that have the same number of protons within the nucleus but have different numbers of neutrons.
- Some nuclei of isotopes have too many neutrons or too many protons for stability.
- Radioactive isotopes spontaneously undergo changes or transformations to rectify their unstable arrangement.
- Rapidly dividing cells that are well oxygenated are very radiosensitive.
- When cells are radiosensitive, cancerous growths or tumors can be either eliminated, or at least controlled, by irradiation of the area containing the growth.
- Therapeutic isotopes generally have relatively long half-lives compared with diagnostically employed isotopes.

- Fast electrons emitted from a nucleus are called beta radiation.
- Gamma rays and x-ray photons differ only in their point of origin.
- Iodine-125 decays with a half-life of 59.4 days by a process called *electron capture*.
- The most practical radiation protection to follow for patients having therapeutic prostate seed implants is use of the concepts of distance and time.
- When iodine-131 is being administered to treat a hospitalized patient for thyroid cancer, a large, up to 2.5 cm or 1-inch thick, rolling lead shield can be positioned between the patient and any attending personnel for protection.
- Residual unused nonreturned radioisotopes, as well as radioactively contaminated items, must be held

in a secure, shielded, and posted storage area for a period of 10 half-lives of the isotope before being able to be discarded in ordinary trash. Proper record keeping is to be kept of storage and disposal.

- Diagnostic techniques in nuclear medicine typically make use of short-lived radioisotopes as radioactive tracers.
- Technetium-99m is the most common radioisotope used in diagnostic nuclear medicine.
- Positron emission tomography (PET) makes use of annihilation radiation events.
- When matter–antimatter annihilation occurs, a positron and an electron relatively at rest interact destructively and disappear. Their respective masses are converted into energy that will be carried off by two photons emerging from the annihilation site in opposite directions, each with a kinetic energy of 511 keV.
- A neutrino is a particle that has almost negligible mass and no electric charge but carries away any excess energy from the nucleus of the atom in processes such as beta and positron decay.
- Fluorine-18 is the most important isotope used for PET scanning.
- PET is an important imaging modality because it can examine metabolic processes within the body.
- Fluorodeoxyglucose (FDG) is a radioactive tracer that is taken up or metabolized by cancerous cells and that reveals their location through positron emission decay and subsequent generation of oppositely traveling annihilation photons.
- A PET-CT scanner can detect the presence of regions of abnormally high glucose metabolism, thus providing evidence of cancer metastasis to other body areas, and at the same time can obtain detailed information about the location and size of these lesions or growths.
- Positron emitters result in the production of high-energy radiation, and for this reason, the design of a PET-CT imaging suite involves significant radiation safety concerns.
- Diagnostic reference levels (DRLs) refer to the amount of activity in megabecquerels (MBq) (or traditionally in millicuries [mCi]) of a particular radionuclide compound of the radioactive material that is administered (through injection or by swallowing) to the patient. In nuclear medicine, DRLs are essentially a tool which is related to the expected radiation dose received by an average-sized patient undergoing a given ionizing radiation imaging examination.

- The term *theranostics* is a cancer treatment method associated with the combination of both diagnostic imaging at the molecular level and cellular targeted radiation therapy with specially configured radionuclides. As such it is a 2-step process that includes a diagnostic examination using a nuclear medicine scanning device followed by a tumor specific therapeutic component (radioimmunotherapy) performed by injection or IV infusion.
- Radioimmunotherapy (RIT) is a specific treatment protocol for cancer by cytotoxic radioisotopes conjugated to specialized immune system antibodies.
- Monoclonal antibodies are antibodies that are made by identical immune cells that are all clones of a unique parent cell.
- Organs of the human body that are part of the immune system include organs such as the liver, thymus gland, bone marrow, lymph nodes, spleen, and tonsils.
- Radioimmunotherapy (RIT) is a combination of radiation therapy and immunotherapy and the success of RIT depends on the selective accumulation of cytotoxic radioisotopes at the affected areas.
- One of the most intriguing advantages of RIT over external x-ray beam therapy is the ability to attack not only the primary tumor but also lesions systemically metastasizing or spreading.
- Most hospitals have elaborate crisis plans for handling emergency situations involving radioactive contamination.
- A radioactive dispersal device, or "dirty bomb," is a radioactive source mixed with conventional explosives, the actual long-term health effects of which will most likely be minimal.
- If radioactive material from a dirty bomb remains in a small area, only a few people may be seriously affected.
- Conversely, if enough explosives are used to spread the same amount of radioactive material over a broad area, radioactivity will be diluted and may not be much higher than background levels.
- If a dirty bomb were to explode with the same force as the explosion at Chernobyl, the actual number of radiation injuries could actually be quite small.
- The United States currently has emergency responders who are prepared and equipped to monitor and assess personnel exposure on-site in an emergency situation.

- After an explosion of a dirty bomb, externally contaminated individuals can be decontaminated by removal of tainted clothing and immersion in a shower.
- Geiger–Müller (GM) detectors may be used by trained emergency personnel to monitor contamination levels.
- During an emergency situation, individuals engaged in nonlifesaving activities are to work under a dose limit of 50 mSv per event, whereas those persons performing lifesaving activities have a dose limit of 250 mSv.

- If surface contamination is suspected, emergency personnel should protect themselves by wearing gowns, masks, and gloves while working with the patient.
- Handling of patients with internal contamination varies depending on the clinical and radiologic form of contamination. Strategies may include dilution and blocking absorption in the gastrointestinal tract. Potassium iodide can be administered to block further uptake of radioactive iodine in the thyroid gland.

GENERAL DISCUSSION QUESTIONS

1. Why do isotopes that have too many neutrons or too many protons spontaneously undergo changes or transformations?
2. What causes cancerous growths or tumors to be eliminated or controlled by irradiation?
3. What difference exists between gamma rays and x-ray photons?
4. What are the best radiation safety practices to follow for patients having therapeutic prostate seed implants?
5. While caring for a hospitalized patient receiving iodine-131 therapy for cancer, what can hospital personnel do to minimize occupational exposure?
6. What radiation safety concerns are associated with the design of a PET/CT imaging suite, and how is radiation protection provided to meet these concerns?
7. What is a radioactive dispersal device, or "dirty bomb," and what are the possible consequences if such a device is detonated?

8. If a wound contains radioactive material, what should be done to decontaminate the wound?
9. What dose level may an individual engaged in lifesaving activities during a radiation emergency receive?
10. If surface contamination is suspected, what should medical personnel wear when working with a contaminated patient?
11. What is the meaning of diagnostic reference levels and where are they most useful?
12. Where does the development of all cells of the immune system begin?
13. What is radioimmunotherapy?
14. Upon what does the success of radioimmunotherapy depend?
15. What professional individuals are usually involved in radioimmunotherapy procedures?
16. For what groups of patients if radioimmunotherapy an important choice?
17. What is the concept of theranostics?

REVIEW QUESTIONS

1. Well-oxygenated rapidly dividing cells are:
   A. Very insensitive and are not damaged by radiation
   B. Very sensitive to damage by radiation
   C. Moderately sensitive to damage by radiation
   D. Somewhat sensitive to damage by radiation
2. PET/CT refers to which of the following?
   A. A procedure for whole body imaging
   B. A method to image cancer activity and detailed anatomical location simultaneously
   C. Using pair production for curing brain cancer
   D. Photodisintegration coupled with ordinary x-ray therapy

3. Diagnostic reference levels correspond to:
   A. Using the highest dose administration of a radionuclide for best imaging
   B. Information gathered for using the lowest dose administration of a radionuclide that will still yield a satisfactory diagnosis
   C. Only using large amounts of radiation for imaging in severe reference cases
   D. None of the above

4. Theranostics consist of:
   A. External multi-fractional x-ray therapy
   B. Utilization of multiple fractions of iodine-131 to cure thyroid cancer
   C. A combination of specific area radionuclide imaging with succeeding infusion of specialized area-targeted cell-killing radioisotopes
   D. High-energy x-ray beams directed by cone beam CT imaging

5. Antibodies that are made by identical immune cells that are all clones of a unique parent cell are known as:
   A. Antigen antibodies
   B. Conjugated antibodies
   C. Monoclonal antibodies
   D. Pathogen antibodies

6. One of the most intriguing advantages of radioimmunotherapy over external x-ray beam radiotherapy is the ability to attack:
   A. Not only the primary tumor but also lesions systemically metastasizing or spreading
   B. Only the primary tumor cells
   C. Only lesions systemically metastasizing or spreading
   D. Only the primary tumor cells and all the noncancerous cells surrounding the primary tumor

7. Which of the following steps should be taken for external decontamination from radioactive materials?
   1. Removal of contaminated clothing
   2. Immersion of contaminated person in a shower
   3. Monitoring of the contaminated individual with a Geiger–Müller detector
   A. 1 and 2 only
   B. 1 and 3 only

C. 2 and 3 only
D. 1, 2, and 3

8. What dose level may an individual who is engaged in nonlifesaving activities during a radiation emergency safely receive?
   A. 10 mSv per event
   B. 30 mSv per event
   C. 50 mSv per event
   D. 250 mSv per event

9. All of the following statements are true *except*:
   A. In dealing with patients with acute radiation syndrome (ARS), some estimate of the amount of exposure they have received helps predict the clinical course of the syndrome.
   B. If beta-emitting radioactive material settles on a patient's skin, the dose is very deep and skin grafts will not be successful.
   C. Gamma-emitting radioactive materials can produce a deep dose that may interfere with healing.
   D. Current strategy for an ARS patient is to administer drugs that stimulate any remaining bone marrow.

10. Some of the strategies used to treat internal radiation contamination include:
    1. Dilution (forcing fluids)
    2. Blocking absorption in the gastrointestinal tract (administration of emetics, charcoal, laxatives)
    3. Administration of potassium iodide to block further uptake in the thyroid if the radionuclide is iodine and no more than a few hours have elapsed since the contamination
    A. 1 only
    B. 2 only
    C. 3 only
    D. 1, 2, and 3

Relationships Between Systems of Units

As has been shown throughout this textbook, various quantities are necessary for describing physical processes. Well-known examples of such quantities are length, mass, force, energy, and time. If one also includes electric charge, then virtually all of the fundamental characteristics of nature can be found to be included within combinations of these physical quantities or, more precisely, *the units associated with them.* The purpose of this appendix is to tabulate quantities and units, including those that pertain to ionizing radiation that may be encountered by the student. It should be emphasized that a concerted effort has long been underway to just have one system of units in place throughout the world, namely the Systeme International, or SI. There are strong pockets of resistance to this, especially in the United States, which is firmly wedded to the English system. However, in official areas such as radiation protection regulations and registry and licensing examinations, SI units have become the norm, and they have been used in this text as much as possible.

Three basic systems of physical units have been in existence for a long time and are familiar to varying degrees, depending on what part of the world one lives in and perhaps one's field of work. They are the English system, the CGS (centimeter-gram-second) system, and the MKS (meter-kilogram-second) or SI system. The following tables specify for each important physical quantity the corresponding associated fundamental unit in each of the three systems and the relationship among these units when possible. Boxes demonstrating calculations for conversions among units and for equivalent and effective radiation doses are also provided.

English System

Quantity	Unit
Length	Foot, inch
Force (weight)	Pound (lb)
Mass	Slug (an object of mass 1 slug weighs 32 lb on the surface of the Earth)
Energy	Foot-pound
Power	Horsepower (hp)
Pressure	Lb/in^2
Time	Second
Electric charge	Coulomb
Temperature	Degrees fahrenheit (°F)
Absorbed dose	No specific unit
Exposure	Roentgen

CGS System

Quantity	Unit
Length	Centimeter (cm)
Force (weight)	Dyne (1 gm-cm/sec^2)
Mass	Gram (g)
Energy	Erg (1 gm-cm^2/sec^2)
Power	Ergs per second
Pressure	Barye (Ba) (1 Ba = 1 dyne/cm^2)
Time	Second
Electric charge	Statcoulomb or ESU (ESU means electrostatic unit of charge)
Temperature	Degrees centigrade (celsius) (°C)
Absorbed dose	Rad (1 rad = 100 ergs/gram)
Equivalent dose	Rem

MKS (SI) System

Quantity	Unit
Length	Meter (m)
Force (weight)	Newton (1 N = 1 kg-m/sec^2)
Mass	Kilogram (kg)
Energy	Joule (1 J = 1 kg-m^2/sec^2)
Power	Watt (1 W = 1 joule/sec)
Pressure	N/m^2
Time	Second
Electric charge	Coulomb (C)
Temperature	Degrees centigrade (°C) (celsius), degrees Kelvin (K)
Absorbed dose	Gray (Gy) (1 Gy = 1 J/kg)
Equivalent dose	Sievert (Sv)

Relationships Among Units

Quantity	Unit Conversions
Length	1 m = 100 cm = 39.37 inches; 2.54 cm = 1 inch
Force (weight)	1 N = 0.225 lb = 10^5 dynes
Mass	1 kg = 1000 g; 1 slug = 14.6 kg
Energy	1 J = 10^7 ergs = 0.738 ft-lb
Power	1 W = 0.738 ft-lb/sec; 1 hp = 550 ft-lb/sec = 746 W = 0.746 kW
Pressure	1 N/m^2 = 1.45(10)$^{-4}$ lb/in^2 =10 Ba; 1 atmosphere = 14.7 lb/in^2 = 1.013(10)^5 N/m^2
Time	1 second = 1/3600 hour = approximately 1/100,000 day
Electric charge	1 ESU = 1 statcoulomb = 3.34(10)$^{-10}$ C
Temperature	$T_F = \frac{9}{5}T_C + 32$, $T_K = T_C + 273$
Exposure	1 coulomb/kg = 1/2.58(10)$^{-4}$ C/kg per R = 3876 R (a very large exposure)
Absorbed dose	1 Gy = 100 rad, 1 cGy = 1 rad
Equivalent dose	1 Sv = 100 rem, 10 mSv = 1 rem 1 mSv = 0.1 rem = 100 mrem

Determining and Expressing Effective Dose (EfD) in Rem

Example: The W_R for x-radiation is 1 (see Table 4.2), and the W_T for the gonads is 0.20 (see Table 4.3). If the gonads receive an absorbed dose (D) of 10 cGy from exposure to x-radiation, what is the EfD in rem?
Answer:

$$EfD = D \times W_R \times W_T$$
$$= 10 \times 1 \times 0.20$$
$$= 2 \text{ rem}$$
$$= 2/100 = 0.02 \text{ Sv} = 20 \text{ mSv}$$

Traditional and SI Equivalents

1 roentgen (R) equals	2.58 × 10^{-4} C/kg of air
1 milliroentgen (mR) equals	$^1/_{1000}$ R or 10^{-3} R
1 rad equals	100 erg/g
	$^1/_{100}$ J/kg
	$^1/_{100}$ Gy
	1 cGy
1 millirad equals	10^{-3} rad
1 rem equals	$^1/_{100}$ J/kg (for x-radiation, Q = 1)
	$^1/_{100}$ Sv
	1 cSv
	10 mSv
1 millirem equals	$^1/_{1000}$ rem

Image Gently Pledge and Image Wisely Pledge

Pledges begin on January 1 of each year and expire on December 31 of the same year. It is up to the radiographer to renew the pledges each year.

IMAGE GENTLY PLEDGE

Yes, I want to **image gently**.

Recognizing that every member of the health care team plays a vital role in caring for the patient and wants to provide the best care, I pledge:

- To make the image gently message a priority in staff communications this year
- To review the protocol recommendations and, where necessary, implement adjustments to our processes
- To respect and listen to suggestions from every member of the imaging team on ways to ensure changes are made
- To communicate openly with parents

Thank you for committing to the goal to image gently when you image or treat children.

Spread the word in your department, practice, hospital, or clinic.

Take the pledge at https://radsociety.wufoo.com/forms/image-gently-pledge/.

image gently℠

This certificate is completed online by the individual (named here) _____ who has pledged to "*image gently*." In doing so, he/she pledges:

- to make the *image gently* message a priority in staff communications this year
- to review the protocol recommendations and, where necessary, implement adjustments to practice processes
- to respect and listen to suggestions from every member of the imaging team on ways to ensure changes are made
- to communicate openly with parents

The Alliance for Radiation Safety in Pediatric Imaging thanks those who commit to the goal to "*image gently*" in the imaging of children. Spread the word in your department, practice, hospital or clinic.

Name/Practice Address

Date

The Image Gently Campaign is a message from the Alliance for Radiation Safety in Pediatric Imaging.

Visit the website at www.imagegently.org for more information

This certificate is not an accreditation document from the Image Gently campaign. It is a sign of the voluntary pledge taken by the named individual.

From The Image Gently Alliance, www.imagegently.org.

IMAGE WISELY PLEDGE

Pledge for Imaging Professionals

Yes, I want to ***image wisely.***

  I wish to optimize the use of radiation in imaging patients and thereby pledge:

1. To *put my patients' safety, health, and welfare first* by optimizing imaging examinations to use only the radiation necessary to produce diagnostic-quality images
2. To *convey the principles of the Image Wisely program* to the imaging team in order to ensure that my facility optimizes its use of radiation when imaging patients
3. To *communicate optimal patient imaging strategies to referring physicians* and to be available for consultation
4. To *routinely review imaging protocols* to ensure that the least radiation necessary to acquire a diagnostic-quality image is used for each examination
5. To *monitor examination radiation dose indices* to enable comparison to established diagnostic reference levels

  Take the pledge at http://www.imagewisely.org/Pledge/Imaging-Professionals-Pledge.

Standard Designations for Metric System Lengths, Electron Volt Energy Levels, and Frequency Spectrum Ranges

Metric System Equivalents for Length[a]

Length	Symbol	Power of 10 Fractional Form	Power of 10 Decimal Form	Scientific Notation
Yottameter	Ym	1,000,000,000,000,000,000,000,000	1,000,000,000,000,000,000,000,000	10^{24} (m)
Zettameter	Zm	1,000,000,000,000,000,000,000	1,000,000,000,000,000,000,000	10^{21} (m)
Exameter	Em	1,000,000,000,000,000,000	1,000,000,000,000,000,000	10^{18} (m)
Petameter	Pm	1,000,000,000,000,000	1,000,000,000,000,000	10^{15} (m)
Terameter	Tm	1,000,000,000,000	1,000,000,000,000	10^{12} (m)
Gigameter	**Gm**	1,000,000,000	1,000,000,000	10^{9} (m)
Megameter	**Mm**	1,000,000	1,000,000	10^{6} (m)
Kilometer	**km**	1000	1000	10^{3} (m)
Hectometer	**hm**	100	100	10^{2} (m)
Dekameter	**dam**	10	10	10^{1} (m)
Meter	**m**	1	1	10^{0} (m)
Decimeter	**dm**	1/10	0.1	10^{-1} (m)
Centimeter	**cm**	1/100	0.01	10^{-2} (m)
Millimeter	**mm**	1/1000	0.001	10^{-3} (m)
Micrometer	**μm**	1/1,000,000	0.00001	10^{-6} (m)
Nanometer	**nm**	1/1,000,000,000	0.000000001	10^{-9} (m)
Picometer	pm	1/1,000,000,000,000	0.000000000001	10^{-12} (m)
Femtometer	fm	1/1,000,000,000,000,000	0.000000000000001	10^{-15} (m)
Attometer	am	1/1,000,000,000,000,000,000	0.000000000000000001	10^{-18} (m)
Zeptometer	zm	1/1,000,000,000,000,000,000,000	0.000000000000000000001	10^{-21} (m)
Yoctometer	ym	1/1,000,000,000,000,000,000,000,000	0.000000000000000000000001	10^{-24} (m)

[a]Bold print indicates those metric system equivalents for length that are most frequently used.

Electron Volt Common Energy Designations

The abbreviation *eV* stands for *electron volt*; 1 eV is defined as the energy acquired by an electron when it is moved through a 1-V potential difference by a battery or some other mechanism.

The following terms designate various powers of 10 multiples of 1 eV:

1 KeV = 1000 eV = 10^{3} eV

1 MeV = 1,000,000 eV = 10^{6} eV

1 GeV = 1,000,000,000 eV = 10^{9} eV

The following terms designate various powers of 10 fractions of 1 eV:

$1\ meV = 0.001\ eV = 10^{-3}\ eV$

$1\ \mu eV = 0.000001\ eV = 10^{-6}\ eV$

$1\ neV = 0.000000001\ eV = 10^{-9}\ eV$

Common Frequency Spectrum Designations

The abbreviation *Hz* stands for *hertz,* which is the standard unit for frequency; 1 Hz is, by definition, equal to one repeatable cycle of a phenomenon or event (e.g., a water wave rising from flat to crest, descending to trough, and returning to flat) occurring in 1 second.

Ten hertz corresponds to 10 such cycles occurring every second, whereas 0.1 Hz corresponds to only 1/10th of a cycle occurring each second.

The following terms designate frequency ranges that constitute various powers of 10 multiples of 1 Hz:

$1\ KHz = 10^3\ Hz$

$1\ MHz = 10^6\ Hz$

$1\ GHz = 10^9\ Hz$

$1\ THz = 10^{12}\ Hz$

$1\ PHz = 10^{15}\ Hz$

$1\ EHz = 10^{18}\ Hz$

Periodic Table of Elements

Legend

- Z — Atomic number
- X — Chemical symbol
- M — Atomic weight

Metals
- Alkali metals
- Alkaline earth metals
- Transition metals
- Posttransition metals

Metalloids

Nonmetals
- Noble gases
- Halogens
- Other nonmetals

1	2	3	4	5	6	7	8	9	10	11	12	13	14	15	16	17	18
1 H 1.008																	**2 He** 4.003
3 Li 6.941	**4 Be** 9.012											**5 B** 10.81	**6 C** 12.01	**7 N** 14.01	**8 O** 16.00	**9 F** 19.00	**10 Ne** 20.18
11 Na 22.99	**12 Mg** 24.31											**13 Al** 26.98	**14 Si** 28.09	**15 P** 30.97	**16 S** 32.07	**17 Cl** 35.45	**18 Ar** 39.95
19 K 39.10	**20 Ca** 40.08	**21 Sc** 44.96	**22 Ti** 47.88	**23 V** 50.94	**24 Cr** 52.00	**25 Mn** 54.94	**26 Fe** 55.85	**27 Co** 58.93	**28 Ni** 58.69	**29 Cu** 63.55	**30 Zn** 65.39	**31 Ga** 69.72	**32 Ge** 72.64	**33 As** 74.92	**34 Se** 78.97	**35 Br** 79.90	**36 Kr** 83.79
37 Rb 85.47	**38 Sr** 87.62	**39 Y** 88.91	**40 Zr** 91.22	**41 Nb** 92.91	**42 Mo** 95.95	**43 Tc** (97)	**44 Ru** 101.1	**45 Rh** 102.9	**46 Pd** 106.4	**47 Ag** 107.9	**48 Cd** 112.4	**49 In** 114.8	**50 Sn** 118.7	**51 Sb** 121.8	**52 Te** 127.6	**53 I** 126.9	**54 Xe** 131.3
55 Cs 132.9	**56 Ba** 137.3	**57 La** 138.9	**72 Hf** 178.5	**73 Ta** 180.9	**74 W** 183.9	**75 Re** 186.2	**76 Os** 190.2	**77 Ir** 192.2	**78 Pt** 195.1	**79 Au** 197.0	**80 Hg** 200.5	**81 Tl** 204.4	**82 Pb** 207.2	**83 Bi** 209.0	**84 Po** (209)	**85 At** (210)	**86 Rn** (222)
87 Fr (223)	**88 Ra** (226)	**89 Ac** (227)	**104 Rf** (267)	**105 Db** (270)	**106 Sg** (269)	**107 Bh** (270)	**108 Hs** (270)	**109 Mt** (278)	**110 Ds** (281)	**111 Rg** (281)	**112 Cn** (285)	**113 Nh** (286)	**114 Fl** (289)	**115 Mc** (289)	**116 Lv** (293)	**117 Ts** (293)	**118 Og** (294)

Lanthanides

57 La 138.9	58 Ce 140.1	59 Pr 140.9	60 Nd 144.2	61 Pm (145)	62 Sm 150.4	63 Eu 152.0	64 Gd 157.2	65 Tb 158.9	66 Dy 162.5	67 Ho 164.9	68 Er 167.3	69 Tm 168.9	70 Yb 173.0	71 Lu 175.0

Actinides

89 Ac (227)	90 Th 232.0	91 Pa 231	92 U 238	93 Np (237)	94 Pu (244)	95 Am (243)	96 Cm (247)	97 Bk (247)	98 Cf (251)	99 Es (252)	100 Fm (257)	101 Md (258)	102 No (259)	103 Lr (262)

From Murray RL, Holbert KE: *Nuclear energy: an introduction to the concepts, systems, and applications of nuclear processes*, ed 8, Philadelphia, 2020, Elsevier.

Relationship Among Photons, Electromagnetic Waves, Wavelength, and Energy

Before 1900, all attempts to use current theories and concepts in physics to explain the measured energy distribution of radiation from a heated body failed grievously. In that year, a German physicist, Max Planck, introduced the concept of a "quantum," or discrete unit of energy, to resolve these discrepancies. According to Planck's theory, whenever radiation is emitted or absorbed by a hot object, the energy of that radiation is not emitted or absorbed continuously but rather in discrete amounts, which he called *quanta*.

Mathematically, a single such amount or energy quantum is given by the following equation:

$$E = hf$$

where f is the frequency of the radiation and h is a proportionality constant called, appropriately, *Planck's constant*. This quantum of energy has since received the name *photon*. Thus, the energy of a photon varies directly with the frequency of the associated radiation. Because the frequency f and the wavelength w of any type of radiation are related by the simple expression

$$c = fw$$

where c is the speed of light (300,000,000 m/sec in a vacuum), then

$$E = hf = hc/w$$

This result shows that the energy of a photon decreases as the wavelength of the radiation increases (e.g., photons of infrared light are less energetic than those of ultraviolet light because infrared wavelengths are longer than ultraviolet wavelengths). Einstein used these ideas to successfully explain the emission of electrons from a metallic surface when visible-light radiation was directed at it. This process is called the *photoelectric effect*. The incident light-produced electrons, or photoelectrons, were found to have *energies that depended on the wavelength of the focused light* but were completely independent of the intensity or brightness of that light. This phenomenon could not be explained by traditional physics. However, it was fully explicable in terms of the new concept of radiation energy (quanta or photons) and the energy relation given in the last equation. That relation contains *no reference to the brightness of the light* and, instead, shows that the incident light's energy, and consequently its ability to eject electrons from the metallic surface, is mainly dependent on the light's wavelength. For his work in this area, Einstein received the Nobel Prize in Physics in 1921.

To summarize, photons are the particles associated with the electromagnetic (EM) radiation spectrum (within which visible light and x-rays are included). When energy is transferred from an EM wave through interaction with matter, the energy is transferred by photons in discrete, or integral, amounts. Each such discrete amount is directly proportional to the frequency of the EM radiation or inversely proportional to its wavelength.

Electron Shell Structure of the Atom

Other than the hydrogen atom, all atoms contain more than one electron. The purpose of this appendix is to describe, without delving too extensively into the details of modern physics, specifically quantum mechanics, how electrons are arranged—that is, ordered—in multielectron atoms. To accomplish this, two discovered principles that serve as the foundations for this discussion must be introduced. These are, simply, that electrons in undisturbed or stable atoms are always distributed in the lowest overall energy configuration or energy states, and that no two electrons can ever occupy the exact same energy level (in more precise terminology, no two electrons in an atom can exist in the exact same quantum state). The latter restriction was postulated from careful analysis of observed atomic spectral lines by the German physicist Wolfgang Pauli in 1925 and has since been known as the *Pauli Exclusion Principle.*

Early in the 20th century, it was discovered that the distribution of electrons within an atom relative to the nucleus is not continuous or equally spaced but rather is specifically "discrete." This means that atomic electrons are not located in a uniform way about the nucleus as marbles in a bowl or stack up one right after the other according to distance from the nucleus. Rather it was determined that their "most probable" allowable locations are in certain concentric "shells" of limited capacity that radially fan out from the nucleus. The existence of these electron shells was first determined experimentally from x-ray absorption studies—that is, missing spectral lines (absent wavelengths or frequencies) that are observed as black segments in an atom's energy spectrum after a beam of x-rays is passed through samples of that atom or element. This has been found to be true for all elements. These missing wavelengths (w) or frequencies (f) are directly related to the energies of x-ray photons ($E = hf = hc/w$) that have been absorbed by the atoms within the target samples. Through examination of such spectra in detail, it became possible to map out the actual pattern of electron energy levels within various atoms. This led to a direct correlation between the Bohr solar system model of the atom, in which groups of electrons were believed to orbit the nucleus at certain distances, and the concept of electron shells that were formed by these orbiting electron groups. Each electron shell was associated with a particular orbital radius at which some electrons were *most likely* to be found. The smaller the radius, the more tightly these electrons held in their orbits about the nucleus, or in terms of energy, the greater their binding energy and, consequently, the effort needed to free them from the attraction of the nucleus. For electron groups or electron shells farther away from the nucleus, the binding energies progressively decreased with distance until one reached the outermost shell, in which electrons needed only a few electron volts of additional energy to escape the atom. These electrons are therefore the predominant category of atomic electrons removed by ionizing radiation and also, quite importantly, the electrons most often involved in chemical reactions. For this reason, they are given the special name "valence" electrons.

The electron shells were labeled in order of increasing distance from the nucleus with capital letters, beginning with the letter K, designating the innermost electron shell, and progressing through L, M, N, O, P, and Q. Again, from exhaustive spectral analysis, it was found that each electron shell except for the K shell was composed of multiple subshells labeled with lowercase letters s, p, d, f, g, h, and i, and these subshells were limited in the maximum number of electrons they could contain (s, 2; p, 6; d, 10; f, 14; g, 18; h, 22; i, 26). The theoretical rules that govern this are beyond the scope of this appendix. The following table demonstrates the electron shell occupancies for a number of atoms.

Atom	Atomic Number	Electron Shells	Electron Subshells and Electron Occupancy	
Hydrogen	1	K	s	1
Helium	2	K	s	2
Lithium	3	K	s	2
		L	s	1
Carbon	6	K	s	2
		L	s	2
			p	2
Oxygen	8	K	s	2
		L	s	2
			p	4
Sodium	11	K	s	2
		L	s	2
			p	6
		M	s	1
Argon	18	K	s	2
		L	s	2
			p	6
		M	s	2
			p	6
Calcium[a]	20	K	s	2
		L	s	2
			p	6
		M	s	2
			p	6
		N	s	2
Krypton	36	K	s	2
		L	s	2
			p	6
		M	s	2
			p	6
			d	10
		N	s	2
			p	6

[a]Because the electrons in an unexcited atom will always be arranged in the lowest overall energy configuration, there will be situations in which small subshells of higher shells will begin filling up before large subshells of lower shells are completely filled.

Compton Interaction

The principle of conservation of mass–energy is that for an isolated system (i.e., a system on which no external energy source or energy drain is active), the total mass plus energy of all the particles comprising the system remains constant. This restraint, however, does not prevent mass–energy transfers between individual particles within the system.

The *linear momentum* of a particle is defined as the product of its mass and its velocity. A photon, which is the particle associated with electromagnetic radiation, moves at the speed of light; consequently, according to Einstein's theory of relativity, a photon must be a massless entity. Because of the equivalence between mass, m, and energy, E, given by the famous relation,

$$E = mc^2$$

where c is the speed of light in a vacuum, one can associate with the photon a mass equivalent given by

$$E/c^2$$

Then the photon can be considered to have a linear momentum given by the product of the "mass equivalent" and the velocity of the photon.* The principle of conservation of linear momentum states that, for an isolated system, the sum of the linear momenta of all its particles is constant. Exchanges of linear momentum between particles within the system can, of course, occur.

The Compton interaction is, most simply, a billiard ball–like collision between an incident x-ray photon and the weakly bound outer electron of a target atom. Application of the principles of conservation of mass–energy and the conservation of linear momentum to the x-ray photon and outer electron system leads to equations that can be used to predict the energies and angles of scattering of both particles after their collision. If the energy of the incident photon is E, the following energy balance relation can be written:

$$E = E' + K$$

where E′ is the photon's energy after the collision and K is the recoil kinetic energy of the "struck" electron.

Several important types of Compton interactions will now be described. These effects depend on the magnitude of the photon's incident energy, E, and the angle at which the photon interacts with the electron.

Case 1: The photon makes a head-on collision with the electron

Result: The ejected electron travels or scatters directly forward, and the photon travels or scatters backward (180-degree scatter angle).

Energy Situations:

a. $E \ll 511$ keV (low energy range):
   E′ is approximately equal to E
   K is almost zero

b. $E = 511$ keV:
   E′ = E/3
   K = (2/3) E

c. $E \gg 511$ keV (high energy range):
   E′ is approximately zero
   K = E to good approximation

---

*Linear momentum = mass times velocity
Photon mass equivalent = E/c^2
Magnitude of photon velocity = speed of light, c
Photon linear momentum, p, therefore, is given by
$$\mathbf{p} = (E/c^2)\,(c) = \mathbf{E/c}$$
Since E = hc/w (see Appendix E), we can also write that
$$\mathbf{p} = E/c = (hc/w)/c = \mathbf{h/w}$$

Case 2: The photon grazes the electron

Result: The photon emerges from the collision nearly undeflected from its initial direction, and the struck outer electron scatters at right angles.

Energy situation result:

E' is approximately equal to E.

K is approximately zero.

Collisions of this nature, in which the incident photon loses little or no energy, are especially important in the planning of radiation shielding for therapeutic x-ray suites.

NCRP 10CFR Part 35.50 Training for Radiation Safety Officer and Associate Radiation Safety Officer

§ 35.50 TRAINING FOR RADIATION SAFETY OFFICER AND ASSOCIATE RADIATION SAFETY OFFICER

Except as provided in § 35.57, the licensee shall require an individual fulfilling the responsibilities of the Radiation Safety Officer or an individual assigned duties and tasks as an Associate Radiation Safety Officer as provided in § 35.24 to be an individual who—

(a) Is certified by a specialty board whose certification process has been recognized by the Commission or an Agreement State and who meets the requirements in paragraph (d) of this section. The names of board certifications that have been recognized by the Commission or an Agreement State are posted on the NRC's Medical Uses Licensee Toolkit web page. To have its certification process recognized, a specialty board shall require all candidates for certification to:

  (1) (i) Hold a bachelor's or graduate degree from an accredited college or university in physical science or engineering or biological science with a minimum of 20 college credits in physical science;

    (ii) Have 5 or more years of professional experience in health physics (graduate training may be substituted for no more than 2 years of the required experience) including at least 3 years in applied health physics; and

    (iii) Pass an examination administered by diplomates of the specialty board, which evaluates knowledge and competence in radiation physics and instrumentation, radiation protection, and mathematics pertaining to the use and measurement of radioactivity, radiation biology, and radiation dosimetry; or

  (2) (i) Hold a master's or doctor's degree in physics, medical physics, other physical science, engineering, or applied mathematics from an accredited college or university;

    (ii) Have 2 years of full-time practical training and/or supervised experience in medical physics—

      (A) Under the supervision of a medical physicist who is certified in medical physics by a specialty board recognized by the Commission or an Agreement State; or

      (B) In clinical nuclear medicine facilities providing diagnostic or therapeutic services under the direction of physicians who meet the requirements for authorized users in §§ 35.57, 35.290, or 35.390; and

    (iii) Pass an examination, administered by diplomates of the specialty board, that assesses knowledge and competence in clinical diagnostic radiological or nuclear medicine physics and in radiation safety; or

(b) (1) Has completed a structured educational program consisting of both:

    (i) 200 hours of classroom and laboratory training in the following areas—

      (A) Radiation physics and instrumentation;

      (B) Radiation protection;

      (C) Mathematics pertaining to the use and measurement of radioactivity;

      (D) Radiation biology; and

      (E) Radiation dosimetry; and

(ii) One year of full-time radiation safety experience under the supervision of the individual identified as the Radiation Safety Officer on a Commission or an Agreement State license or permit issued by a Commission master material licensee that authorizes similar type(s) of use(s) of byproduct material. An Associate Radiation Safety Officer may provide supervision for those areas for which the Associate Radiation Safety Officer is authorized on a Commission or an Agreement State license or permit issued by a Commission master material licensee. The full-time radiation safety experience must involve the following—

    (A) Shipping, receiving, and performing related radiation surveys;

    (B) Using and performing checks for proper operation of instruments used to determine the activity of dosages, survey meters, and instruments used to measure radionuclides;

    (C) Securing and controlling byproduct material;

    (D) Using administrative controls to avoid mistakes in the administration of byproduct material;

    (E) Using procedures to prevent or minimize radioactive contamination and using proper decontamination procedures;

    (F) Using emergency procedures to control byproduct material; and

    (G) Disposing of byproduct material; and

(2) This individual must obtain a written attestation, signed by a preceptor Radiation Safety Officer or Associate Radiation Safety Officer who has experience with the radiation safety aspects of similar types of use of byproduct material for which the individual is seeking approval as a Radiation Safety Officer or an Associate Radiation Safety Officer. The written attestation must state that the individual has satisfactorily completed the requirements in paragraphs (b)(1) and (d) of this section, and is able to independently fulfill the radiation safety-related duties as a Radiation Safety Officer or as an Associate Radiation Safety Officer for a medical use license; or

(c) (1) Is a medical physicist who has been certified by a specialty board whose certification process has been recognized by the Commission or an Agreement State under § 35.51(a), has experience with the radiation safety aspects of similar types of use of byproduct material for which the licensee seeks the approval of the individual as Radiation Safety Officer or an Associate Radiation Safety Officer, and meets the requirements in paragraph (d) of this section; or

(2) Is an authorized user, authorized medical physicist, or authorized nuclear pharmacist identified on a Commission or an Agreement State license, a permit issued by a Commission master material licensee, a permit issued by a Commission or an Agreement State licensee of broad scope, or a permit issued by a Commission master material license broad scope permittee, has experience with the radiation safety aspects of similar types of use of byproduct material for which the licensee seeks the approval of the individual as the Radiation Safety Officer or Associate Radiation Safety Officer, and meets the requirements in paragraph (d) of this section; or

(3) Has experience with the radiation safety aspects of the types of use of byproduct material for which the individual is seeking simultaneous approval both as the Radiation Safety Officer and the authorized user on the same new medical use license or new medical use permit issued by a Commission master material license. The individual must also meet the requirements in paragraph (d) of this section.

(d) Has training in the radiation safety, regulatory issues, and emergency procedures for the types of use for which a licensee seeks approval. This training requirement may be satisfied by completing training that is supervised by a Radiation Safety Officer, an Associate Radiation Safety Officer, authorized medical physicist, authorized nuclear pharmacist, or authorized user, as appropriate, who is authorized for the type(s) of use for which the licensee is seeking approval.

From the United States Nuclear Regulatory Commission, Washington, D.C. https://www.nrc.gov/reading-rm/doc-collections/cfr/part035/part035-0050.html.

Consumer-Patient Radiation Health and Safety Act of 1981*

SUBTITLE I—CONSUMER-PATIENT RADIATION HEALTH AND SAFETY ACT OF 1981

Short Title

[42 USC 10001.] note
SEC. 975. This subtitle may be cited as the "consumer-patient radiation health and safety act of 1981."

Statement of Findings

[42 USC 10001.]
SEC. 976. The congress finds that—
(1) it is in the interest of public health and safety to minimize unnecessary exposure to potentially hazardous radiation due to medical and dental radiologic procedures;
(2) it is in the interest of public health and safety to have a continuing supply of adequately educated persons and appropriate accreditation and certification programs administered by state governments;
(3) the protection of the public health and safety from unnecessary exposure to potentially hazardous radiation due to medical and dental radiologic procedures and the assurance of efficacious procedures are the responsibility of state and federal governments;
(4) persons who administer radiologic procedures, including procedures at federal facilities, should be required to demonstrate competence by reason of education, training, and experience; and

---

*Modified from Consumer-Patient Radiation Health and Safety Act of 1981, Chapter 107, Secs. 10001-8 (Aug. 13, 1981).

(5) the administration of radiologic procedures and the effect on individuals of such procedures have a substantial and direct effect on United States interstate commerce.

Statement of Purpose

[42 USC 10002.]
SEC. 977. It is the purpose of this subtitle to—
(1) provide for the establishment of minimum standards by the federal government for the accreditation of education programs for persons who administer radiologic procedures and for the certification of such persons; and
(2) ensure that medical and dental radiologic procedures are consistent with rigorous safety precautions and standards.

Definitions

[42 USC 10003.]
SEC. 978. Unless otherwise expressly provided, for purposes of this subtitle, the term—
(1) "radiation" means ionizing and nonionizing radiation in amounts beyond normal background levels from sources such as medical and dental radiologic procedures;
(2) "radiologic procedure" means any procedure or article intended for use in—
　(A) the diagnosis of disease or other medical or dental conditions in humans (including diagnostic X-rays or nuclear medicine procedures); or
　(B) the cure, mitigation, treatment, or prevention of disease in humans that achieves its intended purpose through the emission of radiation;

(3) "radiologic equipment" means any radiation electronic product that emits or detects radiation and is used or intended for use to—

    (A) diagnose disease or other medical or dental conditions (including diagnostic X-ray equipment); or

    (B) cure, mitigate, treat, or prevent disease in humans that achieves its intended purpose through the emission or detection of radiation;

(4) "practitioner" means any licensed doctor of medicine, osteopathy, dentistry, podiatry, or chiropractic who prescribes radiologic procedures for other persons;

(5) "persons who administer radiologic procedures" means any person, other than a practitioner, who intentionally administers radiation to other persons for medical purposes and includes medical radiologic technologists (including dental hygienists and assistants), radiation therapy technologists, and nuclear medicine technologists;

(6) "Secretary" means the Secretary of Health and Human Services; and

(7) "State" means the several states, the District of Columbia, the Commonwealth of Puerto Rico, the Commonwealth of the Northern Mariana Islands, the Virgin Islands, Guam, American Samoa, and the Trust Territory of the Pacific Islands.

Promulgation of Standards

[Regulation. 42 USC 10004.]
SEC. 979.

(a) Within 12 months after the date of enactment of this act, the Secretary, in consultation with the Radiation Policy Council, the Administrator of Veterans' Affairs, the Administrator of the Environmental Protection Agency, appropriate agencies of the States, and appropriate professional organizations, shall by regulation promulgate minimum standards for the accreditation of educational programs to train individuals to perform radiologic procedures. Such standards shall distinguish between programs for the education of (1) medical radiologic technologists (including radiographers), (2) dental auxiliaries (including dental hygienists and assistants), (3) radiation therapy technologists, (4) nuclear medicine technologists, and (5) such other kinds of health auxiliaries who administer radiologic procedures as the Secretary determines appropriate. Such standards shall not be applicable to educational programs for practitioners.

[Regulation.]

(b) Within 12 months after the date of enactment of this act, the Secretary, in consultation with the Radiation Policy Council, the Administrator of Veterans' Affairs, the Administrator of the Environmental Protection Agency, interested agencies of the States, and appropriate professional organizations, shall by regulation promulgate minimum standards for the certification of persons who administer radiologic procedures. Such standards shall distinguish between certification of (1) medical radiologic technologists (including radiographers), (2) dental auxiliaries (including dental hygienists and assistants), (3) radiation therapy technologists, (4) nuclear medicine technologists, and (5) such other kinds of health auxiliaries who administer radiologic procedures as the Secretary determines appropriate. Such standards shall include minimum certification criteria for individuals with regard to accredited education, practical experience, successful passage of required examinations, and such other criteria as the Secretary shall deem necessary for the adequate qualification of individuals to administer radiologic procedures. Such standards shall not apply to practitioners.

Model Statute

[42 USC 10005.]
SEC. 980. In order to encourage the administration of accreditation and certification programs by the states, the Secretary shall prepare and transmit to the states a model statute for radiologic procedure safety. Such model statute shall provide that—

(1) it shall be unlawful in a state for individuals to perform radiologic procedures unless such individuals are certified by the state to perform such procedures; and

(2) any educational requirements for certification of individuals to perform radiologic procedures shall be limited to educational programs accredited by the state.

Compliance

[42 USC 10006.]
SEC. 981.

(a) The Secretary shall take all actions consistent with law to effectuate the purposes of this subtitle.

(b) A state may utilize an accreditation or certification program administered by a private entity if—

  (1) such state delegates the administration of the state accreditation or certification program to such private entity;

  (2) such program is approved by the state; and

  (3) such program is consistent with the minimum federal standards promulgated under this subtitle for such program.

(c) Absent compliance by the states with the provisions of this subtitle within 3 years after the date of enactment of this act, the Secretary shall report to the Congress recommendations for legislative changes considered necessary to ensure the states' compliance with this subtitle.

[Report to Congress.]

(d) The Secretary shall be responsible for continued monitoring of compliance by the states with the applicable provisions of this subtitle and shall report to the Senate and the House of Representatives by January 1, 1982, and January 1 of each succeeding year the status of the states' compliance with the purposes of this subtitle.

(e) Notwithstanding any other provision of this section, in the case of a state that has, prior to the effective date of standards and guidelines promulgated pursuant to this subtitle, established standards for the accreditation of educational programs and certification of radiologic technologists, such state shall be deemed to be in compliance with the conditions of this section unless the Secretary determines, after notice and hearing, that such state standards do not meet the minimum standards prescribed by the Secretary or are inconsistent with the purposes of this subtitle.

Federal Radiation Guidelines

[42 USC 10007.]

SEC. 982. The Secretary shall, in conjunction with the Radiation Policy Council, the Administrator of Veterans' Affairs, the Administrator of the Environmental Protection Agency, appropriate agencies of the states, and appropriate professional organizations, promulgate Federal radiation guidelines with respect to radiologic procedures. Such guidelines shall—

(1) determine the level of radiation exposure due to radiologic procedures that are unnecessary and specify the techniques, procedures, and methods to minimize such unnecessary exposure;

(2) provide for the elimination of the need for retakes of diagnostic radiologic procedures;

(3) provide for the elimination of unproductive screening programs;

(4) provide for the optimum diagnostic information with minimum radiologic exposure; and

(5) include the therapeutic application of radiation to individuals in the treatment of disease, including nuclear medicine applications.

Applicability to Federal Agencies

[42 USC 10008.]

SEC. 983.

(a) Except as provided in subsection (b), each department, agency, and instrumentality of the executive branch of the federal government shall comply with standards promulgated pursuant to this subtitle.

[Regulations.]

[38 USC 101 *et seq.*]

(b) (1) The Administrator of Veterans' Affairs, through the Chief Medical Director of the Veterans' Administration, shall, to the maximum extent feasible consistent with the responsibilities of such Administrator and Chief Medical Director under subtitle 38, United States Code, prescribe regulations making the standards promulgated pursuant to this subtitle applicable to the provision of radiologic procedures in facilities over which the Administrator has jurisdiction. In prescribing and implementing regulations pursuant to this subsection, the Administrator shall consult with the Secretary in order to achieve the maximum possible coordination of the regulations, standards, and guidelines, and the implementation thereof, which the Secretary and the Administrator prescribe under this subtitle.

[Report to congressional committees.]

(2) Not later than 180 days after standards are promulgated by the Secretary pursuant to this subtitle, the Administrator of Veterans' Affairs shall submit to the appropriate committees of Congress a full report with respect to the regulations (including guidelines, policies, and

procedures thereunder) prescribed pursuant to paragraph (1) of this subsection. Such report shall include—

(A) an explanation of any inconsistency between standards made applicable by such regulations and the standards promulgated by the Secretary pursuant to this subtitle;

(B) an account of the extent, substance, and results of consultations with the Secretary respecting the prescription and implementation of regulations by the Administrator; and

(C) such recommendations for legislation and administrative action as the Administrator determines are necessary and desirable.

[Publication in Federal Register.]

(3) The Administrator of Veterans' Affairs shall publish the report required by paragraph (2) in the Federal Register.

REFERENCES

CHAPTER 1

1. Leasure EL, Jones RR, Meade LB, et al.: There is no "i" in teamwork in the patient-centered medical home: defining teamwork competencies for academic practice, *Acad Med* 88(5):585–592, 2013.
2. Interprofessional Education Collaborative Expert Panel: *Core competencies for interprofessional collaborative practice: report of an expert panel,* Washington, DC, 2011. https://ipecollaborative.org/uploads/IPEC-2016-Updated-Core-Competencies-Report_final_release_.PDF.
3. Sexton JB, Thomas EJ, Helmreich RL: Error, stress, and teamwork in medicine and aviation: cross sectional surveys, *Br Med J* 320:745, 2000.
4. Havyer RDA, Wingo MT, Comfere NI, et al.: Teamwork assessment in internal medicine, *J Gen Intern Med* 29(6):894–910, 2014.
5. Kohn LT, Corigan JM, Donaldson MS, editors: *To err is human: building a safer health system*, Washington, DC, 1999, National Academies Press.
6. Health Risks from Exposure to Low Levels of Ionizing Radiation, BEIR VII PHASE 2, Committee to Assess Health Risks from Exposure to Low Levels of Ionizing Radiation, Board on Radiation Effects Research, Division on Earth and Life Studies, National Research Council of The National Academies, The National Academies Press, Washington, DC.
7. Gollnick DA: *Basic radiation protection technology*, ed 6, Altadena, CA, 2011, Pacific Radiation Corporation.
8. National Council on Radiation Protection and Measurements (NCRP): *Research needs for radiation protection, report No. 117*, Bethesda, MD, 1993, NCRP, pp 51.
9. Ng K-H, Cameron JR: Using the BERT concept to promote understanding of radiation, International conference on the radiological protection of patients organized by the International Atomic Energy Agency, Malaga, Spain, 2011, C&S Paper Series 7/P, Austria, Vienna, pp 784–787.
10. Preston DL, Cullings H, Suyama A, et al.: Solid cancer incidence in atomic bomb survivors exposed in utero or as young children, *J Natl Cancer Inst* 100:428, 2008.
11. Doody MM, Lonstein JE, Stovall M, et al.: Breast cancer mortality after diagnostic radiography: findings from the U.S. Scoliosis Cohort Study, *Spine* 25:2052, 2000.
12. National Academy of Sciences Committee on Biological Effects of Ionizing Radiation: *Report VII: health risks from exposure to low levels of ionizing radiation*, Washington, DC, 2005, National Academy Press.
13. The Joint Commission. http://www.jointcommission.org/diagnosticimaging-standards/.
14. Nationwide Evaluation of X-Ray Trends (NEXT). http://www.fda.gov/radiation-emittingproducts/radiationsafety/nationwideevaluationofx-raytrendsnext/default.htm.
15. Conference of Radiation Control Program Directors (CRCPD). http://crcpt.org/contact_information.aspx.
16. Hausleiter J, Meyer T, Hermann F, et al.: Estimated radiation dose associated with cardiac CT angiography, *JAMA* 301(5):500–507, 2009.
17. Hricak H, Brenner DJ, Adelstein SJ, et al.: Managing radiation use in medical imaging: a multifaceted challenge, *Radiology* 258(3):889–905, 2011.
18. Image Wisely Website Guide to Diagnostic Reference Levels. http://www.imagewisely.oirg/~/media/ImageWisely%20Files/Medical%20Physicist%20Articles/IW%20McCullough%20Diagnostic%20Reference%20Levels.pdf.
19. American College of Radiology. http://www.ncradiation.net/xray/documents/acrreflevelsfluoro.pdf.
20. Lång K, Josefsson V, Larsson A, et al.: Artificial intelligence-supported screen reading versus standard double reading in the mammography screening with artificial intelligence trial (MASAI): a clinical safety analysis of a randomized, controlled, non-inferiority, single-blinded, screening accuracy study, *Lancet Oncol* 24(8):936–944, 2023.

CHAPTER 2

1. Environmental Protection Agency: Ionizing and nonionizing radiation. http://www.epa.gov/radiation/understand/.
2. Bushong SC: *Radiologic science for technologists: physics, biology, and protection*, ed 11, St. Louis, 2017, Elsevier.
3. Broadhead B: *The health effects of radon in layman's terms*, 2008, WPB Enterprises, Inc.
4. Broadhead B: *Thoron measurements and health risk*, 2008, WPB Enterprises, Inc.
5. Read AB: Radon gas: the invisible threat, *RT Image*, 1992 5(12).
6. National Council on Radiation Protection and Measurements (NCRP): *Exposure of the population in the United*

States and Canada from natural background radiation, Washington, DC, 1987, NCRP Report No. 94.

7. News Release: *Surgeon general release national health advisory on radon*, 2005. https://adph.org/radon/assets/surgeon.general.radon.pdf.

8. National Aeronautics and Space Administration (NASA): *Solar flares*, 2012. http://solarscience.msfc.nasa.gov/flares.shtml.

9. Pratt L, Strekel A: Prepare for take-off: the risk of cosmic radiation associated with air travel, *RT Image*, 2007 20(34).

10. National Council on Radiation Protection and Measurements (NCRP): *Ionizing radiation exposure of the population of the United States*, Bethesda, MD, 1987, NCRP Report No. 93.

11. Cusick M: *40 years after a partial nuclear meltdown, a new push to keep Three Mile Island open*, 2019, North County Public Radio.

12. Geraghty J: *What separates Chernobyl from Three Mile Island and Fukushima*, 2019. National Review, The Corner. https://www.nationalreview.com/corner/what-separateschernobyl-from-three-mile-island-and—fukushima/.

13. United States Nuclear Regulatory Commission, NRC: *Three Mile Island—Unit 2"*, https://www.nrc.gov.

14. Sholtis B: *Three Mile Island nuclear power plant shuts down*, 2019, *National Public Radio*.

15. Putting a lid on Chernobyl. http://www.washingtonpost.com/wp-dyn/article/A49461-2002Dec28.htm.l

16. Chernobyl: The end of a three-decade experiment, BBC News, Science & Environment, February 14, 2019. https://bbc.com/news/science-enviroment-47227767.

17. *Fifteen years after the Chernobyl accident: lessons learned*, Executive Summary, Kiev, April 2001.

18. Swiss Agency for Development Cooperation, Chernobyl. info. https://www.chernobyl.info/.

19. World Health Organization: *Health risk assessment from the nuclear accident after the 2011 great East Japan earthquake and tsunami based on a preliminary dose estimation*, 2013, World Health Organization.

20. World Health Organization: *Health effects of the Chernobyl accident: an overview*, Fact Sheet No. 303, April 2006. http://www.who.int/ionizing_radiation/chernobyl/backgrounder/en/index.html.

21. Chesser RK, Baker RJ: Growing up with Chernobyl, *Am Sci* 94(6):542–549, 2006.

22. Stone R: Living in the shadow of Chernobyl, *Science* 292:420, 2001.

23. Walker SJ: *Permissible dose: a history of radiation protection in the twentieth century*, Berkeley, 2000, University of California Press.

24. Otto Hug Strahleninstit: Information, Ausgabe 9/2001 K, 2001.

25. Chernobyl Children's Project International. https://www.chernobyl-international.org/documents/chernobylfacts2.pdf.

26. : Conclusions of 3rd international conference, health effects of the Chernobyl accident, *Int J Radiation Med* 3:3–4, 2001.

27. Romanenko A, Bebeshko V, Hatch M, et al.: The Ukrainian-American study of leukemia and related disorders among Chornobyl cleanup workers from Ukraine: I. Study methods, *Radiat Res* 170(6):691–697, 2008.

28. Batts V, *The Fukushima legacy: More than just cancer, diabetes diagnoses have increased six-fold*, 2018. https://fukushima.news/2018-05-07-fukushima-more-thancancer-diabetes-diagnoses-have-increased-six-fold.html.

29. Nova: *Japan's killer quake, An eyewitness account and investigation of the epic earthquake, tsunami, and nuclear crisis*. Aired on February 29, 2012, on PBS, originally aired March 30, 2011. http://www.pbs.org/wgbh/nova/earth/japan-killer-quake.html.

30. Myixler E: *Japan acknowledges first radiation-linked death from the Fukushima nuclear disaster*, September 6, 2018, Time.com.

31. Ionizing radiation, Frequently asked questions on health risk assessment. 2013. www.who.int/ionizing_radiation/pub_meet/faqs_fukushima_risk_assessment/en/.

32. Becker R: *Robot squeezes suspected nuclear fuel debris in Fukushima reactor*. The Verge.com, February 15, 2019. https://www.theverge.com/2019/2/15/18225233/robotnuclear-fuel-debris-fukushima-reactor-japan.

33. National Council on Radiation Protection and Measurements (NCRP): *Medical radiation exposure of patients in the United States*, Bethesda, MD, 2019, NCRP Report No. 184.

CHAPTER 3

1. Bohren CF, Fraser AB: Colors of the sky, *Phys Teach* 23:267–272, 1985.

CHAPTER 4

1. National Council on Radiation Protection and Measurements (NCRP): *Limitation of exposure to ionizing radiation*, Report No. 116, Bethesda, MD, 1993, NCRP.

2. Sprawls P: Radiation quantities and units, sprawls educational foundation. The physical principles of medical imaging online. http://www.sprawls.org/ppmi2/RADQU/.

3. Carlton RR, Adler AM, Balac V: *Principles of radiographic imaging: an art and a science*, ed 6, New York, 2019, Cengage Learning.
4. The 2007 Recommendations of the International Commission on Radiological Protection, ICRP publication 103, *ICRP* 37:2–4, 2007.

CHAPTER 5

1. National Human Genome Research Institute: *The human genome project*, 2019. https://www.genome.gov/human-genome-project.
2. Ventner JC: The sequence of the human genome, *Science* 291:1304–1351, 2001.
3. NIH Fact Sheet. https://www.nigms.nih.gov/education/fact-sheets/Pages/studying-cells.aspx
4. National Library of Medicine. https://ghr.nlm.nih.gov/primer/therapy/genotherapy, 2019.
5. Stöppler MC: Electrolytes. https://www.medicinenet.com/electrolytes/article.htm, 2019.
6. Dowd SB, Tilson ER: *Practical radiation protection and applied radiobiology*, ed 2, Philadelphia, PA, 1999, Saunders.

CHAPTER 6

1. Bushong SC: *Radiologic science for technologists: physics, biology, and protection*, ed 11, St. Louis, 2017, Elsevier.
2. Forshier S: *Essentials of radiation biology and protection*, Albany, NY, 2002, Delmar.
3. Hall EJ: *Radiobiology for the radiologist*, ed 5, Philadelphia, 2000, Lippincott Williams & Wilkins.
4. Travis EL: *Primer of medical radiobiology*, ed 2, Chicago, 1989, Mosby.
5. Puck TT, Marcus PI: Action of x-rays on mammalian cells, *J Exp Med* 103:653, 1956.
6. Bergonié J, Tribondeau L: De quelquesrésultats de la radiothérapie et assai de fixation d'une technique rationelle, *CR Acad Sci (Paris)* 143:983, 1906.
7. United Nations Scientific Committee on the Effects of Atomic Radiation (UNSCEAR): Ionizing radiation sources and biologic effects, Report E.82.IX.8. New York, 1992, United Nations.
8. International Commission on Radiological Protection (ICRP): Non-stochastic effects of ionizing radiation, ICRP Publication No. 41. Oxford, 1984, Pergamon.
9. Upton AR: Cancer induction and non-stochastic effects, *Br J Radiol* 60:1, 1987.
10. Lushbaugh CC, Ricks RC: Some cytokinetic and histopathologic consideration of irradiated male and female gonadal tissue. In Vath JM, editor: . Basel, 1972, Karger.
11. Lushbaugh CC, Casarett GW: The effects of gonadal irradiation in clinical radiation therapy: a review, *Cancer* 37:1111, 1976.

CHAPTER 7

1. Finch SC: Acute radiation syndrome, *JAMA* 258:666, 1987.
2. Gale RP: Immediate medical consequences of nuclear accidents: lessons from Chernobyl, *JAMA* 258:625, 1987.
3. Perry AR, Iglar AF: The accident at Chernobyl: radiation doses and effects, *Radiol Technol* 61:290, 1990.
4. Linnemann RE: Soviet medical response to Chernobyl nuclear accident, *JAMA* 258:639, 1987.
5. Bushong SC: *Radiologic science for technologists: physics, biology and protection*, ed 11, St. Louis, 2017, Elsevier.
6. Fry RJM: Acute radiation effects. In Wagner LK, Fabrikant JI, Fry RJM, editors: *Radiation bioeffects and management: test and syllabus*, Reston, VA, 1991, American College of Radiology.
7. American Academy of Oral and Maxillofacial Radiology. Biography of Herbert Rollins. 2005 https://www.aaomr.org/index.php?option=com_content&view=article&id=112:william-h-rollins-award&catid=32:awards-abstracts.
8. New York Times, Volunteer Around the U.S. Submitted to Radiation, October 24, 1986, Section A, Page 20. https://www.nytimes.com/1986/10/24/us/volunteers-around-us-submitted-to-radiation.html.
9. Advisory Committee on Human Radiation Experiments (ACHRE) report: Chapter 9: The Oregon and Washington experiments. http://www.hss.energy.gov/healthsafety/ohre/roadmap/achre/chap9_2.html, 1994.
10. Forshier S: *Essentials of radiation biology and protection*, Albany, NY, 2002, Delmar.
11. Sigurdson AJ, Bhatti P, Preston DL, et al.: Routine diagnostic x-ray examinations and increased frequency of chromosome translocations among U.S. radiologic technologists, *Cancer Res* 68:8825, 2008. http://www.ncbi.nlm.nih.gov/pubmed/18974125.
12. University of Minnesota, Health ScienceSection: U.S. Radiologic Technologists Study2, Minneapolis, 2004, University of Minnesota.
13. University of Minnesota, Health Studies Section: *U.S. Radiologic Technologists Study*. https://www.radtechstudy.org, 2020.
14. M'kacher R, Violot D, Aubert B, et al.: Premature chromosome condensation associated with fluorescence in situ hybridization detects cytogenic abnormalities after a CT scan: evaluation of the low-dose effect, *Radiat Prot Dosimetry* 103:35, 2003.
15. Sakane H, Ishida M, Shi L, et al.: Biological effects of low-dose chest CT on chromosomal DNA, *Radiology* 295:439–445, 2020.

CHAPTER 8

1. Travis EL: *Primer of medical radiobiology,* ed 2, Chicago, 1989, Mosby.
2. Straume T, Dobson RL: Implications of new Hiroshima and Nagasaki dose estimates: cancer risks and neutron RBE, *Health Phys* 41:666, 1981.
3. Webster EW: *Critical issues in setting radiation dose limits, Proceedings No. 3,* Washington, DC, 1982, National Council on Radiation Protection and Measurements (NCRP).
4. Hendee WR, editor: *Health effects of low-level radiation,* Norwalk, CT, 1984, Appleton-Century-Crofts.
5. Health Physics Society. Doses from medical x-ray procedures. http://hps.org/physicians/documents/Doses_from_Medical_X-Ray_Procedures.pdf, 2021.
6. International Commission on Radiological Protection (ICRP): Recommendations of the International Commission on Radiological Protection, ICRP publication No. 60, *Ann ICRP* 21:1–3, 1991.
7. National Research Council, Commission of Life Sciences, Committee on Biological Effects on Ionizing Radiation (BEIR V), Board on Radiation Effects Research: *Health effects of exposure to low levels of ionizing radiations,* Washington, DC, 1989, National Academies Press.
8. Tilke B: Navajo miners battle long-term effects of radiation, *Adv Radiol Technol* 3:3, 1990.
9. Berrington de Gonzalez A, Ntowe E, Kitahara CM, et al.: Long-term mortality in 43,763 U.S. radiologists compared with 64,990 U.S. psychiatrists, *Radiology* 381(3):847–857, 2016.
10. Dowd SB, Tilson ER: *Practical radiation protection and applied radiobiology,* ed 2, Philadelphia, 1999, Saunders.
11. Sinclair WK: Radiation protection recommendations on dose limits: the role of the NCRP and the ICRP and future developments, *Int J Radiat Oncol Biol Phys* 131:387–392, 1995.
12. Hall EJ: *Radiobiology for the radiologist,* ed 5, Philadelphia, 2000, Lippincott Williams & Wilkins.
13. Bushong SC: *Radiologic science for technologists: physics, biology and protection,* ed 11, St. Louis, 2017, Elsevier.
14. WGBH Transcript: *Back to Chernobyl,* Nova No. 1604, Boston, 1989 (television program originally broadcast on PBS on February 14, 1989).
15. Balter M: Children become the first victims of fallout, *Science* 272:357, 1996.
16. United Nations Scientific Committee on the Effects of Atomic Radiation (UNSCEAR): 2000 report to the General Assembly, with Scientific Annexes, UNSCEAR 2000: *sources and effects of ionizing radiation,* New York, 2000, United Nations.
17. Williams N: Leukemia studies continue to draw a blank, *Science* 272:358, 1996.
18. University of Minnesota, Health Studies Section *U.S. radiologic technologists study* 2, 2004, Minneapolis.
19. University of Minnesota, Health Studies Section: *U.S. radiologic technologists study,* 2020. www.radtechstudy.org.
20. Bouffler S, Ainsbury E, Gilvin P, Harrison J: Radiation-induced cataracts: the Health Protection Agency's response to the ICRP statement on tissue reactions and recommendation on the dose limit for the eye lens, *J Radiol Prot* 32(4):479–488, 2012.
21. International Commission on Radiological Protection, *Statement on tissue reactions,* ICRP ref. 4825-3093-1464, April 21, 2011.
22. Stewart A, et al.: A survey of childhood malignancies, *Br Med J* 1:1495, 1958.
23. Otto Hug Strahleninstit: Information, Ausgabe 9/2001 K 2001.
24. International Atomic Energy Agency. Frequently asked Chernobyl questions. https://www.iaea.org/newscenter/focus/chernobyl/faqs.
25. United Nations Scientific Committee on the Effects of Atomic Radiation (UNSCEAR): *Biological effects of prenatal irradiation, 35th session of UNSCEAR, Vienna, April 1986, New York,* 1986, United Nations.
26. Webster EW the Biological Effects Committee of the American Association of Physicists in Medicine (AAPM): *A primer on low-level ionizing radiation and its biological effects, AAPM Report No. 18, New York,* 1986, American Institute of Physics (published for the American Association of Physicists in Medicine).
27. Crow JF: Genetic effects of radiation, *Bull At Sci* 14:19, 1958.

CHAPTER 9

1. International Commission on Radiological Protection (ICRP): ICRP: *structure and organization.* http://www.icrp.org, 2021.
2. National Council on Radiation Protection and Measurements (NCRP): *Background information.* https://www.ncrp.com/info.html, 2015.
3. National Council on Radiation Protection and Measurements (NCRP): *Ionizing radiation exposure of the population of the United States,* Bethesda, MD, 2009, NCRP report no. 160.
4. National Council on Radiation Protection and Measurements (NCRP): *Medical radiation exposure of patients in the United States,* Bethesda, MD, 2019, NCRP report no. 184.

5. FDA White Paper: *Initiative to reduce unnecessary radiation exposure from medical imaging*, 2010, Center for Devices and Radiological Health, U.S. Food and Drug Administration. http://www.fda.gov/Radiation-EmittingProducts/RadiationSafety/RadiationDoseReduction/ucm199994.htm.

6. Recommendations of the International Commission on Radiological Protection. ICRP Publication 26, http://www.icrp.org, Ann ICRP 1977.

7. 1990 Recommendations of the International Commission on Radiological Protection. ICRP Publication 60, http://www.icrp.org, Ann ICRP 1991.

8. ICRP 118—*ICRP statement on tissue reactions/early and late effects of radiation in normal tissues and organs—threshold doses for tissue reactions in a radiation protection context*, ICRP Publication 118, Ann ICRP 41 (1/2), 2012.

9. NCRP 168—*radiation dose management for fluoroscopically guided interventional procedures*, NCRP Report No. 168, 2010, National Council on Radiation Protection and Measurements, www.ncrponline.org.

10. NCRP Statement 11—*outline of administrative policies for quality assurance and peer review of tissue reactions associated with fluoroscopically guided interventions*, NCRP Statement No. 11, 2014, National Council on Radiation Protection and Measurements, www.ncrppublications.org.

11. National Council on Radiation Protection and Measurements (NCRP): *Basic radiation protection criteria*, Washington, DC, 1971, NCRP report no. 39.

12. National Council on Radiation Protection and Measurements (NCRP): *Recommendations on limits for exposure to ionizing radiation*, Bethesda, MD, 1987, NCRP report no. 91.

13. Committee on Biological Effects of Ionizing Radiation, National Research Council, Commission of Life Sciences, Board of Radiation Research: *Health effects of exposure to low levels of ionizing radiation (BEIR V Report)*, Washington, DC, 1989, National Academies Press.

14. Doss M: Linear no-threshold model vs. radiation hormesis, *Dose Response* 11:480–497, 2013.

15. Doss M: Shifting the paradigm in radiation safety, *Dose Response* 10:562–583, 2012.

16. See References 14 and 15.

17. Feinendegen LE, et al.: Hormesis by low dose radiation effects: low dose cancer risk modelling must recognize up-regulation of protection. In Baum RP, editor: *Therapeutic nuclear medicine*, Berlin, 2013, Springer.

18. Boice J: Health Physics Society News, 2014. http://ncrponline.org/wp-content/themes/ncrp/PDFs/BOICE-HPnews/24_The_Eyes_Have_It_May2014.pdf

CHAPTER 10

1. Bushong SC: *Radiologic science for technologists: physics, biology and protection*, ed 11, St. Louis, 2017, Elsevier.

2. Long BW, Rollins JH, ed 13Smith BJ: Merrill's atlas of radiographic positioning and procedures1, St. Louis, 2016, Elsevier.

3. Carlton RR, Adler AM: *Principles of radiographic imaging: an art and a science*, ed 5, Albany, NY, 2013, Delmar Cengage Learning.

4. Kebart RC, James CD: Benefits of increasing focal film distance, *Radiol Technol* 62:434, 1991.

5. National Council on Radiation Protection and Measurements (NCRP): *Medical x-ray, electron beam and gamma ray protection for energies up to 50 MeV: equipment design, performance, and use, Report No. 102*, Bethesda, MD, 1989, NCRP.

6. Bushong SC: *Radiologic science for technologists: physics, biology and protection*, ed 8, St. Louis, 2004, Mosby.

7. Johnston JN, Fauber TL: *Essentials of radiographic physics and imaging*, ed 3, St. Louis, 2020, Elsevier.

8. Seeram E: Digital image processing, *Radiol Technol* 75:6, 2004.

9. Cullinan AM, Cullinan JE: *Producing quality radiographs*, ed 2, Philadelphia, PA, 1994, Lippincott.

10. Seibert JA. appliedradiology.com/digital-radiography-the-bottom-line-comparison-of-cr-and-dr-technology, 2009.

11. Office of the Federal Register: *Federal register August 15, 1972 (37 FR 16461)*, Washington, DC, 1972, U.S. Government Printing Office.

CHAPTER 11

1. Dutton AG, Ryan T: *Torres'patient care in imaging technology*, ed 9, Philadelphia, 2019, Wolters Kluwer.

2. American Association of Physicists in Medicine (AAPM): *Position statement on the use of patient gonadal and fetal shielding*, 2019, AAPM. Policy 32-A. https://www.aapm.org/org/policies/details.asp?id=468&typr=PP.

3. Bushong SC: *Radiologic science for technologists: physics, biology and protection*, ed 11, St. Louis, 2017, Elsevier.

4. DeMaio DN, Herrmann T, Noble LB, et al.: *White paper: best practices in digital radiography*, 2019, American Society of Radiologic Technologists. https://www.asrt.org/docs/default-source/research/whitepapers/asrt12.

5. Gray J, Winkler NT, Stears J, et al.: *Quality control in diagnostic imaging*, 2002, Medical Physics Publishing AAPM Report No. 74.

6. Hendee WR, Chaney EL, Rossi RP: *Radiologic physics equipment and quality control*, Chicago, IL, 1977, Mosby.

7. McKinney W: *Radiographic processing and quality control*, Philadelphia, PA, 1995, Lippincott.

8. Carter CE, Veale BL: *Digital radiology and PACS, ed 3*, St. Louis, MO, 2010, Elsevier.

9. Hofmann B, Rosanowsky TB, Jensen C, et al.: Image rejects in general direct digital radiography, *Acta Radiol Open*, 2015 4 2058460115604339.

10. American College of Radiology: *Chest x-rays before surgery: when you need one and when you don't*, 2016. https://www.choosingwisely.org/patient-resources/chest-x-rays-before-surgery/.

11. Haynes K, Curtis T: Fluoroscopic vs. blind positioning: comparing entrance skin exposure, *Radiol Technol* 81:1, 2009.

12. American Society of Radiologic Technologists: *ASRT organizational issues: fluoroscoping for positioning*, 2019. http://www.org/docs/governance/hodpositionstatements66FE1F374C63.pdf.

13. American Registry of Radiologic Technologists: *ARRT standards of ethics*, 2020. http://org/pdfs/Governing-Documents/Standards-of-Ethics.pdf.

14. Adler A, Carlton R, Wold B: An analysis of radiographic repeat and reject rates, *Radiol Technol* 63:308, 1992.

15. Leeming BW, Hames OS, Gould RG, et al.: A comparison of fluoroscopically controlled patient positioning and conventional positioning, including comparative dosimetry, *Radiology* 124:231, 1977.

16. Reynold FB: Prepared remarks for the October 20, 1976. In *American college of radiology press conference*.

17. National Council on Radiation Protection and Measurements (NCRP): *Medical x-ray, electron beam and gamma-ray protection up to 50 MeV (equipment design, performance and use)*, Bethesda, MD, 1989, NCRP Report No. 102.

18. National Council on Radiation Protection and Measurements (NCRP): *Medical exposure of pregnant and potentially pregnant women*, Washington, DC, 1977, NCRP Report No. 54.

19. Ozasa K, Shimizu Y, Suyama A, et al.: Studies of the mortality of atomic bomb survivors, report 14, 1950–2003: an overview of cancer and noncancer diseases, *Radiat Res* 177(3):229–243, 2012.

20. National Council on Radiation Protection and Measurements (NCRP): *Radiation protection in pediatric radiology*, Washington, DC, 1981, NCRP Report No. 68.

21. Lampignano J, Kendrick L: *Bontrager's textbook of positioning and related anatomy, ed 9*, St. Louis, MO, 2016, Elsevier.

22. Alliance for Radiation Safety in Pediatric Imaging, 2019. https://www.imagegently.org/About-Us/The-Alliance.

23. Black DM: DXA imaging in nontypical populations, *Radiol Technol* 89(4):371–387, 2018.

24. Berry ME: Nonroutine DXA scanning, *Radiol Technol* 90(1):68–75, 2018.

25. AlgaeCal Inc. *What is a bone density test?* 2002–2019. https://www.algaecal.com/osteoporosis-treatment/dexa-scan/.

26. Berry ME: Using DXA to identify and treat osteoporosis in pediatric patients, *Radiol Technol* 89(3):312–321, 2018.

CHAPTER 12

1. National Council on Radiation Protection and Measurements (NCRP): *Limitation of exposure to ionizing radiation, Report No. 116*, Bethesda, MD, 1993, NCRP.

2. Bushong SC: *Radiologic science for technologists: physics, biology and protection, ed 10*, St. Louis, 2013, Elsevier.

3. Femia J: It pays off in safety to know your C-arm, *Adv Imaging Radiat Ther Prof*, 2007 20(19).

4. Marx MV: *Interventional procedures: risks to patients and personnel, in radiation risk*, Reston, VA, 1996, American College of Radiology Commission on Physics and Radiation Safety.

5. Center for Devices and Radiological Health, U.S. Food and Drug Administration: White paper: Association for Medical Imaging Management, 2011.

6. National Council on Radiation Protection and Measurements (NCRP): *Structural shielding design for medical x-ray imaging facilities, Report No. 147*, Bethesda, MD, 2004, NCRP.

7. National Council on Radiation Protection and Measurements (NCRP): *Structural shielding design and evaluation for medical use of x-rays and gamma rays with energies up to 10 meV, Report No. 49*, Washington DC, 1976, NCRP.

8. Conference of Radiation Control Program Directors. Suggested State Regulations for Control of Radiation. http://www.crcpd.org/page/SSRCRs.

CHAPTER 13

1. Landauer, Inc, Glenwood, IL. http://www.landauer.com.

2. Wernli C, Kahilainen J: Direct ion storage dosimetry systems for photons, beta, and neutron radiation with instant readout capabilities, radiation protection dosimetry, *Nucl Technol* 96(1–3):255–259, 2001.

3. Kiuru A, Hahilainen H, Vartiainen E: Comparison between direct ion storage and thermoluminescence dosimetry individual monitoring systems, and internet reporting. radiation protection dosimetry, *Nuc Technol* 96(1–3):231–233, 2001.

4. Gollnick DA: *Basic radiation protection technology, ed 4*, Altadena, CA, 2000, Pacific Radiation Corporation.

5. Frame P: *The nicknames of early survey meters*, Oak Ridge, TN, 1999, Oak Ridge Associated Universities.

http://www.orau.org/ptp/collection/surveymeters/nicknamessurveymeters.htm.

REFERENCES **379**

CHAPTER 14

1. Long BW, et al: *Merrill's atlas of radiographic positioning and procedures* (vol 3). ed 13, St. Louis, 2016, Elsevier/ Mosby.
2. Schimmöller L, et al.: Evaluation of automated attenuation-based tube potential selection in combination with organ-specific dose reduction for contrast-enhanced chest CT examinations, *Clin Radiol* 69:721–726, 2014.
3. Leswick DA, et al.: Thyroid shields versus z-axis automatic tube current modulation for dose reduction at neck CT, *Radiology* 249:572–580, 2008.
4. Servaes S, Zhu X: The effects of bismuth breast shields in conjunction with automatic tube current modulation in CT imaging, *Pediatr Radiol* 43:1287–1294, 2013.
5. Shuman WP, et al.: Model-based iterative reconstruction versus adaptive statistical iterative reconstruction and filtered back projection in liver 64-MDCT: focal lesion detection, lesion conspicuity, and image noise, *AJR Am J Roentgenol* 200(5):1071–1076, 2013.
6. Kanal KM, et al.: Impact of operator-selected image noise index and reconstruction slice thickness on patient radiation dose in 64-MDCT, *AJR* 189(1):219–225, 2007.
7. Pooley RA: Is it possible for a patient with a pacemaker to undergo MRI? *AJR* 206:230, 2016.
8. Lutz M, et al.: Automated tube voltage selection in thoracoabdominal computed tomography at high pitch using a third-generation dual-source scanner: image quality and radition dose performance, *Invest Radiol* 50:352–360, 2015.
9. Mayo-Smith, et al.: How I do it: managing radiation dose in CT, *Radiology* 273(3):657–672, 2014.
10. smarter dose reduction tool, Toshiba America Medical Systems, Inc: http://medical.toshoba.com/downloads/ct-aq-one-fam-wp-sureexposure. Toshiba, 2014.
11. European Union, EUR 16262 EN: *European guidelines on quality criteria for computed tomography*, 1999. http://w3.tue.nl/fileadmin/sbd/Documenten/Leergang/BSM/European_Guidelines_Quality_Criteria_Computed.Tomography_Eur_16252.pdf.
12. Preston DL, et al.: Solid cancer incidence in atomic bomb survivors: 1958–1998, *Radiat Res* 168:1–64, 2007.
13. Ozasa K, et al.: Studies of the mortality of atomic bomb survivors: report 14, 1950–2003—an overview of cancer and noncancer diseases, *Radiat Res* 177:229–243, 2012.
14. United Nations Scientific Committee on the Effects of Atomic Radiation (UNSCEAR): Report of the United Nations Scientific Committee Nations Scientific Committee on the Effects of Atomic Radiation (UNSCEAR). New York, NY; 2012.

15. The 2007 recommendations of the International Commission on Radiological Protection: ICRP publication 103, *Ann ICRP* 37:1–332, 2007.
16. Health Physics Society Website: *Radiation risk in perspective, position statement of the Health Physics Society* (PS010-1). http://hps.org/documents/riskps010-2.pdf. 2010.
17. American Association of Physicists in Medicine website: *AAPM position statement on radiation risks from medical imaging procedures*: Policy no. pp 25-A. www.aapm.org/org/policies/details.asp?id=318&type=pp. 2011.
18. Goldman LW: Principles of CT: multislice CT, *Nucl Med Technol* 36(2):57–68, 2008.
19. Raman SP, Mahesh M, Blasko RV, et al.: CT scan parameters and radiation dose: practical advice for radiologists, *J Am Coll Radiol* 10(11):840–846, 2013.
20. Prokop M: Multislice CT: technical principles and future trends, *EUR Radiol* 13:3–13, 2003 Erratum in: General principles of MDCT, Eur J Radiol 45 [Suppl 1]: S4–S10.
21. Kanal KM: MDCT Technology, ACMP Annual Meeting 2008, Seattle, WA.
22. Haliburton S, Arbab-Zadeh A, Dey D, et al.: State of the art in CT hardware and scan modes for Cardiovascular CT, *J Cardiovasc Comput Tomogr* 6(3):154–163, 2012.
23. National Heart, Lung, and Blood Institute. http://www.nhlbi.nih.gov/health-topics/how–heart–works, 2021.
24. American Heart Association: A scientific statement retrieved from the AHA, *Circulation*, 133(25), 2016.
25. Mahesh M, Cody DD: AAPM/RSNA physics tutorial for residents: physics of cardiac imaging with multiple-row detector CT, *Radiographics* 27(5):1495–1509, 2007.
26. Goldman LW: Principles of CT: multislice CT, *J Nucl Med Technol* 36(2):57–68, 2008.
27. Cardiology Teaching Packages and Cardiac Conduction System Learning Resources, School of Health Sciences, University of Nottingham, United Kingdom.
28. Desjardins B, Kaztrooni EA: ECG-gated cardiac CT, *AJR* 182(4):993–1010, 2004.
29. Lin E, Alessio A: What are the basic concepts of temporal, contrast, and spatial resolution in cardiac CT? *J Cardiovasc Comput Tomogr* 3(6):403–408, 2009.
30. AAPM Report #137: *Comprehensive methodology for the evaluation of radiation dose in x- ray computed tomography*, 2010, American Association of Physicists in Medicine.
31. Dixon RL, *The physics of CT dosimetry: CTDI and Beyond,* CRC Press, 2019.
32. Srinivasan K, Mohammadi M, Shepherd J: Applications of linac-mounted kilovoltage cone-beam computed

tomography in modern radiation therapy: a review, *Pol J Radiol* 79:181–193, 2014.

33. Kan MWK, Leung LHT, Wong W, et al.: Radiation dose from cone beam computed tomography for image-guided radiation therapy, *Int J Radiat Oncol Biol Phys* 70(1):272–279, 2008.

CHAPTER 15

1. deGroot JE, Highnom R, Chan A, et al.: Mammographic compression—a need for mechanical standardization, WoutjanBranderhorstab, *Eur J Rad* 84(4):596–602, 2015.

2. Huda W, et al.: Radiation doses due to breast imaging in Manitoba: 1978–1988, *Radiology* 177:813, 1990.

3. Ritenour ER, Hendee WR: Screening mammography: a risk vs. risk decision, *Invest Radiol* 24:17, 1989.

4. Taubes G: The breast-screening brawl, *Science* 275:1056, 1997.

5. Office of the Federal Register: Federal Register 67FR (5446) subpart B, section 900.12, e5 (vi), Feb 6, 2002, Washington, DC, U.S. Government Printing Office.

6. Yaffe M, Mawdsley GE: Equipment requirements and quality control for mammography, in specification, acceptance testing and quality control of diagnostic x-ray imaging equipment. In Siebert JA, Barnes GT, Gould RG, editors: *American Association of Physicists in medicine medical physics monograph, No. 20*, College Park, MD, 1994, American Association of Physicists in Medicine.

7. Carlton RR, Adler AM: *Principles of radiographic imaging: an art and a science*, ed 5, Albany, NY, 2013, Delmar Cengage Learning.

8. Baldelli P, Phelan N, Egan G: Investigation of the effect of anode/filter materials on the dose and image quality of a digital mammography system based on an amorphous selenium flat panel detector, *Br J Radiol* 83(988):290–295, 2010.

9. Williams MB, et al.: Optimization of exposure parameters in full field digital mammography, *Med Phys* 36:2414–2423, 2008.

10. Reiser I, Sechopoulos I: A review of digital breast tomosynthesis, *Med Phys Int J*, 2014 2.

11. Tagliafico A, Houssami N, Calabrese M: *Digital breast tomosynthesis a practical approach*, Switzerland, 2016, Springer International.

12. Mertlemeier T. https://radiologykey.com/The Physics of Digital Breast Tomosynthesis, Chapter 2/Thomas.

13. Hall FM: Digital mammography versus full-field digital mammography, *AJR* 198:240, 2012.

14. Shift-and-add technique for general tomosynthesis image reconstruction. Reprinted from *Advances in Digital Radiography: RSNA Categorical Course in Digital Radiography*, Oak Brook, IL: Radiological Society of North America; 200357.

15. Chawla AS, Lo JY, Baker JA, et al.: Optimized image acquisition for breast tomosynthesis in projection and reconstruction space, *Med Phys* 36:4859–4869, 2009.

16. Rangarajan K, Hari S: Artifacts in digital breast tomosynthesis, *ECR*, 2013. doi:10.1594/ecr2013/C-1711.

17. : *Kopans D: Breast imaging*, ed 3, Philadelphia, PA, 2007, Lippincott Williams & Wilkins.

18. Lindner M: *Tomosynthesis and contrast-enhanced mammography improve cancer detection*, 2018, Siemens Healthineers.

19. Mertelmeier T, Ludwig J, Zhao B, et al: Optimization of tomosynthesis acquisition parameters: angular range and number of projections, Proceedings of the 9th International Workshop on Digital Mammography, Springer Berlin Heidelberg, pp. 220–227, 2008.

20. Agasthya GA, D'Orsi E, Kim YJ, et al.: Can breast compression be reduced in digital mammography and breast tomosynthesis? *AJR* 209(5):W322–W332, 2017.

21. Saunders RS, Samei E, Lo JY, et al.: Can compression be reduced for breast tomosynthesis? Monte Carlo study on mass and microcalcification conspicuity in tomosynthesis, *Radiology* 251:673–682, 2009.

22. Kundel HL, Revesz G: Lesion conspicuity, structured noise, and film reader error, *AJR* 126(6):1233–1238, 1976.

23. Sechopoulos I: A review of breast tomosynthesis. Part I. the image acquisition process, *Med Phys*, 2013 40(1):014301.

24. Machida H, Yuhara T, Mori T: Optimizing parameters for flat-panel detector digital tomosynthesis, *Radio Graphics* 30:549–562, 2010.

CHAPTER 16

1. ICRP 73: Radiological Protection and Safety in Medicine.

2. ICRP 135: Diagnostic reference levels in medical imaging, *AnnICRP*, 2017.

3. Brink JA, et al: Reference levels and achievable doses in medical and dental imaging: recommendations for the United States, NCRP Report No. 172, 2012.

4. BEIR VII: Phase II, health risks from exposure to low levels of ionizing adiation, 2006.

5. Martin M: Pet-CT planning and shielding design. American College of Medical Physics Meeting, Scottsdale, AZ, 2004.

6. Sedlack AJH, Meyer C, Mench A, et al.: Essentials of theranostics: a guide for physicians and medical physicists, *Radiographics*, 44(1):e230097, 2024.

7. www.primaryimmune.org

8. Kawashima H: Radioimmunotherapy: a specific treatment protocol for cancer by cytotoxic radioisotopes conjugated to antibodies, *Sci World J*, 2014:492061 2014.

9. Siegel J: Immunogenicity. www.gene.com/stories/immunogenicity, 2015.

10. Hendrix CS, de Leon C, Dillman RO: Radioimmunotherapy for non-Hodgkin's lymphoma with yttrium 90 ibritumomab tiuxetan, *Clin J Oncol Nurs* 6(3):144–148, 2002.

11. Nuclear Regulatory Commission Publication: NUREG - 1556, 9(2), Appendix U

12. Nuclear Regulatory Commission Publication: 10 CFR, Part 35.75

13. Mettler FA, Voelz GL: Major radiation exposure: what to expect and how to respond, *N Engl J Med* 346:1554, 2002.

14. National Council on Radiation Protection and Measurements (NCRP): *Management of terrorist events involving radioactive material,* Report No. 138, Bethesda, MD, 2001, NCRP.

15. Gusev I, et al, editor: *Medical management of radiation accidents*, ed 2, Boca Raton, FL, 2001, CRC Press.

16. Jarrett D, editor: *Medical management of radiation casualties: handbook, AFRRI Special Publication 99-92*, Bethesda, MD, 1999, Armed Forces Radiobiology Research Institute. Available from: www.afrri.usuhs.mil.

17. The International Commission on Radiation Units and Measurements, Prepared Jointly with the European Radiation Dosimetry Group, *Journal of the International Commission on Radiation Units and Measurements*, ICRU Report 94 Methods for Initial-Phase Assessment of Individual Doses Following Acute Exposure to Ionizing Radiation, 19(1), 2019. Available from: www.icru.org.

18. Ross JR, Case C, Confer D, et al.: Radiation injury treatment network (RITN): healthcare professionals preparing for a mass casualty radiological or nuclear incident, *Int J Radiat Biol* 87(8):748–753, 2011.

GLOSSARY

A

Aberration Deviation from normal development or growth; a lesion or anomaly.

Absolute risk Model predicting that a specific number of excess cancers will occur as a result of exposure to ionizing radiation.

Absorbed dose (D) The amount of energy per unit mass absorbed by an irradiated object (e.g., the patient's body tissue). This absorbed energy is responsible for any biological damage resulting from the tissues being exposed to radiation. The gray (Gy) is the SI unit of this radiation quantity.

Acids Hydrogen-containing compounds that can attack and dissolve metal (e.g., HNO_3, nitric acid).

Action limits Limits for occupational exposure that are set by the medical facility well below the regulatory values as they appear in state or federal regulations. These limits are set at levels, typically a tenth of the action limit, that are not routinely exceeded by personnel. They are meant to trigger an investigation that should uncover the reason for any unusually high exposure.

Acute Something that begins suddenly and runs a short but severe course (e.g., an acute disease).

Acute radiation syndrome (ARS) Radiation sickness, or early somatic tissue reactions, occurring in humans soon after whole-body reception of large doses of ionizing radiation delivered over a short period.

Added filtration Sheets of aluminum (or its equivalent) of appropriate thickness interposed outside the glass window of the x-ray tube housing above the collimator shutters.

Adenine (A) One of two purine bases found in both DNA and RNA.

Agreement states Individual states of the United States that have entered into an agreement with the Nuclear Regulatory Commission (NRC) to assume responsibility for enforcing radiation protection regulations through their respective health departments.

Air gap technique An alternative procedure to the use of a radiographic grid for reducing scattered radiation during certain examinations.

Air kerma SI quantity that can be used to express radiation energy transferred to a point, such as the surface of a patient's or radiographer's body. Air kerma is kinetic energy released in a unit mass (kilogram) of air and is expressed in metric units of joule per kilogram (J/kg).

ALARA concept/principle Precept holding that occupational exposure of the patient, occupationally exposed persons, and the general public should be kept "as low as reasonably achievable." Radiation exposure should always be kept ALARA for all medical imaging procedures.

Alkali A member of a group of elements that includes lithium, sodium, and potassium.

Alkaline earth A member of a group of elements including calcium, magnesium, and strontium.

Alliance for Radiation Safety in Pediatric Imaging A partnership of medical societies, founded in 2007, whose overall common purpose is to reduce dose for pediatric patients.

Alpha particle A positively charged particle of radiation that is emitted from nuclei of very heavy elements such as uranium and plutonium during the process of radioactive decay. An alpha particle contains two protons and two neutrons and therefore carries an electric charge of plus two.

Aluminum oxide (Al_2O_3) Sensing material found in optically stimulated luminescence dosimeters.

American Association of Physicists in Medicine (AAPM) Professional organization that is the primary scientific and educational body for medical physicists and is also responsible for accrediting laboratories that calibrate instruments used to measure radiation exposure in medical radiology.

American College of Radiology (ACR) Major professional organization of radiologists in the United States.

American Registry of Radiologic Technologists (ARRT) Nongovernmental credentialing organization that tests and certifies radiologic technologists on a national level. The intention is to "seek and ensure quality patient care in radiologic technology."

American Society of Radiologic Technologists (ASRT) The "premier professional association" of persons employed in medical imaging and radiation therapy. It provides education, advocacy, and research for the membership.

Amino acids The structural units of protein.

Amorphous selenium A noncrystalline grouping of silicon atoms in which, rather than a regular geometric pattern, the silicon atoms are distributed in a continuous random fashion.

Amorphous silicon thin-film technology A non-crystalline shapeless form of silicon that can be fabricated into very thin sheets and used to create solar cells. Amorphous silicon has become the material of choice for the active layer in thin-film transistors (TFTs), which are most widely used in large-area electronics applications, mainly for liquid-crystal displays (LCDs) and low energy x-ray detectors.

Ampere The SI unit of electrical charge. One ampere represents the quantity of electrons amounting to a charge of 1 coulomb crossing unit area per second.

Analog image A nondigital visible image produced by x-radiation on a developed radiographic film or other viewing media.

Anaphase The phase of mitosis during which the duplicate centromeres migrate in opposite directions along the mitotic spindle and carry the chromatids to opposite sides of the cell.

Anemia A condition characterized by a lack of vitality and caused by a decrease in the number of red blood cells in the circulating blood.

Anion A negatively charged ion.

Annihilation radiation Radiation in the form of two oppositely moving 511 keV photons generated as the result of the mutual annihilation of matter and antimatter (i.e., an electron and a positron).

Annual occupational effective dose (EfD) limit An upper boundary limit for radiation workers for yearly whole-body exposure (excluding personal medical and natural background exposure) of 50 millisieverts (mSv). There is also an added recommendation that the lifetime EfD in mSv should not exceed 10 times the occupationally exposed person's age in years.

Anode The positively charged target in the x-ray tube.

Antibodies Materials developed by the body in response to the presence of foreign bodies, called *antigens*, such as bacteria or a virus. Once the skin is penetrated, it provides a primary defense mechanism against antigens.

Antigens Any substance that causes an immune system to produce antibodies against it; usually a foreign substance, such as a toxin or a component of a virus, bacterium, or parasite.

Antimatter Matter composed of the counterparts of ordinary matter that does not exist freely in the universe and is unstable in the presence of ordinary matter.

Aplastic anemia Anemia resulting from bone marrow failure.

Apoptosis A nonmitotic or nondivision form of cell death that occurs when cells die without attempting division during the interphase portion of the cell life cycle. Also known as *programmed cell death* (formerly called *interphase death*).

Artifact A structure or an appearance that is not normally present on a radiograph and is produced by artificial means.

Artificial Intelligence (AI) Popular name attached to a rapidly advancing field in computer science that describes the growing ability of computers to realistically simulate human intelligence in performing tasks and/or solving problems.

Artificial radiation See *human-made radiation.*

Ataxia An inability to coordinate voluntary muscular movements.

Atom The smallest portion of an element that has all of its chemical properties.

Atomic number The number of protons (Z) contained within the nucleus of an atom.

ATP (adenosine triphosphate) A type of molecule found in every cell. Its function is to store and supply the cell with energy.

Atrophy A shrinkage of any body part that may follow substantial partial-body radiation exposure.

Auger effect When an inner-shell vacancy occurs in an atom, the energy liberated when this vacancy is filled can be transferred to another electron of the atom, thereby ejecting the electron. The process is known as the *Auger effect*, and the emitted electron is known as an *Auger electron.*

Automatic collimation See *Positive beam limitation (PBL).*

Automatic Exposure Control (AEC) A system used to consistently control the amount of radiation reaching an image receptor by *terminating the length of exposure* when a satisfactory precalibrated level of exposure is registered by one or more detectors. When using AEC systems, the radiographer generally must still use individual experience and discretion to select an appropriate kVp, mA, image receptor, and grid.

Axial CT scan A type of CT scan that is a result of an in-plane step-and-shoot sequence of the scanner table and the x-ray, respectively. For this, the pitch is equal to one.

Axon A long, single tentacle from the nerve cell body that carries impulses away from it.

B

Background equivalent radiation time (BERT) Method to compare the amount of radiation received from a radiologic procedure with natural background radiation received over a specified period such as days, weeks, months, or years.

Backscatter Photons that have interacted with the atoms of an object and as a result are deflected backward (toward the x-ray tube).

Bases In general, any substance in water solution is slippery to the touch, tastes bitter, reacts with acids to form salts, and promotes certain chemical reactions. In chemistry, a *base* is a chemical species that donates electrons, accepts protons, or releases hydroxide (OH-) ions in an aqueous solution. In the cell, bases (adenine, thymine, guanine, and cytosine or uracil) serve as the major compounds of DNA and RNA forming the rungs of the ladder present in these cellular nuclear macromolecules.

Beam direction factor See *Use factor (U).*

Becquerel The SI unit of radioactivity. It is equal to 1 disintegration (decay) per second.

Beta decay The process wherein a nucleus relieves instability by a neutron transforming itself into a combination of a proton and an energetic electron (called a *beta particle*). There is also the emission of another particle called a *neutrino*, which has negligible mass and no electric charge but carries away any excess energy.

Beta particles High-speed electrons ejected from a nucleus that undergoes beta decay. They are also known as *beta rays.*

Binding energy Force that holds the components of an atom or a nucleus together.

Biologic dosimetry A method of dose assessment in which biologic markers or effects of radiation exposure are measured and the dose to the organism is inferred from previously established dose–effect relationships. Examples include white blood cell counts and chromosomal aberrations.

Blebs Tiny membrane-enclosed structures that are produced when cells shrink in apoptosis.

Blood plasma Blood plasma is a fluid component of blood that contains in suspension the blood cells of whole blood. It is essentially the agent that carries cells and proteins throughout the body. It makes up about 55% of the body's total blood volume.

Bone marrow syndrome See *Hematopoietic syndrome.*

Brachytherapy The treatment of cancer by the insertion of radioactive materials or implants either temporarily or permanently directly into the cancerous tissue and its immediate vicinity.

Bragg–Gray theory Relates the ionization produced in a small cavity within an irradiated medium or object to the energy absorbed in that medium as a result of its radiation exposure.

Bremsstrahlung Polyenergetic ionizing electromagnetic radiation that is produced when a beam of electrons in an x-ray tube undergoes deceleration by interaction with the nuclei of the x-ray tube target atoms.

Broad beam x-ray transmission factor (B) The ratio of air kerma (K_a) behind a barrier of material thickness "x" to the value of K_a at the same location with no intervening barrier.

Bucky grid An assembly of moving lead strips resembling a Venetian blind, placed between a patient being x-rayed and the image receptor to improve the collimation and reduce scatter radiation on the detector.

Bucky slot shielding device A protective device made of at least 0.25-mm lead equivalent that automatically covers the Bucky slot opening in the side of the x-ray table during a fluoroscopic examination when the Bucky tray is positioned at the foot end of the table. This protects the radiographer and the radiologist from gonadal radiation exposure.

Bureau of Radiological Health (BRH) See *Center for Devices and Radiological Health (CDRH)*.

C

Calibrated instrument Any device that is compared with a generally accepted (nationally or internationally) standard device so that its accuracy is determined. Radiation survey instruments are usually calibrated annually.

Candela SI unit used to describe the degree of luminance. One candela corresponds to 3.8 million billion photons per second being emitted from a light source through a cone-like field of view. A common wax candle emits light with a luminous intensity of roughly one candela.

Carbohydrates Compounds, also known as *saccharides*, composed of only carbon, hydrogen, and oxygen. Carbohydrates such as sugars and starches are involved in energy-releasing processes in animals and plants.

Carbon Nonmetallic element that is *the basic constituent of all organic matter.*

Carbon fiber Material used in the tops of radiographic tables. It has a lower x-ray absorption potential when compared with materials such as aluminum but has the strength to support adult patients. The use of carbon fiber results in lower radiographic techniques for producing the recorded image, thereby lowering patient dose.

Carcinogenesis The production or origin of cancer.

C-arm fluoroscope A portable device for producing real-time images of areas of patient anatomy. The opposite ends of the C-shaped support arm are respectively the x-ray tube and the image receptor.

Catabolism The breaking down in living organisms of more complex molecules into simpler ones, with the release of energy.

Catalyst Agent that affects the speed of a chemical reaction without being altered itself.

Catalytic failure The inability to influence the speed of a required chemical reaction (e.g., during protein synthesis).

Cataract Opacity of the lens of the eye.

Cataractogenesis The production or origin of cataracts.

Cathode A negative electrode. The cathode is the source of the high-speed electrons in an x-ray tube.

Cation A positively charged ion.

Cell division The process whereby one cell divides to form two or more cells.

Cell membrane The frail, semipermeable, flexible structure encasing and surrounding the human cell. It functions as a barricade to protect cellular contents from their outside environment and controls the passage of water and other materials into and out of the cell.

Cell metabolism The series of chemical reactions that modifies foods for cellular use.

Cell survival curve A graphical method of displaying the sensitivity of a particular type of cell to lethal effects of radiation.

Cells The basic units of all living matter.

Cellular life cycle The passage of a cell through the phases G1, S, G2, and M.

Center for Devices and Radiological Health (CDRH) Known before 1982 as the *Bureau of Radiological Health (BRH)*, this agency is responsible for conducting an ongoing electronic product radiation control program.

Centigray (cGy) One one-hundredth of a gray (1/100 Gy), previously known as a *rad*.

Centrioles A pair of small, hollow, cylindrical structures oriented at right angles to each other and embedded in a material mass of more than 100 proteins. They play a significant role in the formation of the mitotic spindle during cell division.

Centromere A clear region on a chromosome serving as a joining point; it is actually the center of the chromosome.

Centrosomes Structures, located in the center of the cell near the nucleus at each end of the mitotic spindle, that contain the centrioles.

Cerebrovascular syndrome Form of acute radiation syndrome that results when the central nervous system and cardiovascular system receive doses of 50 Gy_t

or more of ionizing radiation. A dose of this magnitude can cause death within a few hours to 2 or 3 days after exposure.

Characteristic photon A quantum or quantity of radiant energy given off by an atom when an electron from an outer-shell drops down to fill an inner-shell vacancy. The energy of a characteristic photon is equivalent to the difference in energy level between the two electron shells. Also known as *characteristic x-ray* or *fluorescent radiation*.

Characteristic radiation Radiation consisting of characteristic photons. In a general-purpose x-ray tube characteristic radiation comprises about 10% of the primary radiation beam for tube voltages between 80 and 100 kVp.

Charge-coupled device (CCD) A device that, when struck by visible light, produces electrical signals in proportion to the brightness of the light. CCDs are used in indirect types of digital x-ray detectors. Indirect digital detectors use a phosphor to convert the x-ray energy to visible light, after which the CCD converts the visible light into electrical signals.

Chromatid A highly coiled strand; one of the two duplicate portions of DNA in a replicated chromosome that appear during cell division.

Chromatid aberrations Deviation from normal development or growth. Lesions that result when irradiation of individual chromatids occurs later in interphase after DNA synthesis has taken place.

Chromatin The substance distributed in the nucleus of a cell that condenses to form chromosomes during cell division.

Chromosome aberrations Deviation from normal development or growth. Lesions that result when irradiation occurs early in interphase before DNA synthesis takes place.

Chromosome breakage The segmenting of a chromosome due to the breaking of one or both of the sugar–phosphate chains of a DNA ladder-like structure, which is a potential outcome when ionizing radiation interacts with a DNA macromolecule.

Chromosomes Tiny, rod-shaped bodies that contain genes.

Chronic Something that continues for a long time (i.e., a chronic disease).

Classical scattering See *Coherent scattering*.

Clear lead shields Transparent lead–acrylic material that has been impregnated with approximately 30% lead by weight. It is used for viewing windows and pull-down or roll-away x-ray room shielding.

Cleaved chromosome A broken chromosome.

Code of Standards for Diagnostic x-ray Equipment Effective August 1, 1974, this code applies to complete x-ray systems and their major components manufactured after that date.

Coherent scattering The process wherein a low-energy photon (typically less than 10 keV) interacts with an atom of human tissue and does not lose its energy. The atom responds by releasing the energy it has received in the form of a scattered photon that has the same wavelength and energy as the original incident photon. The emitted photon changes direction by 20 degrees or less. No ionization of the biologic atom occurs. Also known as *classical scattering, elastic scattering, unmodified scattering, and Rayleigh scattering. Thompson scattering,* which involves a free electron and not an atom, is another type of coherent scattering.

Collective effective dose (ColEfD) Designated for use in the description of a population or group exposed to different individual amounts of ionizing radiation. It is equal to the sum of all of the doses times the number of individuals exposed and would be expressed in units such as person-sievert.

Collimation Limiting all the margins of the useful x-ray field to a specific size and shape to confine the beam to the anatomic area of interest. This reduces the dose that a patient receives and improves the contrast of the radiographic image.

Committed effective dose equivalent (CEDE) A measure of the probabilistic health effect on an individual as a result of intake of radioactive material into the body. It takes into account the length of time that the radioactive material may stay within the body.

Compensating filter A material such as aluminum, lead–acrylic, or other suitable material inserted between the x-ray source and the patient to modify the quality (penetrating power, spectrum) of the beam across the field of view.

Compton scattered electron An energetic electron dislodged from the outer shell of an atom of the irradiated object

as a result of a Compton interaction with an incoming x-ray photon. Also known as a *secondary,* or *recoil, electron.*

Compton scattered photon x-ray photon of weaker energy emerging from an atom, usually in a new direction, following a Compton interaction with that atom.

Compton scattering An interaction between an incoming x-ray photon and a loosely bound outer-shell electron of an atom in the irradiated object. The photon surrenders a portion of its energy to dislodge the electron from its outer-shell orbit, thereby ionizing the atom, and then continues in a new direction. This process accounts for most of the scattered radiation produced during diagnostic procedures. Also known as *incoherent scattering, inelastic scattering,* or *modified scattering.*

Computed axial tomography (CAT) See *Computed tomography (CT).*

Computed radiography (CR) Process in which an image is captured on a removable digital storage cassette, using storage phosphor technology. The cassette is then taken to a "reader" that interprets the stored signal and transfers it in a digital matrix to a picture archiving and communication system (PACS) system. CR has been largely replaced by digital radiography, or DR.

Computed tomography (CT) "The process of creating a cross-sectional tomographic plane of any part of the body." This computer-reconstructed image of a patient is created by "an x-ray tube and detector assembly rotating 360 degrees about a specified area of the body." CT has also been referred to as *computerized axial tomography (CAT).*

Cone beam computed tomography (CBCT) CBCT is an imaging technique that uses a broad kilovoltage x-ray beam that covers the entire length range of the patient that is to be scanned. This beam is directed through the volume of interest (VOI) at a large rectangular detector (also known as a flat panel detector), and *all volumetric data about the patient is gathered in a single rotational pass* of the x-ray tube and detector.

Congenital abnormalities Defects existing at birth that are not inherited but rather acquired during development in utero.

Console See *Control panel.*

Consumer-Patient Radiation Health and Safety Act of 1981 Provides federal legislation requiring the establishment of minimal standards for accreditation of educational programs for persons who perform radiologic procedures and the certification of such persons.

Contrast media (negative) The use of air or gas to enhance visualization of body structures during a radiologic procedure.

Contrast media (positive) A liquid solution containing an element with a higher atomic number than surrounding tissue (e.g., barium or iodine) that is either ingested or injected into biologic tissues or structures to be visualized.

Contrast Resolution A measure of the ability to distinguish small x-ray attenuation differences in a CT image.

Control-booth barrier A permanent secured protective barrier for imaging personnel that is located in an x-ray room that contains housing for permanent or nonportable radiographic equipment. It may be regarded as a secondary protective barrier, since the primary x-ray beam is never directed toward it.

Control monitor Dosimeter provided by the monitoring company with each batch of dosimeters to serve as a basis for comparison with the remainder of the dosimeters after they have been returned to the monitoring company for processing. The control monitor determines whether the batch of dosimeters has been exposed to radiation in transit to or from the health care facility.

Control panel Site where technical exposure factors such as milliamperes (mA) and peak kilovoltage (kVp) are selected and visually displayed. Also called a *console.* Besides having buttons for initiating the exposure, it indicates the conditions of exposure and shows when the x-ray tube is energized.

Controlled area A region that is occupied only by occupationally exposed personnel and others under their direct supervision.

Coronary heart disease (CHF) Malady caused by various anatomical changes or defects that adversely affect the usual function of the heart.

Cosmic radiation (cosmic rays) Very-high-energy particles and photons. They result from immense energy emitting processes that have taken place throughout the universe, including the sun and other stars in this galaxy.

Coulomb (C)   Basic SI unit of electrical charge. It represents the quantity of electrical charge flowing past a point in a circuit in 1 second when an electrical current of 1 ampere is used.

Coulomb per kilogram (C/kg)   SI unit of radiation exposure: 1 coulomb per kilogram (C/kg) of air equals 1 SI unit of exposure, or $1/(2.58 \times 10^{-4}) = 3.88 \times 10^3$ R. C/kg (traditional unit: roentgen). Both of these units can be used for x-ray equipment calibration.

Covalent bond   A chemical union or cross-link created between atoms by the sharing or transfer of one or more electrons.

Crookes tube   Partially evacuated electrical discharge tube used by Wilhelm Conrad Roentgen when he discovered x-rays.

Crossover   Process occurring during meiosis in which the chromatids exchange some chromosomal material (genes).

CT Angiography (CTA)   A CT examination of the chest that is used to diagnose and evaluate blood vessel disease or related conditions, such as ruptures or narrowing or blockage. Performed either with or without the insertion of contrast material.

CTDI'   CT dose index (CTDI) is a standardized measure of radiation dose output of a CT scanner that allows the user to characterize the radiation output of CT scanners for various protocol technique settings. It refers to the dose to a standard 16-cm (head) or 32-cm (body) plastic phantom as measured by an inserted 10 cm long pencil-like ionization chamber.

Cumulative effective dose (CumEfD) limit   A radiation worker's lifetime EfD must be limited to their age in years times 10 mSv. This limit pertains to the whole body.

Cumulative timing device   A required resettable device on a fluoroscopic x-ray unit that measures the elapsed x-ray beam-on time and sounds an audible alarm after the fluoroscope has been activated for 5 minutes.

Curie   The standard unit of radioactivity in use before the SI system of units was established. One curie is defined as being equal to 3.7×10^{10} nuclear disintegrations per second (dps).

Cutie pie   Nickname for an *ionization chamber–type survey meter*.

Cyclotrons   Units that, with the aid of a strong static magnetic field and rapidly oscillating electric fields, produce in a circular evacuated cavity beams of high-energy charged particles such as 150-MeV proton beams.

Cytogenetics   The study of cell genetics with emphasis on analysis of chromosomes.

Cytoplasm   The protoplasm that exists outside of the cell's nucleus.

Cytoplasmic organelles   Miniature cellular components present in the cytoplasm that enable the cell to perform normal functions.

Cytosine (C)   One of two pyrimidine bases found in both DNA and RNA.

D

Daughter cell   A cell resulting from the division of a prior cell (called a parent cell).

Dead-man–type fluoroscopic exposure switch   A fluoroscopic exposure switch (operated by foot pressure) that requires continuous pressure from the operator. If the operator becomes incapacitated, the exposure automatically terminates.

Deep equivalent dose   External whole-body absorbed dose determined by a personnel dosimeter at a tissue depth of 1 cm (1000 mg/cm^2).

Deep learning (DL)   A machine (computer) that processes training sets of data to find patterns that predict useful output without specific instructions.

Deletion   When a part of the chromosome or chromatid is lost at the next cell division, thus creating an aberration known as an *acentric fragment*. This will result in a cell mutation.

Dendrites   Tentacle like or short branched extensions of a nerve cell (neuron), along which impulses or electrical signals received from other cells are transmitted to the cell body.

Deoxyribonucleic acid (DNA)   A type of nucleic acid (very large biomolecules) that carries the genetic information necessary for cell replication and regulation of cellular activity needed to direct protein synthesis. It is often referred to as the *master chemical* in the cell because it contains all the information that the cell needs to function and reproduce.

Deoxyribose   A five-carbon sugar molecule ($C_5H_{10}O_4$), derived from the sugar

ribose by the loss of one oxygen atom, that helps form the phosphate backbone of *DNA* molecules.

Dermis   Middle layer of skin composed of connective tissue.

Desquamation   Shedding or flaking off of the outer layer of skin; can occur after high fluoroscopic radiation doses.

Detector configuration   In CT scanning, detector configuration refers to the number of data channels (i.e., detector rows) being used in the z-axis direction and the effective detector thickness of each data channel. For example, a detector configuration described as 128×0.5 mm would signify the use of 128 data channels along the z-axis, each of which has an effective thickness of 0.5 mm.

Diagnostic efficacy   The degree to which a diagnostic study accurately reveals the presence or absence of disease in the patient.

Diagnostic reference levels (DRLs)   An optimization tool for both radiation safety and image quality for medical imaging procedures using ionizing radiation. They give an indication of the expected radiation dose received by an average-sized patient undergoing a given imaging procedure.

Diagnostic-type protective tube housing   The lead-lined metal housing enclosing the x-ray tube that protects both the radiographer and the patient from leakage radiation by predominantly restricting the emission of the x-rays to the area of the useful, or primary, beam.

Dicentric chromosomes   Chromosomes that have two centromeres.

Diffusion   The motion of liquid, gas, or solid particles from an area of relatively high concentration to an area of lower concentration.

Digital breast tomography (DBT)   An imaging technique which involves multiple brief radiation exposures occurring while the x-ray tube rotates within a limited arc about a patient's stationary compressed breast. It is often called 3D mammography because this tomographic image acquisition method adds a third dimension (z-axis) that provides depth resolution to the breast image.

Digital breast tomosynthesis   The process whereby multiple planar images or image slices of the breast are reconstructed or synthesized from a series of mammographic exposures taken at multiple gantry angles relative to the plane of the compressed breast.

Digital fluoroscopy   A technique in which the fluoroscopic image is produced in digital form in the image acquisition process. In nondigital fluoroscopy, a standard image intensifier is employed whose output is transmitted to an analog television camera which displays the image.

Digital image   An image, generated by a computer, composed of picture elements or pixels, each with finite, discrete quantities of numeric information for its intensity or brightness.

Digital radiography   The use of a flat panel detector to record a radiographic image and render it in digital form without a film developing process or the scanning of the image receptor.

Digital subtraction angiography   A fluoroscopic technique used in interventional radiology for visualizing blood vessels. Radiopaque structures such as bone are eliminated by digitally subtracting them using an initial reference image or *mask* from subsequent images, thus allowing for isolated depiction of the blood vessels.

Direct action   Biologic damage that occurs as a non secondary process of ionization of atoms on essential molecules, which may cause these molecules to become either inactive or functionally altered.

Direct radiation   See *Primary radiation*.

Direct transmission   Primary x-ray photons that traverse a patient without interacting.

Dirty bomb   See *Radioactive dispersal device*.

Distance   A very important *method of protection* from ionizing radiation. Imaging personnel receive significantly less radiation exposure by standing farther away from a source of radiation because an inverse square law governs the decrease in the radiation level with increased distance.

DNA synthesis   The building up of DNA macromolecules.

Dominant mutation   A genetic mutation that will probably be expressed in offspring. A genetic trait is considered *dominant* if it is expressed in a person who has only one copy of that gene as opposed to a *recessive* trait which will be expressed in offspring only when two copies of the recessive gene are present.

Doppler shift   Refers to the apparent change in the frequency of any wave (e.g., its pitch if it is a sound wave) as the observer and the source move toward or away from each other.

Dose   The amount of radiant energy absorbed by an irradiated object per unit mass.

Dose area product (DAP)   The sum total of air kerma over the exposed area of the patient's surface.

Dose commitment   The total dose that could ultimately be delivered from a given intake of radionuclide that may remain in the body for some time.

Dose length product (DLP)   A measure of the radiation dose for an entire CT scan. It is mathematically equal to the product of the volume CTDI and the scan length. It has the units of mGy-cm.

Dose rate constant   Also known as the specific gamma ray constant " Γ," it is the dose rate, usually specified in mSv/hr (rem/hr in traditional units) at a specified distance from a source of activity given either in MBq/hr or mCi/hr. For example, in SI units the radioisotope Tc^{99m} has a Γ value approximately equal to: $2 (10)^{-5}$ mSv/hr per MBq at one centimeter.

Double-strand break   The ionization of a DNA macromolecule that results in the rupture or breakage of both of the two sugar–phosphate chains of the DNA ladder-like molecular structure. This results in splintering of a chromosome.

Doubling dose   The radiation dose that causes the number of spontaneous mutations occurring in a given generation to increase to two times their original number.

Dual Energy x-ray Absorptiometry (DEXA, or DXA Scan)   A noninvasive x-ray procedure that can quantitively predict the risk of bone fracture(s). For this scan two different low-energy level x-ray beams are directed toward bony areas of interest and the ratio of their relative degrees of absorption are compared with established normal ratio value ranges.

E

Early somatic tissue reactions   Reactions in biologic tissues that are dependent on the duration of time after the exposure to ionizing radiation. They appear within minutes, hours, days, or weeks of the time of exposure. These reactions are precipitated by cell death.

Edema   Swelling caused by excess fluid trapped in body tissue.

Effective atomic number (Zeff)   A composite Z value for when multiple chemical elements comprise a material.

Effective dose (EfD)   Quantity that is used for radiation protection purposes to provide a measure of the overall risk of exposure to humans from ionizing radiation. Effective dose takes into account the dose from all types of ionizing radiation (e.g., alpha, beta, gamma, x-ray) to various irradiated organs or tissues in the human body (skin, gonadal tissue, thyroid). By including a specific weighting factor for each of those parts of the body mentioned, EfD takes into account the chance or risk of each of those body parts to develop a radiation-induced cancer (or in the case of the reproductive organs, the risk of genetic damage).

Effective dose (EfD) limit   Concerns the upper boundary dose of ionizing radiation that results in a negligible risk of bodily injury or hereditary damage. These limits may be expressed for whole-body exposure, partial-body exposure, and exposure of individual organs. Separate limits are set for occupationally exposed individuals and for the general public.

Effective dose (EfD) limiting system   The current method for assessing radiation exposure and associated risk of biologic damage to radiation workers and the general public. It is a set of numeric dose limits that are based on calculations of the various risks of cancer and genetic effects to tissues or organs exposed to radiation.

Effective CT dose (EfD)   The product of the scan DLP and the EfDLP.

EfDLP   The normalized EfD associated with a specific scan region of the body (also known as the "k" factor).

Effective half-life (T$_{eff}$)   The actual half-life of a radioactive material in a patient's body resulting from a combination of natural decay and physical removal by bodily functions.

Elastic scattering   Most simply, this signifies an interaction between two particles in which the kinetic energy of each particle remains unchanged but their directions of motion are changed.

Elective examinations   Nonurgent x-ray examinations that can be scheduled at an appropriate time to meet patient needs and safety requirements.

Electric charge   The physical property of matter that causes it to experience a force when placed in an electromagnetic field. There are two types of electric charges: positive and negative. Like charges repel, and unlike charges attract.

Electrical potential difference (voltage difference)   A potential difference or applied voltage is used to add kinetic energy to charged particles. The total energy acquired by an electric charge when it is placed in a potential difference of one volt is equal to one *electron-volt (eV)* of energy. An electron in a potential difference of 100,000 volts can acquire an energy of 100,000 eV or 100 keV.

Electrical potential energy   The energy attained by a charged particle as a result of the voltage difference to which it is exposed. Electrical potential energy may be measured in units of joules or electron-volts. When an x-ray tube uses an applied voltage of 100,000 volts, it accelerates electrons toward its anode with an energy of 100 keV.

Electrocardiogram (ECG)   A graphical tracing or readout of the pulses or electrical activity with time that occur during the heart cycle of contraction and relaxation.

ECG gated imaging   An imaging method whereby the CT scanner is electronically linked to the patient's real-time electrocardiogram. CT image acquisition and reconstruction can then be coordinated with the quiescent heart phases associated with particular magnitude electrical pulses, thereby removing or minimizing motion artifacts.

Electrolytes   See *Salts*.

Electromagnetic radiation   Radiation composed of interacting, varying electric and magnetic fields that propagate through space at the speed of light. Examples include radio waves, microwaves, visible light, ultraviolet rays, x-rays, and gamma rays.

Electromagnetic spectrum   The full range of frequencies and wavelengths of electromagnetic waves.

Electromagnetic wave   Electric and magnetic fields that fluctuate rapidly as they travel through space, including radio waves, microwaves, visible light, and x-rays.

Electrometer   A device used to measure the quantity of electrical charge.

Electron capture   A process wherein an inner-shell electron is captured by one of the nuclear protons, followed directly by the two combining to produce a neutron.

Electrons   Negatively charged fundamental particles.

Element   A substance made up of atoms that all have the same atomic number and hence the same chemical properties.

Embryologic effects   Damage to an organism that occurs as a result of exposure to some agent (such as ionizing radiation) during the embryonic stage of development. Also known as *birth defects*.

Endoplasmic reticulum   A vast, irregular network of tubules and vesicles spreading and interconnecting in all directions throughout the cytoplasm, thus enabling the cell to intercommunicate throughout the extranuclear environment and transfer food from one part of the cell to another.

Energy   The ability to do work.

Enhanced natural sources   Natural sources of ionizing radiation that grow larger because of accidental or deliberate human actions.

Entrance exposure   Quantity of radiation, specified in SI units (coulombs per kilogram) or traditional units (roentgens), incident on an object.

Entrance skin exposure (ESE)   x-ray exposure to the skin of the patient.

Entrance skin exposure dose (ESE$_d$) rates   Limited by federal standards of general-purpose intensified fluoroscopic units to a maximum of 88 mGy$_a$ per minute. Measured at tabletop with the image intensifier entrance surface at a prescribed 30 cm above the tabletop.

Environmental Protection Agency (EPA)   US government agency that facilitates the development and enforcement of regulations pertaining to the control of radiation in the environment. It directs federal agencies, oversees the general area of environmental monitoring, and has authority over specific areas such as determining the action level for radon.

Enzymatic proteins   Proteins that control the cell's various physiologic activities by functioning as catalysts. Also known as *enzymes*.

Epidemiology   "Science that deals with the incidence, distribution, and control of disease in a population."

Epidermis   Outer layer of skin.

Epilation   Loss of hair by various means. The resultant effect, if permanent, is known as *alopecia*.

Epithelial tissue   A substance that lines and covers body tissue; the cells that comprise this tissue are highly radiosensitive because the body constantly regenerates this tissue.

Equivalent dose (EqD)   A radiation quantity used for radiation protection purposes when a person receives exposure from various types of ionizing radiation. This quantity attempts to numerically specify the differences in transferred energy and therefore potential biologic harm that are produced by different types of radiation. EqD is the product of the average absorbed dose in a tissue or organ in the human body and its associated radiation weighting factor chosen for the type of radiation in question. Equivalent dose enables the calculation of the effective dose (EfD).

Erg   A unit of energy and work that is equal to 10^{-7} joules.

Erythema   Diffused redness over an area of skin after irradiation.

Erythroblasts   Red blood stem cells.

Erythrocytes   Red blood cells without a nucleus that contain the protein hemoglobin which, besides imparting the red color to blood, facilitates the transport of oxygen from the lungs to all body tissues and cells as blood circulates.

Europium-activated barium fluorohalide   The most commonly employed photostimulable phosphor used in computed radiography imaging plates as the image receptor.

Excess cancers   Cancers that would not have occurred in a population without exposure to ionizing radiation.

Excitation   The addition of energy to a system, thereby transforming it usually from a ground, or lowest energy, state to an excited, or higher-energy state.

Exit, or image formation, radiation   All the x-ray photons that reach their destination (the image receptor) after passing through the patient being radiographed; previously known as *remnant radiation*.

Exposure   The total electric charge of one sign, either all pluses or all minuses, per unit mass that x-ray and gamma ray photons with energies up to 3 million electron volts (MeV) generate in dry (i.e., nonhumid) air at standard temperature and pressure (760 mmHg or 1 atmosphere at sea level and 22°C); the amount of ionizing radiation that may strike an object, such as the human body, when in the vicinity of a radiation source. In the SI system it can be measured in coulombs per kilogram (C/kg) and in traditional units as roentgens.

Exposure linearity Consistency in output radiation intensity at any selected kVp when x-ray generator settings are changed from one milliamperage and time combination to another. Mathematically, it is the ratio of the difference in mR/mAs values between two successive x-ray unit generator stations to the sum of those mR/mAs values. It must be less than 0.1. When changing from one mA station to a neighboring mA station, the most that linearity can vary is 10%.

Exposure rate dose Given in units of mGy_a per hour; the same quantity as air kerma rate.

Exposure reproducibility Consistency in output in radiation intensity for identical generator settings from one individual exposure to subsequent exposures. This means that the x-ray unit must have the ability to duplicate certain radiographic exposures for any given combination of peak kilovolts (kVp), milliamperes (mA), and time. A variance of 5% or less is acceptable.

Extremity dosimeter A device that monitors the equivalent dose of radiation to the hands.

Eye equivalent dose Radiation equivalent dose to the lens of the eye at a tissue depth of 0.3 cm.

F

Fallout Radiation produced as a consequence of nuclear weapons testing.

Fats Compounds composed of long chains of carbon, hydrogen, and oxygen, with the ratio of hydrogen atoms to oxygen atoms being much greater than 2:1; a rich energy source (see *Lipids.*).

Fatty acids Compounds formed when fat combines with an acidic group of atoms (e.g., the carboxyl group: COOH); also, a constituent of amino acids from which proteins are built.

Fetus A developing human in utero.

Fiber A protracted, thread-like structure.

Fibrils Minute fibers or strands that are frequently part of a compound fiber.

Fibrosis Abnormal formation of fibrous tissue.

Filtration Elements that are part of or added to the x-ray tube to reduce exposure to the patient's skin and superficial tissue

by absorbing most of the lower-energy photons from the produced heterogeneous beam and thereby increasing the mean energy, or quality, of the x-ray beam.

Fission The splitting of the nuclei of atoms whereby some mass is converted into energy.

Fixed radiographic equipment Radiologic equipment that is installed in and cannot be moved from a specific location or room in an imaging facility. It may also be referred to as *stationary equipment*.

Flat contact shield Uncontoured lead strip or lead-impregnated material 1 mm thick placed directly over the patient's reproductive organs to provide protection from exposure to ionizing radiation.

Fluorescent radiation See *Characteristic photon* or *Characteristic radiation*.

Fluorescent yield The number of characteristic x-rays emitted by an atom per inner-shell vacancy.

Fluorine-18 Radioactive isotope used for positron emission tomography (PET) scanning. It decays by positron emission (to: $_8O^{18}$) and has a half-life of 110 minutes.

Fluorodeoxyglucose (FDG) Radioactive tracer chemical compound containing Fluorine-18 that is very similar in chemical behavior to ordinary glucose and so will be taken up or metabolized by cancerous cells. As such it will reveal their locations through its positron emission decay and subsequent generation and the detection of oppositely traveling annihilation photons.

Fluoroscopic-guided positioning (FGP) The practice of using fluoroscopy to determine the exact location of the central ray with respect to the patient's anatomy before taking a diagnostic exposure.

Fluoroscopy Process in which an x-ray examination is performed that demonstrates dynamic, or active, motion of selected anatomic structures by producing a temporary image of these structures on a television monitor working in conjunction with an image intensifier system or with a digital detector and computer monitor.

Focal spot The area on the anode of the x-ray tube from which the x-rays emanate.

Follicle In the female reproductive system, an ovarian follicle is a fluid-filled sac that contains an immature egg, or *oocyte*.

Food and Drug Administration See *US Food and Drug Administration* (FDA).

Foot-candle An English or non-SI unit that refers to the degree of illuminance (brightness) on a surface that is everywhere *1 foot distant* from a uniform point source of light of intensity equal to a standard wax candle. Full daylight typically equals about 1000 foot-candles. On the other hand, twilight produces just 1 foot-candle, while a night with a full moon has 0.01 foot-candle.

Forward scatter Photons that have interacted with the atoms of an object and consequently are deflected forward (toward the radiographic image receptor) (see also *Small-angle scatter*).

Free air ionization chamber An instrument used in a standard accredited calibration laboratory to obtain a precise measurement of exposure from x-radiation.

Free radicals Solitary atoms, or most often a combination of altered atoms, that are very chemically reactive as a result of the presence of unpaired electrons.

Frequency The number of vibrations or cycles per second (given in units of hertz [Hz]) (1 Hz = 1 cycle per second).

Full field digital mammography (FFDM) A digital mammography system in which previously used multiple sized screen-film image receptors are replaced by a single *large x-ray field capture array* of many tiny solid-state detectors similar to those used by a digital camera. These detectors convert x-rays into electrical signals.

G

Gamma camera A mechanically mounted large rectangular device suspended over a patient's region of medical interest that is able to detect scintillations (flashes of light) produced when gamma rays, resulting from radioactive decay of a single photon emitting radioisotope that had been injected into a patient, interact with a sodium iodide crystal located at the front of the device's detection assembly.

Gamma rays High-energy electromagnetic waves emitted by the nuclei of radioactive substances. Although they are generally shorter in wavelength, and therefore of higher energy, than radiographic x-rays and have a different point of origin, their other characteristics are identical to those of diagnostic x-rays.

Gastrointestinal (GI) syndrome   A form of acute radiation syndrome that appears in humans at a rapidly received whole-body threshold dose of approximately 6 Gy_t and that peaks after a dose of 10 Gy_t.

Geiger–Müller (GM) detector   A device that detects individual radioactive materials emitting photons and/or electrons and that also serves as the primary portable radiation survey instrument for area monitoring in nuclear medicine facilities.

Genes   Segments or portions of DNA that serve as the basic units of heredity.

Genetic cells (germ cells)   Cells of the human body associated with reproduction.

Genetic code   The *set of rules* by which information encoded within genetic material (DNA or mRNA sequences) is translated into proteins by living cells.

Genetic damage   Radiation damage to generations yet unborn.

Genetic death   See *Mitotic death*.

Genetic effects   Biologic effects of ionizing radiation on future generations due to irradiation of germ cells in previous generations. Also known as *hereditary effects*.

Genetic mutations   See *Mutations*.

Genetically significant dose (GSD)   Concept used to assess the net impact of gonadal dose to an entire population due to gonadal radiation received by a segment of that population. Specifically, GSD is the equivalent dose to the reproductive organs that, if received by every human, would be expected to bring about an identical gross genetic injury to the total population, as does the sum of the actual doses received by exposed individual members of the population. For the US population, this dose is estimated to be about 0.20 mSv (20 mrem).

Germ cells   Male and female reproductive cells.

Glow curve   A graphic plot that demonstrates the relationship of light output to temperature variation for a thermoluminescent (glowing upon heating up) (TL) material, such as is used in a TL dosimeter (TLD).

Glucose   A form of sugar that is the primary energy source for the cell. It has the chemical form: $C_6H_{12}O_6$.

Glycerine   A sweet, colorless, odorless, syrupy liquid obtained from fats that are soluble in water; often used as a moistening agent.

Glycoproteins   Proteins with a sugar attached to them. They give structural support to cells, help form connective tissues, and are key molecules involved in immune response within the immune system.

Golgi apparatus   Minute vesicles that extend from the nucleus to the cell membrane. They consist of tiny sacs located near the nucleus. The Golgi apparatus unites large carbohydrate molecules and then combines them with proteins to form glycoproteins. These minute pouches transport enzymes and hormones through the cell membrane so that they can exit the cell, enter the bloodstream, and be carried to the areas of the body where they are required.

Gonadal dose   Radiation exposure received by the male and female reproductive organs.

Gonads   Male and female reproductive organs.

Gram (g)   A unit of mass of the metric system. An object near the earth's surface that has a mass of 454 grams will weigh 1 pound.

Granules   Small, insoluble, nonmembranous particles found in cytoplasm.

Granulocyte   A scavenger type of white blood cell that fights bacteria.

Gray (Gy)   SI unit of absorbed dose and air kerma. One Gy equals an energy absorption of one joule (J) per kilogram (kg) of matter in the irradiated object. In the traditional system of units 100 rad equals one Gy.

Grayscale   The number of different shades of gray color that can be stored in memory and subsequently displayed.

Grenz rays   x-rays in the energy range of 10 to 20 kVp.

Grid ratio   The height of the lead strips divided by the distance between each strip.

Guanine (G)   One of two purine bases found in both DNA and RNA.

H

Half-life   *Statistical* quantity equal to the amount of time due to natural processes associated with a 50% decrease in the radioactivity of a sample containing many radioactive atoms.

Half-value layer (HVL)   The thickness of a designated absorber (customarily a metal such as aluminum) required to decrease the intensity of the primary x-ray beam by 50% of its initial value.

Helical CT   See *Spiral computed tomography*.

Hematopoietic syndrome   A form of acute radiation syndrome that occurs when humans receive in a short time span (several hours or less) whole-body doses of ionizing radiation ranging from 1 to 10 Gy_t and in which the reduction of the number of blood cells in the circulating blood results in a loss of the body's ability to clot blood and fight infection; also called *bone marrow syndrome*.

Hematopoietic system   Blood-forming system.

Hemoglobin   A protein inside red blood cells (erythrocytes) that carries oxygen from the lungs to tissues and organs in the body and carries carbon dioxide back to the lungs. It has a reddish pigment because it is an iron-containing biomolecule.

Hemorrhage   Abnormal escape of blood; heavy bleeding.

Hereditary effects   See *Genetic effects*.

High contrast resolution   The ability of a system to make two closely adjacent objects visually distinguishable. It is usually specified in resolvable line pairs per millimeter.

High-LET radiation   Includes particles that possess substantial mass and charge such as alpha particles, ions of heavier nuclei, and charged particles released from interactions between neutrons and atoms. Low energy neutrons, which carry no electric charge, are also high linear energy transfer (LET) radiation.

High-level control fluoroscopy (HLCF)   An operating mode for state-of-the-art fluoroscopic equipment in which patient entrance exposure rates are substantially higher than normally allowed for routine procedures. The higher exposure rate allows visualization of smaller and lower contrast objects that do not usually appear during standard fluoroscopy. HLCF is also known as *"boost"* mode.

High-speed image receptor system   A relative term that describes an image receptor that requires less radiation exposure to obtain a response.

Highly differentiated cells   Mature or more specialized cells.

Holistic approach to patient care   Treating the whole person, rather than just an area of concern.

Homeostasis   A state of equilibrium between the different elements of an organism or a tendency toward such a state; the ability of the body to return to and maintain normal functioning despite the changes it has undergone.

Hormones Chemical secretions manufactured by various endocrine glands and carried by the bloodstream to influence activities of other parts of the body, such as regulating growth and development.

Human genome The total amount of genetic material (DNA) contained within the chromosomes of a human being.

Human-made radiation Ionizing radiation created by humans for various uses, including nuclear fuel for generation of power, consumer products containing radioactive material, air travel security, and medical radiation. Also called *artificial radiation*.

Hydrocephaly An abnormal buildup of cerebrospinal fluid (CSF) in the ventricles of the brain which can compress and damage the brain. In infants, it is characterized by head enlargement.

Hydroperoxyl radical A substance toxic to the cell that can result from the radiolysis of water.

Hyperbaric oxygen High-pressure oxygen sometimes used in conjunction with radiation therapy treatment of certain types of cancerous tumors to increase their radiosensitivity.

Hypodermis A subcutaneous layer of fat and connective tissue.

Hypoxic cells Cells that lack an adequate amount of oxygen.

I

Image guided radiation therapy (IGRT) IGRT is a method used in radiation therapy employing CBCT to precisely position a patient's desired treatment volume prior to delivering each radiation treatment.

Image intensification fluoroscopy Use of an image intensifier to enormously increase the brightness of the real-time image produced on a fluorescent screen during fluoroscopy.

Image intensifier An "electronic device that receives the image forming x-ray beam and converts it into a visible light image of high intensity" (e.g., a gain of 5000 or more is possible).

Image matrix The array of pixels that comprises a digital image. Examples of matrix sizes are 512 × 512 and 1024 × 1024.

Image receptor Any device that captures a radiographic image. Examples include phosphorescent screens and digital detectors.

Immune system A network of cells, tissues, organs, and the substances they make that helps the body fight infections and other diseases. The components of the immune system function collaboratively to provide rapid attack responses to foreign agents.

Immunoglobulin (Ig G) A large, Y-shaped protein, produced mainly by plasma cells, that is employed by the immune system to neutralize germs such as pathogens, bacteria and viruses.

Incoherent scattering See *Compton scattering.*

Indirect action The damaging effect, on key molecules, produced by free radicals that are created by the interaction of radiation with water molecules; cell death can result.

Indirect transmission Primary photons that undergo Compton and/or coherent interactions and are scattered or deflected while passing through a patient and then still reach the image receptor.

Inelastic scatter Any scattering interaction between fundamental particles or a particle and an atom in which energy is lost by one object and gained by another.

Inherent filtration The glass envelope (0.5-mm aluminum equivalent) encasing the x-ray tube, the insulating oil surrounding the tube, and the glass window in the tube housing all taken together.

Inorganic compounds Compounds that do not contain carbon. The inorganic compounds found in the human body occur in nature independent of living things.

Instant cell death Instant death of large numbers of cells occurs when a volume is irradiated with an x-ray or gamma ray dose of about 1000 Gy_t in a period of seconds or a few minutes.

Integral dose Product of dose and the volume of tissue irradiated.

Intensity (of radiation) Quantity, or amount, of radiation crossing unit area per unit time.

Intermittent fluoroscopy Discontinuous manual activation of the fluoroscopic tube by the fluoroscopist or automatic periodic activation (also known as *pulsed fluoroscopy*), rather than continuous activation.

Internal contamination Ingestion or inhalation of radioactive material within the body.

Internal radiation Radiation from radioactive atoms that make up a small percentage of the tissues of the human body.

International Commission on Radiological Protection (ICRP) Radiation protection standards organization considered to be the international authority on the safe use of sources of ionizing radiation. The ICRP is responsible for providing clear and consistent radiation protection guidance through its recommendations on occupational and public dose limits.

International system of units (SI or Systeme International) Common units that makes possible a standard system of units among all branches of science throughout the world.

Interphase The period of cell growth that occurs before actual mitosis.

Interphase death See *Apoptosis.*

Interslice scatter Radiation that scatters from the CT slice currently being acquired into adjacent slices.

Interstrand cross-link A cross-link occurs when chemical agents react with two nucleotides of DNA, forming a covalent linkage or connection between them. This can take place between opposite strands of the double-stranded DNA or between entirely different DNA molecules.

Interventional procedures Medical procedures, such as inserting catheters into vessels or tissues for the purpose of drainage, biopsy, or alteration of vascular occlusions, performed by a physician during an imaging procedure such as digital fluoroscopy.

Intrastrand cross-link A cross-link formed between two places on *the same* DNA strand.

Invasive ductal carcinoma (IDC) Also known as *infiltrating ductal carcinoma*, this is a type of cancer that begins growing in a mammary milk duct from which it will eventually emerge and invade the fibrous or fatty tissue of the breast outside of the duct. IDC is the most common form of breast cancer, representing 80% of all breast cancer diagnoses.

Inverse square law (ISL) Expresses the relationship between distance and intensity (quantity) of radiation. The law states: "The intensity of radiation is inversely proportional to the square of the distance from the source."

Investigational levels   Defined as level I and level II in the ALARA concept. These are personnel monitoring reading levels at which the Radiation Safety Officer investigates the reason for such a degree of exposure even though the excess is still within legal limits. In the United States, these levels are traditionally one tenth to three tenths the applicable regulatory limits.

Iodine-123 (^{123}I)   Unstable isotope of the element iodine (Z = 53, $T_{1/2}$ = 13.2 hours) used for monitoring thyroid gland function.

Iodine-125 (^{125}I)   A radioactive isotope of the element iodine with a half-life of approximately 60 days. It decays by the method of electron capture, emitting a low energy gamma ray and a low energy characteristic photon in the process.

Iodine-131 (^{131}I)   An unstable isotope of the element iodine with 78 neutrons in its nucleus causing it to undergo beta decay with a half-life of 8 days. It is used to treat thyroid cancer.

Ionization   The conversion of a neutral atom to a charged entity, called an ion, by removing one or more electrons from the atom or, in some cases by adding an electron to a neutral atom.

Ionization chamber   A device that measures the amount of electric charge resulting from the ions produced by irradiation of a volume of air.

Ionization chamber–type survey meter ("cutie pie")   This instrument is both a rate meter device used for area surveys and an accurate integrating or cumulative exposure or dose measurement instrument for x-radiation and gamma radiation and, if equipped with a suitable window, for recording beta radiation as well.

Ionizing radiation   Radiation that produces positively and negatively charged particles (ions) when passing through matter.

Ion pair   Two oppositely charged particles.

Isotopes   Atoms that have the same number of protons within the nucleus but have different numbers of neutrons (e.g., helium-3 and helium-4, whose nuclei contain one and two neutrons, respectively). Radioactive isotopes of atoms that make up biologic materials may be used in medical imaging nuclear medicine studies.

Iterative reconstruction   For producing a high-quality final image, CT scan data can be reconstructed, modified, reconstructed again, modified, etc., until an image with the best quality and lowest noise that is possible for the current situation is obtained.

J

Joule (J)   The SI unit of energy. The work done or energy expended when a force of 1 newton acts on an object along a distance of 1 meter.

K

Karyotype   A chromosome map that consists of a *photomicrograph*, that is taken of the human cell nucleus during metaphase, when each chromosome can be individually perceived. It is used to provide a cytogenetic analysis of chromosomes.

Kiloelectron volt (keV)   A unit used to specify the kinetic energy of an individual electron in the electron beam within the x-ray tube; equivalent to 1000 electron volts. This unit is also used to specify the energies of x-rays.

Kinetic energy   Energy of motion.

L

Last image hold feature   An equipment feature in current fluoroscopy units in which the most recent fluoroscopic image remains in view as a guide to the radiologist when the x-ray beam is not activated. The use of this feature leads to dose reduction for the patient and is required by the FDA on all fluoroscopes manufactured for use in the United States.

Late stochastic (probabilistic) somatic effects   Late effects that do not have a threshold, that occur in an arbitrary or probabilistic manner, whose severity does not depend on dose, and that occur months or years after high level and possibly even after low level radiation exposure.

Late tissue reactions   Nongenetic consequences of radiation exposure that appear months or years afterward. These effects may be either stochastic or tissue reactions.

Latent period   The period of about 1 week after the prodromal stage of acute radiation syndrome, during which no visible symptoms of radiation exposure occur.

Law of Bergonié and Tribondeau   The radiosensitivity of cells is directly proportional to their reproductive activity and inversely proportional to their degree of differentiation.

LD 50/30, 50/60, 100/60   A quantitative measurement signifying the whole-body dose of radiation that can be lethal to 50% of the exposed population within 30 days, or can be lethal to 50% of the exposed population within 60 days, or can be lethal to 100% of the exposed population within 60 days.

Lead-equivalent   Thickness of some other radiation absorbing material that produces an attenuation equivalent to that which would be accomplished by a specified amount of lead.

Leakage radiation   Radiation generated in the x-ray tube that does not exit from the collimator opening but partially penetrates the protective tube housing and, to some degree, the sides of the collimator.

LET   See *Linear energy transfer*.

Leukemia   Neoplastic (abnormal) overproduction of white blood cells.

Leukocytes   White blood cells.

Leukopenia   An unnatural decrease of white blood corpuscles, usually to less than 5000/mm^3.

Lifetime effective dose limit   Dose in millisieverts that does not exceed 10 times the occupationally exposed person's age in years, or for the dose in rem, the age of the person.

Light-localizing, variable-aperture rectangular collimator   An x-ray beam limitation device that permits the equipment operator to adjust the size and shape of the x-ray beam either automatically or manually.

Linear dose–response curve   A model used to calculate the occurrence of cancer at low doses by extrapolating from information associated with high levels of radiation. The linear dose–response curve describes current high dose information satisfactorily but exaggerates the actual risk or danger at low doses and dose rates.

Linear energy transfer (LET)   The mean quantity of energy deposited by ionizing radiation in an object per unit length of track as it passes through the object. It is expressed in units of keV/μm.

Linear nonthreshold curve of radiation dose–response   An extrapolated (*from high dose* values) graph which implies that the chance of a biologic response to ionizing radiation is directly proportional to the dose received no matter how low the dose is. The use of this curve is recommended or has been adopted conservatively for most types of cancers.

Linear-quadratic dose–response curve A nonstraightline model used to calculate the occurrence of cancer by extrapolating from information associated with high levels of radiation to determine the risk associated with low doses. This model fits the current high dose information satisfactorily but *may underestimate* risk at low doses.

Linear, threshold dose–response relationship The relationship between dose and response is such that a biologic response does not occur below a specified level of radiation dose.

Lipids Water insoluble, organic macromolecules that consist only of carbon, hydrogen, and oxygen; lipids store energy in the body for long periods. Also known as *fats*.

Lithium fluoride (LiF) The sensing material of the thermoluminescent ring dosimeter (TLD).

Local tissue damage A response in irradiated biologic tissue that can occur where any part of the human body receives a high radiation dose.

Log, or logarithmic, scale A method used to graph data that cover several orders of magnitude (the powers of 10; e.g., 1, 10, 100, 1000, etc. would be the increments on either the x-or y-axis of a graph).

Long scale of radiographic contrast Radiographic contrast containing many shades of gray. A wide range of exposures will produce a wide range of or many shades of gray when a long scale image receptor or display is used.

Low-LET radiations External radiations such as x-rays and gamma rays that produce sparse ionization per unit length of path (LET = linear energy transfer).

Lumen The SI derived unit of luminous flux, equal to the amount of light emitted per second passing into a solid angle of one steradian from a uniform source of one candela. One *lumen* is about the same brightness as a normal birthday candle at a distance of one foot. A foot-candle is equal to one lumen per square foot.

Luminance A scientific term referring to the brightness of a surface. Luminance quantifies the intensity of a light source.

Lux An SI unit of brightness equal to one lumen *per square meter*. In photometry, this is used as a measure of the intensity, as perceived by the human eye, of light that hits or passes through a surface. Because of the different systems of units, approximately 10.76 lux amount to one foot candle.

Lymphocytes A subgroup of white blood cells that play an active role in producing immunity for the body by producing agents called antibodies to combat disease. Lymphocytes are the most radio-sensitive blood cells in the human body.

Lymph A colorless fluid containing white blood cells that bathes the tissues and ultimately drains into the bloodstream.

Lymph nodes Small, *bean-shaped organs* important in the function of the immune response and that also store special cells that can trap cancer cells or bacteria that are traveling through the body through the lymph.

Lymphoma A type of cancer that can develop when lymphocytes (white blood cells that fight infection) grow out of control.

Lysosomes Small, pealike sacs or single membrane spherical bodies that are of great importance for digestion within the cytoplasm. Their primary function appears to be the breaking down of large molecules.

M On a personnel monitoring report, this letter signifies that an equivalent dose below the minimum measurable quantity of radiation has been received during the interval of time covered by the report. Doses less than 0.1 mSv (10 mrem) are not usually detected and are reported as (M) on a personnel monitoring report.

Machine learning (ML) Subset of AI that allows a machine to acquire information and make predictions based on its experience (i.e., its accumulated data in the area of interest). In short, ML is a process that allows computers to pursue a task or objective without explicitly being programmed for that task.

Macromolecule Large molecule built up from smaller chemical structures.

Magnification mode (*Mag mode*) Refers to a selectable smaller but enhanced field of view of an area displayed on a video device by the output phosphor of an image intensification system or by the detector output onto a computer monitor.

Mammography Radiographic study of the breast employing low energy (typically, a mean energy <25 KeV) x-rays in either a fixed angular beam orientation or an arc angular rotational mode.

Manifest illness The stage of acute radiation syndrome when symptoms that affect the hematopoietic, gastrointestinal, and cerebrovascular systems become visible again after a latent period.

Mask image A non-iodinated anatomical image that will be subtracted from sequential iodinated images obtained as the iodinated contrast agent progresses through a selected portion of the patient's anatomy.

Mass density Quantity of matter per unit volume. It is generally specified in units of kilograms per cubic meter (kg/m^3) or grams per cubic centimeter (g/cc).

Mass number (A) The total number of protons and neutrons within the nucleus of an atom.

Master molecule A molecule vital to the survival of the cell that maintains normal cell function. It is also referred to as a *key molecule*.

Maximum permissible dose (MPD) A term used *in the past* to indicate the maximum dose equivalent of ionizing radiation that an occupationally exposed person could absorb in a specified time period without sustaining appreciable bodily injury.

Mean energy The average energy of an x-ray beam.

Mean glandular dose The average dose to the glandular tissue, considered the "tissue at risk," within a breast. For a 4.2-cm compressed breast, consisting of 50% fat and 50% glandular tissue, the maximum permitted dose is 3 mGy (0.3 cGy) per x-ray projection.

Mean marrow dose "The average radiation dose to the entire active bone marrow." Also known as *bone marrow dose*.

Megakaryocytes A large bone marrow cell responsible for the production of blood thrombocytes (platelets), which are necessary for normal blood clotting. They may also be described as *platelet stem cells*.

Meiosis The process of germ (genetic) cell division that reduces the number of chromosomes in each daughter cell to half the number of chromosomes in the parent cell.

Meningitis   An inflammation of the membranes (meninges) surrounding the brain and spinal cord.

Mesons   Penetrating, unstable, subatomic particles that are components of cosmic radiation.

Messenger RNA (mRNA)   The substance that directs the process for making proteins out of amino acids.

Metabolism   Chemical reactions that modify foods for cellular use. Metabolism enables the cell to perform the vital functions of synthesizing proteins and producing energy.

Metaphase   The phase of cell division during which the mitotic spindle is completed. It is also the phase of cell division in which chromosome damage caused by radiation exposure can be evaluated.

Microcalcifications   Small calcium deposits in breast tissue that on a mammogram look like white specks. When seen in a cluster, a biopsy is required. About 80% of microcalcifications are benign. However, they are sometimes an indication of precancerous changes or existing invasive cancer in the breast.

Microcephaly   Abnormally small head circumference.

Microwaves   An electromagnetic wave with a wavelength in the range 0.001 to 0.3 meters, shorter than that of a normal radio wave but longer than those of infrared radiation.

Milliampere-seconds (mAs)   The product of electron tube current (mA) and the amount of time in seconds that the x-ray tube is activated.

Mineral salts   See *Salts*.

Mitochondria   Large, double-membranous, oval or bean-shaped structures containing highly organized enzymes in their inner membranes that supply the energy for cells. Because of this they are referred to as "powerhouses" of the cell.

Mitosis   The process of somatic cell division wherein a parent cell divides to form two daughter cells identical to the parent cell.

Mitotic death   Cell death that occurs when a cell dies after one or more divisions. This can happen after irradiation. Mitotic death is also known as *genetic death*.

Mitotic delay   The failure of a cell to start dividing on time; this can occur when a cell is exposed to as little as 0.01 Gy_t of ionizing radiation just before it begins dividing.

Mitotic spindle   The delicate fibers attached to the centrioles and extending or fanning out from one side of the cell to the other while coming back together at each end.

Mobile C-arm fluoroscopic unit   A portable fluoroscopic x-ray unit that is C-shaped and can be multiply geometrically oriented. It has an x-ray tube attached to one end of its arm and an image intensifier attached to the other end.

Mobile radiographic equipment   Manually movable basic radiographic equipment.

Modified scattering   See *Compton scattering*.

Molecular change   An alteration in the basic structure of a molecule caused by some type of energetic interaction, such as exposure to ionizing radiation. Molecular damage results in the formation of structurally changed molecules that may impair cellular function.

Molecular lesions   See *Point lesions*.

Molecule   The smallest unit of a specific substance composed of one or more atoms.

Monitoring   A means of overseeing occupational radiation exposure to ensure that such exposure is kept well below the annual effective dose limit.

Monoclonal antibodies (MAB)   Antibodies or specific immune system cells that preferentially bind always to a specific part of an antigen (e.g., cancer cell) that is recognized by the antibody,

Monomers   A solitary molecule that can combine with others of the same kind to form a large repetitive molecule called a polymer. Glucose molecules, for example, are monomers that can combine to form the polymer cellulose.

Multidetector Computed Tomography (MDCT)   CT scanning that employs multiple rows of detectors for each image acquisition unlike SSCT scanners which only use one.

Muscle tissue   Tissue that contains fibers that affect movement of an organ or part of the body; muscle tissue does not divide and is relatively insensitive to radiation.

Mutagenesis   Birth defects that can be caused by irradiation of reproductive cells (sperm and ova) before conception.

Mutagens   Agents that increase the frequency of occurrence of mutations, such as elevated temperatures, ionizing radiations, viruses, and chemicals.

Mutation frequency   The number of spontaneous or mutagen-caused mutations that occur in a given generation.

Mutations   Changes in genes caused by the loss or change of a nitrogenous base on the DNA chain. It is generally the result of the direct or indirect interaction of high-energy radiation with a DNA molecule.

Myeloblasts   Precursors of granulocytes, a type of white blood cell.

N

NARM   Stands for "naturally occurring and/or accelerator produced materials."

National Academy of Science/National Research Council Committee on the Biological Effects of Ionizing Radiation (NAS/NRC-BEIR)   An advisory group that reviews studies of the biologic effects of ionizing radiation and risk assessment and provides the information to other organizations for evaluation.

National Council on Radiation Protection and Measurements (NCRP)   In the United States the NCRP is a nongovernmental, nonprofit, private corporation that reviews the recommendations formulated by the International Commission on Radiological Protection (ICRP). The NCRP determines the way ICRP recommendations are incorporated into US radiation protection criteria; recommendations are published in the form of various NCRP Reports.

National Institute of Standards and Technology (NIST)   Professional organization responsible, among other measures and standards tasks, for accrediting calibration laboratories that calibrate instruments used to measure radiation exposure and absorbed dose in medical radiation imaging and therapy.

Nationwide Evaluation of x-ray Trends (NEXT) Program   Conducted by the US Food and Drug Administration and the Conference of Radiation Control Program Directors and most state health departments to provide data on systems as they exist in the United States on the latest survey. These groups have compiled reference values for patient dose. They are usually based on large-scale surveys of actual measurements of x-ray machines in hospitals.

Natural background radiation   Ionizing radiation from environmental sources, including radioactive materials in the earth, cosmic radiation from space, and radionuclides deposited in the human body via the food chain.

Necrosis   Death of areas of tissue or bone surrounded by healthy parts.

Negative contrast media   Agents such as air or gas that result in areas of increased intensity on a completed radiographic image.

Negatron   A normal electron carrying a negative electric charge.

Negligible individual dose (NID)   An annual effective dose that provides a low exposure cutoff level such that regulatory agencies may consider the associated level of individual risk negligible.

Neonatal death   Death at birth.

Neoplasm   An abnormal mass of tissue that forms when cells grow and divide more than is normal or do not die when they should. Neoplasms may be benign or malignant.

Nervous tissue   Conductive tissue found in the brain and spinal cord.

Neural nets   The fundamental structure of a DL machine is a multidimensional grid containing many thousands of, or greater, nodes. Neural nets are usually organized into multiple layers or planes of such nodes (as many as 50 such in the latest systems), and data moves through them in only one direction.

Neuron   A nerve cell consisting of a cell body and two kinds of very fine, string-like tissue segments, called processes, that extend outward, namely, dendrites and the axon.

Neuron organogenesis   In the embryo-fetus, a period of development and change of the nerve cells that extends into the beginning of the fetal period.

Neutrino   A particle that has no electric charge but carries away excess energy during beta decay and has an almost negligible mass. The neutrino shows an exceedingly small tendency to interact with any type of matter and is therefore nearly impossible to detect.

Neutron   An electrically neutral particle located within the nucleus of the atom; one of the fundamental constituents of the atom. It has approximately the same mass as a proton.

Neutrophils   Leukocytes that fight infection.

Newton   Unit of force in the SI system of physical units. One newton corresponds to approximately one-fourth of a pound.

Nit   A *nit* is another term used to describe a brightness of 1 candela per square meter (cd/m^2). Since an average candle produces roughly 1 candela, then that amount of light, spread over a square meter comprises one *nit*.

Nitrogen   A tasteless, odorless, colorless, gaseous chemical element found free in the air and comprising about 78% of it; integral part of protein and nucleic acids and thus found in every living cell.

Nitrogenous bases   An organic molecule, containing multiple interconnected nitrogen, hydrogen, oxygen, and carbon atoms, that acts as a *base* in chemical reactions. The nitrogen *bases* are also called *nucleobases* because they play a major role as building blocks for both DNA and RNA.

Noble gas   Any of rare gases that include helium, neon, argon, krypton, xenon, and usually radon and that exhibit great stability and extremely low reaction rates—also called *inert gases*.

Nodes   Components of layers of a deep learning system that reset connections to other nodes as data from training sets are processed repeatedly and compared to known outcomes.

No-threshold dose concept   That any radiation dose has the capability of producing a biologic effect. No radiation dose can be considered absolutely safe.

Nonagreement states   Individual US states in which both the state departments of environmental protection and the Nuclear Regulatory Commission (NRC) separately enforce radiation protection regulations. These states have decided to maintain their own designed independent radiation protection programs for radioactive materials.

Nonionizing radiation   Radiation that does not have sufficient energy to eject electrons from atoms.

Nonoccupational exposure   Radiation exposure received by members of the general population who are not employed as radiation workers (i.e., nonoccupational personnel).

Nonverbal messages   Unconscious actions, or body language. Very important when handling patients, especially those who may be compromised.

Nuclear medicine   Branch of medicine that employs radioisotopes to study organ function in a patient, to detect the spread of cancer into bone, and to treat certain types of diseases.

Nuclear medicine procedure   In general, the administration, either orally or intravenously, of a radioactive isotope for the purpose of conducting a diagnostic study of a body area.

Nuclear reactor   A mechanism for creating and continuing a controlled nuclear chain reaction in a fissionable fuel for the production of energy or supplementary fissionable material.

Nuclear Regulatory Commission (NRC)   A federal agency (formerly known as the *Atomic Energy Commission*) that has the authority to control the possession, use, and production of atomic energy in the interest of national security. This agency also has the power to set and enforce radiation protection standards for the usage of reactor produced radioisotopes.

Nucleic acids   Very large, complex macromolecules made up of nucleotides.

Nucleolus   A small body in the nucleus of a cell that contains protein and RNA and is the site for the synthesis of ribosomal RNA and for the formation of ribosomal subunits.

Nucleoplasm   A gelatinous liquid within the nucleus that surrounds the chromosomes and the nucleoli.

Nucleotides   Units formed from the following: a nitrogenous base such as adenine, guanine, cytosine, or thymine; a five-carbon sugar molecule, *deoxyribose*; and a phosphate molecule. Long chains of nucleotides are the basic building blocks of a nucleic acid such as DNA or RNA.

Nucleus   The center of the cell; a spherical mass of protoplasm containing the genetic material (DNA), which is stored in its molecular structure.

O

Occupancy factor (T)   A factor used to modify the shielding requirement for a particular barrier by taking into account the fraction of the work week during which the space beyond the barrier is occupied.

Occupational and nonoccupational dose limits   Upper boundary doses of ionizing radiation for which there is a negligible risk of bodily injury or genetic damage.

Occupational exposure   Radiation exposure received by radiation workers (occupationally exposed persons) in the course of exercising their professional responsibilities.

Occupational risk   (1) The probability of injury, ailment, or death resulting from an activity that takes place in the workplace; (2) the possibility of developing a radiogenic cancer or the induction of a genetic defect as a consequence of the radiation exposure received.

Occupational Safety and Health Administration (OSHA)   A monitoring agency functioning in places of employment, predominantly in industry, OSHA regulates occupational exposure to radiation.

Off-focus radiation   x-rays emitted from parts of the x-ray tube other than the focal spot. Also called *stem radiation.*

Oncology   Branch of medicine dealing with cancer.

Oocytes   Immature female germ cells.

Oogonium   Female germ cell.

Optically stimulated luminescence (OSL) dosimeter   A device for monitoring occupational exposure that contains an aluminum oxide detector. The dosimeter is "read out" by using laser light at selected frequencies. When such laser light is incident on the sensing material, it becomes luminescent in proportion to the amount of radiation exposure that was received.

Organic acids   Organic compounds containing the carboxyl (COOH) molecular group.

Organic compounds   All compounds that always contain quantities of carbon, hydrogen, and oxygen.

Organogenesis   (1) Period of gestation that corresponds to approximately 10 days to 12 weeks after conception. During this time, the nerve cells in the brain and spinal cord of the fetus are most susceptible to radiation-induced congenital abnormalities; (2) the stage in which undifferentiated cells are implanted in the uterine wall.

Osmosis   When water tends to move across cell surfaces or membranes into areas in which a high concentration of potassium ions is present.

Osmotic pressure   The force created when a semipermeable membrane separates two solutions of different concentrations.

Osteogenic sarcoma   Bone cancer.

Osteoporosis   Decalcification of the bone.

Ovum   The mature reproductive cell of female animals and human females produced in the ovaries. Also called the *egg,* the ovum contributes one chromosome of each pair to the fertilized cell.

Oxidation   Most simply, the combining of a substance with oxygen. The definition of oxidation, however, has been broadened to include reactions in which electrons are lost by an atom.

Oxygen enhancement ratio (OER)   The ratio of the radiation dose required to cause a particular biologic response of cells or organisms in any oxygen-deprived environment to the radiation dose required to cause an identical response under normally oxygenated conditions.

Oxygen fixation   Refers to *nonreparable* DNA lesions produced by x-rays with the chemical participation of oxygen.

P

PACS   Picture archiving and communication system imaging technology providing both storage and convenient remote access to images from multiple modalities.

Pair production   Interaction between an incoming photon of at least 1.022 MeV and an atom in which the photon approaches, strongly interacts with the nucleus of the atom and disappears. In the process, the energy of the incoming photon is transformed into two new particles—a negatron and a positron—after which these particles exit from the atom and carry away some of the momentum of the absorbed photon when the photon's energy is greater than 1.022 MeV.

Parenchymal cells   The specific cells of a gland or organ, contained in and supported by the connective tissue framework.

Particulate radiation   As opposed to x-rays and gamma rays, which are electromagnetic radiations, particulate radiation is a form of radiation that includes alpha particles (nuclei of helium), beta particles (electrons), neutrons, and protons.

Peak kilovoltage (kVp)   The highest energy level of photons in the x-ray beam and the maximum voltage directed across an x-ray tube.

Peptic or peptide bond   A chemical bond formed between two molecules when the carboxyl group of one molecule reacts with the amino group of the other molecule, releasing a molecule of water (H_2O). Also described as a chemical bond connecting two amino acids.

Personnel dosimeter   A personnel device that determines occupational exposure by detecting and measuring the quantity of ionizing radiation to which the dosimeter has been exposed over a period of time.

Personnel monitoring report   A written report of occupational radiation exposure of personnel prepared by a monitoring company.

Person-sievert   SI unit for the radiation quantity: collective effective dose (ColEfD).

PET/CT scanner   A large physical system in which a positron emission tomography (PET) scanner is mechanically joined in a tandem configuration with a computed tomography (CT) scanner to produce a single imaging device. This unit can detect the presence of abnormally high regions of glucose metabolism, yielding evidence of cancer spread (metastasis) in other body areas, but also, at the same time, obtain detailed information about the anatomic location and extent of these lesions or growths.

Photodisintegration   An interaction that occurs above 10 MeV in high-energy radiation therapy treatment machines. In this interaction, a high energy photon collides with the nucleus of an atom, which directly absorbs all the photon's energy. This energy excess in the nucleus creates an instability that in most cases is alleviated by the emission of a neutron from the nucleus. Also, if sufficient energy is absorbed by the nucleus, another type of emission is possible, such as a proton or proton–neutron combination (deuteron) or even an alpha particle.

Photoelectric absorption   Process whereby the energy of the incident photon is completely absorbed as it interacts with an atom and ejects an inner-shell electron from its orbit about the nucleus.

Photoelectron   An electron emitted from an atom by interaction with a photon, especially an electron emitted from a solid surface by the action of light.

Photomultiplier tube and detector   Useful for light detection of very weak signals. This is a device in which the absorption of a photon results in the emission of an electron. The electronics within the device then amplify the electrons generated by a photocathode exposed to the photon flux. In computed radiography (CR) it represents an electron tube that converts the computed radiography stored latent image, transforming visible light photons into an amplified electronic signal.

Photon   A particle associated with electromagnetic radiation that has neither rest mass nor electric charge but has momentum and always moves at the speed of light.

Photostimulable phosphor (PSP)   The image receptor of a computed radiography (CR) system. When struck by x-rays, electrons within the phosphor become trapped at energy levels that are quasi-stable. When a laser beam imparts additional energy to the surface of the phosphor. visible light is emitted in proportion to the x-ray exposure that had been received by the phosphor. A photomultiplier tube then amplifies and records the visible light intensity, which corresponds to the brightness of a picture element, or pixel, in the CR image.

Phototiming   See *Automatic Exposure Control.*

Pitch (pitch ratio)   CT table advance in one 360-degree gantry rotation divided by beam collimation. For example, if the table traveled 5 mm in one rotation and the beam collimation was 5 mm, then pitch equals 5 mm/5 mm = 1.0.

Pixels   The smallest unit or building block of a digital image that can be displayed on a digital display device. *Pixels* are combined to form a complete image, video, text or any visible thing on a computer display. Higher resolution implies the presence of a greater number of pixels and therefore smaller in size making up the image. A *pixel* is also known as a picture element.

Platelets   Circular or oval disks found in the blood of all vertebrates. Platelets initiate blood clotting and prevent hemorrhage.

Pluripotential stem cell   A single precursor cell from which all of the cells of the hematopoietic system develop.

Point lesions   Altered locations in macromolecules caused by the breaking of a single chemical bond.

Point mutations   Genetic mutations at the molecular level. The chromosome is not broken, but the DNA within it is damaged (see *Single-strand break*).

Polymer   A large molecule, or macromolecule, composed of many repeated subunits called *monomers.*

Polysaccharides   Polymeric carbohydrate molecules composed of long chains of monosaccharides (simple carbohydrates).

Positive beam limitation (PBL)   A feature of radiographic collimators that automatically adjusts them so that the radiation field size matches the size of the image receptor. Also known as *automatic collimation.*

Positive contrast media   Solutions containing elements that have a higher atomic number than surrounding soft tissue (e.g., barium or iodine based) that are either ingested or injected into the body tissues or structures to enhance their visualization.

Positron   A positively charged electron, which is a form of antimatter.

Positron emission tomography (PET)   A nuclear medicine imaging technique that produces a three-dimensional picture of functional processes within the body. It does this with a detection system or camera that records pairs of oppositely traveling photons (annihilation radiation) indirectly produced by a positron-emitting radionuclide attached to glucose. Images in three-dimensional space of heightened metabolic activity can be generated using mathematical reconstruction techniques similar to those employed by x-ray computed tomography.

Precursor cells   See *Stem cells.*

Preimplantation stage   Approximately 0 to 9 days after conception. In this stage the fertilized ovum divides and forms a ball-like structure containing undifferentiated cells.

Primary protective barrier   (1) A barrier designed to prevent primary, or direct, radiation from reaching personnel or members of the general public on the other side of the barrier; (2) a barrier located perpendicular to the undeflected line of travel of the primary x-ray beam.

Primary radiation beam   Well confined radiation that emerges directly from the x-ray tube collimator and moves without deflection toward a wall, door, viewing window, and so on. Also called *direct radiation* or the *useful beam.*

Probabilistic effects   See *Stochastic effects.*

Prodromal syndrome   The first stage of acute radiation syndrome, which occurs within hours after a whole body absorbed dose of 1 Gy_t or more; characterized by nausea, vomiting, diarrhea, fatigue, and leukopenia. Also called the *initial stage of ARS.*

Programmed cell death   See *Apoptosis.*

Prophase   The first phase of cell division, during which the nucleus and the chromosomes enlarge and the DNA begins to take structural form.

Proportional counter   A radiation survey instrument generally used in a laboratory setting to detect alpha and beta radiation and small amounts of other types of low-level radioactive contamination.

Prospective Gating   When the ECG voltage signal level regains a value associated with a specific part of the diastole phase, the CT scanner will be triggered to image the next section of the heart and scan until another voltage pulse is received that will stop the radiation and advance the table position. This delayed or future gating technique is called prospective gating and is essentially a *step and shoot* process, since for most facility scanners the detectors' limited longitudinal extent mandates that the scanner advances the table in between several quiescent phases of the heart and then shoot or produce radiation in order to cover the full z-axis extent of the heart.

Protective apparel   Special garments such as aprons, gloves, and thyroid shields that are conventionally made of lead-impregnated vinyl and worn during fluoroscopic and certain selective radiographic procedures.

Protective barrier   Any medium of adequate composition and thickness that absorbs primary and/or secondary radiation, thereby reducing the exposure of persons located on the other side of the barrier.

Protective curtain   A sliding panel with a minimum of 0.25-mm lead equivalent that can be positioned between the fluoroscopist and the patient to intercept scattered radiation above the tabletop.

Protective eyeglasses   Eyeglasses with optically clear lenses that contain a minimum lead-equivalent protection of 0.35 mm.

Protective shielding   A structure or device made of certain materials such as concrete, lead, or lead-impregnated material, or heavy metals (e.g., nonradioactive or depleted uranium) that will adequately attenuate ionizing radiation.

Protein   Amino acids linked in various patterns and combinations. Proteins are very large molecules always containing carbon, hydrogen, nitrogen, oxygen, and occasionally other elements, such as sulfur. Proteins are the most elementary building blocks of cells.

Proton   One of the three main constituents of an atom, the proton carries a positive electric charge equal in magnitude to that of an electron and is slightly less massive than a neutron.

Protoplasm   The chemical building material for all living things, protoplasm consists of inorganic substances, such as water and mineral salts, and organic substances, including proteins, carbohydrates, lipids, and nucleic acids.

Pulsed fluoroscopy   See *Intermittent fluoroscopy.*

Purines   A class of nitrogenous bases found in DNA and RNA. These bases include adenine (A) and guanine (G).

Pyrimidines   A class of nitrogenous bases found in DNA and RNA. These bases include cytosine (C), thymine (T), and, in the case of RNA, uracil (U), which replaces thymine.

Q

Quality control program:

Radiographic   An organized method used in imaging departments to ensure standardization in image acquisition and processing of those images. It includes monitoring and maintenance of all radiation producing equipment in the facility.

Quality factor   An adjustment multiplier that was used in the calculation of dose equivalence to more accurately quantify the ability of a dose of any kind of ionizing radiation to cause biologic damage. Also known as a *modifying factor.*

Quantum noise (mottle)   Faint blotches (image noise) in the recorded radiographic image produced by an intrinsic or quantum fluctuation in the incident photon intensity. This effect can degrade the radiographic image.

R

Rad (radiation absorbed dose)   The traditional unit that has been used to indicate the amount of radiant energy per gram transferred to an irradiated object

by any type of ionizing radiation. The rad is equivalent to an energy transfer of 100 ergs per gram to an irradiated object and numerically is equal to 1/100 gray or one centigray.

Radiant energy   Energy that moves in the form of a wave and is transmitted by radiations such as x-rays and gamma rays.

Radiation   Energy that passes from one location to another; a transfer of energy that results from either a change occurring naturally within an atom (See *Radiation decay*) or a process caused by the interaction of a particle with an atom.

Radiation biology   The science concerned with the effects of ionizing radiations on living systems.

Radiation Control for Health and Safety Act of 1968   Law passed by the US Congress to protect the public from the hazards of unnecessary radiation exposure resulting from electronic products such as microwave ovens, color televisions, and diagnostic x-ray equipment.

Radiation decay   A naturally occurring process in which atoms with unstable nuclei relieve that instability by various types of nuclear spontaneous transformations and/or emissions, including charged particles, uncharged particles, and photons.

Radiation dose   The amount of energy per unit mass transferred to atoms in biologic tissue by ionizing radiation is the basis of this concept.

Radiation dose–response curve   A graph that maps out the *effects* of radiation observed in relation to the dose of radiation received. The information plotted can be used to attempt to predict the risk of occurrence of malignancies in human populations exposed to low levels of ionizing radiation.

Radiation emergency plan   General plan that hospitals can implement for handling emergency situations involving radioactive contamination within the facility or from radio-contaminated persons brought to the facility.

Radiation hormesis   Effect that is a beneficial consequence of radiation for populations continuously exposed to moderately higher levels of radiation than ordinary background.

Radiation monitoring device   A device worn by diagnostic imaging personnel to indicate occupational exposure by recording the quantity of radiation to which it has been exposed over time.

Radiation permeability   The ability of a structure to be penetrated by radiation.

Radiation protection   Effective measures employed by radiation workers to safeguard patients, personnel, and the general public from unnecessary exposure to ionizing radiation.

Radiation safety committee (RSC)   Group that assists in the development of the radiation safety program in a health care facility, provides guidance for the program, and facilitates its ongoing operation.

Radiation safety officer (RSO)   An individual such as a medical physicist, health physicist, radiologist, or other individual qualified through adequate training and experience in the safe usage of radiation. It is the responsibility of the RSO to ensure that state, federal, and internationally accepted guidelines for radiation protection are accurately followed in the facility.

Radiation safety program   An effective and detailed program practiced and adhered to in facilities that provide imaging services to ensure adequate radiation safety of patients and radiation workers and the general public.

Radiation survey instruments   Area monitoring devices that detect and/or measure radiation levels as well as radiation exposure rates.

Radiation therapy   Use of x-rays or gamma rays as well as particulate radiations such as electrons and protons, usually with energies much greater than those employed for diagnostic purposes, to destroy the cells comprising a tumor while sparing the surrounding nontumor tissues.

Radiation weighting factor (W_R)   A dimensionless factor (a multiplier) that was chosen for radiation protection purposes to account for differences in biologic impact among various types of ionizing radiations. This factor places risks associated with biologic effects on a common scale.

Radiation-induced malignancy   Cancerous (malignant) neoplasm caused by exposure to ionizing radiation.

Radicals   Groups of atoms that remain together during a chemical change and behave almost like a single atom. Usually, these entities are very chemically reactive. Atoms in a radical are held together by covalent bonding.

Radioactive contamination Radioactive material that is attached to or associated with dust particles or is in liquid form on various surfaces. Removal of the liquid or dust accomplishes removal of the radioactive material. Radioactive contamination may consist of surface, internal (inhaled, ingested), internal wound, or external wound contamination.

Radioactive dispersal device A radioactive source mixed with conventional explosives. When detonated, this device explodes, spreading radioactive material through a specific area and causing contamination; also called a *dirty bomb*.

Radioactive tracers Generally, short half-life radioisotopes (e.g., Tc-99m) linked to various chemical compounds which permit specific physiological processes to be scrutinized. They can be given by injection, inhalation, or orally.

Radioantibody A radioactive isotope (typically a short-range, high-energy beta-emitter) that is chemically bound to a target-specific monoclonal antibody forming a radioactive *conjugate* or team.

Radiodermatitis Reddening of the skin caused by exposure to ionizing radiation.

Radiographer A person qualified through formal education and certification to practice medical imaging procedures that make use of ionizing radiation and also provide relevant patient care.

Radiographic beam–light beam coincidence Both physical size (length and width) and alignment between the radiographic beam and the localizing light beam must correspond to within 2% of the source-to–image distance (SID).

Radiographic contrast Differences in gray levels between adjacent anatomic structures on a completed image. Image receptor contrast and subject contrast combined produce radiographic contrast.

Radiographic fog Undesirable additional signal intensity on a completed radiographic image caused by scattered radiation reaching the image receptor.

Radiographic grid A device made of parallel radiopaque lead strips alternately separated with low-attenuation strips such as aluminum or plastic. The grid is placed between the patient and the radiographic image receptor to remove scattered x-ray photons that emerge from the patient before they reach the image receptor. Use of a grid improves radiographic contrast and visibility of detail, but it also increases patient dose.

Radiographic image receptor Phosphor plate, digital radiography detector, or previously, but now discontinued, radiographic film.

Radioimmunotherapy (RIT) A specific treatment protocol for cancer by cytotoxic (cell killing) radioisotopes chemically combined with specialized immune system antibodies.

Radioisotopes Isotopes of a particular element that are unstable because of their neutron–proton configuration.

Radiologist A qualified physician who specializes in diagnosis and sometimes interventional treatment through the use of radiant energy.

Radiolucent Transparent to radiation; a material that allows radiation to pass through it.

Radiolysis of water Ionization interaction of radiation with water molecules resulting in a separation into oxygen and hydrogen components.

Radionuclide An unstable nucleus that emits one or more forms of ionizing radiation to achieve stability. The emissions may include alpha particles, beta particles, and gamma rays.

Radiopaque A classification for objects that block radiation rather than allow it to pass through. Lead is the most common example.

Radiosensitivity Comparable sensitivity of human cells, tissues, and organs to the injurious action of ionizing radiation.

Radio waves Electromagnetic waves which have frequencies from 300 GHz to as low as 3 kHz, and corresponding wavelengths from 1 millimeter to as large as 100 kilometers. Their range of frequencies and wavelengths is very extensive.

Radium This element (Z = 88, A = 226) has an unstable nucleus and decays with a half-life of 1622 years by alpha particle emission to the radioactive element radon (Z = 86, A = 222).

Radon (Z = 86, A = 222) The first decay product of radium. Radon is a colorless, odorless, heavy radioactive gas ($T_{1/2}$ = 3.8 days) that, along with its own decay products, polonium-218 and polonium-214 (solid form), is always present to some degree in the air. It comprises the largest component of natural background radiation and is predominantly an alpha particle emitter during its decay sequence.

Rayleigh scattering See *Coherent scattering*.

Recessive mutation A genetic mutation that probably will not be expressed for several generations because both parents must possess the same genetic characteristic.

Recoil electron See *Compton scattered electron*.

Reconstruction interval This refers to the selected generated or displayed spacing between adjacent slices being a chosen amount (gapping) or being contiguous (no spacing) or overlapping.

Relative biologic effectiveness (RBE) Describes the relative capabilities of radiation with differing linear energy transfers (LETs) to produce a particular biologic reaction. Simply defined, it is the ratio of the dose of a reference radiation (conventionally, 250 kVp x-rays) to the dose of radiation of the type in question that is necessary to produce the same biologic reaction in a given experiment. The reaction is produced by a dose of the test radiation delivered under the same conditions.

Relative risk Model predicting that the number of excess cancers will increase as the natural incidence of cancer increases with advancing age in a population.

Rem (radiation equivalent man) Traditional unit for the radiation quantity equivalent dose (EqD); defined as the dose that is equivalent to any type of ionizing radiation that produces the same biologic effect as 1 rad (radiation absorbed dose) of x-radiation.

Remnant radiation See *Exit*, or *image formation, radiation*.

Repair enzymes Enzymes that can mend damaged molecules and are therefore capable of helping the cell recover from a small amount of radiation-induced damage.

Repeat analysis program An attempt to record the various causes of inadequate quality on occasions when an image has to be retaken (i.e., a repeat image).

Reproductive cells Male and female germ cells (relatively radiosensitive).

Reproductive death The permanent loss of a cell's ability to divide because of exposure to doses of ionizing radiation in the range of 1 to 10 Gy. The cell itself does not die but continues to metabolize and synthesize nucleic acids and proteins.

Restitution   A process in which chromosome breaks rejoin in their original configuration with no visible damage.

Retina   A curved sheet or layer at the rear of the eyeball containing cells that are sensitive to light (rods and cones) and that trigger nerve impulses that pass via the optic nerve to the brain where a visual image is formed.

Ribonucleic acid (RNA)   Type of nucleic acid that carries genetic information from the DNA in the cell nucleus to the ribosomes located in the cytoplasm.

Ribose   A simple sugar and carbohydrate with molecular formula $C_5H_{10}O_5$.

Ribosomal RNA (rRNA)   Type of RNA that assists in the linking of messenger RNA (mRNA) to the ribosome to facilitate protein synthesis.

Ribosomes   Very small, spherical, cytoplasmic organelles that attach to the endoplasmic reticulum; they are the assembly sites where mRNA and tRNA combine amino acids into proteins. They are the cell's "protein factories."

Right-to-Know Act (Employee)   A series of statutes passed by individual states requiring that employees be made aware of the hazards in the workplace. This act covers hazardous substances, infectious agents, ionizing radiation, and nonionizing radiation.

Risk   In general terms, the probability of injury, ailment, or death resulting from an activity. In the medical industry with reference to the radiation sciences, risk is the possibility of inducing a radiogenic cancer or genetic defect after irradiation.

Road mapping   A method of digital image subtraction in which the frame that contains the greatest amount of contrast material in vessels is identified and is then subtracted from all subsequent images. Live fluoroscopic images of the catheter moving through the vasculature can then be seen even after the vessels contain less contrast.

Roentgen (R)   Internationally accepted traditional unit of measurement of exposure to x-radiation and gamma radiation. One roentgen is the photon exposure that under standard conditions of pressure and temperature produces a total positive or negative ion charge of $2.58 \times (10)^{-4}$ coulombs per kilogram of dry air.

Rung   A step in the DNA ladder-like structure composed of a pair of nitrogenous bases.

S

Saccharides   See *Carbohydrates*.

Salts   Chemical compounds resulting from the action of an acid and a base on each other. They are sometimes referred to as *electrolytes*.

Sarcophagus   Large concrete shelter constructed by the Soviet Union atop the remains of the Reactor 4 building after the Chernobyl nuclear accident to provide protection from radiation exposure.

Scan direction collimation   The product of the number of data channels or detector rows used during one axial acquisition (N) and the size or width of a data channel or individual detector (T).

Scattered radiation   All the deflected radiation that arises from the interaction of an x-ray beam with the atoms of a patient or any other object in the path of the beam.

Scintillator   A substance that undergoes atomic transitions causing it to emit visible radiation or "glow" when hit by high-energy particles or photons.

Scotopic vision   Rod vision (night vision).

Scout view   A preliminary radiographic image of a desired portion of a patient's anatomy in either the coronal or sagittal direction obtained before performing a CT scan in that region.

Secondary electron   See *Compton scattered electron*.

Secondary protective barrier   A barrier that affords protection from secondary radiation (leakage and scattered radiation) only; as such, it is not designed to intercept the direct x-ray beam or to provide adequate attenuation of the beam.

Secondary radiation   The radiation that results from the interaction between primary radiation and the atoms of the irradiated object and the off-focus, or leakage, radiation that penetrates the x-ray tube protective housing.

Semipermeable membrane   A structure that permits the passage of a pure solvent such as water but does not allow material dissolved by the solvent to pass through it.

Shadow shield   A shield of radiopaque material suspended from above the radiographic beam-defining system; these shields are positioned at some distance above the patient to cast a radiation protection shadow in the primary beam over the area spanned by the patient's reproductive organs.

Shallow equivalent dose   The external exposure of the skin or extremity at a tissue depth of 0.007 cm averaged over an area of 1 cm^2.

Shaped contact shield   A cup-shaped radiopaque shield, containing 1 mm of lead that is contoured to enclose the scrotum and penis to protect the male reproductive organs from exposure to ionizing radiation.

Shielding   Radiation-absorbent barrier of appropriate thickness used to provide protection from radiation. The most common materials used for structural barriers are lead and concrete. Accessory devices such as aprons, gloves, and thyroid shields are made of lead-impregnated vinyl to provide shielding from radiation exposure when individuals cannot remain behind a protective structural barrier during certain imaging procedures.

Shift and add algorithm (SAA)   The conventional method of image reconstruction used in digital breast tomosynthesis to generate in-focus slice images by shifting and then adding projection images of registered structures in the breast acquired at multiple viewing angles.

Side scatter   Photons that interact significantly with the atoms of an object and consequently are deflected to the side.

Sievert (Sv)   The SI unit of measure for the radiation quantities, equivalent dose (EqD), and effective dose (EfD). It is the product of the absorbed dose and the radiation weighting factor. For x-radiation (Q = 1), 1 sievert equals 1 joule of energy absorbed per kilogram of tissue. This unit is used *only* for radiation protection purposes. It provides a common scale whereby varying degrees of biologic damage caused by equal absorbed doses of different types of ionizing radiation (Q equals one or greater) can be compared with the degree of biologic damage caused by the same amount of x-radiation or gamma radiation. In the traditional system, 100 rem equals 1 sievert.

Sigmoid or "S-shaped" (nonlinear), threshold curve of radiation dose–response   Generally employed in radiation therapy to demonstrate high-dose cellular response. This curve indicates the existence of a threshold. Different effects require different minimal doses.

Signal-to-noise ratio (SNR)   The comparison of the average computed tomography (CT) number in a region with the statistical variation of CT number in that region.

Single-photon emission computed tomography (SPECT)   A nuclear medicine tomographic imaging technique using gamma rays emitted from radionuclides injected into a patient. Unlike a planar imager such as a gamma camera, it is able to provide true 3D information by rotating its detector about a patient.

Single-strand break   The ionization of a DNA macromolecule resulting in a break of one of its chemical bonds, thereby severing one of the sugar–phosphate chain side rails or strands of the ladder-like DNA molecular structure.

Skin dose   In general represents the absorbed dose to the most superficial layers of the skin.

Skin erythema dose   The received quantity of radiation, amounting roughly to an absorbed dose of several gray to a portion of skin surface, that causes diffused redness over an area of skin usually at some short period of time after irradiation.

Small angle scatter   Photons that pass through the patient being radiographed, interact with the atoms of the body, and are deflected at such a small angle that they can reach the image receptor, thereby degrading the completed radiographic image by introducing small amounts of off focus signal or *fog*.

Solid angle   A measure of the amount of the field of view from some particular point that a given object covers. That is, it is a quantification of how large the object appears to an observer looking from that point. The dimensionless unit of solid angle is the *steradian*, with 4π steradians covering or encompassing a full sphere field of view.

Somatic cells   All the cells in the human body other than female and male germ cells.

Somatic tissue reactions   Biologic reactions in tissues of the body that were irradiated that can be directly related to the dose of ionizing radiation received. These are cell-killing responses that exhibit a threshold dose below which the reactions are absent and above which the severity of the early tissue reactions increases as the radiation dose increases.

Source-to–image receptor distance (SID)   The distance from the x-ray tube anode focal spot to the radiographic image receptor or detector.

Source-to-skin distance (SSD)   The distance from the anode focal spot of an x-ray tube to the skin of the patient.

Spacer bar   A device that projects down from the housing of some collimators to prevent the collimators from being closer than 15 cm to the patient.

Spatial Resolution   The ability to distinguish between closely spaced objects. Often quantitatively described in terms of the number of clearly resolved line pairs per millimeter.

Specific area shielding   The use of lead or lead-impregnated material to protect selective body areas from exposure to ionizing radiation.

Spermatocytes   Sperm cells at their infancy. They divide by *meiosis* to produce cells with half the number of chromosomes.

Spermatogonium   The male germ cell.

Spiral computed tomography   In computed tomography (CT), a data acquisition method that combines a continuous gantry rotation with a table advance movement to form a spiral path of acquired scan data. It is also known as *helical CT*.

Spontaneous mutations   A natural phenomenon involving alterations in genes and DNA. These mutations occur at random and without a known cause.

Standardized dose reporting   A system of standardizing or regulating a patient's radiation dose by having the dose dictated into the patient's report and then tracking the dose amount for any subsequent similar procedures.

Stem cells   Immature or precursor cells.

Stem radiation   See *Off-focus radiation*.

Stent   A tubular support that can be placed inside a blood vessel, canal, or duct to open up a previously obstructed or narrowed pathway.

Steradian   The SI unit of solid angle. It is the angle at the center of a sphere generated by a portion of the surface area of the sphere equal to the square of its radius.

Stochastic effects   Mutational or randomly occurring biologic changes, independent of dose, in which the chance of occurrence of the effect rather than the severity of the effect is proportional to the dose of ionizing radiation. These effects occur months or years after high level, and possibly also after low level, radiation exposure. Examples include cancer and genetic effects. Also called *probabilistic effects*.

Structural proteins   Those proteins from which the body acquires its shape and form. They also are a source of heat and energy.

Sunspots   Temporary phenomena on the Sun's photosphere (visible surface of the Sun) that appear as spots darker than the surrounding areas. They are regions of reduced surface temperature caused by concentrations of magnetic field flux that inhibit normal heat convection. This can induce a sudden explosion of energy called a solar flare. Solar flares are sometimes accompanied by a mass ejection comprised of huge bubbles of radiation and particles.

Surface contamination   External contamination of the skin or clothing of an individual with radioactive material.

Surface integral dose   The total amount of radiant energy transferred by ionizing radiation to the human body surface or superficial skin area during a radiation exposure.

Syndrome   A collection of symptoms.

Systole and diastole   Two phases of the cardiac compression/relaxation cycle. *Systole* occurs when the heart contracts to pump blood out, and *diastole* occurs when the heart relaxes or returns to its normal volume after contraction.

T

Target theory   Concept of radiation damage resulting from discrete and random events. If a critical location on the master molecule (believed to be DNA) is a target receiving multiple hits from ionizing radiation, it may well be inactivated. Normal cell function will then cease, and the cell will die. If, on the other hand, it receives only a single hit, then the master molecule most likely will still be operational. The target theory concept may be useful for explaining cell death and nonfatal cell abnormalities caused by exposure to radiation.

Technetium-99m (^{99m}Tc)   A gamma-emitting radioisotope with a 6-hour half-life that is produced from the beta decay of another unstable isotope, molybdenum-99. Technetium-99m is the most common radioisotope used in nuclear medicine studies.

Telangiectasia   Dilation of capillaries and sometimes of terminal arteries of an organ.

Telophase   The phase of mitosis during which cell division is completed with the formation of two new daughter cells, each of which contains exactly the same genetic material as the parent cell.

Temporal resolution   The ability to distinctly resolve (i.e., remove blur from) fast-moving objects.

Teratogenesis   Birth effects induced by irradiation in utero.

Terrestrial radiation   Long-lived radioactive elements such as uranium-238, radium-226, and thorium-232 that emit densely ionizing radiations (alpha particles) as part of their decay processes. These sources are present in variable quantities in the crust of the earth.

Theranostics   A combination of the terms therapeutics and diagnostics. Theranostics is the term used to describe the combination of using one radioactive drug to identify (diagnose) and a second radioactive drug to deliver therapy to treat a primary tumor and any metastatic tumors.

Therapeutic ratio   The ratio obtained by dividing the effective therapeutic dose by the minimum lethal dose; a comparison of the amount of a therapeutic agent that causes the therapeutic effect to the amount that causes toxicity. In radiotherapy, the therapeutic ratio denotes the relationship between the probability of tumor control and the likelihood of normal tissue damage.

Thermal neutron   Nominally classified as a neutron whose kinetic energy is approximately equal to 1 eV. Typically, these are neutrons whose kinetic energy has been significantly degraded as a result of multiple energy loss collisions.

Thermoluminescent dosimeter ring (TLD)   A personnel monitoring device that most often contains a crystalline form of lithium fluoride as its sensing material. When this device is placed in a TLD analyzer and heated, the crystals emit visible light in proportion to the amount of radiation to which the TLD dosimeter ring was exposed. A graphic plot of this light intensity (also known as *thermoluminescence intensity*) versus the heating temperature is known as a "glow curve." The glow curve represents a unique signature of the exposure received by the TLD dosimeter ring.

Thin film transistors (TFT)   TFT is constituted by a stack of insulators and semiconductors in the form of thin films. The active material of these transistors has usually been silicon.

Thompson scattering   The elastic scattering of an x-ray photon by a free electron.

Thoron   A radioactive decay product of an isotope of radon, namely radon-220, with a half-life of 54.5 seconds. It is given the name *thoron* because radon-220 was itself derived from the radioactive decay of thorium-232, a naturally occurring material.

Threshold   (1) The point at which a response or reaction to an increasing stimulation first occurs; (2) with reference to ionizing radiation, this means that below a certain radiation level or dose, no biologic effects are observed.

Thrombocytes   See *Platelets*.

Thrombocytopenia   A disorder in which there is a relative decrease of thrombocytes, commonly known as *platelets*, present in the blood. A normal human platelet count ranges from 150,000 to 450,000 platelets per microliter of blood.

Thymine (T)   A pyrimidine base found only in DNA.

Thymus gland   An organ of the lymphatic system, located in the mediastinal cavity anterior to and above the heart. It plays a critical role in the body's defense against infection.

Thyroid gland   A gland located in the neck just below the larynx. The hormone produced by this gland helps regulate the body's metabolic rate and the process of growth.

Thyroid shield   See *Protective apparel*.

Time   A method of radiation protection that reflects the fact that the amount of radiation a worker receives is directly proportional to the length of time that the individual is exposed to ionizing radiation.

Time interval difference   A method of digital image subtraction in which each image is subtracted from an image a few frames in advance. This technique reveals vessels containing contrast material and suppresses soft tissue in the images. It is less sensitive to patient motion than when the first image (also known as a "mask") is subtracted from all successive images.

Tissue reactions   Any radiation effects on organ or organ systems that increase with increasing dose, and below a certain dose level, the effect rarely or never occurs. They may occur as early effects, immediately after irradiation, or late effects, after some latent period.

Tissue weighting factor (W_T)   A value that denotes the percentage of the summed stochastic (cancer plus genetic) risk stemming from irradiation of specific tissues to the all-inclusive risk when the entire body is irradiated in a uniform fashion.

Title 10 of the Code of Federal Regulations, Part 20   A document prepared and distributed by the US Office of the Federal Register. The rules and regulations of the Nuclear Regulatory Commission (NRC) and fundamental radiation protection standards governing occupational radiation exposure are included in this document.

TLD ring badge   See *Extremity dosimeter*.

Tolerance dose   A radiation dose to which occupationally exposed persons could be continuously subjected without any apparent harmful acute effects, such as erythema of the skin.

Tomosynthesis   A method of obtaining a three-dimensional x-ray image of an object by combining multiple obtained in-focus planar images each obtained at different depths using an x-ray beam that moves in a limited arc about the object with a center of rotation for each arc at the desired imaging depth. Planar depths above and below the center of rotation plane will be blurred. This technique, modified so that isocenter changes are not needed and with the application of specialized computer image reconstruction algorithms, can also be successfully applied to digital mammography.

Total effective dose equivalent (TEDE)   A system of units and quantities used to monitor occupationally exposed personnel such as nuclear medicine technologists and interventional radiologists. TEDE is the sum of effective dose equivalent from external radiation exposures and the committed effective dose equivalent (CEDE) from internal sources. It is designed to take into account all possible causes of radiation exposure.

Total filtration Inherent filtration plus added filtration.

Traditional units Long established fundamental units associated with radiation protection and dosimetry, namely, the roentgen and the rad.

Transfer RNA (tRNA) Type of RNA that combines with individual amino acids from different areas of the cell and attaches or transfers them to the ribosomes.

Trimester A 3-month period of embryo/fetal gestation or development (i.e., first, second, and third trimesters).

Tubules Minute tubes which are a major transport component of the cell's endoplasmic reticulum.

Tungsten A metal with a high melting point (greater than 3400°C or 6100°F) and a high atomic number (Z = 74). In an x-ray tube, tungsten is a major component of both the filament (cathode) and the target (anode).

Tungsten rhenium (W/Rh) A metal alloy with a high melting point (greater than 3000°C) and a high atomic number. The anode of a general purpose x-ray tube is usually made of this alloy.

U

Ulceration The process of pus or discharge formation on a surface, such as the skin or a mucous membrane, to form an ulcer.

Umbra See *Primary radiation*.

Uncontrolled area Area such as a nearby hallway or corridor that can be frequented by the general public.

Undifferentiated cells Immature or nonspecialized cells.

Unit A fixed amount of some property or characteristic (e.g., distance in meters, time in seconds, energy in joules) used as a measure for which other amounts of that property or characteristic can be precisely described.

United Nations Scientific Committee on the Effects of Atomic Radiation (UNSCEAR) A group that plays a prominent role in the formulation of radiation protection guidelines. This group

evaluates human and environmental ionizing radiation exposure from a variety of sources and research conclusions to derive radiation risk assessments for radiation-induced cancer and for genetic (hereditary) effects.

Unmodified scattering See *Coherent scattering*.

Unnecessary radiologic procedure Any radiation examination that does not benefit a person in terms of the diagnostic information obtainable and thus for which there is no sufficient justification to subject a patient to the risk of the absorbed radiation dose resulting from the procedure.

Uracil (U) A pyrimidine base found only in RNA. It replaces thymine (T) as the nitrogenous base in ribonucleic acid.

US Code of Federal Regulations Document prepared and distributed by the US Office of the Federal Register that contains the rules and regulations of the Nuclear Regulatory Commission (NRC) and the radiation protection standards governing occupational radiation exposure.

Use factor (U) For primary radiation, the use factor represents the portion of beam-on time that the x-ray beam is targeted or directed at a particular barrier during the week. Also known as *beam direction factor*.

Useful beam See *Primary radiation*.

V

Vacuum discharge tube A glass tube containing a gas and two electrodes sealed through its walls. When a substantial electrical potential difference is established between the two electrodes and the pressure of gas in the tube is reduced enough, a situation will be reached at which a current flows through it, and energetic interactions occur such that the gas begins to glow.

Variable rectangular collimator A box-shaped device containing the radiographic beam-defining system; the device is most often used to define the size and shape of the radiographic beam.

Vasculitis An inflammation of the blood vessels. It causes changes in the walls of blood vessels, including thickening, weakening, narrowing, and scarring. These changes obstruct or hamper blood

flow, leading eventually to organ and tissue damage.

Vesicle Small cavities or sacs containing liquid.

Volt (V) SI unit of electrical potential and potential difference.

Voltage Electrical potential at a point or position relative to ground potential.

Voluntary motion Motion controlled by will (i.e., skeletal muscle).

Voxel A unit of graphic information that defines a region in three-dimensional space. Unlike a *pixel* (picture element) which defines an area in two-dimensional space with its x and y coordinates, a *voxel* also includes a third dimension or z coordinate and therefore defines a volume element.

W

Wavelength Distance between two consecutive crests or troughs in a wave (given in meters or some fraction thereof).

Wave-particle duality Electromagnetic radiation can travel and interact with matter in the form of a wave or a particle. For this reason, x-rays may be described as both waves and particles.

Window level Sets the midpoint of the range of densities visible on a digital image.

Workload (W) Essentially the radiation output weighted time that an x-ray machine is actually delivering radiation during the week. It is specified either in units of milliampere-seconds (mAs) per week or milliampere-minutes (mA-min) per week.

World Health Organization The authority that directs and coordinates for health within the United Nations system.

X

x-ray beam limitation device Any device that limits the dimensions of the useful beam to a designated size and shape before it enters the area of clinical interest.

x-rays (x-ray photons) Electromagnetic radiation that emerges from the anode of an x-ray tube after bombardment by high-speed electrons in a highly evacuated glass tube or from an atom that has experienced a photoelectric interaction. The latter are typically called *characteristic x-rays*.

INDEX

Note: Page numbers followed by "*b*" indicate boxes, "*f*" indicate figures, and "*t*" indicate tables.